ADVANCED PRACTICE NURSING

Essential Knowledge for the Profession

THIRD EDITION

Edited by

SUSAN M. DeNISCO, DNP, APRN, FNP-BC, CNE, CNL
Professor & Director, Doctor of Nursing Practice Program
Sacred Heart University
Fairfield, Connecticut
Family Nurse Practitioner, St. Vincent's Family Health Center
Bridgeport, Connecticut

ANNE M. BARKER, EdD, RN
Professor of Nursing
Sacred Heart University
Fairfield, Connecticut

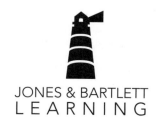

JONES & BARTLETT
LEARNING

World Headquarters
Jones & Bartlett Learning
5 Wall Street
Burlington, MA 01803
978-443-5000
info@jblearning.com
www.jblearning.com

Jones & Bartlett Learning books and products are available through most bookstores and online booksellers. To contact Jones & Bartlett Learning directly, call 800-832-0034, fax 978-443-8000, or visit our website, www.jblearning.com.

Substantial discounts on bulk quantities of Jones & Bartlett Learning publications are available to corporations, professional associations, and other qualified organizations. For details and specific discount information, contact the special sales department at Jones & Bartlett Learning via the above contact information or send an email to specialsales@jblearning.com.

Production Credits
VP, Executive Publisher: David D. Cella
Executive Editor: Amanda Martin
Associate Acquisitions Editor: Rebecca Myrick
Editorial Assistant: Lauren Vaughn
Production Manager: Carolyn Rogers Pershouse
Senior Marketing Manager: Jennifer Stiles
VP, Manufacturing and Inventory Control:
  Therese Connell

Composition: Cenveo Publisher Services
Cover Design: Scott Moden
Rights and Media Manager: Joanna Lundeen
Rights and Media Research Coordinator: Mary Flatley
Media Development Assistant: Shannon Sheehan
Cover Image: © A-R-T/Shutterstock
Printing and Binding: Edwards Brothers Malloy
Cover Printing: Edwards Brothers Malloy

Library of Congress Cataloging-in-Publication Data
Advanced practice nursing (Barker)
  Advanced practice nursing : essential knowledge for the profession / [edited by] Susan M. DeNisco, Anne M. Barker.
—Third edition.
    p. ; cm.
  Includes bibliographical references and index.
  ISBN 978-1-284-07257-0 (pbk.)
  I. DeNisco, Susan M., editor. II. Barker, Anne M., editor. III. Title.
  [DNLM: 1. Advanced Practice Nursing—trends. 2. Nurse's Role. WY 128]
  RT82.8
  610.73—dc23
                                    2014047066

6048
Printed in the United States of America
20 19 18 17   10 9 8 7 6 5

Contents

10 *Microeconomics in the Hospital Firm: Competition, Regulation, the Profit Motive, and Patient Care* **227**

Mary Anne Schultz

11 *Government Regulation: Parallel and Powerful* **251**

Jacqueline M. Loversidge

PART 3 *Quality, Safety, and Information Systems for Advanced Practice Nurses* **281**

12 *Factors Influencing the Application and Diffusion of CQI in Health Care* **285**

William A. Sollecito and Julie K. Johnson

Introduction

Advanced practice nursing education has been rapidly evolving over the past decade, with much attention given to the unique differences between "advance practice nursing" and the four traditional advanced practice roles—that is, certified registered nurse anesthetists (CRNAs), certified nurse-midwives (CNMs), clinical specialists (CNSs), and nurse practitioners (NPs)—as direct care providers. The third edition of this book was conceived in response to several new national initiatives including the evolution of the doctor of nursing practice (DNP) degree and the American Association of Colleges of Nursing's (AACN) recently revised *Essentials of Master's Education for Advanced Practice Nursing* (2011). These initiatives, which were developed in response to healthcare reform legislation and the focus on patient safety and quality care, have provided curricular guidance to master's programs transitioning to the doctoral level for advanced practice. The content of this book was then cross-referenced with the *Essentials of Doctoral Education for Advanced Nursing Practice* (AACN, 2006). The task force that developed the Doctoral Essentials built their work on the former Master's Essentials. **Table I-1** displays the new essential core curriculum content for both the master's and doctoral programs. The last column lists the chapters in this book that address this content.

The publisher, Jones & Bartlett Learning, under the guidance of editors Susan M. DeNisco and Anne M. Barker embarked on a quest to produce a third editon of an advanced practice text book that would compile selected chapters from existing books in the Jones & Bartlett Learning collection. The strength of this approach is that experts in each of the content areas author each chapter in the book.

The revision of this textbook comprehensively addresses the core curriculum content requirements of the MSN and DNP Essentials, recognizing that broad content areas and role competencies cannot be covered in separate courses due to credit limitations. In addition, this book addresses

TABLE I-1	Comparison of Master's Essentials, Doctoral Essentials, and Book Content

Master's Essentials 2011	Doctoral Essentials	Book
I. Scientific and Humanistic Background for Practice	I. Scientific Underpinnings for Practice	Chapter 19
II. Organizational and Systems Leadership	II. Organizational and Systems Leadership for Quality Improvement and Systems Thinking	Chapters 9–11
III. Quality Improvement and Safety	II. Organizational and Systems Leadership for Quality Improvement and Systems Thinking; IV. Information Systems/Technology and Patient Care Technology for the Improvement and Transformation of Health Care	Chapters 12–14
IV. Translating and Integrating Scholarship into Practice	III. Clinical Scholarship and Analytical Methods for Evidence-Based Practice	Chapters 20–22
V. Informatics and Healthcare Technologies	IV. Information Systems/Technology and Patient Care Technology for the Improvement and Transformation of Health Care	Chapters 15–17
VI. Health Policy and Advocacy	V. Health Care Policy for Advocacy in Health Care	Chapters 7–11, 26, and 27
VII. Interprofessional Collaboration for Improving Patient and Population Health Outcomes	VI. Interprofessional Collaboration for Improving Patient and Population Health Outcomes	Chapters 6 and 25
VIII. Clinical Prevention and Population Health for Improving Health	VII. Clinical Prevention and Population Health for Improving the Nation's Health	Chapters 7, 8, and 23–25
IX. Master's-Level Nursing Practice	VIII. Advanced Nursing Practice	Chapters 1–6 and 28–30

an audience of nurses in a variety of advanced practice nurse roles, including nurse executives, nurse educators, and entrepreneurs—not just those nurses who provide direct clinical care.

This book is divided into six parts that are meant to be read in sequence:

1. Professional Roles for the Advanced Practice Nurse
2. Healthcare Delivery and Health Policy for Advanced Practice: Core Knowledge
3. Quality, Safety, and Information Systems for Advanced Practice Nurses
4. Theoretical Foundations, Research, and Evidence-Based Practice
5. The Role of Race, Culture, Ethics, and Advocacy in Advanced Nursing Practice
6. Leadership and Role Transition for the Advanced Practice Nurse

The goal of the book is to provide core knowledge that all nurses in advanced practice roles require, regardless of their specialty or functional focus. This knowledge can then be built upon as graduate students proceed into their specialty foci.

New to this edition are the following topic and content areas:

- Focus on both direct and indirect provider roles
- Role of the clinical doctorate in advanced practice nursing
- Reimbursement and credentialing issues for nurse practitioners
- Federal and state regulation of advanced practice nursing
- Budgeting and finances for advanced practice
- Electronic health records and clinical informatics
- Continuous quality improvement strategies to optimize clinical practice
- Evidence-based practice and clinical scholarship
- Global health, diversity, and healthcare disparities for special populations
- Role transition and professional development

The content of this book has been carefully selected based on the editors' collective 60 years of experience as primary care providers, educators, and administrators. This content is essential to all levels of graduate nursing preparation. With the recent revision and sophistication of the Master's Essentials, there is closer application in each content area to the Doctoral Essentials. Thus the book can be used in both master's-level and postbaccalaureate doctoral programs in the beginning core courses to lay a foundation for advanced nursing practice. As with any textbook, additional scholarly readings, especially research- and evidence-based articles, will enhance the content.

As previously mentioned, some confusion exists regarding the terminology "advanced nursing practice" versus "advanced practice nursing." Over time, the terms "advanced

practice nursing" and "advanced practice nurses" have become commonly used to indicate master's-prepared nurses who provide direct clinical care and include the roles of clinical nurse specialist, nurse practitioner, certified nurse–midwife, and certified registered nurse anesthetist, with the last three roles requiring a license beyond the basic RN license to practice. This book has adopted a broader, more inclusive definition (AACN, 2004), which reflects the current thinking about advanced practice. Advanced practice nursing is defined as follows:

> Any form of nursing intervention that influences health care outcomes for individuals or populations, including direct care of individual patients, management of care for individuals and populations, administration of nursing and health care organizations, and the development and implementation of health policy. (p. 2)

In this book, nurses in advanced practice are defined as any nurse who holds a master's degree or higher in nursing and whose role is consistent with this definition. "Advanced practice nursing," "advanced practice nurses," and "advanced nursing practice" are used interchangeably throughout the book.

Currently, several major professional forces are influencing graduate education in nursing and promise to have dramatic effects on nursing education both today and into at least the next decade:

- The 2010 Affordable Care Act represents the broadest healthcare overhaul legislation passed since the 1965 creation of the Medicare and Medicaid programs.
- The Institute of Medicine report *The Future of Nursing: Leading Change, Advancing Health* (2010) positions nurse regulators to provide leadership on the critically important challenge of assigning accountability for quality and patient safety at the state and local levels.
- The clinical doctorate, designated as a doctor of nursing practice (DNP), has been mandated as the entry to advanced nursing

practice (see the introduction to Part 1 for more details).

- A consensus model for advanced practice nurse regulations has been developed through work by the Advanced Practice Registered Nurse Consensus group (2008) and the National Council of State Boards of Nursing (NCSBN).

- A new role in nursing, the clinical nurse leader (CNL), has been introduced. This role is designed to address many of the problems currently evident in health care, including the nursing shortage, patient safety and medical errors, and fragmentation of the healthcare system. The AACN (2007) provides this definition of the CNL:

The CNL functions within a microsystem and assumes accountability for healthcare outcomes for a specific group of clients within a unit or setting through the assimilation and application of research-based information to design, implement, and evaluate client plans of care. The CNL is a provider and a manager of care at the point of care to individuals and cohorts. The CNL designs, implements, and evaluates client care by coordinating, delegating, and supervising the care provided by the health care team, including licensed nurses, technicians, and other health professionals. (p. 6)

- CNLs are considered generalists who will be prepared at the master's level and require the same core curriculum knowledge as do other master's-prepared nurses.

In both the Master's Essentials and Doctoral Essentials documents, the AACN lays out the foundation for core knowledge needed by all graduate nursing students. This book provides in one manuscript a foundation for this core knowledge. It does not address any of the specific content needed by the specialties. Moreover, this foundational content should be further integrated and applied throughout the rest of the curriculum.

Contributors

Susan M. DeNisco, DNP, APRN, FNP-BC, CNE, CNL
Professor & Director, Doctor of Nursing Practice Program
Sacred Heart University, Fairfield, Connecticut
Family Nurse Practitioner, St. Vincent's Family Health Center, Bridgeport, Connecticut

Anne M. Barker, EdD, RN
Professor of Nursing
Sacred Heart University
Fairfield, Connecticut

Laurel Ash, RN
Professor
College of Saint Scholastica
Duluth, Minnesota

Emily B. Barey, MSN, RN
Director of Nursing Informatics
Epic Systems Corporation
Madison, WI

Audrey Beauvais, DNP, MSN, MBA, RN-C, CNL
Associate Dean
School of Nursing
Fairfield University
Fairfield, Connecticut

Lisa Astalos Chism, DNP, GNP, BC, NCMP, FAANP
Nurse Practitioner
Alexander J. Walt Comprehensive Breast Center
High Risk Breast Clinic
Karmanos Cancer Institute
Detroit, Michigan

Linda Dayer-Berenson, PhD, MSN, CRNP, CNE, FAANP
Drexel University
College of Nursing and Health Professions
Philadelphia, Pennsylvania

Anita Finkelman, MSN, RN
Visiting Faculty, School of Nursing, Bouvé College of Health Sciences
Northeastern University
Boston, Massachusetts

Pamela J. Grace, RN, PhD, FAAN
Associate Professor
Connell School of Nursing, Boston College
Boston, Massachusetts

John Hidley, MD
Psychiatrist
Ojai, California

Julie K. Johnson, MSPH, PhD
Professor
Department of Surgery Center for Healthcare
    Studies Institute for Public Health and
    Medicine Feinburg School of Medicine
Northwestern University
Chicago, Illinois

Janet W. Kenney, RN, PhD
College of Nursing
Arizona State University
Scottsdale, Arizona

Thomas R. Krause, PhD
Campus President
Fortis Institute
Scranton, Pennsylvania

Philip J. Kroth, MD, MS
Associate Professor
Director, Biomedical Informatics Research,
    Training, and Scholarship
Health Sciences Library and Informatics
    Center
The University of New Mexico Health Sciences
    Center
Albuquerque, New Mexico

Jacqueline M. Loversidge, PhD, RNC-AWHC
Assistant Professor of Clinical Nursing
Ohio State University
Columbus, Ohio

Kathleen Mastrian, PhD, RN
Associate Professor and Program Coordinator
    for Nursing
Pennsylvania State University, Shenango
Sr. Managing Editor, *Online Journal of Nursing
    Informatics (OJNI)*

**Dee McGonigle, PhD, RN, CNE, FAAN,
    ANEF**
Chair, Virtual Learning Environments and
    Professor, Graduate Programs
Chamberlain College of Nursing
Member, Informatics and Technology Expert
    Panel (ITEP)
American Academy of Nursing
Member, Serious Gaming and Virtual Envi-
    ronments Special Interest Group for the
    Society for Simulation in Healthcare (SSH)

Catherine Miller, EdD, RN, CNE
Associate Dean, Nursing
Illinois State University
Normal, Illinois

Karla M. Miller, PharmD, BCPP
Director of Medication Usage and Safety
Hospital Corporation of America
Nashville, Tennessee

Kerry Milner, DNSC, RN
Cardiovascular Critical Care Nursing
Assistant Professor
Sacred Heart University
Fairfield, Connecticut

George D. Pozgar, MBA, CHE, DLitt
Consultant
GP Health Care Consulting
Annapolis, Maryland

Beth L. Rodgers, PhD, RN, FAAN
Professor & Interim Research Chair
College of Nursing, University of New Mexico
Albuquerque, New Mexico

Mary Anne Schultz, PhD, MBA, MSN, RN
Department Chair
California State University
Los Angeles, California

Manisha Shaw, MBA, RCP
Chief Operating Officer
National Patient Safety Foundation
Boston, Massachusetts

Leiyu Shi, DrPH, MBA, MPA
Professor, Johns Hopkins Bloomberg School
of Public Health
Director, Johns Hopkins Primary Care Policy
Center
Baltimore, Maryland

Douglas A. Singh, PhD, MBA
Associate Professor of Management
School of Business and Economics
Indiana University at South Bend
South Bend, Indiana

William A. Sollecito, DrPH
Clinical Professor, Public Health Leadership
Program
Gillings School of Global Public Health,
University of North Carolina
Chapel Hill, North Carolina

Julie G. Stewart, DNP, MPH, MSN, FNP-BC
Associate Professor, Director of FNP Program
Sacred Heart University
Fairfield, Connecticut

Harry A. Sultz, DDS, MPH
Professor Emeritus, Social and Preventative
Medicine
School of Medicine and Biomedical Sciences
State University of New York at Buffalo
Dean Emeritus, School of Public Health and
Health Professions
State University of New York at Buffalo,
Buffalo, New York

Catherine Tymkow, ND/DNP, APRN, WHNP-BC
Professor, DNP Director
Governors State University
Flossmoor, Illinois

Kathryn Waud White, DNP, RN, CRNA
University of Minnesota, School of Nursing
Minneapolis, Minnesota

Kristina M. Young, MS
Instructor, School of Public Health and Health
Professions
State University of New York at Buffalo
Instructor, Canisius College
President, Kristina M. Young & Associates,
Inc., Buffalo, New York

Professional Roles for the Advanced Practice Nurse

The chapters in Part 1 of this book consider the role of the advanced practice nurse from historical, present-day, and future perspectives. This content is intended to serve as a general introduction to select issues in professional role development for the advanced practice of nursing. As students progress in the educational process and develop greater knowledge and expertise, role issues and role transition should be integrated into the entire educational program.

In Chapter 1, the editors define advanced practice nursing from a traditional perspective and trace the history of the role. Traditionally, advanced practice has been limited to clinical roles that include the clinical nurse specialist, nurse practitioner, certified nurse-midwife, and certified registered nurse anesthetist; to practice, the last three roles require a license beyond the basic registered nurse (RN) license. This book, however, uses an expanded definition of advanced practice

nursing that reflects current thinking. As you read this chapter, keep in mind this expanded definition and appreciate the development of the advanced clinical roles for nursing practice. This discussion lays the foundation for a deeper understanding of the historical development, current practice, and future opportunities for advanced practice in nursing.

In Chapter 2, Stewart discusses the tipping point for nurse practitioners as we enter the age of healthcare reform and the role nurse practitioners will play in providing cost-effective, quality primary care to a demographically changing population. Stewart's quantitative and qualitative research resulted in the Stewart Model of Nurse Practitionering, which reflects key attributes that make nurse practitioners unique. Much has transpired related to the role and education of nurses for advanced practice. Most revolutionary is the mandate to have by 2015 the clinical doctorate be the required degree for advanced clinical practice nursing (American Association of Colleges of Nursing, 2004). With this change, many master's programs for advanced practice nurses will transition to the doctoral level. The rationale for this position by the American Association of Colleges of Nursing (AACN) is based on several factors:

- The reality that current master's degree programs often require credit loads equivalent to doctoral degrees in other healthcare professions
- The changing complexity of the healthcare environment
- The need for the highest level of scientific knowledge and practice expertise to ensure high-quality patient outcomes

In an effort to clarify the standards, titling, and outcomes of clinical doctorates, the Commission on Collegiate Nursing Education (CCNE)—the accreditation arm of AACN—has decided that only practice doctoral degrees awarding a Doctor of Nursing Practice (DNP) will be eligible for accreditation. In addition, the AACN has published the *Essentials of Doctoral Education for Advanced Nursing Practice*, which sets forth the standards for the development, implementation, and program outcomes of DNP programs.

Needless to say, this recommendation has not been fully supported by the entire profession. For instance, the American Organization of Nurse Executives (AONE, 2007) does not support requiring a doctorate for managerial or executive practice on the basis of expense, time commitment, and cost benefit of the degree. It also suggests that nurses may migrate toward a master's degree in business, social sciences, and public health in lieu of a master's degree in nursing. Further, AONE suggests there is a lack of evidence to support the need for doctoral education across all aspects of the care continuum. In contrast, doctoral- and master's-level education for nurse managers and executives is encouraged.

For other advanced practice roles, including those of the clinical nurse leader, nurse educator, and nurse researcher, a different set of educational requirements exists. The clinical nurse leader as a generalist remains a master's-level program. For nurse educators, the position of AACN—although not universally accepted within the profession (as demonstrated by the existence of master's programs in nursing education)—is that didactic knowledge and practical experience in pedagogy are additive to advanced clinical knowledge. Nurse researchers will continue to be prepared in PhD programs. Thus, there will be only two doctoral programs in nursing, the DNP and the PhD. It is important for readers to keep abreast of this movement as the profession further develops and debates these issues because the outcomes have implications for their own practice and professional development within their own specialty. The best resource for this is the AACN website and the websites of specialty organizations.

The next three chapters in Part 1 discuss the future of advanced practice nursing and the evolution of doctoral education—in particular, the practice doctorate. Within today's rapidly changing and complex healthcare environment, members of the nursing profession are challenging themselves to expand the role of advanced practice nursing to include highly skilled practitioners, leaders, educators, researchers, and policymakers.

In Chapter 3, Chism defines the DNP degree and compares and contrasts the research doctorate and the practice doctorate. The focus of the DNP degree is expertise in clinical practice. Additional foci include the *Essentials of Doctoral Education for Advanced Nursing Practice* as outlined by the AACN (2004), which include leadership, health policy and advocacy, and information technology. Role transitions for advanced practice nurses prepared at the doctoral level call for an integration of roles focused on the provision of high-quality, patient-centered care.

In Chapter 4, White discusses emerging roles of DNP graduates as nurse educators, nurse executives, and nurse entrepreneurs and advanced practice nurses' increased involvement in public health programming and integrative and complementary health modalities.

In Chapter 5, Barker sets the foundation for advanced practice nurses to recognize and embrace their role as leaders and influencers of practice changes in healthcare organizations. Complexity science, organizational change theory, and transformational leadership are used as a platform for advanced practice nurses to realize their leadership potential and their role as agents of change.

Last, in Chapter 6, Ash and Miller provide an in-depth look at interdisciplinary and interprofessional collaborative teams as a means to effect positive health outcomes. They discuss barriers to successful collaborative teams and factors for successful team development. Advanced practice nurse leaders educated at both the master's and doctoral levels are uniquely positioned to overcome the workforce and regulatory issues that might otherwise diminish the success of collaborative teams—in particular, those involving participants from the nursing and medicine disciplines.

REFERENCES

American Association of Colleges of Nursing (AACN). (2004). *AACN position statement on the Doctorate in Nursing*. Retrieved from http://www.aacn.nche .edu/DNP/DNPPositionStatement.htm

American Organization of Nurse Executives (AONE). (2007). *Consideration of the Doctorate of Nursing Practice*. Retrieved from http://www.aone.org /resources/leadership%20tools/Docs/Position Statement060607.doc

CHAPTER 1

Introduction to the Role of Advanced Practice Nursing

Susan M. DeNisco and Anne M. Barker

CHAPTER OBJECTIVES

1. Describe the four roles used to define advanced practice nursing in the United States.

2. Identify the differences between the clinical nurse leader role and the traditional advanced practice nursing roles.

3. Recognize factors that currently influence the supply and demand of nurse educators.

4. Discuss the educational preparation and certification requirements for nurse administrators.

INTRODUCTION

Considerable confusion exists regarding the terminology *advanced nursing practice*, *advanced nurse practice*, and *advanced practice registered nurse*. Based on the definition given by the American Association of Colleges of Nursing (AACN) and other widely accepted usages, the term *advanced practice registered nurse (APRN)* has been used to indicate master's-prepared nurses who provide direct clinical care. This term encompasses the roles of nurse practitioner (NP), certified nurse-midwife (CNM), certified registered nurse anesthetist (CRNA), and clinical nurse specialist (CNS). The first three roles require a license beyond the basic registered nurse (RN) license. The role of the clinical nurse specialist requires a master's degree but does not require separate licensing unless the CNS is applying for prescriptive authority.

Complicating the titling and definition of roles, the AACN (2004) defined advanced practice nursing as follows:

> Any form of nursing intervention that influences health care outcomes for individuals or populations, including direct care of individual patients, management of care for individuals and populations, administration of nursing and health care organizations, and the development and implementation of health policy. (p. 2)

The *Consensus Model for APRN Regulation* is a product of substantial work done by the APRN Consensus Work Group and the National Council of State Boards of Nursing (NCSBN) APRN Advisory Committee in an effort to address the irregularities in regulation of advanced practice registered nurses across states. As defined in the model for regulation, there are four roles: certified registered nurse anesthetist, certified nurse-midwife, clinical nurse specialist, and certified nurse practitioner (CNP). These four roles are given the title of advanced practice registered nurse (APRN). APRNs are educated in one of the four roles and in at least one of the following population foci: family/individual across the life span, adult–gerontology, pediatrics, neonatal, women's health/gender related, and psych/mental health (APRN Consensus Work Group & National Council of State Boards of Nursing APRN Advisory Committee, 2008). Advanced practice registered nurses are licensed independent practitioners who are expected to practice within standards established or recognized by a licensing body. The model further addresses licensure, accreditation, certification, and education of APRNs. **Figure 1-1** depicts the APRN Regulatory Model.

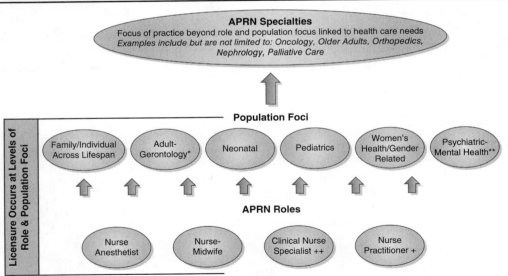

FIGURE 1-1 APRN Regulatory Model.

APRN Specialties
Focus of practice beyond role and population focus linked to health care needs
Examples include but are not limited to: Oncology, Older Adults, Orthopedics, Nephrology, Palliative Care

Population Foci

Licensure Occurs at Levels of Role & Population Foci

Family/Individual Across Lifespan | Adult-Gerontology* | Neonatal | Pediatrics | Women's Health/Gender Related | Psychiatric-Mental Health**

APRN Roles

Nurse Anesthetist | Nurse-Midwife | Clinical Nurse Specialist ++ | Nurse Practitioner +

+The certified nurse practitioner (CNP) is prepared with the acute care CNP competencies and/or the primary care CNP competencies. At this point in time the acute care and primary care CNP delineation applies only to the pediatric and adult-gerontology CNP population foci. Scope of practice of the primary care or acute care CNP is **not setting specific** but is based on patient care needs. Programs may prepare individuals across both the primary care and acute care CNP competencies. If programs prepare graduates across both sets of roles, the graduate must be prepared with the consensus-based competencies for both roles and must successfully obtain certification in both the acute and the primary care CNP roles. CNP certification in the acute care or primary care roles must match the educational preparation for CNPs in these roles.

Source: National Council of State Boards of Nursing: The APRN Consensus Model 2008.

OTHER ADVANCED PRACTICE NURSING ROLES AND THE NURSING CURRICULUM

Consequently, nurse administrators, public health nurses, and policymakers are considered advanced practice nurses albeit they do not provide direct care or obtain advanced practice licensure per the state they practice in. As this text goes to press, there is an initiative to expand and clarify the definition of and requirements for advanced practice nursing. No matter the final outcome of this deliberation, all nurses need the same set of essential knowledge. The Essentials series outlines the necessary curriculum content and expected competencies of graduates of baccalaureate, master's, and doctoral nursing practice programs and the clinical support needed for the full spectrum of academic nursing (AACN, 2006, 2011a, 2011b). Although the terms *advanced practice nursing*, *advanced practice nurses*, *advanced nursing practice*, and *advanced practice registered nurses* are used interchangeably throughout this text, the authors are addressing any students enrolled in master's or doctoral programs that are designed, implemented, and evaluated by the AACN Essentials. Chapter 2 provides an overview of the master's and doctoral essentials.

Clinical Nurse Leaders

Clinical nurse leaders (CNLs) were not considered in the definition of *advanced practice* because the CNL role did not exist when the aforementioned roles were defined. Some argue that the CNL is a generalist, and thus CNL should not be considered an advanced practice role. The authors disagree. The clinical nurse leader role requires advanced knowledge and skill beyond that attained with the baccalaureate degree, and it requires a master's degree for certification.

According to the AACN (2007), the clinical nurse leader is responsible for patient care outcomes and integrates and applies evidence-based information to design, implement, and evaluate healthcare systems and models of care delivery. The CNL is a provider and manager of care at the point of care for individuals and cohorts of patients anywhere healthcare is delivered (AACN, 2007). In fact, as recommended in the AACN white paper on the CNL role, all CNL curricula across the country require graduate-level content that builds on an undergraduate foundation in health assessment, pharmacology, and pathophysiology. In many master's-level programs, NP and CNL students sit side by side to learn these advanced skills. Also, the inclusion of these three separate courses—health assessment, pharmacology, and pathophysiology—facilitates the transition of master's program graduates into Doctor of Nursing Practice degree programs (AACN, 2007). Moreover, the CNL program graduate has completed more than 400 clinical practice hours, similar to number required of NP graduates, and is eligible to sit for the CNL Certification Examination developed by the American Association of Colleges of Nursing.

The clinical nurse leader, similar to the clinical nurse specialist (discussed next), has developed clinical and leadership skills and knowledge of statistical processes and data mining. The CNL brings evidence-based practice to the bedside, creates a culture of safety, and provides quality care. This aligns directly with the American Organization of Nurse Executives' (AONE) guiding principles for the nurse of the future (Haase-Herrick & Herrin, 2007).

Clinical Nurse Specialists

Clinical nurse specialists (CNSs) have been providing care to patients with complex cases across healthcare settings since the 1960s. The CNS role originated largely to satisfy the societal need for nurses who could provide advanced care to psychiatric populations. Since the passage of the National Mental Health Act in 1946, the National League for Nursing (NLN) and the American Nurses Association have supported the CNS role. The first program at Rutgers University educated nurses for the role of psychiatric clinical specialist (McClelland, McCoy, & Burson, 2013). Following this implementation, the usefulness of the role became apparent, and schools of nursing began to educate nurses across specialties, including oncology, medical-surgical, pediatric, and critical care nursing.

The literature of the 1980s and 1990s shows that care provided by clinical nurse specialists produced positive patient outcomes related to self-management and early hospital discharge (Fulton, 2014). More recently, studies show improvement in patient satisfaction and in pain management, and reduced medical complications in hospitalized patients (McClelland et al., 2013).

The recent trend toward hospital and healthcare system mergers and the focus on cost containment force the CNS role into a precarious position. Hospital administrators have a difficult time showing that CNSs decrease hospital costs, and they cannot bill for specialty nursing services. The AACN states that there are significant differences between the CNS and CNL roles; however, few differences are clearly articulated by those being educated in or practicing in these roles or in recent documents created by AACN (National Association of Clinical Nurse Specialists [NACNS], 2005). This has created role confusion and uncertainty regarding the role these nurses should play in the inpatient hospital setting. **Table 1-1** compares role competencies of the CNS and the CNL.

In addition, the APRN Consensus Model states that graduate nursing roles that do not focus on direct patient care will not be eligible for APRN licensure in the future (APRN Consensus Work Group & National Council of State Boards of Nursing APRN Advisory Committee,

TABLE 1-1	Comparison of Select Role Competencies for the CNS and the CNL
Clinical Nurse Specialist	Clinical Nurse Leader
Direct care	Critical thinking/clinical decision making/assessment
Systems leadership	Nursing technology and resource management
Collaboration	Communication
Coaching	
Consultation	
Research	Assimilates and applies research-based information to design, implement, and evaluate client plans of care
Ethical decision making, moral agency, and advocacy	Ethics
	Accountability
	Professional values, including social justice
	Professional development

Sources: American Association of Colleges of Nursing. (2007). *White paper on the role of the clinical nurse leader.* Retrieved from http://www.aacn.nche.edu/aacn-publications/white-papers/cnl-white-paper; National CNS Competency Task Force. (2010). *Clinical nurse specialists core competencies: Executive summary 2006–2008.* Retrieved from http://www.nacns.org/docs/CNSCoreCompetenciesBroch.pdf

2008). This creates further challenges for the CNS, such as variability in state title protection, inconsistency among states grandfathering in the CNS role, lack of a regulatory approach to accepting grandfathered CNSs to practice in other states, and job loss based on misperceptions of the model (NACNS, 2005).

Nurse Educators

The role of nurse educators may be one of the most contentious issues in nursing education. According to the National League for Nursing (2002), the nurse educator role requires specialized preparation, and every individual engaged in the academic enterprise must be prepared to implement that role successfully. Nurse educators are key resources in preparing the nursing workforce to provide quality care to meet the healthcare needs of a rapidly aging and diverse population. Whether in academic or clinical settings, nurse educators must be competent clinicians. However, whereas being a good clinician is essential, some would say it is not sufficient for the educator role. Much of the debate in nursing education centers on the fact that the nurse educator student primarily needs advanced knowledge and skills in clinical practice in order to teach, and therefore graduate education should be directed toward enhancing clinical expertise. According to the AACN (2014), the master's-level curriculum for the nurse educator builds on baccalaureate knowledge, and graduate-level content in the areas of health assessment, pathophysiology, and pharmacology strengthen the graduate's scientific background and facilitate understanding of nursing and health-related information (AACN, 2014). In this model students are required to take courses beyond the graduate core curriculum and that provide content expertise in the "3 Ps" (pharmacology, pathophysiology, and physical assessment), similar to the education of nurse practitioners and clinical nurse leaders. On the other side of the argument, many clinicians who become nurse educators are already clinical experts and are content experts. They need the advanced degree to learn teaching/learning theories and strategies, curriculum development, and student evaluation content.

Nurse Educator Supply and Demand

The Health Resources and Services Administration (HRSA) has projected a large increase in demand for nurses, from approximately 2 million full-time equivalents in 2000 to approximately 2.8 million in 2020. See **Table 1-2.**

TABLE 1-2	Supply, Demand, Shortage of Nurses				
	2000	2005	2010	2015	2020
Supply	1,890,700	1,942,500	1,941,200	1,886,100	1,808,000
Demand	2,001,500	2,161,300	2,347,000	2,569.800	2,824,900
Shortage	(110,800)	(218,800)	(405,800)	(683,700)	(1,016,900)
Supply ÷ Demand	94%	90%	83%	73%	64%
Demand shortfall	6%	10%	17%	27%	36%

Source: Data from U.S. Department of Health and Human Services, 2004.

Meeting this projected demand will require a significant increase in the number of nursing graduates, perhaps by as much as 40%, to fill new nursing positions as well as to account for attrition from an aging workforce. This corresponds to an increase in the demand for nursing faculty. In 2008, approximately 13% of the nation's registered nurses held either a master's or doctoral degree as their highest educational preparation (AACN, 2011b). The current demand for master's- and doctorally prepared nurses for advanced practice, clinical specialties, teaching, and research roles far outstrips the supply.

Consequently, to increase the supply requires a major expansion of nursing faculty and other educational resources. With the "graying" of the current pool of nursing faculty, efforts we make must persuade more nurses and nursing students to pursue academic careers, and to do so at an earlier age. Careers in nursing education are typically marked by long periods of clinical practice prior to being educated for a faculty role. The idea of advanced practice nurses with clinical doctorates versus research doctorates working in academia has been supported by the National Organization of Nurse Practitioner Faculties, NLN, and AACN. The Doctor of Nursing Practice degree may be the answer to imparting advanced knowledge in evidence-based practice, quality improvement, leadership, policy advocacy, informatics, and healthcare systems to clinicians, managers, and educators. The DNP-prepared educator is poised to educate a future nursing workforce that can influence patient care outcomes. The nursing faculty shortage contributes to the problem of nursing programs turning away qualified applicants across graduate and undergraduate programs. See **Figure 1-2**.

This text addresses the essential content that nurses pursuing advanced degrees need to learn to prepare to be nurse educators. Competence as an educator can be established,

---

FIGURE 1-2   Faculty shortage.

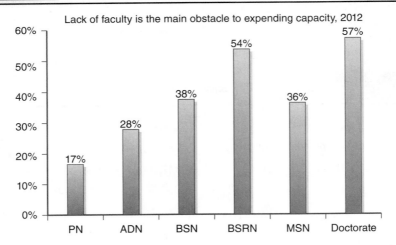

Lack of faculty is the main obstacle to expending capacity, 2012

Source: National League for nursing. 2013. Annual Survey of Schools of Nursing, Fall 2012.
www.nln.org/research/slides/index.htm.

Source: Data from National League for Nursing. (2012). Lack of Faculty Is Main Obstacle to Expanding Capacity, 2012.

recognized, and expanded through master's and doctoral education, post-master's certificate programs, continuing professional development courses, mentoring activities, and professional certification as a faculty member. Each academic unit in nursing must include a cadre of experts in nursing education who provide the leadership needed to advance nursing education, conduct pedagogical research, and contribute to the ongoing development of the science of nursing education.

Nurse Practitioners

Nurse practitioners have been providing care to vulnerable populations in rural and urban areas since the 1960s. The role was born out of the shortage of primary care physicians able to serve pediatric populations. Initial educational preparation ranged from 3 to 12 months, and as the role developed and expanded so did educational requirements. By the 1990s, the master's degree was endorsed as entry-level education for nurse practitioner specialties. In 2004, the AACN took a position recognizing the Doctor of Nursing Practice as the entry-level degree for advanced practice nursing, stating the following:

> Advanced competencies for increasingly complex clinical, faculty and leadership roles . . . enhanced knowledge to improve nursing practice and patient outcomes . . . enhanced leadership skills . . . better match of program requirements . . . provision of an advanced educational credential . . . parity with other health care professionals . . . enhanced ability to attract individuals to nursing from non-nursing backgrounds; increased supply of faculty for clinical instruction; and improved image of nursing. (AACN, 2004, p.7)

Today, nurse practitioners are the largest group of advanced practice nurses. More than 192,000 NPs are licensed and practicing with some level of prescriptive authority in all 50 states and the District of Columbia (American Association of Nurse Practitioners, 2013). Nurse practitioners work, are educated, and hold board certification in a variety of specialty areas, including pediatrics, family, adult-gerontology, women's health, and acute care, to name a few. See **Table 1-3**.

| TABLE 1-3 | Distribution, Mean Years of Practice, Mean Age by Population Focus |

Population	Percentage of NPs	Years of Practice	Age (years)
Acute care	6.3	7.7	46
Adult*	18.9	11.6	50
Family*	48.9	12.8	49
Gerontological*	3.0	11.6	53
Neonatal	2.1	12.2	49
Oncology	1.0	7.7	48
Pediatric*	8.3	12.4	49
Psych/mental health	3.2	9.1	54
Women's health*	8.1	15.5	53

*Primary care

Source: Data from the 2010 AANP National Practice Site Survey.

A federal initiative continues to exist to increase the number of primary care providers in the United States. The 2010 consensus report entitled the *Future of Nursing* developed by the Institute of Medicine (IOM) and the Robert Wood Johnson Foundation (RWJF) calls for a transformative change in nursing education. It calls for nurses to "practice to the full extent of their education and training" and for "nurses to achieve higher levels of education and training through an improved education system" (Institute of Medicine, 2010). This analysis and recommendation coincided with the passage of the legislation for the Patient Protection and Affordable Care Act of 2010, which is estimated to increase the need for qualified primary care providers to 241,200 by 2020. The supply of primary care NPs is projected to increase by 30%, from 55,400 in 2010 to 72,100 in 2020 (Health Resources and Services Administration, Bureau of Health Professions, National Center for Health Workforce Analysis, 2013). This, coupled with a demographically aging and ethnically diverse population, makes the demand for primary care providers, in particular, nurse practitioners, greater than ever. It is well known that nurse practitioners provide high-quality, safe, and cost-effective care. Excellent educational programs are needed to increase this pool of healthcare providers to improve access to care and strengthen care provided for elderly and other vulnerable populations.

Nurse-Midwives

The first nurse-midwifery school was established in 1925 by Mary Breckinridge, who founded the Frontier Nursing Service (FNS) in Hyden, Kentucky, in response to the high maternal and child death rates in rural eastern Kentucky, an area isolated by geography and poverty. The midwives were educated to provide family health services, as well as childbearing and delivery care, at nursing centers in the Appalachian Mountains. As reported by the FNS (2014), by the late 1950s the FNS nurse-midwives had attended more than 10,000 births, and maternal and infant outcome statistics in rural Kentucky were better than those for the whole country during the nurse-midwives first three decades of service. The most significant differences were in maternal mortality rates (9.1 per 10,000 births for FNS compared with 34 per 10,000 births for the United States as a whole) and low birth weights (3.8% for FNS compared with 7.6% for the country).

Today, all nurse-midwifery programs are housed in colleges and universities. There are multiple entry paths to midwifery education, but most nurse-midwives graduate at the master's degree level, and several programs culminate in the DNP degree. These programs must be accredited by the Accreditation Commission for Midwifery Education (ACME) for graduates to be eligible to take the national certification examination offered by the American Midwifery Certification Board (AMCB). Midwifery practice as conducted by certified nurse-midwives (CNMs) and certified midwives (CMs) is the autonomous primary care management of women's health, focusing on pregnancy, childbirth, the postpartum period, care of the newborn, family planning, and gynecologic needs of women.

CNMs are licensed, independent healthcare providers who have prescriptive authority in all 50 states, the District of Columbia, American Samoa, Guam, and Puerto Rico. CNMs are defined as primary care providers under federal law. Although midwives are well known for attending births, 53.3% of CNMs identify reproductive care and 33.1% identify primary care as their main responsibilities in their full-time positions (Fullerton, Schuiling, & Sipe, 2010). Examples include performing annual exams; writing prescriptions; providing basic nutrition counseling, parenting education, and patient education; and conducting reproductive health visits. According to the American Midwifery Certification Board, there are 13,071 CNMs and 84 CMs in practice in the United States. Since 1991, the number of midwife-attended births in the United States has nearly doubled. In 2012,

CNMs or CMs attended 313,846 births—a slight increase despite a decrease in total U.S. births compared with births in 2011 (ACNM, 2014).

In 2012, CNMs or CMs attended 91.7% of all midwife-attended births, 11.8% of all vaginal births, and 7.9% of total U.S. births (Martin, Hamilton, Osterman, Curtin, & Mathews, 2013). **Figure 1-3** shows birth data from 2000 to 2012. Whereas the majority of midwife-attended births occurs in hospitals, some occur at home and in freestanding birth centers. See **Figure 1-4**.

Allowing CNMs to have hospital privileges as full, active members of the medical staff would promote continuity of care, and birth certificate data would more accurately reflect provider type and outcomes (Buppert, 2012).

Medicaid reimbursement for midwifery care is mandatory in all states and is 100% of the physician fee schedule under the Medicare Part B fee schedule. The majority of states also mandates private insurance reimbursement for midwifery services. It is clear that nurse-midwives have improved primary healthcare services for women in rural and inner-city areas. It is imperative that nurse-midwives be given a larger role in delivering women's health care for the greater good of society.

Nurse Anesthetists

According to the American Association of Nurse Anesthetists (AANA), nurses have been providing anesthesia services to patients in the

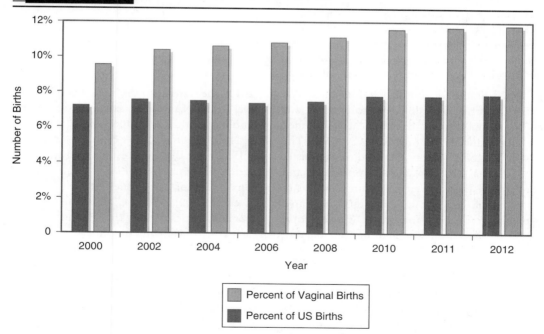

FIGURE 1-3 Percentage of births attended by certified nurse-midwives and certified midwives, 2002–2012.

Legend:
- Percent of Vaginal Births
- Percent of US Births

Source: Martin, J., Hamilton, B., Osterman, M., Curtin, S., & Mathews, T. (2013). Births: Final data for 2012. *National Vital Statistics Reports, 62*(9). Retrieved from http://www.cdc.gov/nchs/data/nvsr/nvsr62/nvsr62_09.pdf

FIGURE 1-4   Site of births attended by certified nurse-midwives and certified midwives, 2012.

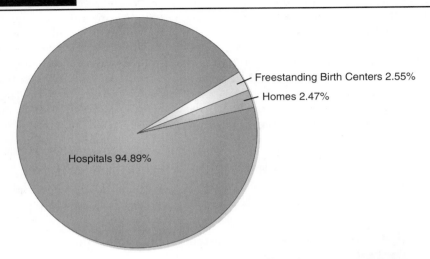

Freestanding Birth Centers 2.55%

Homes 2.47%

Hospitals 94.89%

Source: Martin, J., Hamilton, B., Osterman, M., Curtin, S., & Mathews, T. (2013). Births: Final data for 2012. *National Vital Statistics Reports, 62*(9). Retrieved from http://www.cdc.gov/nchs/data/nvsr/nvsr62 /nvsr62_09.pdf

United States for more than 150 years. The first anesthesia administered to patients was chloroform, used for the treatment of wounded soldiers during the American Civil War. The shortages of physicians qualified to administer anesthesia during wartimes continued, and nurse anesthetists were the main providers of anesthesia care for U.S. military personnel on the front lines for World War I, World War II, the Korean War, and the Vietnam War; nurse anesthetists also provide care in the current conflicts in the Middle East (Keeling, 2009).

Historically, nurse anesthetists have been the primary providers of anesthesia care in rural America, enabling healthcare facilities in medically underserved areas to offer obstetrical, surgical, pain management, and trauma stabilization services. In some states, CRNAs are the sole providers in nearly 100% of rural hospitals. According to the U.S. Bureau of Labor Statistics

(2013), the states with the highest employment level for CRNAs are Texas, Tennessee, North Carolina, Florida, and Ohio.

The credential CRNA came into existence in 1952 when the AANA established an accreditation program to monitor the quality and consistency of nurse anesthetist education (Keeling, 2009). Today, CRNAs safely administer anesthetics in more than 34 million cases each year in the United States, according to the AANA 2012 Practice Profile Survey. There are more than 44,000 CRNAs practicing in the United States (AANA, 2011). The scope and standards of practice for CRNAs are similar to those for other advanced practice registered nurses. Nurse anesthetists are licensed as independent practitioners, and they provide care autonomously and in collaboration with surgeons, dentists, podiatrists, and anesthesiologists, among other healthcare professionals. CRNAs provide evidence-based anesthesia and pain care services to patients at all acuity levels in a variety of settings for procedures, including, but not limited to, surgical, obstetrical, diagnostic, therapeutic, and pain management (AANA, 2013). Currently, CRNAs are qualified and have the legal authority to administer anesthesia without anesthesiologist supervision in all 50 states, the District of Columbia, Puerto Rico, and the Virgin Islands; however, some states have put into place restrictions and supervisory requirements in some settings (Joel, 2013).

NURSE ADMINISTRATORS

The term *nurse administrators* is being used to simplify the following discussion. This includes roles such as the nurse executive, supervisor, director, nurse manager, and so forth. Because individuals in these roles are responsible for leading a successful work environment, it is ironic that educational requirements for nurse administrators are not as demanding as those for other advanced practice roles. The knowledge, skills, and attitudes needed to be successful as a nurse administrator are not included in nursing baccalaureate programs, let alone associate degree/diploma programs, yet some of these exams are offered to experienced nurse managers without a baccalaureate and/or master's degree, as noted in **Table 1-4**.

There are two organizations that certify nurse administrators: the American Nurses Credentialing Center and the American Organization of Nurse Executives. Both offer certification exams in basic and advanced nursing administration. Table 1-4 includes the educational requirements for each organization. Years and levels of experience vary for each certification exam and can be accessed on their websites (American Nurses Credentialing Center, 2014; American Organization of Nurse Executives, 2014).

Further complicating the preparation of nurse administrators are the practices of many organizations of the following:

- Promoting good "bedside" nurses to managerial positions without assessing or developing their leadership abilities
- Weak orientation/on-the-job training for new nurse administrators
- No requirements for an advanced degree for the position

TABLE 1-4	Educational Requirements for Nurse Administrator Certifying Organizations	
	American Nurses Credentialing Center	**American Organization of Nurse Executives**
Basic certification	Hold a bachelor's or higher degree in nursing	Associate degree Diploma Bachelor's degree
Advanced certification	Hold a master's or higher degree in nursing, or hold a bachelor's degree in nursing and a master's in another field	Master's degree or higher

Source: Data from American Nurses Credentialing Center (ANCC). (2014). ANCC certification center. Retrieved from http://www.nursecredentialing.org/Certification; American Organization of Nurse Executives (AONE). (2014). About AONE credentialing center. Retrieved from http://www.aone.org/resources/certification/about_certifications.shtml

CONCLUSION

A national initiative exists to improve access to quality health care while reducing costs. This mandate will require the emergence of many new roles not yet imagined for nurses. Recently, new roles to serve as coordinators of care, such as nurse navigators and healthcare coaches, have been established. In the future, these roles may require advanced degrees and certification. Opportunities for nurses to coordinate care throughout the continuum of care are likely to abound. The aging population will require nurses to be "chronic disease specialists" and "wellness coaches." Population health, gender-specific health care, and global health specialties will become the norm. An understanding of the healthcare delivery system, healthcare policy, and care transition will need to be incorporated into graduate curricula. As this book goes to press, there is a push to expand and clarify the definition of and requirements for advanced practice nursing. No matter the final outcome of this deliberation, all nurses need the same set of essential knowledge and the ability to think outside the box.

DISCUSSION QUESTIONS _____

1. What are the differences between the terms *advanced practice nursing* and *advanced practice registered nurse*?
2. What emerging roles should be considered when describing advanced practice nursing?
3. Why was the APRN Consensus Model developed and what does it hope to do for the provision of health care?

REFERENCES _____

American Association of Colleges of Nursing (AACN). (2004). *AACN position statement on the practice doctorate in nursing.* Retrieved from http://www.aacn.nche.edu/DNP/pdf/DNP.pdf

American Association of Colleges of Nursing (AACN). (2006). *The essentials of doctoral education for advanced nursing practice.* Washington, DC: Author.

American Association of Colleges of Nursing (AACN). (2007). *White paper on the role of the clinical nurse leader.* Retrieved from http://www.aacn.nche.edu/aacn-publications/white-papers/cnl-white-paper

American Association of Colleges of Nursing (AACN). (2011a). *The essentials of master's education in nursing.* Washington, DC: Author.

American Association of Colleges of Nursing (AACN). (2011b). *2010–2011 enrollment and graduations in baccalaureate and graduate programs in nursing.* Washington, DC: Author.

American Association of Colleges of Nursing (AACN). (2014). *Essentials series.* Retrieved from http://www.aacn.nche.edu/education-resources/essential-series

American Association of Nurse Anesthetists (AANA). (2011). *CRNAs and the AANA fact sheet for patients.* Retrieved from http://www.aana.com/forpatients/Documents/crnas_aana.pdf

American Association of Nurse Anesthetists (AANA). (2013). *Professional practice documents: Scope of nurse anesthesia practice.* Retrieved from http://www.aana.com/resources2/professionalpractice/Pages/Scope-of-Nurse-Anesthesia-Practice.aspx

American Association of Nurse Practitioners (AANP). (2013). NP fact sheet. Retrieved from http://www.aanp.org/all-about-nps/np-fact-sheet

American College of Nurse-Midwives (ACNM). (2014). *Fact sheet: Essential facts about midwives.* Retrieved from http://www.midwife.org/ACNM/files/ccLibraryFiles/FILENAME/000000004001/EssentialFactsAboutMidwives-2014_FINAL.pdf

American Nurses Credentialing Center (ANCC). (2014). ANCC certification center. Retrieved from http://www.nursecredentialing.org/Certification

American Organization of Nurse Executives (AONE). (2014). About AONE credentialing center. Retrieved from http://www.aone.org/resources/certification/about_certifications.shtml

APRN Consensus Work Group & National Council of State Boards of Nursing APRN Advisory Committee. (2008, July 7). *Consensus model for APRN regulation: Licensure, accreditation, certification and education.* APRN Joint Dialogue Group Report. Retrieved from http://www.aacn.nche.edu/education-resources/APRNReport.pdf

Buppert, C. (2012). Hospital privileges. In C. Buppert (Ed.), *Nurse practitioner's business practice and legal guide* (pp. 247–253). Burlington, MA: Jones & Bartlett.

Frontier Nursing Service (FNS). (2014). A brief history of the Frontier Nursing Service. Retrieved from https://www.frontiernursing.org/History/HowFNSbegan.shtm

Fullerton, J., Schuiling, K., & Sipe, T. A. (2010). Findings from the analysis of the American College of Nurse-Midwives' membership surveys: 2006–2008. *Journal of Midwifery and Women's Health, 55,* 299–307.

Fulton, J. S. (2014). Evolution of the clinical nurse specialist role and practice in the United States. In J. S. Fulton, B. L. Lyon, K. A. Goudreau (Eds.), *Foundations of clinical nurse specialist practice* (2nd ed., pp. 1–16). New York, NY: Springer.

Haase-Herrick, K., & Herrin, D. (2007). The American organization of nurse executives' guiding principles and American Association of Colleges of Nursing's clinical nurse leader. *Journal of Nursing Administration, 37*(2), 55–60.

Health Resources and Services Administration, Bureau of Health Professions, National Center for Health Workforce Analysis. (2013). *Projecting the supply and demand for primary care practitioners through 2020.* Retrieved from http://bhpr.hrsa.gov/healthworkforce/supplydemand/usworkforce/primarycare/projectingprimarycare.pdf

Institute of Medicine. (2010). *The future of nursing: Leading change, advancing health.* Retrieved from http://www.iom.edu/Reports/2010/the-future-of-nursing-leading-change-advancing-health.aspx

Joel, L. (2013). *Advance practice nursing: Essentials of role development* (3rd ed.). Philadelphia, PA: F. A. Davis.

Keeling, A.W. (2009). A brief history of advance nursing practice in the United States. In A. B. Hamric, J. A. Spross, & C. M. Hanson (Eds.), *Advanced practice nursing: An integrative approach* (4th ed., pp. 3–32). St. Louis, MO: Elsevier.

Martin, J., Hamilton, B., Osterman, M., Curtin, S., & Mathews, T. (2013). Births: Final data for 2012. *National Vital Statistics Reports, 62*(9). Retrieved from http://www.cdc.gov/nchs/data/nvsr/nvsr62/nvsr62_09.pdf

McClelland, M., McCoy, M., & Burson, R. (2013). Clinical nurse specialists: Then, now, and the future of the profession. *Clinical Nurse Specialist, 27*(2), 96–102.

National Association of Clinical Nurse Specialists (NACNS). (2005). *Statement on clinical nurse specialist practice and education* (2nd ed.). Harrisburg, PA: Author.

National CNS Competency Task Force. (2010). *Clinical nurse specialists core competencies: Executive summary 2006–2008.* Retrieved from http://www.nacns.org/docs/CNSCoreCompetenciesBroch.pdf

National League for Nursing (NLN). (2002). *Position.* Retrieved from http://www.nln.org/aboutnln/PositionSTatements/prepofnursed02.htm

National League for Nursing (NLN). (2012). Annual surveys of schools of nursing, fall 2011. Retrieved from http://www.nln.org/researchgrants/slides/topic_admissions_rn.htm

U.S. Bureau of Labor Statistics. (2013). *Occupational employment and wages 29-1151 nurse anesthetists.* Retrieved from http://www.bls.gov/oes/current/oes291151.htm#st

CHAPTER 2

© A-R-T/Shutterstock

The Nurse Practitioner: Historical Perspectives on the Art and Science of Nurse Practitionering

Julie G. Stewart

CHAPTER OBJECTIVES

1. Identify factors that contributed to the evolution of the nurse practitioner role in the United States.
2. Describe the key attributes that make the nurse practitioner role unique.
3. Identify the different educational pathways that are shaping the curriculum in nurse practitioner programs.

These are heady days to be a nurse. With a 2-year-old mandate from the Institute of Medicine calling for us to practice at the highest level of our profession, achieve independence from physician oversight as we diagnose, prescribe, treat sick patients, and care for patients with increasingly complex cases, nurses are poised like never before to continue their march toward the center of healthcare delivery.

It's high time. More and more of us are turning to nurse practitioners for our primary care. And it's not just because they're easier to get appointments with (they are), spend dramatically more time with patients (they do), and have much of the same prescriptive powers as physicians (though not, as yet, in Virginia). It's not even because they get excellent training as healthcare generalists or that advanced practice nurses, like NPs, are everywhere, with some 9,000 new ones graduating each year and joining the ranks of the nation's roughly 140,000.

It's because the care that advanced practice nurses give—at physician-led offices, minute clinics, rural healthcare centers, and bustling urban hospitals—is second to none.

—Reprinted by permission of Dr. Dorrie Fontaine, Dean, University of Virginia School of Nursing, 2012

Nurse practitioners (NPs) have reached a tipping point as a profession (Buerhaus, 2010). Malcolm Gladwell (2000) states that the "tipping point is that magic moment when an idea, trend, or social behavior crosses a threshold, tips, and spreads like wildfire" (p. 12). We are aware that we have reached a time in which nurse practitioners have been given the opportunity to shine and to experience growth professionally. Nurse practitioners provide a solution to some of the issues affecting health care in the United States today. In 2010 the Institute of Medicine (IOM) released a report that identified the need for nurses to be placed at the forefront of health care. The report strongly recommended that advanced practice registered nurses—including nurse practitioners—be allowed to practice to the full scope of their abilities, and that barriers be removed to enable moving forward. The need for NPs is growing as we consider the IOM's recommendation and the large population of aging baby boomers, which is anticipated to increase the use of the healthcare system (Centers for Medicare and Medicaid Services [CMS], 2011; Van Leuven, 2012). In addition, the Patient Protection and Affordable Care Act signed in 2010 instituted comprehensive health insurance reform and has the potential to expand healthcare insurance coverage to 48 million uninsured Americans (Kaiser Family Foundation, 2014). Researchers have validated the cost, quality, and competence of NPs who provide primary care, and patient care outcomes are similar to those of primary care physicians (Hamric, Spross, & Hanson, 2009; Laurant et al., 2005; Mundinger et al., 2000; Wilson et al., 2005). Medical economist and health futurist Jeffrey C. Bauer (2010) reviewed evidence-based data to illustrate how NPs functioning independently can meet the need for cost-effectiveness of healthcare reform while providing high-quality care for patients in multiple settings.

Many important research articles published over a span of 4 decades speak to the excellent quality of care nurse practitioners provide (American Association of Nurse Practitioners [AANP], 2010b). At least 89% of NPs are educated to provide primary care (AANP, n.d.); however, in some states, many NPs do not work in primary care, possibly because of the state's requirements for collaborators and written agreements with physicians. Many states have recognized these barriers and have removed such requirements, and many insurance companies now include NPs in their provider networks. So, will we meet the near-future needs for healthcare providers? The answer appears to be a resounding yes. In an age-cohort regression-based model, RAND Health projected the future workforce of NPs will grow to 244,000 by the year 2025 (Auerbach, 2012). Clearly, there is a need to fully understand the role of the NP in order to advance professionalism and unity of the NP workforce. Pertinent issues must be discussed as part of the education of student NPs as well as among NPs already in practice.

HISTORICAL PERSPECTIVE

The role of the nurse practitioner was developed as a way to provide primary care for the underserved. The role is typically described as having emerged during the 1960s, yet Lillian Wald's nurses of the late 1800s bear a striking resemblance to the NPs of today. The nurses of Wald's Henry Street Settlement House in New York City provided primary care for poverty-stricken immigrants and treated common illnesses and emergencies that did not require referral (Hamric et al., 2009). In 1965 the role of nurse practitioner was formally developed by Loretta Ford, EdD (nurse educator), and Henry Silver, MD (professor of medicine), both of whom were teaching at the University of Colorado (Sullivan-Marx, McGivern, Fairman, & Greenberg, 2010). The nurse practitioner program was developed not only to advance the nursing profession but also to respond to the need for providers in rural, underserved areas. The program was initially funded by a $7,000 grant from the School of Medicine at the University of Colorado (Bruner, 2005; Weiland, 2008). The first program, a pediatric NP program, was based on the nursing model and advanced the clinical practice of students by teaching them how to provide primary care and how to make medical diagnoses.

Whereas NP pioneers focused on advancing the profession, "making a difference," and gaining autonomy (Weiland, 2008, p. 346), in the socioeconomic and political climate of the times, the NP was viewed as a cost-effective way to provide health care to the underserved. During the 1970s, federal funding helped to establish many NP programs to address a shortage of primary care physicians, particularly in underserved areas. In 1971 Idaho was the first state to endorse nurse practitioners' scope of practice to include diagnosis and treatment. The number of NP programs doubled between 1992 and 1997. By the year 2000, 321 institutions offered either a master's-level or a post-master's-level NP program (Health Resources and Services Administration, Bureau of Health Professions, 2004). By 2002, more than 30% of NPs were working with vulnerable populations, including homeless, indigent, chronically ill, and elderly patients (Jenning, 2002). Today there are more than 192,000 nurse practitioners in the United States, with approximately 87% of these professionals in clinical practice as NPs in primary care, acute care, and rural health care (AANP, 2014; Ortiz, Wan, Meemon, Paek, & Agiro, 2010; Pearson, 2011).

With the need for healthcare providers expanding, and the focus on the ability of NPs to fulfill that role, schools are accepting more applicants for the NP track than before. In 2011, more than 14,000 students graduated from approximately 360 NP programs in the United States (AANP, 2014; Pearson, 2011).

NURSE PRACTITIONER EDUCATION AND TITLE CLARIFICATION

In the 1960s, the role of the NP was not warmly welcomed by nurse educators; therefore, many of the educational programs to train nurses in the NP role were continuing education programs rather than university-housed programs (Pulcini, 2013). In the 1980s and 1990s, NP education moved into the university setting as master's-level programs, although confusion arose when efforts were made to interchange the clinical nurse specialist (CNS) and NP roles. Today more than 330 graduate-level NP programs exist. Many offer a clinical doctorate—the Doctor of Nursing Practice (DNP)—for NP education in response to the American Association of Colleges of Nursing (AACN) recommendation that advanced practice nurses be educated at that level by 2015.

In 2008 the *Consensus Model for APRN Regulation: Licensure, Accreditation, Certification and Education* was finalized through the collaborative efforts of the APRN Consensus Work Group and the National Council of State Boards of Nursing APRN Advisory Committee (2008). To clarify who is an advanced practice registered nurse, the document included the following definition:

An advanced practice registered nurse (APRN) is a nurse:

1. Who has completed an accredited graduate-level education program preparing him or her for one of the four recognized APRN roles;

2. Who has passed a national certification examination that measures APRN, role and population-focused competencies, and who maintains continued competence as evidenced by recertification in the role and population through the national certification program;

3. Who has acquired advanced clinical knowledge and skills preparing him or her to provide direct care to patients, as well as

a component of indirect care; however, the defining factor for all APRNs is that a significant component of the education and practice focuses on direct care of individuals;

4. Whose practice builds on the competencies of registered nurses (RNs) by demonstrating a greater depth and breadth of knowledge, a greater synthesis of data, increased complexity of skills and interventions, and greater role autonomy;

5. Who is educationally prepared to assume responsibility and accountability for health promotion and maintenance as well as the assessment, diagnosis, and management of patient problems, which includes the use and prescription of pharmacologic and nonpharmacologic interventions;

6. Who has clinical experience of sufficient depth and breadth to reflect the intended license; and

7. Who has obtained a license to practice as an APRN in one of the four APRN roles: certified registered nurse anesthetist (CRNA), certified nurse-midwife (CNM), clinical nurse specialist (CNS), or certified nurse practitioner (CNP).

Clearly, the NP role is included under the umbrella definition of APRN; however, the title APRN does not clearly define which role and what type of educational background a professional has. Each APRN role differs from the others, and state regulatory agency requirements for licensing vary in each state and, in many cases, for each APRN role.

THE MASTER'S ESSENTIALS

The American Association of Colleges of Nursing prepared the *Essentials of Master's Education in Nursing* (American Association of Colleges of Nursing [AACN], 2011). Nine essentials focus on outcomes for all master's-level programs. In addition, direct patient care provider (APRN) education must offer

three separate courses on the "3 Ps": advanced pharmacology, advanced pathophysiology, and advanced physical assessment. The nine essentials are as follows:

  I. Background for practice from sciences and humanities
 II. Organizational and systems leadership
III. Quality improvement and safety
 IV. Translating and integrating scholarship into practice
  V. Informatics and healthcare technologies
 VI. Health policy and advocacy
VII. Interprofessional collaboration for improving patient and population health outcomes
VIII. Clinical prevention and population health for improving health
 IX. Master's-level nursing practice

Essential IX, master's-level nursing practice, recognizes that nursing practice at the master's level is broadly defined as any form of nursing intervention that influences healthcare outcomes for individuals, populations, or systems. Master's-level nursing graduates must have an advanced level of understanding of nursing and relevant sciences as well as the ability to integrate this knowledge into practice. Nursing practice interventions include both direct and indirect care components (AACN, 2011).

NURSE PRACTITIONER CORE COMPETENCIES

In addition to the AACN, which strives to advance the education of nurses in general, the National Organization of Nurse Practitioner Faculties (NONPF) sets the standards for nurse practitioner programs. NONPF (2012) states that there are core competencies for nurse practitioners in all tracks and specialties. The core competencies are listed here to demonstrate how coursework reflects these competencies.

Scientific Foundation Competencies

1. Critically analyzes data and evidence for improving advanced nursing practice.
2. Integrates knowledge from the humanities and sciences within the context of nursing science.
3. Translates research and other forms of knowledge to improve practice processes and outcomes.
4. Develops new practice approaches based on the integration of research, theory, and practice knowledge.

Leadership Competencies

1. Assumes complex and advanced leadership roles to initiate and guide change.
2. Provides leadership to foster collaboration with multiple stakeholders (e.g., patients, community, integrated healthcare teams, and policymakers) to improve health care.
3. Demonstrates leadership that uses critical and reflective thinking.
4. Advocates for improved access, quality, and cost-effective health care.
5. Advances practice through the development and implementation of innovations incorporating principles of change.
6. Communicates practice knowledge effectively both orally and in writing.
7. Participates in professional organizations and activities that influence advanced practice nursing and/or health outcomes of a population focus.

QUALITY COMPETENCIES

1. Uses best available evidence to continuously improve quality of clinical practice.
2. Evaluates the relationships among access, cost, quality, and safety and their influence on health care.
3. Evaluates how organizational structure, care processes, financing, marketing, and policy decisions impact the quality of health care.

4. Applies skills in peer review to promote a culture of excellence.
5. Anticipates variations in practice and is proactive in implementing interventions to ensure quality.

Practice Inquiry Competencies

1. Provides leadership in the translation of new knowledge into practice.
2. Generates knowledge from clinical practice to improve practice and patient outcomes.
3. Applies clinical investigative skills to improve health outcomes.
4. Leads practice inquiry, individually or in partnership with others.
5. Disseminates evidence from inquiry to diverse audiences using multiple modalities.
6. Analyzes clinical guidelines for individualized application into practice.

TECHNOLOGY AND INFORMATION LITERACY COMPETENCIES

1. Integrates appropriate technologies for knowledge management to improve health care.
2. Translates technical and scientific health information appropriate for various users' needs.
   a. Assesses the patient's and caregiver's educational needs to provide effective, personalized health care.
   b. Coaches the patient and caregiver for positive behavioral change.
3. Demonstrates information literacy skills in complex decision making.
4. Contributes to the design of clinical information systems that promote safe, high-quality, and cost-effective care.
5. Uses technology systems that capture data on variables for the evaluation of nursing care.

POLICY COMPETENCIES

1. Demonstrates an understanding of the interdependence of policy and practice.

2. Advocates for ethical policies that promote access, equity, quality, and cost.

3. Analyzes ethical, legal, and social factors influencing policy development.

4. Contributes in the development of health policy.

5. Analyzes the implications of health policy across disciplines.

6. Evaluates the impact of globalization on healthcare policy development.

Health Delivery System Competencies

1. Applies knowledge of organizational practices and complex systems to improve healthcare delivery.

2. Effects health care change using broad-based skills including negotiating, consensus building, and partnering.

3. Minimizes risk to patients and providers at the individual and systems level.

4. Facilitates the development of healthcare systems that address the needs of culturally diverse populations, providers, and other stakeholders.

5. Evaluates the impact of healthcare delivery on patients, providers, other stakeholders, and the environment.

6. Analyzes organizational structure, functions, and resources to improve the delivery of care.

7. Collaborates in planning for transitions across the continuum of care.

Ethics Competencies

1. Integrates ethical principles in decision making.

2. Evaluates the ethical consequences of decisions.

3. Applies ethically sound solutions to complex issues related to individuals, populations, and systems of care.

Independent Practice Competencies

1. Functions as a licensed independent practitioner.

2. Demonstrates the highest level of accountability for professional practice.

3. Practices independently, managing previously diagnosed and undiagnosed patients.

   a. Provides the full spectrum of healthcare services to include health promotion, disease prevention, health protection, anticipatory guidance, counseling, disease management, palliative care, and end-of-life care.

   b. Uses advanced health assessment skills to differentiate between normal, variations of normal, and abnormal findings.

   c. Employs screening and diagnostic strategies in the development of diagnoses.

   d. Prescribes medications within scope of practice.

   e. Manages the health or illness status of patients and families over time.

4. Provides patient-centered care recognizing cultural diversity and the patient or designee as a full partner in decision making.

   a. Works to establish a relationship with the patient characterized by mutual respect, empathy, and collaboration.

   b. Creates a climate of patient-centered care to include confidentiality, privacy, comfort, emotional support, mutual trust, and respect.

   c. Incorporates the patient's cultural and spiritual preferences, values, and beliefs into health care.

   d. Preserves the patient's control over decision making by negotiating a mutually acceptable plan of care.

The comprehensive nature of the competencies for role development is necessary and useful for developing curricula, evaluating the NP student during the educational training period, and establishing standards to which the practicing NP can be held accountable.

DOCTOR OF NURSING PRACTICE

In 1999 the AACN developed a task force to address the confusion that had arisen around the variety of doctoral degrees available to nurses (Zaccagnini & White, 2011). Until this point, nurses had obtained doctorates in education (EdD), in nursing (ND), in nursing science (DNS/DNSc), and in other disciplines. In 2004, the AACN formally approved the Doctor of Nursing Practice (DNP) degree, which focuses on clinical practice in contrast to the research focus of the PhD. The DNP degree is available as a clinical doctorate for all nurses—not only NPs—who seek to improve healthcare delivery systems and patient outcomes. Although an original goal was to require by 2015 that the DNP degree be an entry requirement for NP education, the complexities associated with the endeavor, particularly at the state licensure level, make this unlikely to occur in such a short time. However, AACN endorses achievement of the DNP degree as a goal for all APRNs (AACN, 2013). The DNP degree is recognized as the terminal practice degree (AACN, 2006).

Why the need for a DNP degree when numerous studies have validated the excellent and cost-effective care provided by MSN-level NPs (AANP, 2010a, 2010b)? Owing to the ever-increasing complexity of health care and healthcare delivery systems, it is optimal to have clinicians who are well educated in the areas of health policy, quality improvement, evidence-based practice, and outcomes evaluation. Currently, MSN-level programs for NPs require 42–50 credits—much more than other MSN tracks, which typically require approximately 30 credits for completion. In addition, most NP programs require at least 500–600 clinical hours to graduate and take certification examinations. The DNP degree offers the NP student additional education and preparation to meet the needs of the complex healthcare system of the near future. Also, NPs work collaboratively with numerous other doctorally prepared clinicians whose education was clinically focused, including pharmacists (PharmD), physical therapists (DPT), physicians (MD), doctors of osteopathy (DO), and naturopaths (ND). To achieve educational

parity, the clinical doctorate (DNP) is recommended for nurse practitioners.

Currently, 184 DNP programs in the United States enroll students, and at least another 101 DNP programs are being developed (AACN, 2013). In 2012 more than 8,900 nurses were enrolled in a DNP program (AACN, 2013). There are differences in the existing programs, particularly as they relate to the scholarship of the terminal project—the title of which in itself has sparked numerous passionate debates among leaders in doctoral-level nursing education. Whether the final scholarly product is called a project, project dissertation, practice dissertation, practice project, or—perhaps more like an MSN terminal project—a capstone, it is crucial that the NP/DNP be fully educated on the various types of research and evidence-based practice approaches to health care on individual and aggregate levels. It is important not to further discredit the clinical practice doctorate by drawing any lines in the sand as to who may or may not conduct research. That being said, it is probably much more appropriate for nursing's PhD colleagues to focus on theory development and for NPs/DNPs to focus on knowledge vital to practice (Dahnke & Dreher, 2011).

The AACN published *The Essentials of Doctoral Education for Advanced Nursing Practice* to shape the education of the DNP student to meet quality indicator criteria. The essentials were developed to build on the baccalaureate and master's essentials. They align with recommendations from the Institute of Medicine (IOM) that emphasize quality in education and evidence-based practice and that advocate nurses practice to the full extent of their scope of practice (Zaccagnini & White, 2011). The DNP essentials are as follows (AACN, 2006):

DNP Essentials

I. Scientific underpinnings for practice

II. Organizational and systems leadership for quality improvement and systems thinking

III. Clinical scholarship and analytical methods for evidence-based practice

IV. Information systems/technology and patient care technology for the improvement and transformation of health care

V. Healthcare policy for advocacy in health care

VI. Interprofessional collaboration for improving patient and population health outcomes

VII. Clinical prevention and population health for improving the nation's health

VIII. Advanced nursing practice

The DNP essentials also contain language that reflects the need for the 3 Ps and the expertise required of APNs, which is in the following paragraphs for ease of access during seminar discussions.

Advanced Practice Nursing Focus

The DNP graduate prepared for an APN role must demonstrate practice expertise, specialized knowledge, and expanded responsibility and accountability in the care and management of individuals and families. By virtue of this direct care focus, APNs develop additional competencies in direct practice and in the guidance and coaching of individuals and families through developmental, health–illness, and situational transitions (Hamric et al., 2009). The direct practice of APNs is characterized by the use of a holistic perspective; the formation of therapeutic partnerships to facilitate informed decision making, positive lifestyle change, and appropriate self-care; advanced practice thinking, judgment, and skillful performance; and use of diverse, evidence-based interventions in health and illness management (Brown, 2005).

APNs assess, manage, and evaluate patients at the most independent level of clinical nursing practice. They are expected to use advanced, highly refined assessment skills and employ a thorough understanding of pathophysiology and pharmacotherapeutics in making diagnostic and practice management decisions. To ensure sufficient

depth and focus, it is mandatory that a separate course be required for each of these three content areas: advanced health/physical assessment, advanced physiology/pathophysiology, and advanced pharmacology. In addition to direct care, DNP graduates emphasizing care of individuals should be able to use their understanding of the practice context to document practice trends, identify potential systemic changes, and make improvements in the care of their particular patient populations in the systems within which they practice. (AACN, 2006, p. 18)

To be clear, the DNP degree does not confer a change in scope of practice. What it does afford nurses is the opportunity to improve health outcomes for patients and populations by supplying the tools to do so. Opportunities abound for the DNP/NP: the ability to clinically practice anywhere; to act in leadership roles in community health centers, larger acute care facilities, solo practice sites, and nurse-managed health centers; to perform research and then apply it in practice; to have joint appointments with educational institutions and healthcare facilities; to be a leader in disease management; and much more. Most importantly, the DNP/NP has the credibility and skills to be outstanding in clinical excellence. So, why become an NP? What is it that makes this role unique?

NURSE PRACTITIONERS' APPROACH TO PATIENT CARE

Sometimes I am asked why I became an NP instead of a doctor. My response is that becoming a nurse practitioner gave me the best of both worlds, nursing and medicine. I support my answer by stating that nursing continues to be one of the top trusted professions in the United States (Gallup Politics, 2012). I also point out that NPs have extremely high patient satisfaction scores, and nurse practitioners have a unique approach to health care (Weiland, 2008). This is not to say that there are no doctors who are amazing, but a common theme I hear from my patient population is that "nurses listen to what I have to say." One study found that only 50% of the patients seen by physicians—compared to more than 80% of NP patients—reported that they felt that the healthcare provider "always" listened carefully (Creech, Filter, & Bowman, 2011). In a study of more than 1.5 million veterans, satisfaction levels were highest in primary care clinics when the healthcare provider was an NP (Budzi, Lurie, Singh, & Hooker, 2010). Budzi and colleagues state that NPs' interpersonal skills in patient teaching, counseling, and patient-centered care contribute to positive health outcomes and patient satisfaction. These researchers concluded their report by encouraging the largest healthcare system in the United States to hire more NPs to increase access to cost-effective, quality care.

Of course, it is important to review and analyze quantitative research that supports the cost-effectiveness and improved health outcomes when NPs provide primary care, but it is also as important (in many cases, more important) to listen to what patients have to say about their experiences with NPs as healthcare providers. See the boxed feature "Stephanie's Story."

CASE STUDY   Stephanie's Story

At the turn of my 25th birthday, life was going well for me. I had just completed my master's degree in elementary education and secured my first job as a head teacher in a local private school. I enjoyed my time during the day with my students, excited to employ the learning strategies I had discovered in graduate school. After school hours and on the weekends, I spent my time exercising outside, traipsing around New York City, and socializing with my friends and family. All of this changed the day I visited my gynecologist seeking treatment for a yeast infection.

Having no relief from an over-the-counter antifungal medication, I turned to my gynecologist—a highly regarded physician who studied at the Chicago School of Medicine. I found Dr. X to be warm, attentive, and funny; she did her best to make me feel comfortable despite the lay-on-your-back-feet-up-in-stirrups position. After confirming my self-diagnosis with a culture, Dr. X prescribed an antifungal suppository cream and sent me on my way home.

At the end of treatment, I still had severe itching and called my gynecologist's office.

After discussing my situation with the nurse, we both assumed that I was fighting off a tough strain. Dr. X prescribed a stronger medication for me, and although I was itchy throughout this course of treatment, I held hope that my symptoms would abate soon after.

Still plagued with itching, I visited Dr. X a week after I finished the latest medicine. She asked me to remind her if diabetes ran in my family. She asked me to have my primary care physician run some blood work to be certain that I had not developed type 2. Throughout this, Dr. X and I still kept our humor about my condition. Although we were puzzled about why it lasted so long, we both assumed that it would clear up shortly.

Unfortunately, we were wrong. For 3 more months, Dr. X examined me at least twice each month as I was still experiencing relentless itching and redness. At each visit, she swabbed my vagina, ran a culture, asked if I was certain that I was not diabetic, and then prescribed me a cream, suppository, or pills. Dr. X explained that I would always test positive for yeast, as it is normal for a small amount to live in the vagina.

(continues)

However, she was surprised that the small amount of cells that I had caused me to be so itchy and red, that I must be sensitive to yeast.

Throughout my treatment with Dr. X, she maintained her warm demeanor; however, her nursing staff grew irritated with me. They became curt with me, sighing on the phone upon hearing my voice and rushing me through procedures at office visits. Through their lack of professionalism, they made it clear that I was not an important patient and that they were skeptical of my condition.

I began to feel worn down, broken. A simple infection had turned into a chronic illness, causing my gregarious nature to fade. I no longer wished to go out with friends. I pushed prospective boyfriends away so I would not have to contend with intimacy. I stopped exercising as body heat and sweat further aggravated my symptoms. I was tired of being sick.

Understanding my discomfort, which seemed to intensify after each round of medication, Dr. X decided to try something that was not a typical course of treatment: gentian violet. This antifungal dye was "painted" onto the outside of my vagina as well as inside the first third of the canal. As with the previous medications, my symptoms worsened. My skin felt raw and burned. And although I thought it impossible at this stage, the incessant itching intensified. Dr. X was all out of ideas and sent me to see a *Candida* specialist located 90 minutes away.

Dr. Y was an older man who entered the exam room while laughing with his nurse. Immediately he acted as though we had known each other for years. He was overly familiar, touching my arm, and doing his best to assure me that there wasn't a patient yet who presented a medical condition he couldn't fix. I quickly regretted taking Dr. X's recommendation to see him.

After Dr. Y questioned me about my condition, he asked me to lie back and then made sure to point out the strategically placed artwork in the room. Above my head on the ceiling was a painting by Georgia O'Keefe. O'Keefe is famous for her floral still lifes that strongly resemble parts of the female anatomy. Dr. Y not only thought this was comical, considering his line of work, but also believed the art helped distract his patients from why they were in the stirrups. Personally, I found this strange, and rather than diverting my attention away from the purpose of my visit, I was forced to stare at a visual reminder while lying down!

Dr. Y separately swabbed the inside of my mouth, vagina, and anus, all the while sharing double-entendre jokes with his nurse. Half-naked and vulnerable, I willed myself to go through with the exam thinking that if I could get through these lousy 10 minutes I could finally have an answer to my problem. Dr. Y sent the swabs off to a lab, and then wrote me a prescription for an antidepressant. He told me that sometimes when a person has an illness as long as I have, it really is no longer a medical condition as much as a psychological one. He told me to take the antidepressant for at least 6 weeks and that it should help get my mind off dwelling on my problem and that he wouldn't be surprised if my symptoms vanished by that time. The nurses at Dr. X's office made me feel as though they didn't believe that I had an actual medical issue, and now this "specialist" was saying the same thing.

Desperate for relief and willing to consider the possibility that my illness was "all in my head," I began the antidepressant. When Dr. X's office called to say that my tests were negative for *Candida*, I continued the antidepressant, now hoping that it was a psychological issue, meaning there would be an end

CASE STUDY Stephanie's Story *(continued)*

eventually. Although my mood had improved a bit, the itching and redness did not. During this time, I had scheduled an appointment with my dermatologist to check a questionable mole. Prior to her exam, Dr. Z asked how I was doing, what was new with me. I opened my mouth to say "fine," but broke down in tears. I had been uncomfortable and frustrated for so long that I couldn't control my emotions. I explained my ordeal—which by this point had been going on for over 6 months—to Dr. Z, and she replied, "I think I know what you have."

Dr. Z. suspected that I had acquired eczema from being overmedicated. A biopsy of my labia proved her correct, and I started a course of steroid treatment that lasted for several months. The relief was immediate! While I was ecstatic that I was on my way back to normal, I was also very angry. Initially, yes, I had a yeast infection. But at some point, the infection cleared and the itching and redness was from the medications. So, having a small amount of yeast cells in the cultures should have been a clue to Dr. X that it was not an infection. Dr. Y could not correctly diagnose my condition either and could only focus on yeast. After my experiences with Drs. X and Y, I lost trust in their capabilities as diagnosticians. I stopped seeing Dr. X and missed a year between my annual exams.

Months after I ended my steroid treatment, I developed what I was certain was a yeast infection. Scared to return to a gynecologist, I called my neighbor, a nurse practitioner, for a recommendation. She referred me to a fellow nurse practitioner who was working at the local Planned Parenthood. The NP was a friendly woman and patiently listened as I told her my recent medical history. She examined me, found a high number of yeast cells in the culture, and then prescribed me an

oral antifungal so as not to cause the eczema to return. Because I had experienced recurring yeast infections, she asked if I was diabetic. Unlike Drs. X and Y, and the nurses at their offices, the NP didn't stop after my reply of no. She then asked if I had a lot of wheat and/or chocolate in my diet as some recent studies have shown a correlation between those foods and yeast infections. Not able to do a thorough evaluation of my diet on the spot, I told her that I didn't think so. She told me to think about it and to give her a call to let her know how I fared with the medication.

On my drive home from Planned Parenthood, I started thinking about what I ate that morning and noon for lunch and couldn't believe how unaware I had been earlier with the NP. My breakfast had consisted of fruit and almond butter on two wheat waffles. Lunch was ham and cheese on whole wheat bread. The more I thought about my eating habits, the more I realized that wheat was in heavy rotation in my daily diet, and chocolate did indeed play a role during my menstrual cycle. I drove past my house and directly to the supermarket to purchase both wheat-free waffles and bread.

In the 8 years since spending those enlightening 30 minutes with the NP, I have had only two yeast infections, both successfully treated with over-the-counter medications. The NP shared invaluable information with me, information that has changed my life. To this day, if one is available, I prefer to see an NP to a doctor. I have found that the NPs tend to think more outside the box to solve a problem. They seem to be more aware of current research and studies and are willing to share this with their patients.

Thanks to my NP, I no longer have a chronic illness.

WHAT NURSE PRACTITIONERS DO

To articulate what nurse practitioners actually do, it is easy to discuss NPs' daily tasks: reviewing laboratory tests, performing physical examinations, charting, writing prescriptions, and ordering radiological procedures. Yet this approach describes only the profession or duties of the NP, and not the actual art of nurse practitionering.

Nurse practitionering—a unique term—incorporates the vital elements of nursing as well as philosophical theories, communication skills, diagnostic skills, coaching and educating activities, and, most importantly, skills for developing reciprocal relationships with patients. The foundation of nursing forms the basis of a holistic approach to the interview, assessment, diagnosis, and collaboration on goals for patient care, which help NPs to engage patients as full partners in aspects of their health care.

Dr. Loretta Ford described what sets NPs apart from primary care physicians as holistically oriented goals for self-care (Weiland, 2008). Florence Nightingale recognized the main difference between nursing and medicine by writing that, whereas medicine focuses on disease, nursing focuses on illness and suffering with the goals of easing suffering and promoting disease prevention (Nightingale, 1859/2009). Physicians are trained in a framework that is different from the one used to educate NPs. In an interesting article titled "The Total Package: A Skillful, Compassionate Doctor," the theme was stated thusly:

> Traditionally, medical school curricula have focused on the pathophysiology of disease while neglecting the very real impact of disease on the patient's social and psychological experience, that is, their illness experience. It is in this intersection that humanism plays a profound role. (Indiana University, 2009)

NPs, with their comprehensive, humanistic nursing background, formulate nurse practitionering in that intersection.

The role of the nurse practitioner is based on a nursing foundation and has integrated segments of the medical model to become the unique profession of nurse practitioner; therefore, differences in the role and practice of nurses and nurse practitioners exist (Haugsdal & Scherb, 2003; Kleinman, 2004; Nicoteri & Andrews, 2003; Roberts, Tabloski, & Bova, 1997). However, there remains confusion among the public and other members of the healthcare professions, as well as among some NP students, as to what NP practice truly is.

It is not surprising that defining nurse practitionering is difficult when one considers that it has historically been difficult to define nursing (Chitty & Black, 2007). Certainly today we have comprehensive definitions of nursing as developed by the American Nurses Association, Royal College of Nursing, and International Council of Nurses; however, it seems that Florence Nightingale wrote the first definition of a holistic approach to patient-centered care that can apply to the concept of nurse practitionering:

> I use the word nursing for want of a better. It has been limited to signify little more than the administration of medicines and the application of poultices. It ought to signify the proper use of fresh air, light, warmth, cleanliness, quiet, and the proper selection and administration of diet—all at the least expense of vital power to the patient. (Nightingale, 1859/2009)

NURSING THEORIES FOR NURSE PRACTITIONERS

Many nursing philosophies, theories, and models exist today, and NPs can and should build their professional practice on these. For example, Henderson (1991) identified the 14 basic needs of the patient (**Box 2-1**), which are needs common to all humankind.

BOX 2-1 The 14 Components of Virginia Henderson's Need Theory

1. Breathe normally.
2. Eat and drink adequately.
3. Eliminate body wastes.
4. Move and maintain desirable postures.
5. Sleep and rest.
6. Select suitable clothes—dress and undress.
7. Maintain body temperature within normal range by adjusting clothing and modifying environment.
8. Keep the body clean and well groomed, and protect the integument.

9. Avoid dangers in the environment and avoid injuring others.
10. Communicate with others in expressing emotions, needs, fears, or opinions.
11. Worship according to one's faith.
12. Work in such a way that there is a sense of accomplishment.
13. Play or participate in various forms of recreation.
14. Learn, discover, or satisfy the curiosity that leads to normal development and health, and use the available health facilities.

Source: Henderson, V. A. (1991). *The nature of nursing: Reflections after 25 years.* New York, NY: National League for Nursing Press, pp. 22–43. Reprinted by permission of National League for Nursing.

Jean Watson's 10 Carative Processes (**Box 2-2**) exemplify the changing relationship between patient and nurse attending to the unification of body, mind, and soul to achieve optimal health. Watson has spent many years as director of the Center for Human Caring at the University of Colorado in Denver. Her Theory of Human Caring was developed by utilizing Carper's four fundamental ways of knowing to conceptualize her theory (Carper, 1978). Reflecting on empirical, personal, ethical, and aesthetic domains, Watson used the metaparadigm of person, environment, nursing, and health to provide a foundation for her theory of caring.

BOX 2-2 Ten Carative Processes

1. Embrace altruistic values, and practice loving kindness with self and others.
2. Instill faith and hope, and honor others.
3. Be sensitive to self and others by nurturing individual beliefs and practices.
4. Develop helping, trusting, and caring relationships.

5. Promote and accept positive and negative feelings as you authentically listen to another's story.
6. Use creative scientific problem-solving methods for caring decision making.
7. Share teaching and learning that addresses the individual needs and comprehension styles.

(continues)

BOX 2-2   Ten Carative Processes *(continued)*

8. Create a healing environment for the physical and spiritual self that respects human dignity.

9. Assist with basic physical,

emotional, and spiritual human needs.

10. Open to mystery, and allow miracles to enter.

Source: Ten Carative Processes, Jean Watson 2007, 2008; www.watsoncaringscience.org; Watson, J. (2008). *Nursing: The philosophy and science of caring* (New rev. ed.). Boulder: University Press of Colorado. Reprinted by permission of Jean Watson.

Hildegard Peplau (1952) focused as well on the relationship between patient and nurse in which the nurse takes on the role of counselor, resource, teacher, technical expert, surrogate, and leader, as needed. Whether an NP practices professionally in the United States or elsewhere in the global arena, to be successful in clinical practice the NP must use transcultural nursing theory, which was founded by Leininger (1995). The NP must use culturally sensitive and aware skills to develop relationships and to assess, diagnose, and treat patients.

King's (1981) framework uses personal, interpersonal, and social interacting systems to form a theory of nursing. Interestingly, upon review one might notice many of the concepts are the same in the *Calgary-Cambridge Guide to the Medical Interview* for physicians in training (Kurtz, Silverman, & Draper, 1998; Silverman, Kurtz, & Draper, 1998). In both of these methods for interacting with patients, the focus is on the concerns of the patient. King's framework gives the NP the ability to see the patient holistically by including the family and community aspects. Both King's framework and the *Calgary-Cambridge Guide* focus on mutual goal setting—taking the time during each step of the interview, assessment, and planning stages to truly understand the patient's issues and perspectives. By eliciting the patient's input frequently, it is easier for the NP to develop mutual understanding and design

interventions and goals for the patient to reach a state of optimal health.

The idea of forming a partnership with the patient is hardly new. Whitlock, Orleans, Pender, and Allan (2002) wrote about this concept in a U.S. Preventive Services Task Force recommendation, "Evaluating Primary Care Behavioral Counseling Interventions: An Evidence-Based Approach." Developing mutually respectful relationships with patients is likely to prevent patients resisting advice on healthy living and behavior change. Also detailed in this recommendation is an approach the National Cancer Institute developed to guide physician intervention in smoking cessation known as the "5 As": assess, advise, agree, assist, and arrange (Whitlock et al., 2002):

- *Assess:* Ask about and assess behavioral health risk(s) and factors affecting choice of behavior change goals/methods.

- *Advise:* Give clear, specific, and personalized behavior change advice, including information about personal health harms/benefits.

- *Agree:* Collaboratively select appropriate treatment goals and methods based on the patient's interest in and willingness to change the behavior.

- *Assist:* Using behavior change techniques (self-help and/or counseling), aid the patient in achieving agreed-upon goals by acquiring the skills, confidence, and social/environmental supports for behavior change, supplemented with adjunctive medical treatments when appropriate (e.g., pharmacotherapy for tobacco dependence, contraceptive drugs/devices).

- *Arrange:* Schedule follow-up contacts (in person or by telephone) to provide ongoing assistance/support and to adjust the treatment plan as needed, including referral to more intensive or specialized treatment.

All of the approaches mentioned in this chapter focus on the need for the healthcare provider to be open to patients' needs, to hear what patients really have to say, to understand what patients really believe is wrong or right, and to let patients collaborate in the development of goals. The NP's ability to be culturally sensitive, flexible, and willing to collaborate and compromise when needed and appropriate helps to form the framework for a successful patient–NP relationship and, most importantly, assists patients to reach a state of optimum health. This is not to say that becoming expert in these skills is easy, or that it can be accomplished in one course; the student NP should start practicing these skills as soon as the educational program begins.

NURSE PRACTITIONERS' UNIQUE ROLE

In a survey seeking to identify barriers to using standardized nursing language (SNL) for documenting nursing practice, researchers found that most NP survey participants—believing that their role was a blending of the nursing and medical models—were not aware of what SNL consisted of (Conrad, Hanson, Hasenau, & Stocker-Schneider, 2012). Jacqueline Fawcett (in Cody, 2013) exhorts nurses to sever our "romance" with medical science and nonnursing professions and, in particular, to stop comparing NPs with physicians providing primary care. Instead, she advises we integrate nursing science as nurse scholars. With this in mind, while clarifying the professional practice of nurse practitioners it is important

to distinguish the profession from that of physicians and physician assistants.

In a qualitative study, Carryer, Gardner, Dunn, and Gardner (2007) interviewed NPs in Australia and New Zealand to illustrate the core role of NPs. Three components were described: dynamic practice, professional efficacy, and clinical leadership. *Dynamic practice* represented the clinical skills and expertise the NPs used in direct patient care, including physical assessment and treatment. *Professional efficacy* was what the researchers called the aspects of NP practice that were highly autonomous and for which NPs were accountable. This level of practice does not exclude the need for collaboration; however, the NP acted as an integral member of the multidisciplinary team. The participants described the overlap in role boundaries of NPs and physicians. Another aspect of professional efficacy was described as part of the patient–NP relationship: integrating the complex components of psychosocial aspects and the concrete physical aspects by taking the time needed in a patient visit to do so, and thus developing the therapeutic link for a significant relationship. Finally, the researchers described the advanced education and clinical experience that the NP brought to the advanced professional role. NPs understood the vital place that nurses need to occupy in healthcare delivery systems and how important it is to be a part of designing and implementing systems that can improve patient access to quality care. Therefore, NP leadership occurred in both the direct practice environment and in the context of the larger healthcare system. This final theme was not recognized at the same level by all participants. Many were still developing in this portion of role identity.

Nicoteri and Andrews (2003) sought to uncover any theory that was unique to understanding the attributes associated with NPs. This integrative review of the literature found that the role of the NP is influenced by many disciplines, especially medicine. The authors posited that an emergence of theory that is unique to NPs and grounded in nursing, medicine, and social science was discovered. They suggested developing the concept of "nurse practitionering" (p. 500). The concept of nurse practitionering as a unique phenomenon has been written about in only a few journal articles. The term itself is not one used in typical conversation between healthcare providers and patients or within the nursing community; thus, there may be confusion with the term. The researchers' goal for this endeavor was not to elevate or denigrate one profession or another, but to better understand the components of nurse practitionering.

Hagedorn (2004) posited that the difference between nurse practitioners and "biomedical practitioners" is related to nurse practitioners' humanistic approach to patient care. According to many theorists such as Jean Watson, Patricia Benner, and Anne Boykin and Savina Schoenhofer, nursing's essence is that of caring (Zaccagnini & White, 2011). The interpersonal focus of nursing within a caring and nurturing framework is the building block of all nursing theories (Brunton & Beaman, 2000; Chinn & Kramer, 1999; Green, 2004; Nicoteri & Andrews, 2003; Visintainer, 1986). If one accepts this as a core element of being a nurse, it would be difficult to imagine one losing this essence when acquiring advanced education that contains skills and competencies associated with the practice of medicine. In fact, NPs should familiarize themselves with

nursing theory in order to use it to guide their practice. By doing so, NPs can practice beyond the medical model, offering a unique approach to the relationship, assessment, and treatment plan.

In an effort to expand on the concept of nurse practitionering, Stewart (2008) conducted a descriptive study of 90 NPs in Connecticut who responded to an online survey about "nurse practitionering" and what they believed it encompassed. Fifty-nine respondents (65.6%) stated that nurse practitionering is a unique term that describes what they do, which is different from practicing solely nursing or medicine. Because many activities of practice overlap and are subjective, participants were not given definitions of nursing activities or medical activities. Regarding how much time they perceived they spent in solely nursing activities, 36.7% of participants believed it was low, between 0% and 25%. In contrast, 34.4% of NP participants stated that the amount of time they spent performing medical activities was between 36% and 50%. These results are included in **Table 2-1**.

The respondents entered key terms and phrases that described providing care to patients as a nurse practitioner. Participants were not given terms or phrases from which to choose; rather, this portion of the survey was

TABLE 2-1	Percentage of Clinical Practice Time Spent in Nursing and Medical Activities (N = 90)	
Time	Nursing Activities	Medical Activities
0–25%	**36.7% (n = 33)***	13.3% (n = 12)
26–50%	30.0% (n = 27)	**34.4% (n = 31)***
51–75%	25.6% (n = 23)	32.2% (n = 29)
76–100%	7.8% (n = 7)	20.0% (n = 18)

*Bold type denotes highest value.

Source: Stewart, J., & DeNisco, S. (2015). Role development for the nurse practitioner. Burlington, MA: Jones & Bartlett.

open-ended. The researcher grouped similar terms when deemed appropriate. The most frequently used key phrases in order of the number of times mentioned were *nurture/care /empathy* (*f* = 31), *educate* (*f* = 30), *assess/diagnose /treat/prescribe* (*f* = 30), *holistic* (*f* = 22), *listener* (*f* = 17), *collaborate* (*f* = 13), *advocate* (*f* = 11), and *coach* (*f* = 5). The frequency of the key phrases and terms used in this pilot study confirms that the core of nurse practitionering is based on the nursing model. Key phrases and terms relating to medical practice included *diagnose /treat/prescribe*, which were used as frequently as the nursing category, except in the area of nurture, care, and empathy, which was slightly higher.

In an effort to expand on the key phrases from the previous study, Stewart (2009) invited 150 NPs in Connecticut to participate in interviews to share their perceptions of nurse practitionering. A total of 14 individual interviews were conducted with a convenience sample of experienced NPs. The 14 participants were all females between the ages of 31 and 70 years who were currently practicing as nurse practitioners. The following four themes were identified after analyzing the interviews: authentic listening, empathy, negotiating, and going above and beyond.

Authentic Listening

The NPs in this study were exemplars of authentic listeners. According to Bryant (2009), listening well involves being present, being interested, spending time, and showing respect. One NP explained:

> I think the biggest reason why people like to come here is they say, "You listen. The docs don't listen to me." It is probably what I do the most and, one of the nurses got very frustrated with me and said, "You nurse practitioners, when a patient comes in to see the doctor and their finger is the problem, the doctor just looks at the finger and the patient is out. You go and you guys talk about everything. You have to talk about everything!"

Another NP described the time she spends teaching patients:

> I prescribed the medications, I go out, I get the inhaler, you know, the sample inhaler and the sample spacer, and I go right back in and I tell the patient, "This is what I am ordering, and this is how you use it," versus the pediatrician or the pulmonologist who says, "Here are your medications. I'll have the nurse come in to teach you how to use it."

Empathy

Empathy is the ability to relate to the patient's thoughts and feelings and develop an understanding of what the patient is experiencing (Baillie, 1996). The NPs in this study were genuinely concerned about the patient's psychosocial well-being, family matters, and future goals and aspirations:

> This woman this morning has lots of what I perceive as small complaints. She's a relatively healthy 28-year-old woman, and I asked her, "Tiffany, are you working?"
>
> She said, "No."
>
> I said, "When was the last time you worked?"
>
> She said, "Oh, 9 years ago, before my daughter was born." Then she said, "It's really hard to get a job."
>
> I asked, "Do you have your high school diploma?"
>
> She said, "No."
>
> So I recommended to her a local learning center program. I encouraged her, and that's where I think the nurse practitioner is different. It was me listening first, caring about what she was telling me, and then offering her something and trying to be an advocate for her.

Empathy enabled another NP to gain a deep understanding of what motivated the patient:

> She has a disabled child at home that needs total care. That's something that I know about her and her situation. That's an example of, I guess, of advocating and coordinating and knowing that a lot of people don't have

transportation. Like if I want to send them to radiology, I'll ask them, "What time of the day is good for you?" because a lot of these people are grandmothers raising grandkids, and they need to arrange their life. Some of them are pretty capable of making appointments for themselves, but others are not. They are scared to or they don't think that they're going to do it right. Maybe we are enabling them by doing it for them, but we will take the extra time and, you know, ask "What's the best day for you to go for that ultrasound? Morning or afternoon?"

Negotiating

Authentic listening and empathy enabled the NPs in this study to communicate more effectively and negotiate with patients when formulating treatment plans. An integrated literature review on communication styles of NPs and the impact on patients found that NPs who are trained to use a patient-centered communication style are most likely to have patients with better understanding of their health and treatment options and who are more likely to follow the treatment plan, thereby having better health outcomes (Charlton, Dearing, Berry, & Johnson, 2008). This same result was found in this study in NPs who involved patients in the decision-making process and actively negotiated with patients:

> One of the things here that we do well, I think, is negotiate with the patients. Part of when I see people I'm not going to be paternalistic and tell them you have to do this, this, and that. I have a woman I saw this morning; she came in for follow-up of her labs. She has hypertension, and the first time she had a hemoglobin A1C of 6, and she has a family history of diabetes, so we talked. She's not a dummy; she is a registered nurse. She just became a registered nurse, just got out of school, and I said "Let's talk about this new thing that's coming up. Do you have diabetes? Or are you prediabetic? Let's discuss it." So we negotiated what she was going to do next. I didn't want to say to her, "You have to start on more meds today." Her fasting sugars

have been normal, the A1C was 6, and she is a woman that takes care of herself, pretty much. Now she may go on metformin in 3 months, but I know she doesn't like to take pills. She cares about a healthy lifestyle, so we negotiated: try lifestyle changes for 3 months and check the A1C in 3 months; if it goes up, then we'll talk about starting medication.

Going Above and Beyond

NPs describe going beyond what is expected or required of the role of primary care provider. The NPs in the study were motivated to do more for their patients and ensure that patients were satisfied with their care.

> My patient that came in this morning was status posthospitalization. When she was in the hospital, they did a big cardiac and neuro workup. I had sent her out by ambulance the week before, and they kept her for 4 days because they did a really good workup on her, but they didn't do a stress test, so she needed to have that done. And so, I coordinated today for her to have a stress test, and I picked a Spanish-speaking cardiologist for her because I thought she would be more comfortable with that. And then they also recommended that she see a therapist because she's on an antidepressant, so we talked about that today, and I coordinated that for her.

Another NP described her ability to take on a difficult patient and gain his trust, thereby improving his adherence to the treatment plan and reducing costs of overuse of the emergency room.

> Treating marginalized patients with multiple comorbidities is challenging. This challenge is amplified by mental illness and substance abuse, combined with mistrust of the healthcare system. An example of this begins with the discharge of a difficult patient from a clinic for threatening front desk staff and a few nurses. He was belligerent, and when he felt he was not being respected, he threatened staff members, including his physician. He had been followed in the medical resident clinic for his chronic medical illnesses but was not addressing his anger management, cocaine abuse, obsessive

compulsive disorder, and depression, and ultimately he was not adherent to medications or medical appointments either. The patient had been fired by multiple agencies in the town he lives in for the same behaviors, and at this point was about to be fired from the only medical provider left within walking distance. He does not own a car and could not afford to travel by bus. Final discharge from the clinic and care would render this man with no primary care locally, except the emergency room.

A final attempt was made to have the patient receive his care with a nurse practitioner, as she could at least provide continuity, if he showed up for the appointment, and she was not afraid. But really, the NP provided more than the same face in the clinic each visit. The NP provided this man with a milieu of empathy and teamwork between patient and care provider. Her approach to practice sparked a level of trust of the practitioner. The patient recognized the NP's genuine interest in providing him individualized care and respect. She built upon this practitioner–patient relationship. The NP helped the patient realize his control of his healthcare commitment and his role in his health outcome. This empowerment and trust lead to successful engagement in following through for his routinely scheduled medical visits as well as medication adherence. When the patient was ready to address his mental health and addiction, he asked the NP to be his advocate.

The NP's commitment to holistic patient-centered care led to reinstatement of his mental health services. And today, this patient is significantly healthier, drug free, treating his medical and mental illness, and is one less person sitting in the emergency room.

Another NP described the impact one can have when going the extra step for a patient:

While at a precollege arts experience, a teen came to the clinic to ask for help with a sore throat. While assessing her I began discussing her comfort with being away from home for the first time. She mentioned that she was really surprised that having three meals a day made her feel so comfortable. (Students eat in the college cafeteria during the program.)

Further questioning revealed that she rarely ate except at school as she qualified for free lunch because "There is an empty refrigerator in my house." When asked if her school had a breakfast program, she said that they did but her mom "was too busy to apply—says it is too complicated." Her strep culture was positive, so I prescribed antibiotics and had the resident assistant pick them up from the pharmacy. Meanwhile, I asked the young lady if she would like to speak to the nurse practitioner at her school to contact social services for assistance with not only the breakfast program but also what else the assessment would allow. At that point I learned that her mom was in rehab and unable to be reached—that this student had been assigned a foster care person—who I contacted regarding care and treatment for the strep throat and confirmed the rest of the story. Activation of social services through contact with the NP at the school-based health center started the process in motion. Additional contact with her throughout the 5 weeks proved to positively impact this child's life.

The NPs in this study expressed how much they loved being nurse practitioners. They believed in the added value and unique contributions of the NP to health care and got a lot of gratification from putting in extra time and effort. This finding is supported by a similar study that showed NPs believe that their lives are enhanced and cite experiencing internal rewards and gratification from their interactions with patients:

I think the most gratifying thing is when I sit down with them and explain their disease and really spend the time with them that they need. I feel like they really understand the necessity for the treatment plan that I recommend, and I really feel like if I spend the time with them that they are so grateful because they feel like you've really invested in them. . . . I think that most nurse practitioners will probably say something to this effect, but when they sit down with their patients, they try to treat them like they would want one of their family members treated. And so when people really see that you're really doing that for them, and distinguish it from the way that they feel like they've been treated by other providers in the past or when they really recognize the amount of energy and the amount of giving—when they really see that—there's nothing more gratifying than that. (Kleinman, 2004)

These quantitative and qualitative pilot studies validate similar components uncovered by Kleinman (2004) regarding nurse practitioners and their relationships with patients. Essential meanings in her phenomenological study included "openness, connection, concern, respect, reciprocity, competence, time, and professional identity" (p. 264).

Based on research, review of the literature, and both formal and informal interviews, a concept map depicting nurse practitionering was developed (**Figure 2-1**). From that, the Stewart Model of Nurse Practitionering was developed to depict this model of nurse practitioner practice (**Figure 2-2**). This model has as its core the nursing model—the foundation of NP practice. As the NP student evolves through the educational program, scientific knowledge and attributes of the medical model are incorporated in order to provide accurate assessment, medical diagnoses, and appropriate evidence-based treatment modalities to patients who need health care. The circles within the larger circle represent unity and wholeness.

FIGURE 2-1   Model of nurse practitioner practice.

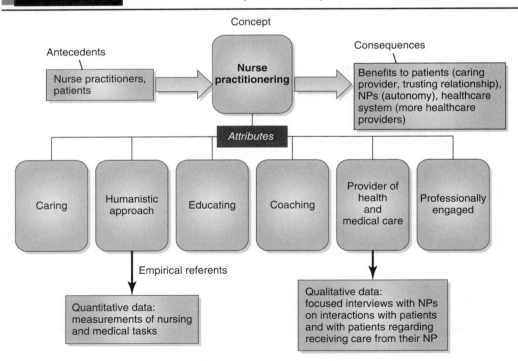

Source: Stewart, J., & DeNisco, S. (2015). *Role development for the nurse practitioner.* Burlington, MA: Jones & Bartlett.

| FIGURE 2-2 | The Stewart Model of Nurse Practitionering. |

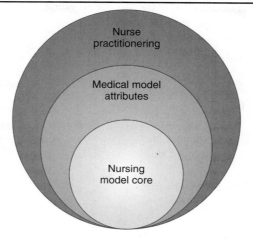

Source: Stewart, J., & DeNisco, S. (2015). *Role development for the nurse practitioner.* Burlington, MA: Jones & Bartlett.

It is evident that to function successfully within this model, the NP must retain the crucial interpersonal skills required to provide education surrounding health promotion and disease management. Brykczynski (2012), in an article discussing qualitative research that looked at how NP faculty keep the nurse in the NP student, suggested that holistically focused healthcare providers consider thinking of "patient diagnoses" instead of either medical or nursing diagnoses (p. 558). Nurse practitioner students and novice NPs need to beware of minimizing the importance of nursing as the core foundation from which excellence in practice develops. Rather, all NPs should emphasize the art and science of nursing and nursing philosophies and theories as the building blocks of providing health care to patients. It is these very qualities that make NPs unique—what engenders trust and confidence, as well as positive patient–NP

relationships, which is the circle labeled in Figure 2-2 as "nurse practitionering."

An opinion article in *The New York Times* clearly noted that nurse practitioners approach patient care differently from how physicians do, and that research has proven that the NP approach is as effective and "might be particularly useful for treating chronic disease, where so much depends on the patients' behavioral choices" (Rosenberg, 2012, para. 5). Sullivan-Marx and colleagues (2010) posited that the NP encompasses both the holistic nursing caring model and the physician's curing model—that NPs have a paradigm flexible enough to be able to move between the two. Who better than NPs/DNPs to tackle the inequities in health that have been tied to variations in socioeconomic status, racial and ethnic discrimination and stressors, and policies relating to social and economic justice?

DISCUSSION QUESTIONS ────────

1. What was the purpose for the initial role of the nurse practitioner? Did that role differ from the role of the nurse practitioner in today's healthcare system?

2. Who are advanced practice registered nurses (APRNs)?

3. What are the master's and DNP essentials, and what are they used for?

4. Describe the NP core competencies as identified by NONPF, and discuss how students can attain basic mastery of those competencies.

5. What are elements of role transition from RN to APN, and what are you currently experiencing in this process?

6. The concept of "nurse practitionering" has been introduced in this chapter. Comment on your responses to this idea.

REFERENCES ────────

American Academy of Nurse Practitioners. (2010a). *Nurse practitioner cost-effectiveness*. Austin, TX: Author.

American Academy of Nurse Practitioners. (2010b). *Quality of nurse practitioner practice*. Austin, TX: Author.

American Association of Colleges of Nursing (AACN). (2006). *The essentials of doctoral education for advanced nursing practice*. Washington, DC: Author.

American Association of Colleges of Nursing (AACN). (2011). *The essentials of master's education in nursing*. Washington, DC: Author.

American Association of Colleges of Nursing (AACN). (2013). *DNP fact sheet*. Washington, DC: Author.

American Association of Nurse Practitioners (AANP). (2014). *Nurse practitioners fact sheet*. Retrieved from http://www.aanp.org/all-about-nps/np-fact-sheet

APRN Consensus Work Group & National Council of State Boards of Nursing APRN Advisory Committee. (2008, July 7). *Consensus model for APRN regulation: Licensure, accreditation, certification and education*. APRN Joint Dialogue Group Report. Retrieved from http://www.aacn.nche.edu/education-resources/APRNReport.pdf

Auerbach, D. I. (2012). Will the NP workforce grow in the future? New forecasts and implications for healthcare delivery. *Medical Care, 50*(7), 606–610.

Baillie, L. (1996). A phenomenological study of the nature of empathy. *Journal of Advanced Nursing, 24*(6), 1300–1308.

Bauer, J. (2010). Nurse practitioners as an underutilized resource for health reform: Evidence-based demonstrations of cost-effectiveness. *Journal of the American Academy of Nurse Practitioners, 22*, 228–231.

Brown, S. J. (2005). Direct clinical practice. In A. B. Hamric, J. A. Spross, & C. M. Hanson (Eds.), *Advanced practice nursing: An integrative approach* (3rd ed., pp. 143–185). Philadelphia, PA: Elsevier Saunders.

Bruner, K. (2005, May). Nurse practitioners' program to celebrate 40th anniversary. Retrieved from http://www.uchsc.edu/news/bridge/2005/may/NP_anniversary.html

Brunton, B., & Beaman, M. (2000). Nurse practitioners' perceptions of their caring behaviors. *Journal of the American Academy of Nurse Practitioners, 12*, 451–456.

Bryant, L. (2009). The art of active listening. *Practice Nurse, 37*(6), 49.

Brykczynski, K. (2012). Clarifying, affirming, and preserving the nurse in nurse practitioner education and practice. *Journal of the American Academy of Nurse Practitioners, 24*, 554–564.

Budzi, D., Lurie, S., Singh, K., & Hooker, R. (2010). Veterans' perceptions of care by nurse practitioners, physician assistants and physicians: A comparison from satisfaction surveys. *Journal of the American Academy of Nurse Practitioners, 22*(3), 170–176. doi:10.1111/j.1745-7599.2010.00489.x

Buerhaus, P. (2010). Have nurse practitioners reached a tipping point? Interview of a panel of NP thought leaders. *Nursing Economics, 28*(5), 346–349.

Carper, B. A. (1978). Fundamental patterns of knowing in nursing. *Advances in Nursing Science, 1*(1), 13–23.

Carryer, J., Gardner, G., Dunn, S., & Gardner, A. (2007). The core role of the nurse practitioner: Practice, professionalism and clinical leadership. *Journal of Clinical Nursing, 16*(10), 1818–1825. doi:10.1111/j.1365-2702.2006.01823.x

Centers for Medicare and Medicaid Services (CMS). (2011). Over $100 million to help states crack down on unreasonable health insurance rate. Retrieved from http://www.cms .gov/CCIIO/Resources/Fact-Sheets-and-FAQs /rate-review09202011a.html

Charlton, C. R., Dearing, K. S., Berry, J. A., & Johnson, M. J. (2008). Nurse practitioners' communication styles and their impact on patient outcomes: An integrated literature review. *Journal of the American Academy of Nurse Practitioners, 20*, 382–388. doi:10.1111/j.1745-7599.2008.00336.x

Chinn, P. L., & Kramer, M. K. (1999). *Theory and nursing: Integrated knowledge development* (5th ed.). St. Louis, MO: Mosby.

Chitty, K., & Black, B. (2007). *Professional nursing: Concepts and challenges*. St. Louis, MO: Saunders.

Cody, W. (Ed.). (2013). *Philosophical and theoretical perspectives for advanced practice nursing* (5th ed.). Burlington, MA: Jones & Bartlett.

Conrad, D., Hanson, P., Hasenau, S., & Stocker-Schneider, J. (2012). Identifying the barriers to use of standardized nursing language in the electronic health record by the ambulatory care nurse practitioner. *Journal of the American Academy of Nurse Practitioners, 24*(7), 443–451.

Creech, C., Filter, M., & Bowman, S. (2011). *Comparing patient satisfaction with nurse practitioner and physician delivered care*. Poster presented at the 26th Annual American Academy of Nurse Practitioners Conference, Las Vegas, NV.

Dahnke, M., & Dreher, H. M. (2011). *Philosophy of science for nursing practice: Concepts and application*. New York, NY: Springer.

Gallup Politics. (2012, December 3). Congress retains low honesty rating. Retrieved from http://www .gallup.com/poll/159035/congress-retains-low-honesty-rating.aspx

Gladwell, M. (2000). *The tipping point: How little things can make a big difference*. New York, NY: Little, Brown.

Green, A. (2004). Caring behaviors as perceived by nurse practitioners. *Journal of the American Academy of Nurse Practitioners, 16*, 283–290.

Hagedorn, M. (2004). Caring practices in the 21st century: The emerging role of nurse practitioners. *Topics in Advanced Practice Nursing eJournal, 4*(4). Retrieved from http://www.medscape.com /viewarticle/496372

Hamric, A., Spross, J., & Hanson, C. (2009). *Advanced practice nursing* (4th ed.). Philadelphia, PA: Saunders.

Haugsdal, C., & Scherb, C. (2003). Using the nursing interventions classification to describe the work of the nurse practitioner. *Journal of the American Academy of Nurse Practitioners, 15*, 87–94.

Health Resources and Services Administration, Bureau of Health Professions. (2004). *A comparison of changes in the professional practice of nurse practitioners, physician assistants, and certified midwives: 1992 and 2000*. Retrieved from http: //bhpr.hrsa.gov/healthworkforce/reports/com-parechange19922000.pdf

Henderson, V. A. (1991). *The nature of nursing: Reflections after 25 years*. New York, NY: National League for Nursing Press.

Indiana University. (2009, January 22). The total package: A skillful, compassionate doctor. Indiana University News Room. Retrieved from http://newsinfo.iu.edu/web/page/normal/9704 .html

Jenning, C. (2002, October 29). Testimony: American Academy of Nurse Practitioners before the National Committee on Vital and Health Statistics. Retrieved from http://www.ncvhs.hhs .gov/021029p3.htm

Kaiser Family Foundation. (2014). *Health reform: How will the uninsured fare under the Affordable Care Act?* Retrieved from http://kff.org/health-reform/fact -sheet/how-will-the-uninsured-fare-under-the -affordable-care-act

King, I. (1981). *A theory for nursing: Systems, concepts, process*. New York, NY: Wiley.

Kleinman, S. (2004). What is the nature of nurse practitioners' lived experiences interacting with patients? *Journal of the American Academy of Nurse Practitioners, 16*(6), 263–269.

Kurtz, S. M., Silverman, J. D., & Draper, J. (1998). *Teaching and learning communication skills in medicine*. Oxford, England: Radcliffe Medical Press.

Laurant, M., Reeves, D., Hermens, R., Braspenning, J., Grol, R., & Sibbald, B. (2005). Substitution of doctors by nurses in primary care. *Cochrane Database of Systematic Reviews, 2*, CD001271.

Leininger, M. (1995). Culture care theory, research and practice. *Nursing Science Quarterly, 9*, 71–78.

Mundinger, M. O., Kane, R. L., Lenz, E. R., Totten, A. M., Tsai, W. Y., Cleary, P. D., . . . Shelanski, M. L. (2000). Primary care outcomes in patients treated by nurse practitioners or physicians: A randomized trial. *Journal of the American Medical Association, 283*(1), 59–68.

National Organization of Nurse Practitioner Faculties. (2012). *Domains and core competencies of nurse practitioner practice*. Washington, DC: Author.

Nicoteri, J. A., & Andrews, C. (2003). The discovery of unique nurse practitioner theory in the literature: Seeking evidence using an integrative review approach. *Journal of the American Academy of Nurse Practitioners, 15,* 494–500.

Nightingale, F. (2009). *Florence Nightingale: Notes on nursing.* New York, NY: Fall River Press. (Original work published 1859)

Ortiz, J., Wan, T. T., Meemon, N., Paek, S. C., & Agiro, A. (2010). Contextual correlates of rural health clinics' efficiency: Analysis of nurse practitioners' contributions. *Nursing Economics, 28*(4), 237–244.

Pearson, L. J. (2011). The Pearson report 2011. *American Journal for Nurse Practitioners, 15*(4).

Peplau, H. (1952). *Interpersonal relations in nursing.* New York, NY: Putnam.

Pulcini, J. (2013). Advanced practice nursing: Moving beyond the basics. In S. DeNisco & A. M. Barker (Eds.), *Advanced practice nursing: Evolving roles for the transformation of the profession* (2nd ed., pp. 19–26). Burlington, MA: Jones & Bartlett.

Roberts, S. J., Tabloski, P., & Bova, C. (1997). Epigenesis of the nurse practitioner role revisited. *Journal of Nursing Education, 36,* 67–73.

Rosenberg, T. (2012, October 24). The family doctor, minus the M.D. *The New York Times.* Retrieved from http://opinionator.blogs.nytimes.com/2012/10/24/the-family-doctor-minus-the-m-d

Silverman, J. D., Kurtz, S. M., & Draper, J. (1998). *Skills for communicating with patients.* Oxford, England: Radcliffe Medical Press.

Stewart, J. G. (2008, 2009). Toward a middle range theory of nurse practitionering. Unpublished manuscripts.

Sullivan-Marx, E., McGivern, D., Fairman, S., & Greenberg, S. (Eds.). (2010). *Nurse practitioners: The evolution and future of advanced practice* (5th ed.). New York, NY: Springer.

Van Leuven, K. (2012). Population aging: Implications for nurse practitioners. *Journal for Nurse Practitioners, 8*(7), 554–559.

Visintainer, M. (1986). The nature of knowledge and theory in nursing. *Image: Journal of Nursing Scholarship, 18,* 32–38.

Weiland, S. (2008). Reflections on independence in nurse practitioner practice. *Journal of the American Academy of Nurse Practitioners, 20*(7), 345–352. doi:10.111/j.1745-7599.2008.00330.x

Whitlock, E., Orleans, T., Pender, N., & Allan, J. (2002). Evaluating primary care behavioral counseling interventions: An evidence-based approach. *American Journal of Preventative Medicine, 22*(4), 267–284.

Wilson, I. B., Landon, B. E., Hirschhorn, L. R., McInnes, K., Ding, L., Marsden, P. V., & Cleary, P. D. (2005). Quality of HIV care provided by nurse practitioners, physician assistants, and physicians. *Annals of Internal Medicine, 143*(10), 729–736.

Zaccagnini, M., & White, K. (2011). *The doctor of nursing practice essentials: A new model for advanced nursing practice.* Sudbury, MA: Jones & Bartlett.

CHAPTER 3

Overview of the Doctor of Nursing Practice Degree

Lisa Astalos Chism

What exactly is a doctor of nursing practice (DNP) degree? As enrollment to this innovative practice doctorate program continues to increase, this question is frequently posed by nurses, patients, and other healthcare professionals both in and out of the healthcare setting. Providing an explanation to this question requires not only defining the DNP degree, but also reflecting on the rich history of doctoral education in nursing. Doctoral education in nursing is connected to our past and influences the directions we may take in the future (Carpenter & Hudacek, 1996). The development of the DNP degree is a tribute to where nursing has been and where we hope to be in the future of doctoral education in nursing.

Understanding the DNP degree requires developing an awareness of the rationale for a practice doctorate. This rationale illustrates the motivation behind the evolution of doctoral education in nursing and provides further explanation of this contemporary degree. The need for parity across the healthcare team, the Institute of Medicine's call for safer healthcare practices, and the need for increased preparation of advanced-practice registered nurses to meet the changing demands of health care are all contributing antecedents of the development of the practice doctorate in nursing (American Association of Colleges of Nursing [AACN], 2006a, 2006b; Apold, 2008; Dracup, Cronenwett, Meleis, & Benner, 2005; Roberts & Glod, 2005). Becoming familiar with the motivating factors behind the DNP degree will aid understanding of the development of this innovative degree.

This chapter provides a definition of the DNP degree and a discussion of the evolution of doctoral education in nursing. The rationale for a practice doctorate is also described. The recipe for the DNP degree, which includes the *Essentials of Doctoral Education for Advanced Nursing Practice* by the AACN (2006b) and the *Practice Doctorate Nurse Practitioner Entry-Level Competencies* by the National Organization of Nurse

Practitioner Faculties (NONPF, 2006), is provided in this chapter as well. The pathway to the DNP degree is also discussed. Providing a discussion of these topics will equip one with the information necessary to become familiar with this innovative degree.

RESEARCH-FOCUSED DOCTORATE AND PRACTICE-FOCUSED DOCTORATE DEFINED

The question, What is a DNP degree? is often followed by the question, What is the difference between a doctor of philosophy (PhD) and a DNP degree? Nurses now can choose between a practice-focused or research-focused doctorate as a terminal degree. Although the academic or research degree, once the only terminal preparation in nursing, has traditionally been the PhD, the AACN now includes the doctor of nursing science (DNS, DNSc, DSN) as a research-focused degree (AACN, 2004). Further, the AACN Task Force on the Practice Doctorate in Nursing has recommended that the practice doctorate be the DNP degree, which will replace the traditional nursing doctorate (ND) degree (AACN, 2006a). Currently ND programs are taking the necessary steps to adjust their programs to fit the curriculum criteria of DNP degree programs.

The practice- and research-focused doctorates in nursing share a common goal regarding a "scholarly approach to the discipline and a commitment to the advancement of the profession" (AACN, 2006b, p. 3). The differences in these programs include differences in preparation and expertise. The practice doctorate curriculum places more emphasis on practice and less on theory and research methodology (AACN, 2004, 2006b). The final scholarly project differs in that a dissertation required for a PhD degree should document development of new knowledge, and a final scholarly project required for a DNP degree should be grounded in clinical practice and demonstrate ways in which research has an impact on practice.

The focus of the DNP degree is expertise in clinical practice. Additional foci include the *Essentials of Doctoral Education for Advanced Nursing Practice* by the AACN (2006b), which include leadership, health policy and advocacy, and information technology. The focus of a research degree is the generation of new knowledge for the discipline and expertise as a principal investigator. Although the research degree prepares the expert researcher, it should be noted that frequently DNP research projects will also contribute to the discipline by generating new knowledge related to clinical practice and demonstrate the use of evidence-based practice. Please refer to **Table 3-1** for the AACN's comparison of a DNP program and PhD, DNS, and DNSc programs.

EVOLUTION OF DOCTORAL EDUCATION IN NURSING

To appreciate the development of doctoral education in nursing, one must understand where nursing has been with regard to education at the doctoral level. Indeed, nursing has been unique in its approach to doctoral preparation since nurses began to earn doctoral degrees. Even today nurses are prepared at the doctoral level through various degrees, including doctor of education (EdD), PhD, DNS, and now DNP. Prior to the development of the DNP degree, the ND was also offered as a choice for nursing doctoral education.

Examining the chronological development of doctoral education in nursing is somewhat complicated because early doctorates were offered outside nursing. These included the EdD degree and the PhD degree in basic science fields, such as anatomy and physiology (Carpenter & Hudacek, 1996; Marriner-Tomey, 1990). The first nursing-related doctoral program was originated in 1924 at Teachers College, Columbia University, and was an EdD designed to prepare nurses to teach at the college level (Carpenter & Hudacek, 1996). Teachers College was unique in that its program was the first to combine

TABLE 3-1	AACN Contrast Grid of the Key Differences Between DNP and PhD/DNS/DNSc Programs	

	DNP	PhD/DNS/DNSc
Program of study	**Objectives:**	**Objectives:**
	Prepare nurse specialists at the highest level of advanced practice	Prepare nurse researchers
	Competencies:	**Content:**
	Based on *Essentials of Doctoral Education for Advanced Nursing Practice* (AACN, 2006b)*	Based on *Indicators of Quality in Research-Focused Doctoral Programs in Nursing* (AACN, 2001)**
Students	Commitment to a practice career	Commitment to a research career
	Oriented toward improving outcomes of care	Oriented toward developing new knowledge
Program faculty	Practice doctorate and/or experience in area in which teaching	Research doctorate in nursing or related field
	Leadership experience in area of specialty practice	Leadership experience in area of sustained research funding
	High level of expertise in specialty practice congruent with focus of academic program	High level of expertise in research congruent with focus of academic program
Resources	Mentors and/or precepts in leadership positions across a variety of practice settings	Mentors/preceptor in research settings
	Access to diverse practice settings with appropriate resources for areas of practice	Access to research settings with appropriate resources
	Access to financial aid	Access to dissertation support dollars
	Access to information and patient-care technology resources congruent with areas of study	Access to information and research technology resources congruent with program of research
Program assessment and evaluation	**Program outcome:**	**Program outcome:**
	Healthcare improvements and contributions via practice, policy change, and practice scholarship	Contributes to healthcare improvements via the development of new knowledge and other scholarly projects that provide the foundation for the advancement of nursing science

(continues)

	AACN Contrast Grid of the Key Differences Between DNP and
TABLE 3-1	PhD/DNS/DNSc Programs *(continued)*

DNP	PhD/DNS/DNSc
Oversight by the institution's authorized bodies (i.e., graduate school) and regional accreditors	Oversight by the institution's authorized bodies (i.e., graduate school) and regional accreditor
Receives accreditation by specialized nursing accreditor	
Graduates are eligible for national certification exam	

*American Association of Colleges of Nursing. (2006). *Essentials of doctoral education for advanced nursing practice.* Retrieved from http://www.aacn.nche.edu/publications/position/DNPEssentials.pdf

**American Association of Colleges of Nursing. (2001). *Indicators of quality in research-focused doctoral programs in nursing.* Retrieved from http://www.aacn.nche.edu/publications/position/quality-indicators

Reprinted with permission from AACN DNP Roadmap Task Force Report, October 20, 2006.

both the "nursing and education needs of leaders in the profession" (Carpenter & Hudacek, 1996, p. 5). EdD degrees continued well into the 1960s to be the mainstay of doctoral education for nursing (Marriner-Tomey, 1990).

The first PhD in nursing was offered in 1934 at New York University. Unfortunately, the next PhD in nursing was not offered until the 1950s at the University of Pittsburgh and focused on maternal and child nursing. Incidentally, this degree was the first to recognize the importance of clinical research for the development of the nursing discipline (Carpenter & Hudacek, 1996). The PhD degrees earned elsewhere continued to be in nursing-related fields, such as psychology, sociology, and anthropology. This trend continued until nursing PhD degrees became more popular in the 1970s (Grace, 1978).

Grace (1978) summarized the progression of nursing education over time. Between 1924 and 1959 doctoral education in nursing focused on preparing nurses for "functional specialty" (p. 22). In other words, nurses were prepared to fulfill functional roles as teachers and administrators to lead the field of nursing toward advancement as a profession. The problem with these programs was that they lacked the substantive content necessary to develop nursing as a discipline and a profession. The next shift in doctoral education attempted to fulfill this need and took place between 1960 and 1969. Within this time period, popularity increased for doctoral programs that were nursing related. This included doctorates (PhDs) that were related to disciplines such as sociology, psychology, and anthropology. Grace (1978) noted that the development of these types of programs provided the basic science and research input necessary for the development of future ND programs. Murphy (1981) concurred that this stage in the development of doctoral education in nursing led to pertinent questions for the discipline of nursing, such as "(1) What is the essential nature of professional nursing? (2) What is the substantive knowledge base of professional nursing? (3) What kind of research is important for nursing as a knowledge discipline? As a field of practice? (4) How can the scientific base of nursing knowledge be identified and expanded?" (1981, p. 646).

In response to these questions, nursing doctoral education again progressed in the 1970s to include doctorate degrees that are actually in nursing (Grace, 1978). This stage also supported the growth of nursing's substantive structure, hence, the growth of the discipline of nursing. This is where nursing's history of doctoral education becomes more complex. In 1960 the DNS degree originated at Boston University and "focused on the development of nursing theory for a practice discipline" (Marriner-Tomey, 1990, p. 135), hence, the development of the first practice doctorate. The notion of a practice-focused doctorate in nursing is not new. Even as early as the 1970s, it was proposed that the research doctorate (PhD) should focus on preparing nurses to contribute to nursing science, and the practice (or professional) doctorate (DNS) should focus on expertise in clinical practice (Cleland, 1976). Newman also suggested a practice doctorate as the preparation of "professional practitioners" (1975, p. 705) for entry into practice. Grace (1978) noted that it was not sufficient to have a core of nursing researchers building the knowledge base (discipline) without also giving attention to the clinical field. It was also suggested by Grace that nurses prepared through a practice doctorate be titled "social engineers" (1978, p. 26). This seems appropriate given what expert clinicians in nursing are called upon to do.

Although the DNS degree was initially proposed as a practice or professional doctorate, over time the curriculum requirements have become very similar to those for a PhD degree (AACN, 2006a; Apold, 2008; Marriner-Tomey, 1990). Research requirements for this degree have eventually become indistinguishable from that of a PhD in nursing. Because of this, it is not surprising that the AACN has characterized all DNS degrees as research degrees (2004). With the DNS and PhD degrees so similar in content and focus, the challenge to develop a

true practice doctorate remained. An attempt toward this was made in 1979 when the ND originated at Case Western Reserve University, followed by the University of Colorado, Rush University, and South Carolina University. The first ND program was developed by Rozella M. Schlotfeldt, PhD, RN. The ND was different in that the research component was not the general focus of the degree. This degree was designed to be a "pre-service nursing education which would orient nursing's approach to preparing professionals toward competent, independent, accountable nursing practice" (Carpenter & Hudacek, 1996, p. 42). This general theme for a practice doctorate remains consistent even today. Unfortunately, this program did not share the same popularity of DNS or PhD degrees in nursing, and it was less common to find a clinician with this preparation. Further, the curricula in these programs were varied and lacked a uniform approach toward a practice doctorate (Marion et al., 2003).

In 2002 the AACN board of directors formed a task force to examine the current progress of practice doctorates in nursing. Their objective also included comparing proposed curriculum models and discussing recommendations for the future of a practice doctorate (AACN, 2004). To accomplish their mission, the AACN task force (2004) took part in the following activities:

- Reviewed the literature regarding practice doctorates in nursing and other disciplines.
- Established a collaborative relationship with NONPF.
- Interviewed key informants (deans, program directors, graduates, and current students) at the eight current or planned practice-focused doctoral programs in the United States.
- Held open discussions regarding issues surrounding practice-focused doctoral education at AACN's Doctoral Education Conference (January 2003 and February 2004).

- Participated in an open discussion with NONPF along with representatives from key nursing organizations and schools of nursing that were offering or planning a practice doctorate.

- Invited an External Reaction Panel, which involved participation from 10 individuals from various disciplines outside nursing. This panel responded to the draft of the *AACN Position Statement on the Practice Doctorate in Nursing.*

In 2004 the AACN published the *AACN Position Statement on the Practice Doctorate in Nursing* and recommended that the DNP degree would be the terminal degree for nursing practice by 2015. According to NONPF, the purpose of the DNP degree is to prepare nurses to meet the changing demands of health care today by becoming proficient at the following (Marion et al., 2003):

- Evaluating evidence-based practices for care
- Delivering care
- Developing healthcare policy
- Leading and managing clinical care and healthcare systems
- Developing interdisciplinary standards
- Solving healthcare dilemmas
- Reducing disparities in health care

Not only is the development of the DNP degree a culmination of today's emerging healthcare demands; the degree also provides a choice for nurses who wish to focus their doctoral education on nursing practice.

Since its inception the growth of this degree has been astonishing. The University of Kentucky's College of Nursing was the pioneer for this innovative degree and admitted the first DNP class in 2001. In spring 2005, 8 DNP programs were offered, and more than 60 were in development. By summer 2005, 80 DNP programs were being considered. In fall 2005, 20 programs offered DNP degrees,

and 140 programs were in development. Today there are 243 DNP programs in the United States (AACN, 2014).

It should also be mentioned that in 1999, Columbia University's School of Nursing was formulating plans for a doctor of nursing practice (DrNP) degree that would build on a model of "full-scope, cross-site primary care that Columbia had developed and evaluated over the past ten years" (Goldenberg, 2004, p. 25). This degree was spearheaded by Mary O. Mundinger, DrPH, RN, dean of Columbia University's School of Nursing. The curriculum of a DrNP program is clinically focused with advanced preparation designed to teach "cross-site, full-scope care with content in advanced differential diagnosis skills, advanced pathophysiology and microbiology, selected issues of compliance, management of health care delivery and reimbursement, advanced emergency triage and management, and professional role collaboration and referrals" (Goldenberg, 2004, p. 25). This expanded clinical component is what seems to differentiate a DrNP degree from a DNP degree. The first DrNP class graduated from Columbia University in 2003.

Since the development of the DrNP degree, the Commission on Collegiate Nursing Education (CCNE), the autonomous accrediting body of the AACN, has decided that only practice ND degrees with the doctor of nursing practice title will be eligible for CCNE accreditation (AACN, 2005). This decision was reached unanimously by the CCNE Board of Directors on September 29, 2005 in an effort to develop a process for accrediting only clinically focused NDs (AACN, 2005). The CCNE's decision is consistent with accrediting organizations for other healthcare professions and helps to ensure consistency with degree titling and criteria. Specific criteria for the DNP degree, including the AACN's *Essentials of Doctoral Education for Advanced Nursing Practice* (2006b) and the *Practice Doctorate Nurse Practitioner Entry-Level Competencies* (NONPF, 2006), are discussed later in this chapter.

WHY A PRACTICE DOCTORATE IN NURSING NOW?

It has already been mentioned that the notion of a practice doctorate is not new, so why the development of the DNP degree now? It has been noted that the development of the DNP is "more than a mere interruption but rather a response to the need within the healthcare system for expert clinical teachers and clinicians" (Marion, O'Sullivan, Crabtree, Price, & Fontana, 2005, para. 1). Healthcare needs are not new, yet the growth of this program has been escalating. The question is therefore posed, What are the drivers of this DNP degree, and why is there such urgency?

The Institute of Medicine's Report and Nursing's Response

In 2000 the Institute of Medicine (IOM) published a report titled *To Err Is Human: Building a Safer Health System* (Kohn, Corrigan, & Donaldson, 2000). This report summarized information regarding errors made in health care and offered recommendations to improve the overall quality of care. It was found that "preventable adverse events are a leading cause of death in the United States" (p. 26). In more than 33.6 million admissions to U.S. hospitals in 1997, 44,000 to 98,000 people died as a result of medical-related errors (American Hospital Association, 1999). It was estimated that deaths in hospitals by preventable adverse events exceed the amount attributable to the eighth leading cause of death in America (Centers for Disease Control and Prevention [CDC], 1999b). These numbers also exceed the number of deaths attributable to motor vehicle accidents (43,458), breast cancer (42,297), and AIDS (16,516) (CDC, 1999a). The total cost of health care is greatly affected by these errors as well, with estimated total national costs (lost income, lost household production, disability, healthcare costs) reported as being between $29 billion and $36 billion for adverse events

and between $17 billion and $29 billion for preventable adverse events (Thomas et al., 1999).

As a follow-up to the *To Err Is Human* report, in 2001 the IOM published *Crossing the Quality Chasm: A New Health System for the 21st Century*. In an effort to improve health care in the 21st century, the IOM (2001) proposed six specific aims for improvement, deeming that health care should have the following attributes:

1. Safe in avoiding injuries to patients from the care they receive
2. Effective in providing services based on scientific knowledge to those who could benefit, but services should not be provided to those who may not benefit
3. Patient centered in that provided care is respectful and responsive to individual patient preferences, needs, and values; all patient values should guide all clinical decisions
4. Timely in that wait time and sometimes harmful delays are reduced for those who give and receive care
5. Efficient in that waste is avoided, particularly waste of equipment, supplies, ideas, and energy
6. Equitable in that high-quality care is provided to all regardless of personal characteristics, such as gender, ethnicity, geographic location, and socioeconomic status

The IOM (2001) emphasized that to achieve these aims, additional skills may be required on the healthcare team. This includes all individuals who care for patients. The new skills needed to improve health care and reduce errors are, ironically, many skills that nurses have long been known to exemplify. Some examples of these skills include using electronic communications, synthesizing evidence-based practice information, communicating with patients in an open manner to enable their decision making, understanding the course of illness that specifically relates to the patient's experience outside the hospital, working collaboratively in teams, and understanding the link between health care and healthy populations (IOM, 2001). Developing expertise in these areas required curriculum changes in healthcare education as well as addressing how healthcare education is approached, organized, and funded (IOM, 2001).

In 2003 the Health Professions Education Committee responded to the IOM's *Crossing the Quality Chasm* report (IOM, 2001) by publishing *Health Professions Education: A Bridge to Quality* (Greiner & Knebel, 2003). The committee recommended that "all health professionals should be educated to deliver patient-centered care as members of an interdisciplinary team, emphasizing evidence-based practice, quality improvement approaches, and informatics" (Greiner & Knebel, 2003, p. 45). To meet this goal, the committee proposed a set of competencies to be met by all healthcare clinicians, regardless of discipline. These competencies include the following: provide patient-centered care, function in interdisciplinary teams, employ evidence-based practice, integrate quality improvement standards, and utilize various information systems (Greiner & Knebel, 2003).

As part of the continued effort to advance the education of healthcare professionals, the Robert Wood Johnson Foundation (RWJF) and the IOM specifically addressed advancing nursing education. In 2008 the RWJF and the IOM "launched a two-year initiative to respond to the need to access and transform the nursing profession" (IOM, 2010a, p. 1). The IOM appointed the Committee on the RWJF Initiative on the Future of Nursing. This committee published a report titled *The Future of Nursing: Focus on Education* (IOM, 2010a). In this report, the IOM concluded that "the ways in which nurses were educated during the 20th century are no longer adequate for dealing with the realities of healthcare in the 21st century" (2010a, p. 2). The IOM reiterated the need for the aforementioned competencies, such as leadership, health policy,

system improvement, research and evidence-based practice, and teamwork and collaboration. In response to the increasing demands of a complex healthcare environment, the IOM recommended higher levels of education for nurses and new ways to educate nurses to better meet the needs of this population.

The IOM included recommendations in the report that specifically address the number of nurses with doctorate degrees. It was noted that although 13% of nurses hold a graduate degree, fewer than 1% hold doctoral degrees (IOM, 2010a). The IOM concluded that "nurses with doctorates are needed to teach future generations of nurses and to conduct research that becomes the basis for improvements in nursing science and practice" (2010a, p. 4). Therefore, recommendation 5 states that "schools of nursing, with support from private and public funders, academic administrators and university trustees, and accreditation bodies, should double the number of nurses with a doctorate by 2020 to add to the cadre of nurse faculty and researchers, with attention to increasing diversity" (IOM, 2010b, p. 4).

The development of the DNP degree is one of the answers to the call proposed by both the IOM's Health Professions Education Committee and the IOM's and the RWJF's Initiative on the Future of Nursing Committee to redefine how healthcare professionals are educated. Nursing has always had a vested interest in improving quality of care and patient outcomes. Since Florence Nightingale, "nursing education has been directed toward the individualized, personalized care of the patient, not the disease" (Newman, 1975, p. 704). To further illustrate nursing's commitment to improve quality of care and patient outcomes, the competencies described by the Health Professions Education Committee are reflected in the AACN's *Essentials of Doctoral Education for Advanced Nursing Practice* (2006b) and NONPF's *Practice Doctorate Nurse Practitioner Entry-Level Competencies* (2006). Preparing nurses at the practice doctorate level who are experts at using information technology, synthesizing and integrating evidence-based practices, and collaborating across healthcare disciplines will further enable nursing to meet the challenges of health care in the 21st century.

Additional Drivers for a Practice Doctorate in Nursing

In a 2005 report titled *Advancing the Nation's Health Needs: NIH Research Training Programs,* the National Academy of Sciences (2005) recommended that nursing develop a nonresearch doctorate. The rationale for this initiative included increasing the numbers of expert practitioners who can also fulfill clinical nursing faculty needs (AACN, 2011). The report specifically states that "the need for doctorally prepared practitioners and clinical faculty would be met if nursing could develop a new non-research clinical doctorate, similar to the MD and PharmD in Medicine and Pharmacy, respectively" (National Academy of Sciences, 2005, p. 74). The initiatives of the National Academy of Sciences regarding doctoral education in nursing are reflected in the AACN's development of the DNP degree.

An additional rationale for a practice doctorate is reflected in nursing's educational history when the practice doctorate was first proposed. Newman noted that "nursing lacked the recognition for what it has to offer and authority for putting that knowledge into practice" (1975, p. 704). Starck, Duffy, and Vogler stated that "for nursing to be accountable to the social mandate, the numbers as well as the type of doctorally prepared nurses need attention" (1993, p. 214). The NONPF Practice Doctorate Task Force summarized the most frequently cited additional drivers for a practice doctorate in nursing (Marion et al., 2005):

- Parity with other professionals who are prepared with a practice doctorate. Disciplines such as audiology, dentistry, medicine, pharmacy, psychology, and physical therapy require a practice doctorate for entry into practice.

- A need for longer programs that both reflect the credit hours invested in master's degrees and accommodate additional information needed to prepare nurses for the demands of health care. Most master's degrees require a similar number of credit hours for completion as the number required for practice doctoral degrees.

- Remedy the current nursing faculty shortages. The development of a practice doctorate will help meet the needs for clinical teaching in schools of nursing.

- The increasing complexity of healthcare systems requires additional information to be included in current graduate nursing programs. Rather than further burden the amount of information needed to prepare nurses at the graduate level for a master's degree, a practice doctorate allows for additional information to be provided and affords a practice doctorate to prepare nurses for the changing demands of society and health care.

WHAT IS A DNP DEGREE MADE OF? THE RECIPE FOR CURRICULUM STANDARDS

The standards of a DNP program have been formulated through a collaborative effort among various consensus-based standards. These standards reflect collaborative efforts among the AACN as the *Essentials of Doctoral Education for Advanced Nursing Practice* (2006b), NONPF as the *Practice Doctorate Nurse Practitioner Entry-Level Competencies* (2006), and more recently the National Association of Clinical Nurse Specialists (NACNS) as *Core Practice Doctorate Clinical Nurse Specialist Competencies* (2009). These organizations' strategies for setting the standards of a practice doctorate in nursing demonstrate interrelated criteria that are congruent with all rationales for a practice doctorate in nursing. It should be noted, however, that while maintaining these consensus-based standards, there may be some variability in content within DNP curricula.

AACN Essentials of Doctoral Education for Advanced Nursing Practice

In 2006 the AACN published the *Essentials of Doctoral Education for Advanced Nursing Practice*. These essentials are the "foundational outcome competencies deemed essential for all graduates of a DNP program regardless of specialty or functional focus" (AACN, 2006b, p. 8). Nursing faculties have the freedom to creatively design course work to meet these essentials, which are summarized in the following sections.

Essential I: Scientific Underpinnings for Practice

This essential describes the scientific foundations of nursing practice, which are based on the natural and social sciences. These sciences may include human biology, physiology, and psychology. In addition, nursing science has provided nursing with a body of knowledge to contribute to the discipline of nursing. This body of knowledge or discipline is focused on the following (adapted from AACN, 2006b; Donaldson & Crowley, 1978; Fawcett, 2005; Gortner, 1980):

■ The principles and laws that govern the life process, well-being, and optimal functioning of human beings, sick or well

■ The patterning of human behavior in interaction with the environment in normal life events and critical life situations

■ The processes by which positive changes in health status are affected

■ The wholeness of health of human beings, recognizing that they are in continuous interaction with their environments

Nursing science has expanded the discipline of nursing and includes the development of middle-range nursing theories and concepts to guide practice. Understanding the practice of nursing includes developing an understanding of scientific underpinnings for practice (the science and discipline of nursing). Specifically, the DNP degree prepares the graduate to do the following (adapted from AACN, 2006b):

■ Integrate nursing science with knowledge from the organizational, biophysical, psychological, and analytical sciences, as well as ethics, as the basis for the highest level of nursing practice

■ Develop and evaluate new practice approaches based on nursing theories and theories from other disciplines

■ Utilize science-based concepts and theories to determine the significance and nature of health and healthcare delivery phenomena, describe strategies used to enhance healthcare delivery, and evaluate outcomes

Essential II: Organizational and Systems Leadership for Quality Improvement and Systems Thinking

Preparation in organizational and systems leadership at every level is imperative for DNP graduates to have an impact on and improve healthcare delivery and patient care outcomes. DNP graduates are distinguished by their ability to focus on new healthcare delivery methods that are based on nursing science. Preparation in this area will provide DNP graduates with expertise in "assessing organizations, identifying systems' issues, and facilitating organization-wide changes in practice delivery" (AACN, 2006b, p. 10). Specifically, the DNP graduate will be prepared to do the following (adapted from AACN, 2006b):

■ Utilize scientific findings in nursing and other disciplines to develop and evaluate care delivery approaches that meet the current and future needs of patient populations

- Guarantee accountability for the safety and quality of care for the patients they care for
- Manage ethical dilemmas within patient care, healthcare organizations, and research, including developing and evaluating appropriate strategies

Essential III: Clinical Scholarship and Analytical Methods for Evidence-Based Practice

DNP graduates are unique in that their contributions to nursing science involve the "translation of research into practice and the dissemination and integration of new knowledge" (AACN, 2006b, p. 11). Further, DNP graduates are in a distinctive position to merge nursing science, nursing practice, human needs, and human caring. Specifically, the DNP graduate is expected to be an expert in the evaluation, integration, translation, and application of evidence-based practices. Additionally, DNP graduates are actively involved in nursing practice, which allows for practical, applicable research questions to arise from the practice environment. Working collaboratively with experts in research investigation, DNP graduates can also assist in the generation of new knowledge and affect evidence-based practice from the practice arena. To achieve these goals, the DNP program prepares the graduate to do the following (adapted from AACN, 2006b):

- Analytically and critically evaluate existing literature and other research to determine the best evidence for practice
- Evaluate practice outcomes within populations in various arenas, such as healthcare organizations, communities, or practice settings
- Design and evaluate methodologies that improve quality in an effort to promote "safe, effective, efficient, equitable, and patient-centered care" (AACN, 2006b, p. 12)
- Develop practice guidelines that are based on relevant, best-practice findings

- Utilize informatics and research methodologies to collect and analyze data, design databases, interpret findings to design evidence-based interventions, evaluate outcomes, and identify gaps within evidence-based practice, which will improve the practice environment
- Work collaboratively with research specialists and act as a "practice consultant" (AACN, 2006b, p. 12)

Essential IV: Information Systems Technology and Patient Care Technology for the Improvement and Transformation of Health Care

DNP graduates have cutting-edge abilities to use information technology to improve patient care and outcomes. Knowledge regarding the design and implementation of information systems to evaluate programs and outcomes of care is essential for preparation as a DNP graduate. Expertise is garnered in information technology, such as web-based communications, telemedicine, online documentation, and other unique healthcare delivery methods. DNP graduates must also develop expertise in utilizing information technologies to support practice leadership and clinical decision making. Specific to information systems, DNP graduates are prepared to do the following (adapted from AACN, 2006b):

- Evaluate and monitor outcomes of care and quality of care improvement by designing, selecting, using, and evaluating programs related to information technologies
- Become proficient at the skills necessary to evaluate data extraction from practice information systems and databases
- Attend to ethical and legal issues related to information technologies within the healthcare setting by providing leadership to evaluate and resolve these issues
- Communicate and evaluate the accuracy, timeliness, and appropriateness of healthcare consumer information

Essential V: Healthcare Policy for Advocacy in Health Care

Becoming involved in healthcare policy and advocacy has the potential to affect the delivery of health care across all settings. Thus, knowledge and skills related to healthcare policy are central to nursing practice and are therefore essential to the DNP graduate. Further, "health policy influences multiple care delivery issues, including health disparities, cultural sensitivity, ethics, the internalization of health care concerns, access to care, quality of care, health care financing, and issues of equity and social justice in the delivery of health care" (AACN, 2006b, p. 13). DNP graduates are uniquely positioned to be powerful advocates for healthcare policy through their practice experiences. These practice experiences provide rich influences for the development of policy. Nursing's interest in social justice and equality requires that DNP graduates become involved in and develop expertise in healthcare policy and advocacy.

Additionally, DNP graduates need to be prepared in leadership roles with regard to public policy. As leaders in the practice setting, DNP graduates frequently assimilate research, practice, and policy. Therefore, DNP preparation should include experience in recognizing the factors that influence the development of policy across various settings. The DNP graduate is prepared to do the following (adapted from AACN, 2006b):

- Decisively analyze health policies and proposals from the points of view of consumers, nurses, and other healthcare professionals
- Provide leadership in the development and implementation of healthcare policy at the institutional, local, state, federal, and international levels
- Actively participate on committees, boards, or task forces at the institutional, local, state, federal, and international levels

- Participate in the education of other healthcare professionals, patients, or other stakeholders regarding healthcare policy issues
- Act as an advocate for the nursing profession through activities related to healthcare policy
- Influence healthcare financing, regulation, and delivery through the development of leadership in healthcare policy
- Act as an advocate for ethical, equitable, and social justice policies across all healthcare settings

Essential VI: Interprofessional Collaboration for Improving Patient and Population Health Outcomes

This essential specifically relates to the IOM's mandate to provide safe, timely, equitable, effective, efficient, and patient-centered care. In a multitiered, complex healthcare environment, collaboration among all healthcare disciplines must exist to achieve the IOM's and nursing's goals. Nurses are experts at functioning as collaborators among multiple disciplines. Therefore, as nursing practice experts, DNP graduates must be prepared to facilitate collaboration and team building. This may include both participating in the work of the team and assuming leadership roles when necessary.

With regard to interprofessional collaboration, the DNP graduate must be prepared to do the following (adapted from AACN, 2006b):

- Participate in effective communication and collaboration throughout the development of "practice models, peer review, practice guidelines, health policy, standards of care, and/or other scholarly products" (AACN, 2006b, p. 15)
- Analyze complex practice or organizational issues through leadership of interprofessional teams

- Act as a consultant to interprofessional teams to implement change in healthcare delivery systems

Essential VII: Clinical Prevention and Population Health for Improving the Nation's Health

Clinical prevention is defined as health promotion and risk reduction–illness prevention for individuals and families, and population health is defined as including all community, environmental, cultural, and socioeconomic aspects of health (Allan et al., 2004; AACN, 2006b). Nursing has foundations in health promotion and risk reduction and is therefore positioned to have an impact on the health status of people in multiple settings. The further preparation included in the DNP curriculum will prepare graduates to "analyze epidemiological, biostatistical, occupational, and environmental data in the development, implementation, and evaluation of clinical prevention and population health" (AACN, 2006b, p. 15). In other words, DNP graduates are in an ideal position to participate in health promotion and risk reduction activities from a nursing perspective with additional preparation in evaluating and interpreting data that are pertinent to improving the health status of individuals (adapted from AACN, 2006b).

Essential VIII: Advanced Nursing Practice

Because one cannot become proficient in all areas of specialization, DNP degree programs "provide preparation within distinct specialties that require expertise, advanced knowledge, and mastery in one area of nursing practice" (AACN, 2006b, p. 16). This specialization is defined by a specialty practice area within the domain of nursing and is a requisite of the DNP degree. Although the DNP graduate may function in a variety of roles, role preparation within the practice specialty, including legal and regulatory issues, is part of every DNP curriculum. With regard to

advanced nursing practice, the DNP graduate is prepared to do the following (adapted from AACN, 2006b):

- Comprehensively assess health and illness parameters while incorporating diverse and culturally sensitive approaches
- Implement and evaluate therapeutic interventions based on nursing and other sciences
- Participate in therapeutic relationships with patients and other healthcare professionals to ensure optimal patient care and improve patient outcomes
- Utilize advanced clinical decision-making skills and critical thinking, and deliver and evaluate evidence-based care to improve patient outcomes
- Serve as a mentor to others in the nursing profession in an effort to maintain excellence in nursing practice
- Participate in the education of patients, especially those in complex health situations.

A Note About Specialty-Focused Competencies According to the AACN

The purpose of specialty preparation within the DNP curricula is to prepare graduates to fulfill specific roles within health care. Specialty preparation and the eight DNP essentials equip DNP graduates to serve in roles within two different domains. The first domain includes specialization as advanced-practice registered nurses who care for individuals (including, but not limited to, clinical nurse specialist (CNS), nurse practitioner, nurse anesthetist, nurse–midwife). The second domain includes specialization in advanced practice at an organizational or systems level. Because of this variability, specialization content within DNP programs may differ (AACN, 2006b). It should also be noted that postmaster's degree DNP preparation includes doctoral-level content exclusively; however, postbaccalaureate DNP preparation includes both advanced-practice specialty content that was previously covered in master's preparation and doctoral-level content.

NONPF Practice Doctorate Nurse Practitioner Entry-Level Competencies

NONPF published *Practice Doctorate Nurse Practitioner Entry-Level Competencies* for nurse practitioner and DNP graduates (2006). These competencies differ somewhat from the AACN's essentials in that they are particular to nurse practitioner roles. However, these competencies are also reflective of the AACN's essentials. The competencies are as follows:

I. Competency Area: Independent Practice
Practices independently by assessing, diagnosing, treating, and managing undifferentiated patients.
Assumes full accountability for actions as a licensed practitioner.

II. Competency Area: Scientific Foundation
Critically analyzes data for practice by integrating knowledge from arts and sciences within the context of nursing's philosophical framework and scientific foundation.
Translates research and data to anticipate, predict, and explain variations in practice.

III. Competency Area: Leadership
Assumes increasingly complex leadership roles.
Provides leadership to foster intercollaboration.
Demonstrates a leadership style that uses critical and reflective thinking.

IV. Competency Area: Quality
Uses best-available evidence to enhance quality in clinical practice.
Evaluates how organizational, structural, financial, marketing, and policy decisions affect cost, quality, and accessibility of health care.

Demonstrates skills in peer review that promote a culture of excellence.

V. Competency Area: Practice Inquiry
Applies clinical investigative skills for evaluation of health outcomes at the patient, family, population, clinical unit, systems, or community levels.
Provides leadership in the translation of new knowledge into practice.
Disseminates evidence from inquiry to diverse audiences using multiple methods.

VI. Competency Area: Technology and Information Literacy
Demonstrates information literacy in complex decision making.
Translates technical and scientific health information appropriate for user need.

VII. Competency Area: Policy
Analyzes ethical, legal, and social factors in policy development.
Influences health policy.
Evaluates the impact of globalization on healthcare policy.

VIII. Competency Area: Health Delivery System
Applies knowledge of organizational behavior and systems.
Demonstrates skills in negotiating, consensus building, and partnering.
Manages risks to individuals, families, populations, and healthcare systems.
Facilitates development of culturally relevant healthcare systems.

IX. Competency Area: Ethics
Applies ethically sound solutions to complex issues.

NACNS Core Practice Doctorate Clinical Nurse Specialist Competencies

In 2006 the NACNS consulted with various nursing organizations and nursing accrediting entities regarding the implications of the DNP degree for CNS practice and education

(NACNS, 2009). A formal task force, including representatives from NACNS and 19 other nursing organizations, was charged with developing competencies for the CNS at the doctoral level (NACNS, 2009). Because traditional CNS education has included a master's degree, "the *Core Practice Doctorate Clinical Nurse Specialist Competencies* should be used with the National CNS Competency Task Force's *Organizing Framework and Core Competencies* (2008) and the AACN *Essentials of Doctoral Education for Advanced Nursing Practice* (2006b) to inform educational programs and employer expectations" (NACNS, 2009, p. 10).

The foci of the *Core Practice Doctorate Clinical Nurse Specialist Competencies* are congruent with the AACN's *Essentials of Doctoral Education for Advanced Nursing Practice* and NONPF's *Practice Doctorate Nurse Practitioner Entry-Level Competencies* (**Figure 3-1**). Specifically, graduates of CNS-focused DNP programs should be prepared beyond traditional CNS competencies to "strengthen the already significant contribution

that CNSs make in ensuring quality patient outcomes through establishing a practice foundation based on advanced scientific, theoretical, ethical, and economic principles" (NACNS, 2009, p. 11). These competencies ensure that doctoral-prepared CNS graduates are prepared to do the following (adapted from NACNS, 2009):

- Generate and disseminate new knowledge
- Evaluate and translate evidence into practice
- Employ a broad range of theories from nursing and related disciplines
- Design and evaluate innovative strategies to improve quality of care and safety in all settings
- Improve systems of care
- Provide leadership that promotes interprofessional collaboration
- Influence and shape health policy

Certified Registered Nurse Anesthetists

As advanced-practice nursing moves toward doctoral preparation for entry into practice, certified registered nurse anesthetists (CRNAs)

FIGURE 3-1 Relationship among the DNP Essentials, the NONPF Competencies, the NACNS Competencies, and the Core Competencies Needed for Healthcare Professionals per the Committee on Health Professions Education.

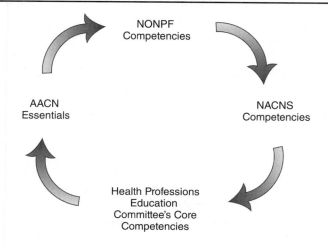

have debated if this progression is appropriate for this advanced-practice specialty. In 2005 the American Association of Nurse Anesthetists (AANA) Summit on Doctoral Preparation for Nurse Anesthetists convened to discuss and identify potential implications of adopting doctoral preparation (Martin-Sheridan, Ouellette, & Horton, 2006). The summit participants concluded that in the future CRNAs may need additional knowledge and skills that include doctoral preparation. Following the summit, the Task Force on Doctoral Preparation of Nurse Anesthetists was formed to develop recommendations regarding doctoral preparation for CRNAs. In 2007 a decision was made by AANA to transition from master's-level education to doctoral-level education by 2025 (AANA, 2007). To date, the *Standards for Accreditation of Nurse Anesthesia Programs Practice Doctorate* state that "students accepted into accredited entry-level programs on or after January 1, 2022, must graduate with doctoral degrees" (Council on Accreditation of Nurse Anesthesia Programs, 2013, p. 2).

The Path to the DNP Degree: Follow the Academic Road

The path to the DNP degree is currently in transition. Previously DNP preparation included exclusively postmaster's degree preparation. Many postmaster's degree students will have already fulfilled several of the criteria listed in the *Essentials of Doctoral Education for Advanced Nursing Practice* and the *Practice Doctorate Nurse Practitioner Entry-Level Competencies* in their master's degree curricula. Further, as mentioned earlier, the specialization content included in the DNP degree curriculum is currently being fulfilled within the master's degree curriculum. However, a shift is occurring to include postbaccalaureate DNP preparation. This option presents many new challenges for both students and schools of nursing.

Each individual's path to the DNP degree may be unique. Prospective students' program content may be individualized to include the learning experiences necessary to incorporate the described requirements for the DNP degree. Please refer to **Figure 3-2** for an illustration of the pathways to the DNP degree.

FIGURE 3-2 Pathways to the DNP degree.

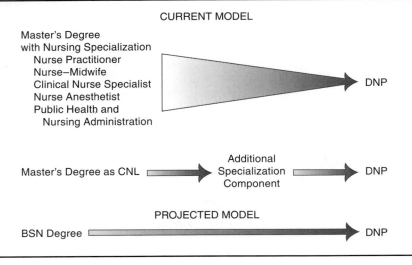

ROLE TRANSITION INTRODUCED

As explained earlier in the chapter, the doctoral-level content of the DNP degree is not intended to provide specialization in nursing practice. The doctoral-level content instead builds on advanced nursing practice specialization and provides additional preparation in the formulation, interpretation, and utilization of evidence-based practices, health policy, information technology, and leadership. Although DNP graduates may function as evaluators and translators of research, health policy advocates, nursing leaders, educators, information specialists, or clinicians, it is entirely likely that these roles will be integrated as well. One DNP graduate may participate in research in addition to practicing as a nurse anesthetist. Another DNP graduate may be a nurse executive in addition to developing health policy. Nursing has always been a profession that involves juggling multiple roles (Dudley-Brown, 2006; Jennings & Rogers, 1988; Sperhac & Strodtbeck, 1997). Within these multiple roles, the fundamental goal of the DNP graduate remains the development of expertise in the delivery of high-quality, patient-centered care, and the graduate utilizes the necessary avenues to provide that care.

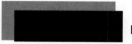

Interview with a DNP Cofounder: Then and Now

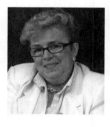

Carolyn A. Williams, PhD, RN, FAAN, is professor and dean emeritus of the University of Kentucky. She was president of the American Association of Colleges of Nursing from 2000 to 2002 and scholar-in-residence at the Institute of Medicine from 2007 to 2008.

THEN ... 2008

Dr. Williams, could you please describe your background and current position?

I began my nursing career as a public health nurse at a public health department in a rural area and practiced for 2 years before returning to graduate school. I then received my master's degree in public health nursing. This was a joint master's degree from both the School of Nursing and the School of Public Health from the University of North Carolina at Chapel Hill (UNC, CH). I then went on to earn a PhD in epidemiology from the School of Public Health at UNC,

CH. This was met with some controversy in that I did not have a large amount of nursing experience before returning to graduate school. Interestingly, the School of Public Health was supportive of my doctoral studies whereas the School of Nursing seemed to think I needed more nursing experience. This is what I call a "pernicious pattern" in nursing education. I actually had to talk faculty [in nursing] into supporting me to earn a doctorate. However, faculty from other disciplines, for example, medicine, psychology, and sociology in the School of Public Health, were very supportive. This is where nursing differs from medicine: we don't build in the experience into our educational programs.

Upon finishing my PhD in epidemiology, I took a faculty position at Emory University's School of Nursing. From there, I was asked to return to Chapel Hill to participate in the development and evaluation of a family nurse practitioner program in the School of Nursing and to teach epidemiology in the School of Public Health. The program in the School of Nursing was one of the first six federally funded family nurse practitioner programs in the country. I remained at

(continues)

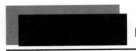 Interview with a DNP Cofounder: Then and Now *(continued)*

Chapel Hill for 13 years before accepting an appointment as dean of the College of Nursing at the University of Kentucky. Last year I retired as dean after 22 years in that position and remained as a faculty member.

This year [2007 to 2008] I am a scholar-in-residence at the Institute of Medicine in Washington, DC. My role here includes development of a project, which happens to be interprofessional collaboration. This stems from the view that improvement in quality care depends on people working together in interprofessional teams. Interprofessional collaboration is happening around the margins of education for health care instead of in the mainstream, particularly core clinical components of undergraduate and graduate education for health care. It may be picked up in passing, but frequently it is not a formal part of the curriculum. Part of my project involves identifying the policy changes [that] are needed at the university level to integrate interprofessional collaboration as part [of] an integral component of education in the health professions. Interprofessional collaboration is a necessary part of practice and therefore needs to be integrated into the preparation of healthcare professionals. This leads me to an issue I have always struggled with: too few clinical faculty in nursing actually practice. This is a problem due to the fact that a practice culture is not as visible as I believe it needs to be in most schools of nursing. Some progress in having nursing faculty engaged in practice was achieved with the nurse practitioner movement that started in the 1970s, but it is still a struggle for nursing faculty to engage in practice as part of their faculty role in a manner similar to what happens in medical education. Some faculty attempt to practice on their own, not as a part of their faculty role, and usually faculty practice is not viewed as a priority in schools of nursing. I feel if we want nursing faculty to provide leadership in practice and develop leaders for practice, each school of nursing

needs to have a core group of faculty who actually engage in practice as part of their faculty role.

Dr. Williams, could you please describe how your vision for a doctor of nursing practice became a reality?
While on the faculty at the University of North Carolina at Chapel Hill and consulting with a number of individuals in practice settings, I developed some ideas of what nursing education to prepare nurse leaders needs to be. Initially, I viewed the degree as what public health nurses could earn to prepare them to face the challenges of public health nursing. I didn't feel that the master's degrees in nursing offered at that time [1970s through early 1980s] were sufficient for the kind of leadership roles nurses were moving in to. I felt a true practice degree at the doctoral level was needed.

When I went to the University of Kentucky as the dean of nursing, I was charged with developing a PhD in nursing program. While at Chapel Hill I had been very involved in research activity, doctoral education in epidemiology, and was active nationally in research development and advocacy in nursing as chair of the American Nurses Association's Commission on Nursing Research and as the president of the American Academy of Nursing. I proceeded to work with the faculty at the University of Kentucky, and we developed the PhD program in nursing. However, I was still interested in the concept of a practice doctorate and promoting stronger partnerships between nursing practice and nursing education.

As time went on it became clearer and clearer to me that to prepare nurses for leadership in practice, something more in tune with preparing nurses to utilize knowledge, not necessarily generate new knowledge, which was expected in PhD programs, was needed. Thus, I began to talk with and work with my faculty colleagues on the concept of a new practice

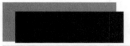

Interview with a DNP Cofounder: Then and Now *(continued)*

degree for nurses to prepare for leadership in practice, not in education or research.

I saw practice as the focus with this degree, not research. Working with my University of Kentucky faculty colleagues, particularly Dr. Marcia K. Stanhope and Dr. Julie G. Sebastian, we developed the initial conceptualization of the degree. These foci included four themes that I feel should be central to a practice doctorate in nursing:

1. Leadership in practice, which included leadership at the point of care. This also includes leadership at the policy level to impact care.

2. A population approach and perspective. This involves a broader view of health care, which recognizes the importance of populations when planning and evaluating care processes.

3. Integration of evidence-based practice to make informed decisions regarding care.

4. The ability to understand change processes and institute positive changes in health care.

These four themes guided the development of the curriculum of the first DNP program at the University of Kentucky, which when we instituted it was the first in the United States. These themes also influenced and are incorporated in what became the AACN's Essentials of Doctoral Education for Advanced Nursing Practice.

To expand on the development of the DNP program at University of Kentucky, the following is the time line:

1994–1998 Informal conversations among faculty, people in practice, and others regarding a practice doctorate in nursing

1998 Professional Doctorate Task Force Committee formed

May 1999 Approval of DNP program by total college faculty

July 1999 Medical Center Academic Council approval

January 2000 University of Kentucky Board of Trustees approved the program

May 2000 Approval by the Kentucky Council of Postsecondary Education

January 2001 The first national paper on the DNP degree at the AACN's

National Doctoral Education Conference (Williams, Stanhope, & Sebastian, 2001)

Fall 2001 Students admitted to the first DNP program in the country.

In 1998, when the University of Kentucky's DNP task force was created, we decided we didn't want this degree to look like anything else currently in nursing education. We also decided on the name of this degree in this committee. We wanted the degree and the name to focus on nursing practice, and we did not want the degree to be limited to preparing for only one particular type of nursing practice. We decided on the doctor of nursing practice because that describes what the degree is: a practice degree in nursing.

One of the most important things that happened during my presidency of the American Association of Colleges of Nursing was the appointment [of] a task force to look at the issue of a practice doctorate. The task force committee was carefully planned. I wanted to have a positive group of people as well as major stakeholders represented. These stakeholders were credible individuals who had an interest in the development of a practice doctorate. Members of the committee included representatives from Columbia University, the University of Kentucky, a representative from an ND program, as well as a representative

(continues)

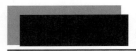

Interview with a DNP Cofounder: Then and Now (*continued*)

from schools that did not have nursing doctoral programs. This committee was chaired by Dr. Elizabeth Lentz, who has written extensively on doctoral education in nursing. As this task force began sorting out the issues, it became the goal that by 2015, the DNP would become the terminal degree for specialization in nursing.

From this point, a group to develop both the essentials of doctoral education in nursing and a roadmap task force were formed. These committees worked together, and we presented together nationally in a series of regional forums. We invited others to engage in discourse regarding the essentials as well as ask questions about the DNP degree. As our presentations across the country came to a conclusion, we noticed an obvious transformation. The DNP degree was beginning to gain more acceptance. By the time we were done, the argument of whether to adopt a practice doctorate in nursing had given rise to how to put this degree in place.

Dr. Williams, are you surprised by the acceptance of the degree and speed with which programs are being developed?
Yes, I am surprised. I thought the DNP degree would be an important development for the field of nursing, and I thought some would adopt a practice doctorate. I certainly did not think things would move so fast. The idea of a DNP really struck a chord with many people.

Dr. Williams, do you think the history of doctoral education in nursing has influenced the development of a practice doctorate in nursing?
Well, we need to have scientists in our field. However, we also need to come to grips with the fact that we are a practice discipline. Over the years, since the late 1970s, many of the leading academic settings in nursing have become increasingly research intensive

and [have] not spent as much effort on developing a complementary practice focus. I feel the development of a practice doctorate has more to do with our development as a discipline than the history of doctoral nursing education. Attraction and credibility from the university setting stem from involvement in research. Therefore, it becomes a struggle when handling this practice piece. If nursing wants acceptance as a discipline, we must have research. But we are a practice discipline, and all practice disciplines struggle to some extent in research-intensive university environments.

Dr. Williams, do you agree that nursing should have both a research- and a practice-focused doctorate?
Of course. The ratio between research-focused and practice-focused doctorates may be tipped toward the practice focus due to the practice focus of our discipline.

Dr. Williams, could you describe what you feel is the future of doctoral education in nursing?
Down the pike, some people may move into DNP programs and then discover they want to be researchers and end up also getting a PhD. This would be very healthy for our profession. Essentially, we have lost talented folks due to offering only a research-focused terminal degree. The DNP allows us to accommodate those folks who don't want a research-focused degree. I also feel we need a more intensive clinical component integrated into the degree. This may be in the form of residency programs integrated within nursing degrees or as a postdoctorate option.

Dr. Williams, could you expand on the grandfathering of advanced-practice registered nurses (APRNs) who don't wish to pursue a DNP degree?
The DNP degree will not be required to practice anytime soon. It took a while to require a master's degree

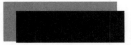

Interview with a DNP Cofounder: Then and Now *(continued)*

to practice as an APRN. There will be a similar transition regarding the DNP degree. If someone is certified and successful as an APRN without a DNP, they should continue to be successful.

Dr. Williams, do you believe the DNP will continue to flourish as a degree option for nursing? If so, what would your advice be regarding nurses earning a DNP degree?
Yes, I do. My advice regarding nurses earning a DNP degree is that it depends on their career choice. Some have been looking for this option for a long time. This may be the right degree for some no matter where they are in practice.

NOW ... 2014

Dr. Williams, we discussed your nursing background and education the last time we spoke. Could you please describe your current position and what types of projects you are currently involved in?
Since I left the deanship of the College of Nursing at the University of Kentucky in the fall of 2006 I have remained on the faculty as a professor in the college and teach in both our DNP and PhD programs. I spent the 2007–2008 academic year at the Institute of Medicine in DC as the American Academy of Nursing–American Nurses' Foundation's scholar-in-residence. During that year I had the opportunity to be a part of the Health Policy seminars designed for the Robert Wood Johnson Foundation's Health Policy Fellows. It was a unique experience to interact with health policy makers and experts in the national arena.

I continue to teach at the University of Kentucky in the areas of health policy, leadership, and ethics, and I work with students on DNP Clinical Projects and Dissertations. I also continue to serve as a consultant and mentor on issues related to graduate education in nursing and leadership in the field.

Dr. Williams, what is your impression of the current progress of the DNP degree? How does the current progress of the DNP degree compare to your original vision of the DNP degree?
The original vision that my colleagues and I at the University of Kentucky's College of Nursing had for the DNP when we opened the first program of study leading to the DNP in the fall of 2001 was that it would be a postmaster's program for those interested in leadership in nursing practice. Further we saw the DNP as a program of study for clinical nurse specialists, nurse practitioners, and nurse administrators. We conceptualized four key areas that we felt were necessary for leadership in practice and which we felt were not sufficiently dealt with in the master's programs at that time. Those four pillars were a population approach; the use of the best evidence possible in clinical decision making; understanding how to guide sustainable changes in practice based on the best evidence possible; and leadership at the unit and system level. Our original program was built around those concepts, and I am pleased that those concepts are clearly evident in the DNP essentials developed by the American Association of Colleges of Nursing (AACN, 2006b). For a program to receive accreditation by the Commission on Collegiate Nursing Education (CCNE) all of the essentials have to be evident in the curriculum. However, one issue that we need to continue to keep in focus and work on, particularly in the emerging BSN-to-DNP programs preparing nurse practitioners, is how to integrate those concepts into the manner in which the nurse practitioner student conceptualizes their practice. This is tricky since students in such programs focus so much of their efforts on getting comfortable with the assessment and management of individual patients, and time in many programs is limited.

The overall growth of DNP programs has been far more rapid than I expected. The latest data from

(continues)

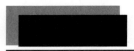

Interview with a DNP Cofounder: Then and Now *(continued)*

AACN obtained during the fall of 2013 is that there are now 243 DNP programs in the United States (AACN, 2014). The good news is that access to a DNP program for those interested in such preparation has markedly increased. For those seeking a program, the challenge is to look carefully at what a given program can provide in terms of faculty expertise in key areas—doctoral education, relevant and current practice, and clinical scholarship. Given the national shortage of faculty with the necessary expertise, the very rapid increase in the number of programs makes it imperative that all involved in approving programs and providing them do all that is possible to ensure the quality of DNP programs.

Dr. Williams, why do you think the DNP degree continues to gain acceptance and momentum?

I believe some of the initial momentum for the DNP, particularly among nurse practitioners, was stimulated by AACN's 2015 target. However, I think much of it stems from the recognition that better-prepared nurses can be key players in improving patient outcomes at various levels of care and that the focus of DNP programs is on target with regard to the knowledge base and skills necessary for leadership in improving the quality of patient care and patient outcomes. Finally, the Institute of Medicine's report, The Future of Nursing *(IOM, 2010b), which in recommendation 5 calls for doubling the number of nurses with a doctorate by 2020, has probably added to the momentum.*

Dr. Williams, when we last spoke, you agreed that nursing needed both a research- and practice-focused doctorate. Do you still agree that a research and practice-focused doctorate are beneficial to the profession?

Absolutely. Until the emergence of the DNP the consensus among academic and research leaders in nurs-

ing was that the PhD was the route to prepare for leadership in both the academic and practice arena. However, that was an unsustainable course for several reasons. First, too few nurses were seeking PhDs, and too few were being produced. Secondly, most of the PhD programs did not provide content or learning opportunities that directly addressed leadership in the practice arena. Finally, leaders in the field were increasingly recognizing that to be competitive in obtaining grant monies to sustain a viable program of research requires a concentrated focus on research; thus the strongest doctoral programs put their emphasis on how to prepare their graduates to be successful in doing research and obtaining grant support for their work. There was little or no time for preparing for leadership in practice.

In a presentation to the Advisory Council of the National Institute for Nursing Research in 2006 I argued that unless we had practice leaders in nursing who appreciated the need for the best evidence to inform clinical decisions and who knew how to guide evidence-based changes designed to improve nursing practice, the successful efforts of National Institute for Nursing research researchers would not have much impact on the quality of care provided to patients (Williams, 2006). I still hold that view.

Dr. Williams, do you believe that a partnership continues to form between PhD and DNP graduates?

I have been happy to observe some of those partnerships, and I look forward to more. I think all of us concerned about increasing the positive impact that nursing can have on patient outcomes need to encourage and foster such collaboration. I believe those who are faculty in schools and have both a DNP program and a PhD program have a special opportunity and an obligation to work on modeling such behavior by developing collaborative endeavors between DNP and PhD faculty

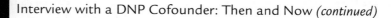

Interview with a DNP Cofounder: Then and Now *(continued)*

and having students in both programs work with them in their collaborative efforts.

Dr. Williams, are you noticing a transition of roles in nursing as more students graduate from DNP degrees and begin their careers? Are there any specific roles you see evolving as more nurses earn their DNP degree?
I have noticed that a year or two after completing a DNP a number of our graduates have moved into roles that involve assuming more responsibility and demand more organizational leadership. These include moving from providing care as a nurse practitioner to developing a new clinic in a rural area and moving from having responsibility as the nurse leading several clinical programs to becoming the vice president of nursing for a hospital. In addition to gaining more recognition as expert practitioners and clinical consultants, in the future I think we will see more of our graduates moving into leadership roles traditionally held by individuals with preparation in other fields, such as medicine and management. These include clinic directors, directors of clinical services, directors of quality assurance programs for various types of healthcare organizations and systems, health officers in large health departments, directors of practice initiatives in large healthcare organizations, and chief operating officers in healthcare organizations.

Dr. Williams, what do you think are the most significant contributions the DNP degree has made to nursing education?
I think it has helped to refocus many of our academic leaders in nursing on the essence of our discipline, which is practice, and realistic ways in which we can prepare graduates to provide leadership in improving nursing practice.

Dr. Williams, how would you recommend we continue to move forward with AACN's recommended target date of the DNP for entry into practice by 2015?
The target date was really an aspiration and it has done its work of fostering momentum. Now I think the emphasis should shift to more attention on continuous efforts to ensure program quality and the competence of the graduates in each of the DNP essential areas. Examples of such initiatives include faculty development related to clinical scholarship and partnerships between schools of nursing and practice settings that provide more opportunities for nursing faculty to have meaningful engagement in practice as a part of their faculty role. The DNP will continue to evolve, but for it to continue to be relevant and cutting edge, core DNP faculty who lead in curriculum development and implementation need to be in touch with and understand practice realities and possibilities.

SUMMARY

- The DNP degree is defined as a practice-focused doctorate that prepares graduates as experts in nursing practice.
- Nursing practice is defined by the AACN as "any form of nursing intervention that influences health care outcomes for individuals or populations, including direct care of individual patients, administration of nursing and health care organizations, and the implementation of health policy" (AACN, 2004, p. 3).
- According to the AACN's (2004) position statement, the DNP degree is proposed to be the terminal degree for nursing practice by 2015.

- A nursing PhD degree is a research-focused degree, and a DNP degree is a practice-focused degree.

- The evolution of doctoral education in nursing illustrates where we have been in doctoral education and the direction nursing is taking in the development of doctoral education.

- The concept of a practice doctorate is not new. The idea began in the 1970s with the development of the DNS degree.

- The AACN now designates the DNS and PhD degrees as research-focused degrees, and the DNP and DrNP degrees are designated as practice-focused degrees.

- In 2002 the AACN board of directors formed a task force to examine the current progress of proposed doctorates in nursing.

- In 2000 the IOM published a report titled *To Err Is Human: Building a Safer Health System*, which summarized errors made in the healthcare system and proposed recommendations to improve the overall quality of care.

- In 2003 the Health Professions Education Committee published *Health Professions Education: A Bridge to Quality*, which outlined a specific set of competencies that should be met by all clinicians.

- In 2008 the IOM appointed the Committee on the RWJF Initiative on the Future of Nursing. This committee published a report in 2010 titled *The Future of Nursing: Focus on Education*, which concluded that "the ways in which nurses were educated during the 20th century are no longer adequate for dealing with the realities of healthcare in the 21st century" (IOM, 2010a, p. 2). This committee also recommended doubling the number of nurses with doctorates by 2020.

- In 2004 the AACN published a position statement regarding a practice doctorate in nursing and recommended that by 2015 all nurses pursuing advanced-practice degrees will be prepared as DNP graduates.

- In 2005 the National Academy of Sciences recommended that a nonresearch ND be developed to meet nursing faculty needs.

- In 2006 the AACN described the *Essentials of Doctoral Education for Advanced Nursing Practice*, which represents the standards for DNP curricula.

- NONPF outlined the *Practice Doctorate Nurse Practitioner Entry-Level Competencies* as standards for DNP curricula.

- In 2009 the NACNS developed *Core Practice Doctorate Clinical Nurse Specialist Competencies*.

- In 2007 the AANA stated that nurse anesthetist education would adopt doctoral education as preparation to enter into practice by 2025.

- The DNP degree includes postmaster's degree programs and postbaccalaureate degree programs.

- Graduate students may follow an individualized path to the DNP degree, depending on their current degree preparation.

- DNP graduates may be involved in many different roles that may include, but are not limited to, research evaluator and translator, leader, healthcare policy advocate, educator, information technology specialist, and clinician.

DISCUSSION QUESTIONS

1. How do you think nursing's history has contributed to the development of the DNP degree?

2. How do you think the IOM report *To Err Is Human: Building a Safer Health System*, along with the follow-up report *Crossing the Quality Chasm: A New Health System for the 21st Century*, contributed to the development of the DNP degree?

3. Explain why you think the IOM and the RWJF concluded, in their report *The Future*

of Nursing: Focus on Education, that nurses need improvement in their educational preparation.

4. Do you think a struggle still exists within nursing today regarding whether doctoral education should be research or practice focused?

5. Do you think nursing doctoral education should be research focused, practice focused, or both?

6. Do you think a DNP degree is the right degree for you?

REFERENCES

Allan, J., Barwick, T., Cashman, S., Cawley, J. F., Day, C., Douglass, C. W., ...Wood, D. (2004). Clinical prevention and population health: Curriculum framework for health professions. *American Journal of Preventive Medicine, 27*(5), 471–476.

American Association of Colleges of Nursing (AACN). (2004). *AACN position statement on the practice doctorate in nursing.* Retrieved from http://www.aacn.nche.edu/DNP/pdf/DNP.pdf

American Association of Colleges of Nursing (AACN). (2005). Commission on Collegiate Nursing Education moves to consider for accreditation only practice doctorates with the DNP degree title. Retrieved from http://www.aacn.nche.edu/news/articles/2005/commission-on-collegiate-nursing-education-moves-to-consider-for-accreditation-only-practice-doctorates-with-the-dnp-degree-title

American Association of Colleges of Nursing (AACN). (2006a). *DNP roadmap task force report.* Retrieved from http://www.aacn.nche.edu/dnp/roadmapreport.pdf

American Association of Colleges of Nursing (AACN). (2006b). *Essentials of doctoral education for advanced nursing practice.* Retrieved from http://www.aacn.nche.edu/publications/position/DNPEssentials.pdf

American Association of Colleges of Nursing (AACN). (2007). *AACN white paper on the education and role of the clinical nurse leader.* Retrieved from http://www.aacn.nche.edu/publications/white-papers/cnl

American Association of Colleges of Nursing (AACN). (2011). *DNP fact sheet: The doctor of nursing practice (DNP).* Retrieved from http://www.aacn.nche.edu/media-relations/fact-sheets/dnp

American Association of Colleges of Nursing (AACN). (2014). *Program directory.* Retrieved from http://www.aacn.nche.edu/dnp/program-directory

American Association of Nurse Anesthetists (AANA). (2007). *AANA position on doctoral preparation of nurse anesthetists.* Retrieved from http://www.aana.com/ceandeducation/educationalresources/Documents/AANA_Position_DTF_June_2007.pdf

American Hospital Association. (1999). *Hospital statistics.* Chicago, IL: Author.

Apold, S. (2008). The doctor of nursing practice: Looking back, moving forward. *Journal for Nurse Practitioners, 4*(2), 101–107.

Carpenter, R., & Hudacek, S. (1996). *On doctoral education in nursing: The voice of the student.* New York, NY: National League for Nursing Press.

Centers for Disease Control and Prevention, National Center for Health Statistics. (1999a). Births and deaths: Preliminary data for 1998. *National Vital Statistics Reports, 47*(25), 1–45.

Centers for Disease Control and Prevention, National Center for Health Statistics. (1999b). Deaths: Final data for 1997. *National Vital Statistics Reports, 47*(19), 1–104.

Cleland, V. (1976). Developing a doctoral program. *Nursing Outlook, 24*(10), 631–635.

Council on Accreditation of Nurse Anesthesia Programs. (2013). *Standards for accreditation of nurse anesthesia programs practice doctorate.* Retrieved from http://www.aana.com/newsandjournal/20102019/educnews-0614-p177-183.pdf

Donaldson, S., & Crowley, D. (1978). The discipline of nursing. *Nursing Outlook, 26*(2), 113–120.

Dracup, K., Cronenwett, L., Meleis, A., & Benner, P. (2005). Reflections on the doctorate of nursing practice. *Nursing Outlook, 53*(4), 177–182.

Dudley-Brown, S. (2006). Revisiting the blended role of the advanced practice nurse. *Gastroenterology Nursing, 29*(3), 249–250.

Fawcett, J. (2005). *Contemporary nursing knowledge: Analysis and evaluation of nursing models and theories* (2nd ed.). Philadelphia, PA: F. A. Davis.

Goldenberg, G. (2004). The DrNP degree. *The Academic Nurse: The Journal of the Columbia University School of Nursing, 21*(1), 22–26.

Gortner, S. (1980). Nursing science in transition. *Nursing Research, 29*(3), 180–183.

Grace, H. (1978). The development of doctoral education in nursing: In historical perspective. *Journal of Nursing Education, 17*(4), 17–27.

Greiner, A. C., & Knebel, E. (Eds.). (2003). *Health professions education: A bridge to quality.* Washington, DC: National Academies Press.

Institute of Medicine (IOM). (2001). *Crossing the quality chasm: A new health system for the 21st century.* Washington, DC: National Academies Press.

Institute of Medicine (IOM). (2010a). *The future of nursing: Focus on education.* Retrieved from http://www.iom.edu/~/media/Files/Report%20Files/2010/The-Future-of-Nursing/Nursing%20Education%202010%20Brief.pdf

Institute of Medicine (IOM). (2010b). *The future of nursing: Leading change, advancing health.* Retrieved from http://www.iom.edu/Reports/2010/The-Future-of-Nursing-Leading-Change-Advancing-Health.aspx

Jennings, B., & Rogers, S. (1988). Merging nursing research and practice: A case of multiple identities. *Journal of Advanced Nursing, 13*(6), 752–758.

Kohn, L. T., Corrigan, J. M., & Donaldson, M. S. (Eds.). (2000). *To err is human: Building a safer health system.* Washington, DC: National Academies Press.

Marion, L., O'Sullivan, A., Crabtree, M. K., Price, M., & Fontana, S. (2005). Curriculum models for the practice doctorate in nursing. *Topics in Advanced Practice Nursing eJournal, 5*(1). Retrieved from http://www.medscape.com/viewarticle/500742_print

Marion, L., Viens, D., O'Sullivan, A., Crabtree, M. K., Fontana, S., & Price, M. (2003). The practice doctorate in nursing: Future or fringe. *Topics in Advanced Practice Nursing eJournal, 3*(2). Retrieved from http://www.medscape.com/viewarticle/453247_print

Marriner-Tomey, A. (1990). Historical development of doctoral programs from the middle ages to nursing education today. *Nursing and Health Care, 11*(3), 132–137.

Martin-Sheridan, D., Ouelette, S. M., & Horton, B. J. (2006). Education news: Is doctoral education in our future? *AANA Journal, 74*(2), 101–104.

Murphy, J. (1981). Doctoral education in, of, and for nursing: An historical analysis. *Nursing Outlook, 29*(11), 645–649.

National Academy of Sciences. (2005). *Advancing the nation's health needs: NIH Research Training Programs.* Washington, DC: National Academies Press. Retrieved from http://www.nap.edu/openbook.php?isbn=0309094275

National Association of Clinical Nurse Specialists (NACNS). (2009). *Core practice doctorate clinical nurse specialist competencies.* Retrieved from http://www.nacns.org/docs/CorePracticeDoctorate.pdf

National CNS Competency Task Force. (2008). *Organizing framework and core competencies.* Retrieved from http://www.nacns.org/docs/CNSCoreCompetenciesBroch.pdf

National Organization of Nurse Practitioner Faculties (NONPF). (2006). *Practice doctorate nurse practitioner entry-level competencies.* Retrieved from http://c.ymcdn.com/sites/www.nonpf.org/resource/resmgr/competencies/dnp%20np%20competenciesapril2006.pdf

Newman, M. (1975). The professional doctorate in nursing: A position paper. *Nursing Outlook, 23*(11), 704–706.

Roberts, S., & Glod, C. (2005). The practice doctorate in nursing: Is it the answer? *The American Journal for Nurse Practitioners, 9*(11/12), 55–65.

Sperhac, A., & Strodtbeck, F. (1997). Advanced practice nursing: New opportunities for blended roles. *The American Journal of Maternal/Child Nursing, 22*(6), 287–293.

Starck, P., Duffy, M., & Vogler, R. (1993). Developing a nursing doctorate for the 21st century. *Journal of Professional Nursing, 9*(4), 212–219.

Thomas, E., Studdert, D., Newhouse, J., Zbar, B., Howard, K., Williams, E., & Brennan, T. A. (1999). Costs of medical injuries in Utah and Colorado. *Inquiry, 36*(3), 255–264.

Williams, C. A. (2006, January 24). The doctorate of nursing practice: An option for leader-ship in nursing practice. Presented to the Advisory Council of the National Institute for Nursing Research, National Institutes of Health, Bethesda, MD.

Williams, C. A., Stanhope, M. K., & Sebastian, J. G. (2001). Clinical nursing leadership: One model of professional doctoral education in nursing. In C. M. Golde & G. E. Walker (Eds.), *Envisioning doctoral education for the future* (pp. 85–91). Washington, DC: AACN.

CHAPTER 4

© A-R-T/Shutterstock

Emerging Roles for the DNP Nurse Educator

Kathryn Waud White

CHAPTER OBJECTIVES

1. Describe nursing leadership roles that are emerging from the Doctor of Nursing Practice (DNP) degree.

2. Explore the impact of the DNP degree on nursing education and healthcare outcomes.

3. Discuss the influence of the DNP on nursing administration and nurse executive roles.

4. Define the characteristics of a nurse entrepreneur.

5. Distinguish between public health and community health nursing and the role of the DNP-prepared nurse as program developer and evaluator.

6. Analyze complementary healthcare modalities and discuss the role of the DNP-prepared nurse as an integrative practitioner.

As the nursing profession moves toward implementation of the American Association of Colleges of Nursing's (AACN's) recommendation that all advanced practice nurses (APNs) be educated in a Doctor of Nursing Practice (DNP) framework (AACN, 2006), the DNP-prepared nurse educator is certain to emerge as a clear and vital component of advanced practice nursing education. The education of APNs focuses on the development of the knowledge and skills to care for patients at the highest level possible and implies the infusion of clinical scholarship into the care of all patients, at all times, and in all practice settings. The role of APNs in health care is receiving national attention (Institute of Medicine [IOM], 2010). The DNP-prepared nurse educator is well suited to teach clinical scholarship in the context of a practice doctorate to help advanced practice nursing students achieve this level of practice.

The notion of advanced practice nursing faculty obtaining practice doctorates versus research degrees is supported by several professional organizations. In 2005, the National Organization of Nurse Practitioner Faculties (NONPF) issued a statement on faculty practice (Blair, Dennehy, & White, 2005). In this statement, the organization asserted that "faculty practice is necessary to maintain competence, a forum for scholarship, and the expectation of professionalism" (p. 2). NONPF has also proposed that the competence of faculty should be evaluated in both the teaching arena and the clinical arena (NONPF, 2000). The board of governors of the National League for Nursing (NLN) issued a position statement in 2002 that states in part that "nurse educators practice in both academic and clinical settings and they must be competent clinicians" (p. 2). It also goes on to state that "while being a good clinician is essential, it is not sufficient for the educator role" (NLN, 2002). The American Nurses Credentialing Center (ANCC, 2012, 2014) and the American Academy of Nurse Practitioners (American Academy of Nurse Practitioners Certification Program, 2012) require advanced practice nurses to document a minimum of 1,000 hours of nursing practice in the specialty and population for which they are prepared every 5 years in order to renew certification. The Commission on Collegiate Nursing Education's (CCNE's) National Task Force on Quality Nurse Practitioner Education's report from 2008 states in Standard I.C, "Institutional support ensures that NP faculty teaching in clinical courses maintain currency in clinical practice" (CCNE, 2008, p. 4). This again supports the role of the educator who is prepared with a practice doctorate rather than a research doctorate.

Nevertheless, a practice doctorate is not necessarily adequate preparation for the role of a nurse educator, nor is a research doctorate (AACN, 2006). Both the NLN and the AACN have suggested that advanced practice nursing faculty should recommend additional course work in curriculum design and evaluation and teaching methodologies. The nursing educator who is prepared with a practice doctorate brings some unique skills to the educational practice.

In examining *Essentials of Doctoral Education for Advanced Nursing Practice*, as delineated by the AACN in 2006, it is clear that the DNP-prepared educator who has mastered these essentials has a unique skill set that enhances the education of APNs (AACN, 2006). The first essential, *scientific underpinnings for practice*, reveals the complexities of nursing practice and the many ways that DNP graduates will be able to quickly integrate science and theory from nursing and other disciplines into practice. A DNP-prepared educator brings the scholarship of integration into the academic setting and uses many different concepts from other disciplines to educate APNs.

Mastery of the second essential, *organizational and systems leadership for quality improvement and systems thinking*, also brings a unique perspective to the education of advanced practice students. Many APN programs exist within large, complex educational organizations. It could be said that there is an analogous situation between the large educational institution and a large healthcare organization. The DNP-prepared nurse educator has the skills to work effectively within the organization to evaluate education delivery and make evidence-based educational recommendations for systems change within these large university settings. The DNP-prepared educator can use the principles of business, finance, economics, and health policy to improve the delivery of the education.

This educator has the advanced communications skills to lead such changes.

Diers (1995) asserted that scholarship is a habit of the mind that begins with observations of the phenomena of health and illness but that then applies the "disciplined habits of analysis and analogy," which brings new comprehension of the phenomena. The DNP-prepared educator who has mastered the third essential, *clinical scholarship and analytical methods for evidence-based practice*, brings those skills and habits of mind into the academic setting. The DNP educator is also a scholar who is in the habit of seeking evidence to support the practice of education and integrating evidence from many fields of study into the solutions to problems in education. As cited by Regal (1990), Jeroslav Pelikan (1984) described the difference between good scholarship and great scholarship: "The difference between good scholarship and great scholarship is, as often as not, the general preparation of the scholar in fields other than the field of preparation. It is the general preparation that makes possible that extra leap of imagination and analogy by which scholarship moves ahead" (p. 291). The broad preparation of the DNP-educated nurse in the areas of foundational science, theory, economics, informatics, advocacy, epidemiology, leadership, and collaboration across professions places this educator in a unique place to use the scholarship of integration in an educational setting.

Technology in education is an emerging tool for teaching and learning, and educators are rapidly learning how to leverage technology to improve education. The DNP-prepared educator who has mastered the fourth essential, *information systems/technology and patient care technology for the improvement and transformation of care*, not only is proficient in the use of technology for patient care but also brings that expertise into the academic environment. Distance education and online teaching are the accepted norms. Simulation experiences for advanced practice students are burgeoning as

well, and these simulation environments can be very technologically sophisticated. The DNP-prepared nurse educator not only can navigate in this technological environment but also can model the use of technology to improve systems and outcomes.

The fifth essential, *health care policy for advocacy in health care*, is another area in which the DNP-prepared nurse educator acquires valuable skills for providing a secure place for nursing in the future. Health policy includes not only healthcare system reform but also those issues that are relevant to the education of APNs. Advocacy for significant federal money to support nursing education is only one area where efforts are needed to secure the future of nursing. This educator also has the skills to effectively advocate for resources within the academic institutions that are experiencing budget cuts from donors and state sources. The DNP-prepared educator has the ability to analyze internal and external policy processes and competently influence policy within and outside academic institutions. He or she can serve as a role model of advocacy for the advanced practice students.

Interprofessional collaboration is an area where the DNP-prepared educator brings unique skills to the academic setting. What better, richer environment for interprofessional collaboration is there than an academic health center? The DNP-prepared educator has the skills to value, model, and implement interprofessional teams in the clinical area as well as the academic area. Team leadership and collaboration are the skills recommended by the IOM report of 2001, *Crossing the Quality Chasm*. The DNP-prepared nurse educator who has mastered the sixth essential, *interprofessional collaboration for improving patient and population health outcomes*, is ready to bring team leadership and collaboration to the academic arena.

The DNP-prepared nurse educator readily recognizes that the student body is a population with its own unique characteristics. Students who are taking classes on a doctoral level, going to clinical rotations, managing personal relationships, trying to remain engaged in family activities, and perhaps working part time are prone to fatigue and are certainly functioning in a stressful environment. The DNP educator who has mastered the seventh essential, *clinical prevention and population health for improving the nation's health*, seeks evidence-based solutions to monitor student stress and interventions to assist students in adopting healthy behaviors.

It is in the last essential, *advanced practice nursing*, that the DNP-prepared nurse educator's skills are most valuable as he or she seeks out specific competencies, formulates a plan for students to become proficient in those areas, and implements evaluation programs to measure progress toward competency. Although clinical competency is the last competency, nursing is a clinical profession that synthesizes evidence from all these essentials into competent evidence-based clinical practice of the highest quality for patient safety and improved outcomes. The measurement of clinical ability and continuous process improvement for the educational program are key to maintaining this high level of performance in the complex, rapidly changing healthcare environment.

The notion of the DNP graduate as a nurse educator has come into its own, but challenges remain. It appears that DNP graduates are no more likely to accept the low salaries in academia as are their PhD faculty colleagues (Kelly, 2010). Kelly refuted the notion that the DNP degree is the solution to the nursing faculty shortage, citing the paucity of evidence that DNP graduates who work in advanced practice roles will choose a career in academics, and thus advocated for a comprehensive approach to the faculty shortages. In addition, the ability of DNP faculty members to attain tenure is a controversial subject. In many large universities, this is not likely at this time because of concerns about the DNP-prepared nurse's ability to produce research and secure grants (Nicholes

& Dyer, 2012). Although Nicholes and Dyer found that the deans of colleges of nursing and the PhD-prepared nursing faculty they surveyed had positive attitudes toward DNP-prepared faculty being eligible for tenure, these concerns reflect the continued undervaluing of the scholarship of application and integration articulated by Boyer in 1990. Boyer's definition of the scholarship of practice as it relates to nursing has been a catalyst for change, except in the academy. Nicholes and Dyer (2012) advocated for an attitudinal expansion of the definition of scholarship, as Boyer suggested in 1990, to embrace the scholarship of practice and thus the work of the DNP.

The DNP course of study confers a set of unique skills that are highly valuable and that add to the academic preparation of APNs. These skills support the education of APNs to the highest level and help to fulfill the promise of the IOM (2010) report for improvements in the education of advanced practice nursing. However, challenges remain for acceptance of the role of the DNP-prepared educator in academia.

THE NURSE ADMINISTRATOR

Mary Jean Vickers

The DNP educational program prepares nurses to lead health care in a tremendously challenging reform atmosphere that demands better access and quality while reducing the costs. During this period of rapid change, it is critical for the administrator to appreciate the many governmental and private influences on healthcare programming. Among these agencies are The Joint Commission, the Centers for Medicare and Medicaid Services (CMS), the National Quality Forum (NQF), the Agency for Healthcare Research and Quality (AHRQ), insurance companies, private businesses, and, specifically for nursing, the American Nurses Credentialing Center Magnet Recognition Program and the National Database for Nursing Quality Indicators (NDNQI). These groups are developing certification programs and quality improvement measures in which hospitals are encouraged and rewarded for participation. Sometimes the improvement projects are educational, but often the projects are redesigns of past processes intended to embrace technology in order to improve efficiency and the metrics related to care delivery. Specific best practices are embedded into the care requirements of common diagnoses to promote standardized care and reduce readmissions. Embracing these best practices is often rewarded with higher reimbursement fees. A DNP-prepared administrator has an appreciation of the delicate balance between cost and quality. He or she has a keen understanding of the interdependencies between providing high-quality patient-centered care and achieving the highest reimbursement rates available.

Change Theory

An administrator is well served by the study of the concepts explored in change theories and the knowledge gained through DNP coursework. There are many change models to explore, and each can be helpful in guiding our decisions and facilitating change assimilation into practice. As a novice nurse, this author was educated about Lewin's change theory (Smith, 2001). The early work of social psychology researcher Kurt Lewin is seminal in understanding how groups process change (Smith, 2001). Kurt Lewin developed a simple theory with three phases: unfreezing, change, and freezing. This theory, in its simplest form, suggests that first you need to prepare those who will change through a process of unfreezing their current view of the issue. Next, you must implement the change and, finally, freeze the new process into place.

Current business literature abounds with books on the subject of leading change and managing change for large organizations. These publications offer a more comprehensive model from which to design project plans. The works of Kotter (1996) and Taylor (2006) are helpful to DNP graduates in administrative positions. These authors provide a useful approach to leading change and managing large projects effectively. A change theory that this section's author has found helpful is the model developed by Kotter (1996). John Kotter is a professor at the Harvard Business School and published *Leading Change* in 1996. His model consists of eight steps:

1. Establishing a sense of urgency
2. Creating a guiding coalition
3. Developing a vision and strategy
4. Communicating the change vision
5. Empowering employees for broad-based action
6. Generating short-term wins
7. Consolidating gains and producing more change
8. Anchoring new approaches in the culture

This model proved to be very useful in leading our nursing education department through several large projects. Establishing the sense of urgency required nurse managers, clinical nurse specialists, staff nurses, and preceptors to become engaged in each project. Nursing executive leadership must also become engaged to help build a guiding coalition for each project. Developing the vision and a strategy is best served by having a collaborative effort among those involved. Ultimately, creating the vision for the implementation of any project often becomes the sole responsibility of the administrator. Empowering the team to follow the plan and implement the change is motivated by this vision.

Communication is constant in any change project. Repeating, reinforcing, and reviewing messages previously delivered are necessary. Refining the process during implementation is critical to the ultimate success of all projects. This refining process merges into the next step, empowering employees for broad-based action.

One of the most difficult tasks of the project leader is relinquishing control over every element of the project. Letting others take ownership of the project and empowering them to help guide the decisions during implementation will serve the DNP-educated nurse leader well during the implementation phase of each project undertaken. Measuring and reporting short-term gains and consolidating those gains are motivational for those employees involved in the project and fuel their enthusiasm. Consolidating gains, producing more change, and ultimately anchoring the change into practice require continued vigilance.

Each model that a leader explores will have some areas of weakness. The one area in which Kotter's (1996) theory is weak is the evaluation phase of the program. Exploring program evaluation methods is a skill found in DNP programs. A review of the literature to find the right tool of evaluation for each project may be time consuming. Many projects undertaken by this section's author have been educational in nature, so alignment of these training projects with the Bersin (2008) model of training measurement and evaluation promotes consistency in how each project outcome is measured. Kotter's theory of change and Bersin's model of training measurement provide useful theoretical frameworks to guide projects in the real world, with real people to motivate and lead.

Leadership Style

Exploring leadership models is another skill that the DNP-prepared administrator gains in the course of study. Throughout this section author's academic career, leadership models have often been a part of the curriculum. The first leadership styles explored were limited to authoritarian, laissez-faire, or democratic (Cherry, 2011). As a staff nurse, this author often experienced the authoritarian style, which was frequently unsatisfying. Nurses experience the decisions of nursing leaders and other administrators daily. They often express the need to be involved in the making of these decisions. Authoritarian leadership styles are autocratic and do not involve other participants in making the decision. This style of leadership can be useful in emergency situations but is limited in relationship building and staff development of those who report to us.

The Magnet Recognition Program encourages more decision-making control by the staff who are served by administrators. Participative management is a form of democratic leadership. This style of leading has always held an attraction for this author. Democratic leaders will allow for group discussion of a problem and the selection of an acceptable solution. This participative leadership style promotes shared responsibility and greater involvement of those who are charged with implementation of the solution. We should not underestimate the importance of dialogue in the workplace. The ability of staff to openly share their concerns, offer ideas for resolving problems, and participate in both the discussion and the selection of resolutions empowers staff toward greater personal and professional satisfaction. This will ultimately result in improved patient outcomes and patient satisfaction.

In the past, when in an academic role as clinical faculty, the desire to intellectually stimulate students, mentor them toward the acquisition of knowledge and skills, and develop their abilities improved this author's leadership competencies. Developing a transformational and transactional leadership style, as suggested by Failla (2008), is a worthy professional goal for all administrators. This article effectively describes the importance of more contemporary leadership models. The five critical strategies of transformational leaders described by Failla (2008) are useful:

- Instill employee pride in the leader's vision and mission.
- Use leader behaviors to demonstrate the values and mission to employees.

- Increase staff awareness and acceptance of the desired mission.
- Intellectually stimulate employees and others to think in new ways.
- Individualize consideration by mentoring and expressing appreciation when the mission and related goals are accomplished.

A publication related to improving the nursing work environment, *Keeping Patients Safe: Transforming the Work Environment of Nurses* (IOM, 2003), supports transformational nursing leadership style for nursing leaders.

The accountabilities of leaders discussed in Stefl (2008) are "communication and relationship management, professionalism, leadership, knowledge of the healthcare system, and business skills and knowledge" (p. 360). Missing from this model are the skills needed to evaluate and improve the competency of followers. Holding others accountable and maintaining the clinical discipline required for the delivery of safe care is an important competency of managers in a healthcare environment. One area for skills growth among many administrators and managers is holding people accountable and motivating them to improved clinical performance. It is beneficial as an administrator to have strong values and high expectations of those you lead and those with whom you need to collaborate. Many times, communicating your expectations clearly leads to accomplishing these goals. Many employees have a strong desire to meet their manager's expectations and even to exceed them. However, if the goals are not clearly communicated, it is not unusual to be disappointed when one's team fails to meet expectations. Being a good coach by spending time with all employees to train them and facilitate their performance at the level expected is a valuable approach. However, it is also wise to understand that the learning curve is steeper for some, and this can create some tension for both the leader and the team.

Evidence-Based Management Practices

The DNP program prepares graduates to embrace evidence-based practice. An administrator also needs to adopt evidence-based management practices. This is accomplished through exploring the literature or delegating this task to those working on projects with the administrator. A review of executive summaries and formal literature reviews, as well as local programs and processes, provide the administrator with the clearest picture of the current situation. Discussions with the team regarding these findings and selection of the best management approaches to achieve the organization's goals can result in improved outcomes. It is not unusual for administrators to set goals that might not be achievable and then to try to force the team to achieve an unrealistic goal. This can be costly and should be avoided unless urgent situations require quick solutions.

Balancing the objectives of many healthcare disciplines can often challenge the administrator. Physicians' need for adequate bed capacity to provide for the care of patients in their specialty and those receiving specialized treatments can challenge the skills and abilities of the available nursing staff. Working in a collaborative manner with the physicians, educators, nurses, and specialists in other disciplines to promote the ability to meet the care needs of patients and to provide for the education that nurses or others need requires patience and commitment. Approaching these situations in a manner that does not address the educational needs of the nurses may result in less than optimal outcomes for patients.

Collaboration

One of the most important skills the DNP-prepared administrator needs is that of collaboration. In its simplest form, collaboration "implies collective action toward a common goal in a spirit of trust and harmony" (D'Amour,

Ferrada-Videla, San Martin-Rodriquez, & Beaulieu, 2005, p. 116). Working well in teams to achieve the goals of the organization requires this level of collaboration. In the experience of this administrator, barriers to achieving good collaborative relationships can be work-related boundary concerns ("it's not my job") and competition. Healthcare reform requires healthy work relationships that use limited resources to provide the best care possible. Working together in healthy teams that put the patient and organizational goals ahead of our own serves us in reducing costs, managing limited resources, and reforming in an efficient and effective manner. Deliberate collaboration can strengthen colleagues of the same discipline and interdisciplinary teams. This approach can lead to improved patient safety and staff satisfaction.

Conclusion

DNP preparation provides an opportunity to explore leadership theories, project management and evaluation techniques, evidence-based practices, and change theories. Lifelong learning and exploring the literature to improve leadership skills must be embraced. The challenge for the administrator is to integrate this academic preparation and lifelong learning into practice to promote innovative approaches to problems in our highly complex healthcare environments. Thinking outside the box, exploring technologies that allow for more efficiency, and embracing new ideas while consistently paying attention to patient safety, patient and staff satisfaction, and cost promote both better patient care and the role of DNP-prepared administrators.

PUBLIC HEALTH NURSE

Carol Flaten
Jeanne Pfeiffer

Dramatic effects on the health of populations have been the work of public health nurses (PHNs) who consider population-level assessment, intervention, and evaluation to influence the health of the communities they serve. This work has improved the quality and quantity of life of individuals and communities. In the 20th century, life expectancy increased from 47.3 years in 1900 to 77.8 years in 2000 (National Center for Health Statistics, 2010). The 10 great public health achievements of the 20th century (Centers for Disease Control and Prevention, 2011) can be credited with this dramatic change in life expectancy. These 10 achievements are (1) immunizations, (2) motor vehicle safety, (3) workplace safety, (4) control of infectious disease, (5) decline in deaths from heart disease and stroke, (6) safer and healthier foods, (7) healthier mothers and babies, (8) family planning, (9) fluoridation of water, and (10) tobacco as a health hazard. PHNs have played a part in all these areas. DNP-prepared PHNs bring a depth of knowledge and an advanced skill set to the healthcare arena, which is becoming ever more complex. These nurses focus their practice and expertise at the community and systems levels. The DNP-prepared PHN is pivotal in this multifaceted, interprofessional work to protect and promote health and prevent disease and disability in our communities. An intervention at the community or system level has the potential to affect the larger community as demonstrated by the 10 great public health achievements of the 20th century.

Public Health Nurse: A Definition

Public health nursing practice is grounded in knowledge from nursing and social and public health sciences. PHN practice is focused on the health of populations rather than the specific health needs of individuals. PHNs are involved in interventions that promote health, prevent disease and disability, and create conditions in which all people can be healthy (Quad Council of Public Health Nursing Organizations, 2005; Stanhope & Lancaster, 2012). According to the American Public Health Association's (1996) definition, a public health nurse has "preparation in public health and nursing science with a primary focus on population-level outcomes" (p. 2). The population may be based on geographical boundaries or characteristics of interest—such as elderly adults or children receiving cancer treatment—or a combination of the two. The underlying ethical principle of public health nursing practice is the theory of utilitarianism, which states, "the greatest good for the greatest number" (Bayer, Gostin, Jennings, & Steinbock, 2007). In addition, the concept of social justice is considered a foundation of public health nursing (Stanhope & Lancaster, 2012).

The terms *community health nursing* and *public health nursing* have historically caused confusion. *Community based* tends to focus on nursing care of individuals and families in the community, typically managing acute or chronic conditions in the community. The terms *community health nurse* and *public health nurse* have been used interchangeably. In this discussion, the term *public health nurse* is used. The primary focus of care is on the population, with the goal of preventing disease and promoting health (Stanhope & Lancaster, 2012).

The IOM (1988) published a report that defined public health as "what we, as a society, do collectively to assure the conditions in which people can be healthy" (p. 1). This definition demonstrates the broad scope of practice and interdisciplinary nature of public health work, within which PHNs play an important role based on scientific principles of public health and public health nursing. Along with these central definitions, the PHN is also a master at developing and maintaining relationships with individuals, communities, and systems. The ability to establish and maintain caring relationships is one of the cornerstones of public health nursing identified by the Minnesota Department of Health (2007).

History of Public Health Nursing

Many nursing leaders have influenced the practice of public health nursing. Florence Nightingale (1820–1910) improved health outcomes of soldiers in Europe during the Crimean War by being aware of environmental conditions that affected health and using basic principles of epidemiology to document outcomes such as mortality rate (Nightingale, 1859/1946). Epidemiology is a foundational science for public health nursing. This notion of population-based nursing and systematically collecting data to inform practice was revolutionary for the time and provided nursing with another dimension to assess the health of a population.

The life and work of Lillian Wald (1867–1940) carried the concept of population-based nursing even further in the late 1800s in the United States. Wald is credited with coining the term *public health nursing*. Wald's impact on nursing and the community in which she practiced was revolutionary for the time. Wald noticed the impoverished conditions and lack of basic necessities among the residents on the Lower East Side of New York City. After seeing firsthand the poor living and health conditions of recent immigrants and their families, Wald, along with several colleagues, established the Visiting Nurse Service. The Visiting Nurse Service provided the beginning model for PHNs interacting with families in their homes and communities. The Henry Street Settlement, which followed a short time later, provided a variety of services to this population. It is important to note that Wald believed in meeting the individual in the home or on the street and emphasized the importance of the environment surrounding the individual. However, it was Wald's capacity to notice and act on behalf of individuals and families at the community and system levels, as well as at the individual level, that has left a legacy of work that many still attempt to achieve today. Wald was very effective as a community organizer, advocate, and leader and effected dramatic changes in the quality of life in the community. In public health nursing, a single intervention at the community or systems level has the potential to affect large numbers of individuals (Jewish Women's Archive, n.d.).

At the population level, Wald's work provides a variety of examples of population-based public health nursing interventions, including (1) developing safe playground spaces for neighborhood children; (2) advocating for the role of school nurses to ensure that children had adequate nutrition and health care; (3) advocating for decent working conditions for women; (4) partnering with the Metropolitan Life Insurance Company to provide health care to policy holders; (5) advocating for safe industrial working conditions; (6) campaigning for the first federal Children's Bureau to abolish child labor; (7) promoting children's health; and (8) supporting children who had dropped out of school. All these examples addressed individual needs, yet the interventions were aimed at the systems level or at the community level to affect programs and develop policy. The entire population benefited from these interventions ultimately aimed at improving the lives of individuals. These accomplishments at the state and federal levels were all made before women had a voice through voting in the United States. Lillian Wald was a reformer of her day who has greatly influenced public health nursing as it is practiced today (Jewish Women's Archive, n.d.).

Foundational Principles of Public Health Nursing

In light of the preceding definition and examples of public health and public health nursing, the core functions of the PHN practice are assessment, policy development, and assurance, along with the 10 essential services of public health (Public Health Functions Steering Committee, 1998). This is illustrated in **Figure 4-1**.

The three core functions that drive public health nursing practice are (IOM, 1988; Stanhope & Lancaster, 2012, p. 7):

Assessment: Systematically collecting data on the population, monitoring the population's health status, and making information available about the health of the community.

Policy development: The need to provide leadership in developing policies that support the health of the population, including the use of the scientific knowledge base in making decisions about policy.

Assurance: The role of the public health nurse in ensuring that essential community-oriented health services are available, which may include providing essential personal health services for those who would not otherwise receive them. Assurance also refers to making sure that a competent public health and personal healthcare workforce is available.

Specific to public health nursing practice, the *intervention wheel* is a model that identifies specific PHN interventions that support the work toward these core functions and 10 essential services (Keller & Strohschein, 2012).

Public Health Nursing National Organizational Framework

The Quad Council of Public Health Nursing is the overarching entity that includes four national nursing organizations that address public health nursing issues: the Association of Community Health Nurse Educators (ACHNE), the American Nurses Association's (ANA's) Congress on Nursing Practice and Economics, the American Public Health Association (APHA) Public Health Nursing Section, and the Association of State and Territorial Directors of Nursing (ASTDN). The purpose of the Quad Council is to promote and stimulate collaboration among the member groups. The Quad Council also includes public health nurse experts who advance the work of public health nursing practice and education at the national level. The Quad Council posted a document, "Quad Council

| FIGURE 4-1 | Action model to achieve Healthy People 2020's overarching goals. |

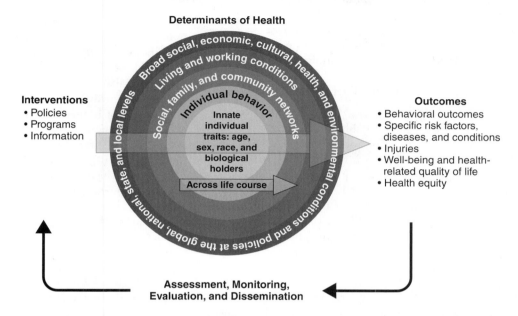

Determinants of Health

Interventions
• Policies
• Programs
• Information

Broad social, economic, cultural, health, and environmental conditions and policies at the global, national, state, and local levels

Living and working conditions

Social, family, and community networks

Individual behavior

Innate
individual
traits: age,
sex, race, and
biological
holders

Across life course

Outcomes
• Behavioral outcomes
• Specific risk factors, diseases, and conditions
• Injuries
• Well-being and health-related quality of life
• Health equity

Assessment, Monitoring, Evaluation, and Dissemination

Source: U.S. Department of Health and Human Services, Secretary's Advisory Committee on Health Promotion and Disease Prevention Objectives for 2010. (2008). *Phase I report: Recommendations for the framework and format of Healthy People 2020* (p. 8). Retrieved from http://healthypeople.gov/2020/about/advisory/PhaseI.pdf

PHN Competencies," in April 2003 that distinguishes between characteristics of the "generalist/staff PHN" and the PHN in a manager/specialist/consultant role. These competencies were intended to be a guide for practice and academic settings in order to facilitate the education of the PHN. The competencies were grouped in eight domains (Quad Council of Public Health Nursing Organizations, 2009):

1. Analytic assessment skills

2. Policy development and program planning skills

3. Communication skills

4. Cultural competency skills

5. Community dimensions of practice

6. Basic public health sciences

7. Financial planning and management skills

8. Leadership and systems thinking skills

At the advanced level of practice, for the most part the PHN is expected to be "proficient" (rather than knowledgeable or aware) in each of the domains. Each domain has specific criteria listed. The AACN supports doctoral education for community/public health nursing. This is noted in Essential VII of doctoral education (AACN, 2006). The Quad Council Competencies and the AACN document complement each other. Both documents recognize the advanced level of practice that is needed in the PHN role and the complexities that this role embraces. Doctoral education is imperative to meet these components of PHN practice in the context of an ever-changing healthcare environment and the demands that the PHN seek doctoral education to practice to the fullest extent of his or her ability and license (Quad Council of Public Health Nursing Organizations, 2009).

National Public Health Performance Standards Program

The office of the Chief of Public Health Practice, Centers for Disease Control and Prevention (CDC), has led a partnership with national public health organizations to develop a program to "improve the practice of public health, the performance of public health systems, and the infrastructure supporting public health actions" (CDC, n.d.). These performance standards are key components of an accreditation process for governmental public health agencies similar to that used in acute care settings. The accreditation process is currently being carried out by the Public Health Accreditation Board (PHAB), and state and local boards of health are in the process of submitting applications (PHAB, 2011).

As the practice of public health moves toward standards for accreditation, the PHN must be educated at an appropriate level and be able to practice in an environment with high expectations to serve the population in an era of growing concern aimed at population-level assessment, interventions, and outcome measures. There is a need for DNP-prepared PHNs to fill roles in this type of environment. The vision, mission, and goals put forth by the National Public Health Performance Standards Program align with the education and practice of a PHN with a DNP degree. This initiative indicates the high standards expected of public health practitioners. The convergence of the PHAB accreditation standards and the emergence of DNP-prepared PHNs speak to the importance of the level of education needed for PHNs to provide leadership and to guide public health nursing practice.

Theoretical Framework for Nursing Practice in Public Health

There are multiple issues to consider in providing good quality care to populations. A strategy that encompasses the multifaceted nature of public health work is the ecological approach (Stanhope & Lancaster, 2012). As noted in the example of Wald's work, multiple factors affect the health of individuals and populations. These multiple factors are termed "determinants of health" and include (1) health, social, economic, cultural, and environmental conditions; (2) family, social, and living conditions; and (3) individual traits and biological factors. The linkages among all these factors are important to consider as interventions are developed to affect the health of populations. The ecological model provides a structure that incorporates these linkages (Quad Council of Public Health Nursing Organizations, 2009).

The diagram in **Figure 4-2** incorporates the ecological approach at the center. This approach illustrates how the goals of the action model for the *Healthy People 2020* initiative converge with the work of PHNs (U.S. Department of Health and Human Services, Secretary's Advisory Committee on National Health Promotion and Disease Prevention Objectives for 2020, 2008).

Two initiatives, one at the global level and one at the national level, highlight these concepts as PHNs work in population-based programs that incorporate the principles of the ecological approach. The Millennium Development Goals (MDGs) were established in 2002 by the Millennium Project commissioned by the United Nations Secretary-General. The charge of this project was to develop a concrete action plan to "reverse the grinding poverty, hunger, and disease affecting billions of people" (United Nations, 2002). There are eight MDGs, which range from reducing extreme poverty by 50% to enhancing environmental stability. All eight goals are associated with the determinants of health described earlier and operationalize the

| **FIGURE 4-2** | *Healthy People 2020* **Vision and Mission Statements.** |

> **Vision**
> A society in which all people live long, healthy lives.
> **Mission**
> To improve health through strengthening policy and practice, Healthy People will:
> • Identify nationwide health improvement priorities;
> • Increase public awareness and understanding of the determinants of health, disease, and disability and the opportunities for progress;
> • Provide measurable objectives and goals that can be used at the national, state, and local levels;
> • Engage multiple sectors to take actions that are driven by the best available evidence and knowledge; and
> • Identify critical research and data collection needs.

Source: U.S. Department of Health and Human Services. Office of Disease Prevention and Health Promotion. Healthy People 2020. Washington, DC. Available at https://www.healthypeople.gov /sites/default/files/Phase1_0.pdf. Accessed December 15th, 2014.

definitions of public health and public health nursing.

On a national level in the United States, the Healthy People initiative has driven public health programs and awareness over the past 40 years. There have been four previous initiatives, in 1979, 1990, 2000, and 2010. *Healthy People 2020* provides goals and objectives to guide national health promotion and disease prevention strategies to improve the health of all people over the next decade. The overarching goals of this initiative for 2020 are to (U.S. Department of Health and Human Services, Secretary's Advisory Committee on National Health Promotion and Disease Prevention Objectives for 2020, 2008):

1. Attain high-quality, longer lives, free from preventable disease, disability, injury, and premature death

2. Achieve health equity, eliminate disparities, and improve the health of all groups

3. Create social and physical environments that promote good health for all

4. Promote quality of life, healthy development, and healthy behaviors across all life stages

Educational Preparation and Credentialing

In today's nursing education environment, baccalaureate programs that prepare beginning practitioners typically include public health nursing content, theory, and clinical practice. This allows the new nurse to practice as a beginning-staff-level PHN. This is similar to the new graduate beginning a medical-surgical position in an acute care setting. Additional orientation time is likely required as the new graduate transitions from the student role to practice. Some states (e.g., Minnesota, California) also have PHN certification for baccalaureate graduates who apply to the state board of nursing. This certification acknowledges the PHN content in the curriculum and allows the individual to use the PHN credentials with his or her title.

Specializing in public health nursing requires an advanced degree. Currently, a master's degree in nursing is required to sit for a certification exam administered by the ANCC (2012). In the future, it is likely that the DNP will be the required prerequisite for taking this certification exam. The 1984 Consensus Conference on the Essentials of Public Health Nursing Practice and Education sponsored by the U.S. Department of Health and Human Services Division of Nursing identified that minimal qualifications for a PHN include a baccalaureate degree in nursing. Specialists in the field hold either a master's or doctorate degree that focuses on public health sciences, and they have the ability to work with populations to assess and intervene at the aggregate level (U.S. Department of Health and Human Services, Health Resources and Services Administration, Bureau of Health Professionals, Division of Nursing, 1984). ACHNE has affirmed this position, and the ANA has also supported this position in *Public Health Nursing: Scope and Standards of Practice* (ANA, 2007; Quad Council of Public Health Nursing Organizations, 2007).

Roles of Advanced Practice PHNs

The roles of advanced practice public and community health nurses have evolved over time. States have the authority to determine the scope of practice of a PHN. For instance, in Virginia, PHN roles reflect the essential elements of the National Association of County Health Officials contained within the *Blueprint for a Healthy Community*. The nine essential elements are (1) conducting community assessments; (2) preventing and controlling epidemics; (3) providing a safe

and healthy environment; (4) measuring performance, effectiveness, and outcome of health services; (5) promoting healthy lifestyles; (6) providing targeted outreach and forming partnerships; (7) providing personal healthcare services; (8) conducting research and innovation; and (9) mobilizing the community for action. Within each of these essential elements, PHNs contribute their expertise and leadership to develop programs to promote health and prevent disease; tools to standardize case definitions, data collection, and analysis; indicators to monitor the health status of the population; regulatory guidelines for the prevention of targeted diseases; community partnerships and resources to promote informed decision making for the health of citizens; direct services for patients for targeted diseases that threaten the health of a community; leadership and advocacy strategies through collaboration, coalition building, and public relations; and healthy community research projects with measurable outcomes (National Association of County Health Officials, 1994).

PHNs with expertise in the field have traditionally been promoted to lead agency-related, population-based health programs as funding is allocated to administer and implement them. PHNs who take on administrative responsibilities write program proposals and testify for the support of these programs at federal and state legislative committees and jurisdictional board meetings. Programs routinely led by PHNs include immunizations; family, maternal, and child health; disease prevention and control; family planning; health promotion; emergency preparedness; school health; senior services; home care refugee health; healthcare services; children with disabilities; women, infants, and children (WIC); chronic disease; adults with disabilities; and environmental health (Association of State and Territorial Directors of Nursing, 2008). Furthermore, advanced practice PHNs who work in the public policy and advocacy arenas serve as executive nurse leaders at departments of health in each state to represent nursing issues within the health department; to ensure effectiveness, efficiency, and quality of programs and services delivered; and to ensure that there is a workforce prepared for the nursing needs of the state, and they collaborate with educational systems to ensure the quality of the future public health nursing workforce (Association of State and Territorial Directors of Nursing, Centers for Disease Control and Prevention, & Partners' Cooperative Agreement, 2009). The roles of advanced practice PHNs, who will benefit from the DNP preparation, continue to develop as the complexity of health care increases in proportion to the growth of the population, particularly in relation to the rate of growth of the senior citizen population in the United States.

Practice Sites

PHNs commonly enter practice within a local public health agency that may be governed by a city or county. Proficient public health nursing leaders discover satisfying careers in diverse practice settings. PHNs with expertise in the field are employed at jurisdictional levels that encompass federal, state, regional, county, and city public health agencies. The federal employer may be the U.S. Public Health Service, the Centers for Disease Control and Prevention, or the American Public Health Association. Advanced PHN expertise is critical to the planning, piloting, and implementation of evidence-based population health programs initiated at the state or federal jurisdiction level. DNP-prepared PHNs support these leaders with the needed skill sets to perform in the complex socioeconomic environment of health promotion and disease prevention in this country. Advanced practice PHNs are employed in academic settings to teach, direct programs, and conduct research. They also work in acute and long-term care systems to manage population-based infection prevention, safety, quality improvement, occupational health, and emergency

preparedness programs (Stanhope & Lancaster, 2012). Within the last decade, PHNs have been hired by health systems that provide a continuum of care to their chronically ill or rehabilitating patients in the community to direct hospice, home care, palliative care, complex medical care, and advanced care directive programs. Insurance companies have also benefited from the skills of DNP-prepared PHNs (Stanhope & Lancaster, 2012). These health-integrated organizations are complex, and their operations (Melnyk & Fineout-Overholt, 2011) need to be informed by practice-based evidence related to client outcomes within each specialty program. The DNP-prepared PHN has the academic preparation to address these growing multifaceted demands in the marketplace.

Evidenced-Based Practice in Population-Based Public Health Nursing

Evidence-based practice (EBP) was introduced into medicine initially to guide professionals' decision making using the best available evidence (Guyatt & Rennie, 2002). Sackett, Straus, and Richardson (2000) later developed the definition for evidence-based medicine that has become an industry standard. This approach seeks to answer a clinical question about an individual patient condition (Guyatt & Rennie, 2002; Sackett et al., 2000). EBP was a seven-step process initiated to make an accurate diagnosis and to prescribe the most appropriate treatment or outcome.

When nursing began implementing EBP, the concentration tended to be related to a collection of patients (Leven, Keefe, & Marren, 2010; Melnyk & Fineout-Overholt, 2011). The application of EBP started in acute care and primary care. There is little in the literature about its application to community settings. Examples of EBP that surface in public health nursing when the literature is searched include (1) the Family Nurse Partnership program, which is designed to help teen mothers make healthy life choices, complete their education, and space future pregnancies (Olds et al., 1997); (2) public health nursing interventions with individuals, families, and the community, and the systems that affect them as modeled by the public health "wheel" (Keller & Strohschein, 2012); (3) survey of the tasks performed and frequencies by PHN participants from local and state health departments in the United States (Association of State and Territorial Directors of Nursing, 2008); (4) mining aggregate electronic data in the public health record for health outcomes to inform practice (Monsen, 2005); and (5) public health nursing competencies as developed by the Quad Council of Public Health Nursing Associations (Quad Council of Public Health Nursing Organizations, 2009). These examples are instrumental in guiding and informing practice, and they form the basis for further PHN research. PHN-initiated research has traditionally been funded by government agencies, such as the National Institutes of Health and the Health Resources and Services Administration, and private foundations, including the Robert Wood Johnson Foundation and the Bill and Melinda Gates Foundation.

The Doctor of Nursing Practice–Prepared Public Health Nurse as Leader

The Association of Community Health Educators (formerly the Association of Graduate Faculty in Community Health Nursing/Public Health Nursing), established in 1978, has promoted the increase in graduate-level programs to prepare the public health nursing leaders of the future. In addition to holding traditional responsibilities, PHNs are assuming high-functioning roles in the complex planning and implementation of health promotion and maintenance programs in the community.

The skill sets that DNP-prepared nurses bring to the multiagency planning groups involve knowledge about EBP related to population health programs, the science of nursing

intervention, policy development, financial astuteness, informatics, patient-centered care, quality improvement, safety, and interprofessional teamwork and collaboration. DNP-prepared public health leaders will be influenced daily by information generated by professional associations and government and nongovernment agencies. These leaders are expected to access and evaluate this information in relation to its role in advocacy for population-based health programs. DNP-prepared nurses advocate for population health initiatives in writing, in public testimony, and within interdepartmental and interagency planning groups. PHN nurses are customarily respected in the community by the clients they serve, but a DNP-prepared PHN is better equipped to articulate strategic population health positions effectively with nonnursing professionals, policy planners, and legislative bodies. The public recognizes the nurse as a trusted professional who is now publicly advocating with confidence for the health of the nation.

INTEGRATIVE PRACTITIONER

Joy Elwell
Kathryn Waud White

Integrative health care is growing as a choice for Americans. The CDC's National Health Statistics Report *Complementary and Alternative Medicine Use Among Adults and Children* (Barnes, Bloom, & Nahin, 2007) revealed that 38% of American adults and 12% of children use alternative or complementary therapies of some type. Integrative health care is just that: the integration of the best concepts of traditional medicine with the best concepts of alternative therapies (Center for Spirituality and Healing, 2008). The skills gained in the DNP program will enhance the practice of the APN in integrative therapy. Essential III states that the DNP program prepares APNs to "critically appraise existing literature and other evidence to implement the best evidence for practice" (AACN, 2006). Essential VI speaks to interprofessional collaboration, which is truly an essential for the practice of this specialty that reaches across so many different healthcare fields (AACN, 2006). Essential VII describes clinical prevention and population health, all facilitated through integrative health care (AACN, 2006). The DNP-prepared integrative health practitioner has much to offer patients.

To address the DNP-prepared APN as an integrative practitioner, it is essential to explore integrative health as a specialty within health care. Integrative health, also known as holistic health, is described as "treating the whole person, helping the person to bring the mental, emotional, physical, social, and spiritual dimensions of his or her being into greater harmony, using the basic principles and elements of holistic healing and, as much as possible, placing reliance on treatment modalities that foster the self regenerative and self reparatory processes of natural healing" (Otto & Knight, 1979, p. 3). Nursing's approach to wellness from a holistic perspective makes nursing and integrative health perfect partners for the APN.

Nurses as Integrative Practitioners

Florence Nightingale may be considered one of the first professional integrative health practitioners in nursing. Nightingale "was a mystic, visionary, healer, reformer, environmentalist, feminist, practitioner, scientist, politician and global citizen" (Dossey, Selanders, Beck, & Attewell, 2005). She looked beyond the era's traditional medical and surgical treatment of disease and injury to include nutrition, sanitation, lighting, and activity. She addressed the mind, body, and spirit connection and paved the way for modern professional integrative practitioners.

Since Nightingale's death in 1910, professional nursing has evolved in numerous ways, including the development of advanced practice nursing roles. Numerous nursing pioneers have explored integrative modalities to assist clients in achieving optimum levels of wellness, alleviating suffering, and facilitating healing.

Founded in 1980, the American Holistic Nurses Association (AHNA) focuses on holistic nursing as "all nursing practice that has healing the whole person as its goal" (AHNA, n.d.). That nurses practice integrative health is not a novel concept. Major nursing theorists incorporate holism into their theories. Dr. Jean Watson's Theory of Human Caring is one example. She identifies caring beliefs and behaviors that benefit not only the client but the nurse as well.

New York University established the first holistic nurse practitioner (NP) program, and others have followed. Within the United States, certain states (e.g., New York) identify holistic health as a specialty (New York State Education Department, Office of the Professions, 2014). There are also clinical nurse specialists in integrative health. The ANA now recognizes holistic nursing as a specialty, and certification can be obtained through the American Holistic Nurses' Credentialing Corporation (AHNCC, 2012). In addition, the American Holistic Nurses Association (AHNA) has articulated standards of practice, core values, a certification curriculum, and requirements for endorsement of holistic nursing programs. A current listing of nursing programs endorsed by the AHNCC can be found at http://ahncc .org/home/endorsedschools.html.

Nurses can pursue educational programs for integrative or holistic modalities at all levels of postlicensure preparation. Certification through the AHNCC reflects the level of academic study in the board certification test administered and the credential conferred on the successful applicant. The general requirements for certification include active practice as a holistic nurse for 1 year (full time) or 2,000 hours in the past 5 years (part time) and 48 contact hours of continuing education in holistic nursing over the preceding 2 years (AHNCC, 2012). Registered nurses who meet the general criteria and who hold a diploma or associate's degree preparation may sit for the Holistic Nurse Board Certification (HN-BC). Those with a baccalaureate degree preparation may sit for the Holistic Baccalaureate Nurse Board Certification (HBN-BC), and those who hold a master's or doctoral degree may sit for the Advanced Holistic Nurse Board Certification (AHN-BC) (AHNCC, 2012). Certain roles within the realm of integrative practitioners, such as chiropractors, acupuncturists, and massage therapists, are licensed and have educational requirements. Nurses who pursue these roles must fulfill those requirements in addition to any nursing curriculum.

Types of Integrative Healing Modalities

Integrative health care includes many healing modalities. There are five different approaches to care as organized by the National Center for Complementary and Alternative Medicine (NCCAM): whole medical systems, manipulative and body-based practices, mind–body medicine, biologically based practices, and energy medicine (NCCAM, 2007). The modalities described here are not intended to be an exhaustive list of every integrative healing modality known. **Table 4-1** lists websites where further information can be found.

Whole Medical Systems

- *Homeopathy:* A medical discipline that facilitates healing through the administration of substances prescribed according to three principles: (1) like cures like, also known as the "law of similars"; (2) the more a remedy is diluted, the greater the potency; and (3) illness is specific to the individual. Homeopathy is based on the belief that symptoms are signs of the body's effort to get rid of disease; treatment is based on the whole person rather than on the symptoms (NCCAM, 2012).

- *Osteopathic medicine:* A form of medicine focusing on the relationship between the structure of the body and its function, identifying that both structure and function are subject to a range of illnesses. In treating the client, osteopathic practitioners use various types of physical manipulation to stimulate the body's self-healing ability, as well as traditional allopathic medical modalities. Osteopathic physicians are licensed to diagnose, treat, and prescribe nationally.

TABLE 4-1	Websites for Further Information on Integrative Health

American Holistic Nurses' Certification Corporation

    http://www.ahncc.org

Center for Spirituality and Healing at the University of Minnesota

    http://www.csh.umn.edu

Life Science Foundation

    http://www.lifesciencefoundation.org/abmain.html

National Center for Complementary and Alternative Medicine (NCCAM)

    http://nccam.nih.gov/sites/nccam.nih.gov/files/d347_05-25-2012.pdf

University of Michigan, Doctor of Nursing Practice Program

    http://nursing.umich.edu/admissions/application-information/requirements
    /doctor-nursing-practice-program

Manipulative Modalities

- *Acupressure:* Pressure by fingers and hands over specific areas of the body, is used to alleviate pain and discomfort and to positively influence the function of internal organs and body systems. Various approaches are used to release tension and restore the natural flow of energy in the body.

- *Acupuncture:* Use of fine-gauged needles inserted into specific points on the body to stimulate or disperse the flow of energy. This ancient Eastern technique is used to alleviate pain or increase immunity by balancing energy flow. Massage, herbal medicine, and nutritional counseling are often used in conjunction with acupuncture.

- *Alexander technique:* This technique, developed by Australian actor Frederick Matthias Alexander, involves learning a series of lessons in rebalancing the body through awareness, movement, and touch. As the student explores new ways of reorganizing neuromuscular function, the body is reintroduced to healthy posture and direct, efficient movement (Trivieri & Anderson, 2002).

- *AMMA therapy:* AMMA therapy is a form of Eastern massage that focuses on the balance and movement of energy within the body.

- *Applied kinesiology:* Originated by chiropractic physician George Goodheart Jr. in the 1960s, applied kinesiology incorporates the principles of a number of holistic therapies, "including chiropractic, osteopathic medicine and acupuncture, and involves manual manipulation of the spine, extremities, and cranial bones in performing its procedures" (Trivieri & Anderson, 2002, p. 71).

- *Aromatherapy:* Aromatherapy incorporates the use of essential oils extracted from plants and herbs to treat physical imbalances and to achieve psychological and spiritual well-being. The oils are inhaled, applied externally, or ingested. According to

Dr. Kurt Schnaubelt, "The chemical makeup of essential oils gives them a host of desirable pharmacological properties, ranging from antibacterial, antiviral, and antispasmodic, to uses as diuretics, vasodilators, and vasoconstrictors. Essential oils also act on the adrenals, ovaries, and thyroid, and can energize, pacify or detoxify, and facilitate the digestive process" (Trivieri & Anderson, 2002, p. 76).

- *Breema bodywork:* Breema bodywork incorporates simple, playful bodywork sequences along with stretch and movement exercises that help create greater flexibility, a relaxed body, a clear mind, and calm, supportive feelings. Developed by chiropractic physician Jon Schraiber, Breema bodywork is based on nine principles: body comfortable, no extra, firmness and gentleness, full participation, mutual support, no judgment, single moment/single activity, no hurry/no pause, and no force (Mann, 2009).

- *Chiropractic medicine:* A healthcare system emphasizing structural alignment of the spine. Adjustments involve the manipulation of the spine and joints to reestablish and maintain normal nervous system functioning. Some chiropractors employ additional therapies, such as massage, nutrition, and specialized kinesiology.

- *Cranial osteopathy:* Gentle and almost imperceptible manipulation of the skull to reestablish its natural configuration and movement. Such correction can have a positive influence on disorders manifested throughout the body.

- *Craniosacral therapy:* Diagnosis and treatment of imbalances in the craniosacral system. Subtle adjustments are made to the system through light touch and gentle manipulations.

- *Dance therapy:* Dance therapy is a modality in which dance and music combine to allow the body, mind, soul, and spirit to be refreshed and uplifted and to experience the freedom that natural bodily movement allows.

- *Feldenkrais method:* The Feldenkrais method is a method of instruction, through movement and gentle manipulation, to enhance self-image and restore mobility. Students are taught to notice how they are using their bodies and how to improve their posture and move more freely.
- *Jin shin jyutsu:* This is a bodywork technique that balances body energy as it travels along specific pathways. Specific combinations of healing points are held with the fingertips to restore balance and harmony.
- *Lymphatic therapy:* Lymphatic therapy is a vigorous form of massage that helps the body release toxins stored in the lymphatic system—excellent for the immune system and rebuilding the body.
- *Massage:* Massage involves the use of strokes and pressure on the body to dispel tension, increase circulation, and relieve muscular pain. Massage can provide comfort and increased body awareness and can facilitate the release of emotional as well as bodily tension.
- *Movement therapy:* This modality involves a guided series of movements and body work to open energy pathways and facilitate healing.
- *Neuromuscular therapy:* Neuromuscular therapy is a massage therapy in which moderate pressure over muscles and nerves, as well as on trigger points, is used to decrease pain and tension.
- *Physical therapy:* Physical therapy includes the treatment of physical conditions of body malfunction, damage, or injury using procedures designed to reduce swelling, relieve pain, strengthen muscles, restore range of motion, and return functioning to the patient.
- *Shiatsu:* Shiatsu is an energy-based system of bodywork using a firm sequence of rhythmic pressure held on specific pressure points on the body, designed to awaken acupressure meridians.
- *Trigger point therapy:* This is a method of compression of sensitive points in the muscle tissue, along with massage and passive stretches, for the relief of pain and tension. Treatment decreases swelling and stiffness and increases range of motion. Exercises may be assigned.

Mind–Body Medicine

- *Art therapy:* Art therapy incorporates the use of basic art materials to discover how to restore, maintain, or improve physical and mental health. Through observation and analysis, the art therapist is able to formulate treatment plans specific to the individual.
- *Color therapy:* Color therapy involves the use of electronic instrumentation and color receptivity, according to the work of Jacob Lieberman (1993), to integrate the nervous system and body–mind. It increases well-being and can be helpful for many acute and chronic ailments.
- *Counseling/psychotherapy:* A broad category of therapies that treat individuals as a whole. Treatments and sessions are focused on integrated care on all levels, for individuals, families, or groups.
- *Eye movement desensitization and reprocessing (EMDR):* EMDR is an accelerated information-processing method using alternating stimuli—either eye movements or sounds—to desensitize and reprocess emotional wounds and install a healthier belief system. EMDR is effective with posttraumatic stress syndrome, childhood trauma, depression, addictions, compulsions, unhealthy patterns, and future-oriented solutions.
- *Guided imagery:* A holistic modality that assists clients in connecting with their inner knowledge at the thinking, feeling, and

sensing levels, thus promoting their innate healing abilities. Together, guide and client co-create an effective way to work with pain, symptoms, grief, and stress management; conflict resolution; and self-empowerment issues; and to prepare for medical or surgical interventions.

- *Hypnotherapy:* A state of focused attention, achieved through guided relaxation, hypnotherapy is used to access the unconscious mind. Hypnosis is used for memory recall, medical treatment, and skill enhancement or personal growth.

- *Interactive imagery:* Fostering active participation, disease prevention, and health promotion, interactive imagery returns the focus of wellness to the individual.

- *Meditation:* A method of relaxing and quieting the mind to relieve muscle tension and facilitate inner peace. There are numerous forms of meditation, taught individually or in group settings, and it is thought that prayer for the self might have an effect similar to meditation. The nonsectarian form of prayer, which is akin to meditation and used for stress reduction, has long been recognized by clinicians to improve one's sense of well-being.

- *Music therapy:* An expressive art form designed to help the individual move into harmony and balance. Through the use of music, individuals explore emotional, spiritual, and behavioral issues. Musical skill is not necessary because the process, rather than technique, is emphasized.

- *Neurolinguistic programming:* A systematic approach to changing behavior through changing patterns of thinking. Its originators, Dilts, Grinder, Delozier, and Bandler (1980), proposed theoretical connections between neurological processes (neuro), language (linguistic), and behavioral patterns that have been learned through experience (programming), which can be organized to achieve specific goals in life.

- *Stress management:* Any therapy or educational practice with the objective of decreasing stress and enhancing one's response to the elements of life that cannot be changed. This broad category may include bodywork, energy work, visualization, and counseling.

- *Tai chi (chuan):* A movement practice and Chinese martial art that enhances coordination, balance, and breathing and that promotes physical, emotional, and spiritual well-being. Tai chi is taught in classes or as private lessons and requires home practice to be effective.

- *Yoga therapy:* The use of yoga postures, controlled breathing, relaxation, meditation, and nutrition facilitates the release of muscular and emotional tension, improves concentration, increases oxygen levels in the blood, and assists the body in healing itself.

Biologically Based Practices

- *Biofeedback:* A relaxation technique involving careful monitoring of vital functions (such as breathing, heart rate, and blood pressure) to improve health. By conscious thought, visualization, movement, or relaxation, one can learn which actions result in desirable changes in these vital functions. Biofeedback is used for medical problems related to stress and for management of many health problems, including pain syndrome, migraine, and irritable bowel syndrome.

- *Herbal therapy:* The use of herbs and their chemical properties to alleviate specific conditions or to support the function of various body systems. Herbal formulas have three basic functions: elimination and detoxification, health management and maintenance, and health building. The scope of herbal medicine is sometimes extended to include fungal and bee products, as well as minerals, shells, and certain animal parts (Acharya & Shrivastava, 2008).

- *Hydrotherapy:* The use of water, ice, steam, and hot and cold temperatures to relieve pain, fever, and inflammation and to maintain and restore health. Treatments include full-body immersion, steam baths, saunas, and the application of hot or cold compresses.

- *Nutritional counseling:* Nutritional counseling is performed by a practitioner who uses diet and supplementation therapeutically as the primary or adjunctive treatment for illness and for maintaining good health. Nutritionists employ a variety of approaches, including food combining, macrobiotics, and orthomolecular theory.

Energy Medicine

- *Chi kung healing touch:* An Eastern method of healing involving breath and gentle movements that follows the Chinese five-element theory and works with the meridian system.

- *Energy work:* A broad category of healing influencing the seven major energy centers (chakras) and the flow of energy around and through these fields.

- *Healing touch:* A therapeutic approach in which touch is used to influence energy systems. Healing touch is employed to affect physical, emotional, mental, and spiritual health and healing.

- *Magnetic therapy:* A modality using magnets to generate controlled magnetic fields. Magnetic therapy is used to improve the functioning of bodily systems and facilitate healing.

- *Reiki:* Using the hands and visualization, the Reiki practitioner directs energy to affected areas of the client's body to facilitate healing and relaxation.

- *Therapeutic touch:* A technique for balancing energy flow in the body through human energy transfer.

The DNP-Educated Nurse as Integrative Practitioner: Unique Aspects of DNP Preparation

The question will be asked, What advantage is there to having DNP preparation for an APN specializing in integrative health? Any professional registered nurse (RN) who takes a course in holistic nursing at the post-RN level should be able to function competently and therapeutically as an integrative practitioner. What, then, does the DNP bring to integrative health? And what is the advantage to seeking DNP preparation for this role?

The AACN addresses the competencies of the doctorally prepared APN (AACN, 2006). The DNP, a practice-focused terminal degree, prepares the APN to serve as an expert in nursing practice. Compared with the PhD and Doctor of Nursing Science (DNS) degrees, which are research-focused degrees, the DNP is unique in providing education in those components of advanced nursing practice that are essential to practice at the highest clinical level. The skills gained in the DNP course of study not only prepare the nurse for clinical competence but also prepare him or her for establishing a successful practice or business.

As DNP programs proliferate in colleges and universities across the nation, certain states (e.g., Alabama and New York) are mandating that the curricula include a significant percentage of clinical content; indeed, some DNP programs (e.g., Columbia University, University of Wisconsin, University of Washington) include a clinical residency in the curriculum. The AACN *Essentials of Doctoral Education* states that DNP programs should require a minimum of 1,000 supervised clinical hours of practice for the baccalaureate to DNP degree course of study in any specialty (AACN, 2006). Including clinical components in the DNP curriculum strengthens the DNP-prepared APN as a clinician. The University of Minnesota's Doctor of Nursing Practice Integrative Health and Healing area of concentration "prepares graduates with skills necessary for working with individuals, families, communities and health systems in developing holistic approaches to health promotion, disease prevention and chronic disease management, with a special emphasis on managing lifestyle changes and incorporating the use of complementary therapies" (University of Minnesota, n.d.). This program fully integrates the specialty courses relevant to integrative practice with those courses designed to meet the requirements of the AACN's Essentials competencies. These courses uniquely position the DNP graduate to succeed on many different fronts of integrative health.

DNP curricula are unique in other areas, in that they include coursework in business finance, health policy, human resource management, change, and leadership (Rush University, n.d.). The APN engaging in integrative health practice benefits from understanding past, current, and future trends in health policy. Healthcare legislation and regulation undergo frequent change, affecting the right to practice; scope of practice; definition of specialty; and related rights, privileges, and responsibilities. Legislation and regulation are influenced by many factors, including political, socioeconomic, and cultural. Advanced coursework in public policy provides the DNP with a firm foundation to clearly view the nuanced political landscape.

The number of APNs owning or directing solo practices remains small, due in part to the expensive and adventurous nature of being an entrepreneur. Because of the lack of research on APNs in private practice, it is not possible to quantify with any specificity the number of APNs who own their own businesses. However, one survey on NPs indicated that 3% are engaged in private practice (Rollet & Lebo, 2007). Given the nature and challenges of integrative health care (e.g., that health insurers do not consistently pay for holistic health services, that clients may be more inclined to

pay for these services with disposable income, and that educated healthcare consumers are becoming increasingly interested in modalities that are more wellness oriented), it is reasonable to speculate that the number of APNs starting integrative health practices will increase. DNP programs provide the APN with education in health economics, financial management, budget creation and management, human resources, practice management, and business models.

In the case of the DNP-prepared nurse as integrative or holistic practitioner, earning the DNP degree provides advantages in the areas of direct delivery of health care, practice development and management, and interpreting and synthesizing research. Although some will posit that enough is learned at the baccalaureate or master's level, the competencies needed to provide health care to increasingly complex populations while managing a practice autonomously, using research for evidence-based care, and advocating for patient access to all relevant forms of interventions that promote wellness are all presented comprehensively in a DNP curriculum and provide the APN with the most optimal level of preparation for practice.

NURSE INFORMATICIST

Sandra McPherson
Mary Zaccagnini
Kathryn White

Nursing informatics is defined by the ANA (2001) as "a specialty that integrates nursing science, computer science and information science to manage community data, information, and knowledge in nursing practice" (p. 73). The APN informaticist can guide practice in both hospitals and private practice settings to meet *meaningful use* criteria and contribute to the delivery of safer patient care.

Recent developments in American health care have promoted the role of the nurse informaticist. Chief among those developments is the meaningful use incentive program developed by the CMS. This CMS program provides incentive payments to eligible professionals, eligible hospitals, and critical access hospitals (CAHs) as they adopt, implement, upgrade, or demonstrate meaningful use of certified electronic health record (EHR) technology. The certification ensures "purchasers and other users that an EHR system or module offers the necessary technological capability, functionality, and security to help them meet the meaningful use criteria. Certification also helps providers and patients be confident that the electronic health IT products and systems they use are secure, can maintain data confidentially, and can work with other systems to share information" (Centers for Medicare and Medicaid Services [CMS], 2012). The DNP-prepared nurse informaticist can help practitioners and facilities achieve meaningful use incentives from the CMS.

The meaningful use criteria were developed and written by physicians, for physicians. Scherger (2010) mentioned that these physicians knew that criteria placed into certain software applications could help prevent some medical errors and possibly save lives. One motivator for this development was the IOM publication *To Err Is Human* (IOM, 1999). This IOM report brought to light that many deaths in the United States are the result of medical errors. In fact, it states that more Americans die from preventable medical errors than from motor vehicle accidents, breast cancer, and AIDS (IOM, 1999). It encouraged development of systems to reduce errors and improve communication between healthcare providers. In addition to the medical influence on meaningful use, nurses and other members of the interdisciplinary health team have made contributions to improve safety and reduce errors.

Despite the good intent of the meaningful use criteria, many hospitals are struggling to meet the criteria and to deal with the impact of an EHR. Many physicians and providers struggle with EHR entries because the output of the electronic record does not resemble a progress note (Baron, 2010), and it is difficult to submit for reimbursement. Another struggle that hospitals are experiencing in meeting the meaningful use criteria involves achieving provider proficiency in navigating the EHR and making accurate, timely entries into the EHR across all specialties. Training of providers is crucial for the success of any software implementation such as the EHR. As clinical practice changes to an electronic, digital workflow, the manual, analog workflow is quickly departing from clinical care areas. Technology is appearing in the basic functions of the nursing role.

In the past, supplies were stored on wire racks or in closets that were open to all providers—and visitors. Now they are stored in electronic cabinets that track utilization and control access. These computerized cabinets associate the patient name with the supplies being accessed. An additional interface sends charges to the patient account once the provider clicks on a button that decrements the inventory. Only authorized providers are allowed to access the cabinet. Intravenous (IV) pumps are another example of emerging technology. Newer IV pumps have a database that allows maximum drug doses to be programmed in order to prevent overdosing. Many of the pumps also have an interface that allows the data collected at the bedside to be automatically entered into the EHR. In addition, the clinical documentation of assessments, flow sheets, care plans, and orders are all electronic, and the hard copy patient paper record is becoming a part of history.

The emerging *informatics DNP* specialty role is a result of the changing demands in health care. The complexity of patient care and the public concern about quality and safety of care are catalysts for the rapid enrollment in these advanced degree programs. Nationwide, enrollment into DNP programs at both the postmaster's and postbaccalaureate level has been steady and competitive (AACN, 2012), including the DNP specialty focused on informatics.

Curriculum/Preparation

The curriculum for the DNP degree builds on the master's-level program and encompasses many areas of practice. Generally, the curriculum has a core set of courses that all DNP-level students, regardless of their nursing specialty, are required to complete. The specialty classes are based on the student's field of practice. Colleges vary greatly with what specialties they offer, and this must be researched prior to enrollment. Additional courses for a DNP degree focused on informatics can include classes on project management, system development life cycle, nursing terminologies, database and technology, knowledge management, decision support systems, and other related technology courses, depending on the institution. These courses fulfill the requirements for the AACN's Essential IV, information systems/technology and patient care technology for the improvement and transformation of health care, and expand the practitioner's knowledge beyond the basics.

Certification

One can obtain many certifications within the field of informatics that complement the education received in the DNP degree course of study. The American Health Information Management Association (AHIMA), the ANCC, and the Health Information Management System Society (HIMSS) offer these specialty certifications. Certificate programs can be found through many colleges both onsite and online. The Project Management Professional (PMP) is another certification that may be obtained through the doctoral study of informatics.

Project Management

Project management is often part of the nursing informatics role. The informaticist may work on or manage a range of projects, from simple customizations of a computer screen, minor upgrades, or an EHR to full systems implementation. Most of these projects include a needs assessment and the full system development life cycle (SDLC). The SDLC includes planning, analysis, design, implementation, and evaluation (Dennis & Wixom, 2003). The DNP program in informatics allows for a deep immersion in all phases of the project life cycle to achieve an organized method of delivering the project.

Work plans, work breakdown structures, project schedules, and project reporting tools can all be part of the project management role for the nursing informaticist. Process improvement activities such as flow mapping can be beneficial to the overall project success when workflows are changed. Project reporting tools can vary depending on the project. The DNP-prepared nurse informaticist uses many tracking tools to facilitate delivery of projects on time and within budget. Pert and Gantt charts are the most commonly used visual charts in project management to display a visual representation of the milestones for the project and the date associated with each milestone. The Gantt chart represents the timeline of the project with estimated task durations and sequences. At a quick glance, it displays the project status and the overall anticipated project duration. A disadvantage of Gantt charts is the inability to show relationships between items or display items that are on the critical path (Luecke, 2004). The critical path items determine the entire project length. Failure to complete critical path items delays overall implementation of the project. The Pert chart shows both the critical path items and the relationships between tasks. This type of chart has a great amount of information. The disadvantage of this chart is that it is not as simplified as the Gantt. The chart does not lend itself to a quick, at-a-glance assessment of the status of the project.

Hybrid Health Records

Because of the rapid pace of technology enhancements and rapidly changing requirements, the literature for EHRs can become out of date within a short period. A common theme that this author found is that many facilities were in a hybrid status with health records: some portions of the record were electronic, whereas others were on paper or possibly in a different electronic system, and the data were not shared. Studies identified the value of sharing documentation as much as possible and removing hybrid systems if feasible, though results of the search and path varied. Some authors have stated that hybrid systems do not work well (Borycki, Lemieux-Charles, Nagle, & Eysenbach, 2009; Dimick, 2008; Hall, 2008), whereas others have claimed that hybrid systems do work well (Hamilton, Round, Sharp, & Peters, 2003; Manchester, Raia, Scott, Emery, & Russo, 1992). Although the literature has conflicting opinions—both for and against—regarding the use of hybrid records, the overall literature supports the use of EHRs to increase access to previous health histories, to enhance patient safety and improve patient outcomes, to increase access to decision support tools, and to increase the speed and accuracy of order processing. This is a role for the DNP-educated informaticist: to bring the hybrid systems into the future of an all-inclusive EHR.

Theoretical Supports for Nursing Informatics

The nursing informatics specialty covers a wide breadth of clinical care areas but offers the flexibility of pulling from many different theory domains: nursing theories, nursing care models, project management theories, systems theory, behavioral theory, information science, computer science, and education theories. All these theories from within and outside nursing may be applicable to nursing informatics. One theory that can easily be used to describe change in the clinical setting is Lewin's change theory. Although Lewin's theory has only three steps, it offers the most flexibility. Lewin's theory consists of unfreezing, making changes, and then refreezing. According to Burnes (2004), Kurt Lewin believed that planned change and learning would enable individuals to resolve conflict and understand their world in order to restructure their perceptions. The first stage is unfreezing. This allows people to recognize the need for change from the original process/procedure and move to another by creating the right environment. In informatics, this may occur when frontline staff get involved with redesigning their workflow as technology changes it. Stage 2 involves the actual change to be made. In informatics, stage 2 might include customization of a computerized documentation system or the implementation of an EHR. Stage 3 is the freezing or refreezing process that allows the new process or procedure to become the new standard and the change to be stabilized and integrated (Boyd, Luetje, & Eckert, 1992). Sometimes there are several iterations of an EHR functionality or a screen display before the final outcome is reached. Lewin's theory is flexible enough to describe these iterations.

Future

The future of the DNP-prepared informaticist can only expand. Requirements for data reporting within the healthcare organization, benchmarking, and documentation of quality measures and patient outcomes all continue to increase. Additionally, meaningful use requirements will continue to evolve.

The Office of the National Coordinator for Health Information Technology (ONC) has articulated national goals to be accomplished by 2014 to encourage the widespread adoption of EHR, to interconnect clinicians so that data and information can be more easily shared, to personalize care through the use of personal health records and telehealth, and to improve public health through accessible information

(NLN, 2008). Such national goals will secure the place of the doctorally prepared nurse informaticist for the future.

NURSE ENTREPRENEUR

Timothy F. Gardner

Definitions

To aid in the understanding of how the DNP degree prepares APNs to become entrepreneurs, we have to begin with definitions. First and foremost, there must be an understanding of what entrepreneurship is, what an entrepreneur does, and what the DNP curriculum covers to prepare a graduate with business savvy.

Entrepreneurship, by definition, "is a proess through which individuals identify opportunities, allocate resources, and create value. This creation of value is often through the identification of unmet needs or through the identification of opportunities for change. Entrepreneurs see 'problems' as 'opportunities,' then take action to identify the solutions to those problems and the customers who will pay to have those problems solved. "Entrepreneurial success is simply a function of the ability of an entrepreneur to see these opportunities in the marketplace, initiate change (or take advantage of change) and create value through solutions" (Watson, 2011).

An entrepreneur is "one who undertakes innovations, finance and business acumen in an effort to transform innovations into economic goods" (Shane, 2004, p. 205). The attributes and abilities of a successful entrepreneur are self-motivation, autonomy, problem solving, leadership, decision making, risk taking, self-confidence, determination, and being ethical (Dayhoff & Moore, 2003).

In comparison, the DNP is the highest clinical degree that exists in the profession of nursing, and it is the terminal practice degree for the profession. The DNP is a practice-focused degree and is designed to prepare experts in a specialized advanced practice role

(AACN, 2006). The DNP educational course of study builds on the generalist foundation of the core knowledge and competencies of the professional nursing undergraduate Bachelor of Science in Nursing (BSN) and the graduate Master of Science in Nursing (MSN) degrees for post-MSN DNP programs (AACN, 2006). When envisioning the DNP, the AACN (2006) identified and developed eight core competencies that the DNP graduate will have mastered upon completing the doctoral course of study. These core competencies are in addition to those attained at the BSN and MSN levels of educational preparation. To address these competencies, programs typically have coursework that covers the fields of epidemiology, economics, business management, organizational systems analysis, health policy, EBP, healthcare information technology, and leadership. The majority of programs require students to plan, develop, implement, and evaluate a scholarly project. The purpose of the scholarly project is for students to synthesize, apply, and demonstrate learned concepts (Sperhac & Clinton, 2008). Students are required to complete advanced didactic and clinical coursework in physiology, pathophysiology, pharmacology, health/physical assessment, and the student's area of specialization, such as acute care, family primary care, midwifery, clinical nurse specialist, nurse anesthetist, and so on (AACN, 2006). Throughout this section, these core essential competencies are identified as they relate to doctoral educational preparation and entrepreneurship.

It should be noted that the DNP-prepared APN is an independently licensed healthcare professional who performs as an independent and interdependent member of an interdisciplinary healthcare team. As a result of professional licensure and educational preparation, the DNP APN is well positioned to independently own and operate a private business venture.

Background

Embedded throughout the nursing educational process is a combination of the three fundamental specialized skills of problem solving, critical thinking, and decision making. This combination is known in the profession as the nursing process. This trifecta of fundamental skills forms the core entrepreneurial skill essentials of the DNP. Because of their educational underpinnings, DNP entrepreneurs are prepared to perform a needs assessment, identify a problem, develop a plan of action, implement evidence-based interventions, evaluate the plan, and start over if needed. These concepts are not unique to the nursing profession. Critical thinking, problem solving, and decision making are also core concepts of, and basic critical skills in, the business world. The procedural steps of the nursing process are very similar to those actions outlined in the business definition of entrepreneurship.

Nursing is, and has always been, an eclectic profession with a scope of practice that overlaps with other professional disciplines such as medicine, pharmacology, public health, psychology, sociology, and business in the effort to provide optimal health care. For example, advanced practice nursing combines the holistic perspective of nursing science with specialized knowledge and skill sets obtained from the biomedical sciences, medicine, and pharmacology to provide healthcare services (AACN Essentials I and II; AACN, 2006). Because of this acquired expanded knowledge, APNs are able to use clinical thinking and skills traditionally associated with medicine to obtain a health history, perform a physical examination, and formulate a diagnosis gleaned from the patient's signs, symptoms, and results of ordered diagnostic/laboratory tests in order to develop a treatment plan, including prescribing pharmaceuticals. It should be noted that the expanded knowledge and skills needed to provide these services are now fundamental to the APN educational process and should no longer require

medical delegation, protocols, supervision, or mandatory written collaboration (Wisconsin Nurses Association, 2011). Similarly, nursing has incorporated other expanded knowledge and specialized skills from the business profession, such as principles of management, elements of accounting, budgeting, and contract negotiation. Given these overlapping scopes of practice, the DNP-prepared APN possesses great entrepreneurial potential.

The Relationship of Entrepreneurship and the DNP Degree

In regard to the relationship of entrepreneurship and the DNP-prepared nurse, doctoral-level education provides the nurse entrepreneur with expanded knowledge and specialized skill sets necessary to navigate and thrive in today's complex healthcare environment, not simply as a clinician possessing "the ability to design and deliver effective care to patients" (Hanson & Bennett, 2005, p. 543). In addition, the "enhanced leadership, policy making and collaboration skills" obtained during the course of study positions the DNP entrepreneur to "make changes at the system and practice setting level" (Hanson & Bennett, 2005, p. 543). This enables the DNP-prepared entrepreneur to function as an administrator, educator, consultant, and community leader and to operate as an agent of change in legislation and policymaking (depending on his or her area of expertise). Doctoral-level education enhances the entrepreneur's ability to analyze and bring evidence-based research from the laboratory and scientific literature to the clinical arena. This area addresses AACN Essential III (AACN, 2006). This is in line with the AACN's position that requires the DNP educational process to be designed to prepare the graduate APN to gain competence in the application of research to practice, to be able to evaluate evidence and research findings for decision making, and to implement potential innovations to change current clinical practice. It is also the AACN's position that during the course of study, significant consideration should be given to programmatic decision making and program evaluation using assessment data collected at the population or cohort level (AACN, 2009, p. 2).

However, in the call for healthcare restructuring by institutions such as the IOM and the National Research Council of the National Academies, the consistent mantra has been "patient-centered care." By definition, patient-centered care is "healthcare that establishes a partnership among practitioners, patients, and their families (when appropriate) to ensure that decisions respect patients' wants, needs, and preferences and that patients have the education and support they need to make decisions and participate in their own care" (American Academy of Family Physicians, American Academy of Pediatrics, American College of Physicians, & American Osteopathic Association, 2010). In patient-centered care, the central theme is that a healthcare provider can provide care for only one individual at a time, and therefore, the tenets of population-based care belong in the public health domain and should not be the guiding principles of an individual healthcare practitioner (Peraino, 2011).

Herein lies a conundrum. How can a doctoral education process that focuses on the tenets of EBP with data obtained from population-based research studies effectively support the call for patient-centered care? The appropriate answer would be through individualizing the findings. However, EBP, as it is currently implemented in health care, does not individualize care; rather, it standardizes care through clinical guidelines, protocols, and best practices. It must be remembered that all research findings are not generalizable. Is it prudent for all healthcare decisions to be based on the cultural health beliefs, values, and behaviors of an individual patient's racial and ethnic background? Isn't this racial profiling and cultural stereotyping? Consequently, this does not constitute patient-centered care; it is providing care based on the patient's culture and ethnicity (Hasnain-Wynia, 2006).

In answering these questions, the doctoral educational process prepares the DNP graduate to obtain population-based information, individualize the findings based on the individual patient's risk assessment, and use this information to provide high-quality, evidence-based, patient-centered care (AACN Essential VII; AACN, 2006). Other provisions of the call for restructuring include providing care that is "safe, effective . . . timely, efficient, and equitable . . . as members of an interdisciplinary team, emphasizing evidence-based practice, quality improvement, and informatics," and the report calls for nursing to have "the best prepared senior level nurses in key leadership positions and participating in executive decisions" (AACN, 2006, p. 6). Again, the doctoral education process prepares the DNP graduate to meet these needs and provide care that addresses all these provisions. DNP-prepared entrepreneurs must have these added competencies to enhance the development of their professional business and to have practice management skills.

Business and Practice Management

Doctoral education prepares the nurse entrepreneur to plan, organize, finance, and operate his or her own business venture. DNP programs typically offer courses that address practice management, economics, management of the client in the healthcare system, healthcare information technology, and project planning and evaluation in order to strengthen business acumen and performance. The DNP core courses and advanced practice specialization provide the nurse entrepreneur with the scientific underpinning for practice and the expert advanced clinical knowledge and skills to provide direct and indirect care in an area of role specialization (AACN Essentials I and VIII; AACN, 2006). Knowledge of direct and indirect care processes is vital for the successful management of healthcare systems, regardless of the organization's size or capacity (Hanson & Bennett, 2005).

Doctoral-level education enables the APN to participate in both direct and indirect care processes within the scope of the role. It prepares the nurse entrepreneur to design and develop healthcare services provided to clients. Providing direct care to clients/patients is a central competency of an APN regardless of the specific specialized role of the practitioner (Tracy, 2005). However, many tasks performed are the same across various specialty APN roles (Tracy, 2005). For example, role specialization prepares the DNP-educated primary care nurse to participate in direct care processes, such as obtaining comprehensive medical histories; performing physical examinations; diagnosing, treating, and managing acute and chronic illnesses and diseases; and performing minor procedures such as suturing, incision and drainage, and IUD insertion. Direct care processes also include providing services such as wound management, pain management, counseling, and education; providing health promotion and disease prevention services (AACN Essential VII; AACN, 2006); and using electronic medical records and e-prescribing (AACN Essential IV; AACN, 2006). Some of these tasks may fall under the role of clinical nurse specialist and other advanced practice nurses (Hanson & Bennett, 2005; Tracy, 2005).

Indirect processes of care include organizational, administrative, and operational systems. The DNP-educated entrepreneur, regardless of area of specialization, has control over, and responsibility for, an increased proportion of indirect processes of care within the specialty role. These may include administration, budgeting, management, inventory and purchasing, quality control, risk management, development of office policies and procedures, supervision of staff, mentoring, medical coding and billing, and reimbursement issues. Other important indirect processes include the assessment and acquisition of appropriate office computer systems and information technology software that requires knowledge of Certification Commission for Health Information Technology–certified EHR programs (AACN Essential IV; AACN, 2006; Hanson & Bennett, 2005).

The scholarly project that is undertaken and completed during the course of DNP study prepares the entrepreneurial nurse with the specialized knowledge and skills of project management and evaluation. Knowledge of these principles enables the nurse to (1) identify a systems-based problem; (2) perform a scholarly literature review; (3) develop process and outcome objectives; (4) develop, plan, and implement evidence-based interventions to address the problem; and (5) develop, implement, manage, and evaluate program outcomes. This again demonstrates the eclectic nature of nursing and its overlapping scope of practice with other professional disciplines such as engineering and project management.

Organizational Systems Leadership and Collaboration

Doctoral education prepares the nurse entrepreneur to assume leadership positions and understand the basic principles of strategic planning, organizational management, systems thinking, and interprofessional collaboration. The DNP-educated entrepreneur has the knowledge necessary to develop the skills to become a successful and effective leader. As a leader, the entrepreneur must be visionary and creative. Doctoral education includes coursework on strategic planning that involves exercises on developing vision and vision statements. Consequently, these exercises instill in the nurse entrepreneur the concept that "any success achieved in life must begin with a vision" (Love, 2005). A vision is defined as forming a detailed mental picture of exactly what you intend to accomplish or produce. "The visionary entrepreneur is able to see exactly what his or her business is going to look like in every detail when it is finished. . . . A visionary entrepreneur constantly thinks in terms of innovation, and continually searches for opportunities for innovation and implementation" (Love, 2005).

Potential opportunities for "innovation come through the creation of a new process" (direct or indirect) or with the redesigning of an existing process to render it more cost effective, efficient, and profitable (Hanson & Bennett, 2005, p. 544). In the effort to be successful and maintain success, it is essential that DNP-educated entrepreneurs "develop, implement, and continuously analyze direct and indirect processes of care" they may use to meet healthcare outcomes for their clients (Hanson & Bennett, 2005, p. 543). More often than not, this will occur when "working within the constraints of available resources and reimbursement" (Hanson & Bennett, 2005, p. 543), especially during these unsettled economic times when healthcare dollars are very sparse.

The DNP-educated entrepreneur exhibits transformational leadership and is capable of clearly conveying the corporate vision to tap into the creativity of other members of the organization as potential sources of new ideas. This entrepreneur uses systems thinking and understands the principles of systems theory, chaos theory, and the butterfly effect as they apply to an organization. The DNP-educated entrepreneur is apt in utilizing other principles of organizational systems thinking and leadership styles, such as team, situational, and participative leadership. Of the three, team leadership is most pertinent in health care today. This is in line with the AACN's (2006) position stating that DNP graduates "have preparation in methods of effective team leadership and are prepared to play a central role in establishing interprofessional teams, participating in the work of the team, and assuming leadership of the team when appropriate" (p. 14).

The entrepreneur is often the major risk taker in a business venture and at times may need to employ alternative leadership styles. The DNP-prepared nurse entrepreneur understands that leadership is about accomplishing critical tasks for the organization, and in some business situations, an autocratic or paternalistic style of decision making may be required. On the other hand, DNP-educated nurse entrepreneurs understand that interprofessional collaboration is essential to practicing effectively (AACN Essential VI; AACN, 2006). According to the AACN's position, "Today's highly complex multi-tiered health care environment depends on the contribution of highly skilled and knowledgeable individuals from multiple professions" and "healthcare professionals must function as highly collaborative teams" (AACN, 2006, p. 14). Doctoral education prepares the entrepreneur to understand both the clinical microcosm and the healthcare macrocosm, which define practice and directly influence their ability to provide care (AACN Essential II; AACN, 2006). The DNP-prepared nurse entrepreneur understands healthcare policies and legislative issues that "facilitate or impede the delivery of health care services or the ability of the provider to engage in practice to address health care needs" (AACN, 2006, p. 13).

Healthcare Policy and Legislative Issues

Doctoral education provides the nurse entrepreneur with the essential skills to function in the arena of political activism. Courses and class activities provide the student with learning experiences that deal with healthcare policy and legislative issues. This addresses AACN Essential V of the DNP educational process, which states that the graduate should possess the ability to "analyze the policy process and . . . to engage in politically competent action" (AACN, 2006, p. 13) and "design, influence, and implement health care policies that frame health care financing, practice regulation, access, safety, quality, and efficacy" (AACN, 2006, p. 13). Now more than ever, it is imperative that nurses, especially nurse entrepreneurs, be able to function competently in the political arena during these very volatile times in health care as critical decisions concerning nursing's scope of practice are being pondered by legislative and judicial systems.

Current and Future Trends

In the current healthcare environment, DNP-prepared entrepreneurs are standing on the threshold of playing key roles as leaders and agents of change at the decision-making tables and in the clinical setting as primary care providers. As stated in the IOM's landmark report on the future of nursing, the DNP-prepared nurse must be capable of functioning "from the bedside to the board room" (IOM, 2010, p. 6). All of this is a result of a perfect storm that is playing out in health care today as fewer medical students pursue careers in general practice, thus increasing the shortage in available primary care physicians. These factors, combined with the soaring costs of health care, an aging population that is living longer, chronic health problems, and the implementation of the Affordable Care Act, indicate a growing need for high-quality, affordable, and available health services. As a result, there is an increased demand for primary care services such as those provided by the healthcare professional role created to address this problem more than 40 years ago: the APN (Robert Wood Johnson Foundation, 2011). These circumstances position the DNP-prepared APN entrepreneur to be a viable complement to the traditional physician internist or primary care provider for the healthcare-seeking consumer. Other precipitating factors, such as lack of appreciation, subordination to physicians, role diminution, low wages, short staffing, poor working conditions, inflexible schedules, frequent schedule changes, and burnout, have reduced the number of experienced professional nurses in the United States, further ripening the field of opportunity for nurse entrepreneurs (American Society of Registered Nurses, 2008; Wood, 2009).

Commercial opportunities abound for DNP-prepared entrepreneurs in private practice, foundations, retail clinics, legal and business consulting, journalism, education, information technology development, pharmaceuticals, and organizational management and administration (American Society of Registered Nurses, 2008). As barriers to practice are eliminated and the national move for true autonomous APN practice progresses, the future is very promising for DNP-prepared entrepreneurs in the business world. This effort has been greatly bolstered by the findings of the IOM's landmark report (IOM, 2010, p. 4), which calls for restructuring of the current healthcare system "to allow nurses to function at the full extent of their educational training" by removing the scope of practice barriers that currently exist in the system. At present, the regulations defining APN scope of practice vary widely from state to state (IOM, 2010, p. 4). This is one major hurdle that must be addressed. Another is the recognition and impaneling of APNs as primary care providers by government agencies, insurance companies, and third-party payers, whether APNs are part of a physicians group or in independent practice. These changes are destined to happen; there is no turning back at this point. Nursing at all levels will play significant supporting and defining roles in the restructuring of the healthcare system that is under way in the United States. During the restructuring, the nursing profession must learn to speak in one voice to address professional issues. By speaking in one voice, the nursing profession, which includes more than 3.1 million nurses (Health Resources and Services Administration, 2010), becomes a very formidable presence in the political arena and at the decision-making tables. The doctorally educated nurse entrepreneur is prepared to accept the challenge of leading change. The profession must not sit idly at the sidelines and allow other professions, agencies, and entities to decide and define what these roles will be.

BIOSKETCHES OF SELECT SUCCESSFUL DNP ENTREPRENEURS

Margaret A. Fitzgerald, DNP, FNP-BC, NP-C, FAANP, CSP, FAAN, Founder, President, and Principal Lecturer, Fitzgerald Health Education Associates, Inc., North Andover, MA, www.fhea.com

Margaret A. Fitzgerald is the founder, president, and principal lecturer at Fitzgerald Health Education Associates (FHEA), an international provider of NP certification preparation and continuing education for healthcare providers. More than 60,000 NPs have used the Fitzgerald review course to successfully prepare for certification.

An internationally recognized presenter, Dr. Fitzgerald has provided thousands of programs for numerous professional organizations, universities, and national and state healthcare associations on a wide variety of topics, including clinical pharmacology, assessment, laboratory diagnosis, and health care and NP practice. For more than 20 years, she has provided graduate-level pharmacology courses for NP students at a number of universities, including Simmons College (Boston, MA), Husson College (Bangor, ME), University of Massachusetts–Worcester, Pennsylvania State University, La Salle University (Philadelphia, PA), and Samford University (Birmingham, AL). She is a family NP at the Greater Lawrence Family Health Center, in Lawrence, Massachusetts, and adjunct faculty for the Greater Lawrence Family Health Center Family Practice Residency Program. She holds a DNP degree from Case Western Reserve University (Cleveland, OH), where she received the Alumni Association Award for Clinical Excellence.

Dr. Fitzgerald is the recipient of the NONPF Faculties' Lifetime Achievement Award, given in recognition of vision and accomplishments in successfully developing and promoting the NP role; the American College of Nurse Practitioners Sharp Cutting Edge Award; and the Outstanding Nurse Award for Clinical Practice by the Merrimack Valley Area Health Education Council. She is also a fellow of the American Academy of Nursing and a charter fellow in the Fellows of the AANP. Dr. Fitzgerald is a professional member of the National Speakers Association and is the first NP to earn the Certified Speaking Professional (CSP) designation in recognition of excellence and integrity as a speaker.

Dr. Fitzgerald is an editorial board member for the *Nurse Practitioner Journal*, *Medscape Nurses*, Lexi-Comp, *American Nurse Today*, and *Prescriber's Letter*. She is widely published, with more than 100 articles, book chapters, monographs, and audio and video programs to her credit. Her book, *Nurse Practitioner Certification Examination and Practice Preparation* (2nd edition), received the *American Journal of Nursing* Book of the Year Award for Advanced Practice Nursing and has been published in English and Korean. She has provided consultation to nursing organizations in the United States, Canada, the Dominican Republic, Japan, South Korea, Hong Kong, and the United Kingdom. Dr. Fitzgerald is an active member of numerous professional organizations at national and local levels.

Providing a description of her business, Dr. Fitzgerald states:

> Fitzgerald Health Education Associates, Inc. (FHEA), an NP-owned company, is the industry leader in NP certification review, as well as a major provider of ongoing NP education and university courseware. FHEA delivers the most up-to-date, evidence-based NP certification exam preparation available, while also providing practicing nurse practitioners and other healthcare providers with the continuing education and resources needed to maintain professional competence.

In regard to her perspective on how the DNP degree has enhanced her current practice and business, Dr. Fitzgerald states:

> The purpose of the Doctor of Nursing Practice study is to provide rigorous education to

prepare clinical scholars who translate science to improve population health through expert leadership that powers innovation in health care. I serve my profession in a number of roles; entrepreneur, scholar, and clinician. As part of my DNP studies at Case Western Reserve University, I developed a business plan for the expansion of Fitzgerald Health Education Associates, Inc., with the project's focus being the NP certification preparation course. The process of developing the business plan afforded the opportunity to delve into areas that would be critical to the company's success and helped me to realize the significant possibilities in this niche market. My capstone project focused on the NP certification marketplace. These products of my DNP studies directly have influenced my business's success. I also practice as a family NP and Adjunct Faculty to the Family Practice Residency at the Greater Lawrence (MA) Family Health Center. As a result of my DNP, my ability to critique healthcare literature has been further enhanced, reinforcing my role as a clinical scholar and teacher.

In sharing her thoughts on nurse entrepreneurship, Dr. Fitzgerald further states:

As a nurse entrepreneur, I quickly realized that nursing practice is business practice. The strong clinical assessment skills of the advanced practice nurse, the ability to analyze a problem, study options to work towards the problem's resolution, development of a plan to address the problem, perform ongoing evaluation, and adjusting intervention to ensure the desired outcome, serve the entrepreneur well. In addition, DNP prepares the nurse leader; leadership is critical to entrepreneurship. The successful entrepreneur must be have expert intrapersonal skills, possess initiative and be risk tolerant; again, these are skills that are developed as part of nursing education and critical to nursing practice. While not all nurses aspire to be entrepreneurs, nurse trailblazers can fulfill the role of the intrapreneur, applying the entrepreneur's skill set within an organization. The nurse intrapreneur [sic] provides the forward-thinking mindset needed, focusing on creativity, innovation and leadership. (Personal communication, December 16, 2011)

David O'Dell, DNP, FNP-BC, Cofounder, Doctors of Nursing Practice, LLC (DNP-LLC), www.doctorsofnursingpractice.org

Dr. David O'Dell is the director of, and associate professor in, the family NP program at South University, Palm Beach County, Florida, and he has a part-time faculty practice in neurology with a special interest in neurocognitive disorders and coordinating family dynamics. Outside of these roles, Dr. O'Dell is the lead member of Doctors of Nursing Practice, an organization founded by a small group of students at the University of Tennessee Health Science Center in 2006, which today has grown from a small website that shared static information about the DNP role to a robust site with many components, features, and benefits. The site has several databases of information describing DNP student projects, DNP programs, and program characteristics, as well as a bibliography and a careers page. The online networking feature specifically aims to build the DNP community and has approximately 3,000 current members and a mailing list of approximately 5,000 APNs and students. The site encourages discussions, forums, blogs, events, and groups as a result of participant interests that have helped to form an identifiable and consequential community. Another important function of the organization is the development and management of an annual national DNP conference.

Dr. O'Dell is a site evaluator for the CCNE. The CCNE, the nation's top nursing school review body, evaluates baccalaureate, graduate, and residency programs in nursing to ensure that they meet the standards set forth by the AACN. Dr. O'Dell purports that the DNP degree has afforded him the opportunity to enhance his clinical, academic, and professional life. The DNP degree and past professional experiences have allowed him to assume his academic role to continue to enhance efforts to grow the profession while bolstering an organization with the mission of DNP growth and development.

He believes these efforts would not have been possible if not for the DNP degree.

Dr. O'Dell believes that, as a result of the DNP degree and the dynamics caused by the growth in DNP graduates, the DNP, LLC, website and online community continue to grow, and the need for community development continues. The need for educational venues and platforms to evaluate the contributions of DNPs also continues and no doubt will expand in the future. He believes these are exciting times to be a nurse and a DNP.

Dr. O'Dell surmises that entrepreneurship has been a natural phenomenon for him. He states that he incorporated his professional life many years ago with the recognition that a business entity has more opportunities to augment and grow than an individual does. He further states:

> I've maintained and plan to always work within my self-created corporate structure. Similarly, the business entity of DNP, LLC, affords many opportunities for growth and development in the profession that individuals could not appreciate in isolation. The opportunities for growth and development of the profession of the discipline as a result of the collective contributions of professional colleagues cannot be underestimated. The creation of the DNP, LLC, organization has evolved into the generation of a foundation—a platform—for others to grow and evolve. This continues to be the goal for this organization into the future.

Dr. O'Dell gives the following alternate perspective on nurse entrepreneurship:

> We are all business people in our own way. All professionals, regardless of the discipline, have something to contribute in whatever environment we choose to flourish. No matter where we are in our professional lives, we all contribute and attempt to enhance the flow and outcomes as a result of our individual and collective efforts. This is an entrepreneurial spirit that can be satisfied within and outside of [an] existing organization. Therefore, we are all *in the same boat* trying to move it upstream.

On a personal note, Dr. O'Dell believes that his own entrepreneurial spirit has allowed him to experience great satisfaction as a business owner and as a developer of a communication system designed to enhance the discipline of nursing through the facilitation of the growth of the professional DNP degree (personal communication, October 10, 2011).

Carol Lisa Alexander, DNP, APRN, ACNS-BC, President and CAO of CAAN Academy of Nursing, Nurse Entrepreneur, Educator, CNS–APRN Healthcare Provider, www.caanacademy3.com/Index.html

Dr. Carol Lisa Alexander is cofounder, president, and CAO of CAAN Academy of Nursing. Over the past 34 years, Dr. Alexander has committed herself to caring for the medically underserved, vulnerable, economically disadvantaged, and at-risk populations. During this period, she actively advanced her education to more effectively accomplish her goals. Those goals are to promote and improve healthcare services within the minority community, thereby decreasing the existing healthcare disparity. Dr. Alexander is a DNP-prepared, board-certified clinical nurse specialist presently serving in the role of NP and providing medical healthcare services for the Aunt Martha's Healthcare Network in Illinois.

Dr. Alexander is the visionary for the Coalition of African American Nurses (CAAN), founded in 2002 in an effort to decrease the existing healthcare disparities in her inner-city community. With the realization that nurses are critical in keeping people healthy and safe, Dr. Alexander cofounded CAAN Academy of Nursing with Rose M. Murray, RN, MS, ACNS-BC, in 2007. Dr. Alexander's vision for CAAN is "to inspire, motivate, cultivate, and educate nurses woven in the moral fibers of care and compassion."

Dr. Alexander serves as the administrator for CAAN and an educator for the CAAN Academy of Nursing. She is an active member of Rotary International and serves on the board of directors for the Illinois Nurses Association (INA) District 20 and the board of directors for the Governors State University (GSU) Alumni Association. Dr. Alexander serves on the advisory board of Southland Healthcare Career Forum and is an active lifetime member of the Chicago Chapter of the National Black Nurses Association (CCNBNA). She is a member of Sigma Theta Tau Nursing Honor Society—Lambda Lambda Chapter GSU, and the Meadow-lake Homeowners Association, to mention a few.

In regard to the synergy of possessing the DNP degree and entrepreneurship, Dr. Alexander states:

> I found the course content from my DNP program an essential aid in the strategic plan in developing our business plan. The program also influenced the building of my character in my assuming the leadership role. The ongoing conceptualization of leadership throughout my DNP program actually gave me a more in-depth initiation to translate evidence-based research into practice "right here" and "right now." The courses guided me in refining my leadership skills most specifically in communicating the vision, the ideas, and the needs of the organization, which proved indispensable in contract negotiations. The concept of communication infiltrated every course, redefining the essentials in negotiating, delegating, planning, and managing financial resources effectively and efficiently.
>
> The structure of my administrative courses allowed me to recognize that it is acceptable to operate at various levels of competencies in the role of leadership. I acknowledge that I have developed many leadership role competencies demonstrated within the following: identifying and meeting my customers/partners' needs and expectations expeditiously. In conducting my business, I have learned the significance in having a strong ethical value system, which provides for obtaining mutual respectable outcomes in negotiations. CAAN is partnered with two other major community organizations. Our company has received grant funding that is supporting our adult

students. One of those partners is Governors State University, the institution where I received my DNP. My DNP program has not only afforded me the academic tools that I need in order to be successful but has extended itself beyond to aid in the financial support of the vision and success of the program. To date, we have 74 students in our adult program and 29 in our high school program. (Personal communication, December 10, 2011)

DISCUSSION QUESTIONS

1. After reflecting on all the possible roles the Doctor of Nursing Practice graduate can assume, where do you see your career in 5 years and 10 years?

2. Select one of the *Healthy People 2020* healthcare goals and propose a community intervention program to meet a minimum of one of the objectives for that goal.

3. Give examples of barriers to and facilitators of advanced practice nurses as entrepreneurs. How can the nurse entrepreneur influence healthcare outcomes?

4. Can an nurse educator with a Doctor of Nursing Practice degree influence curriculum development in nursing education? If so, give examples.

REFERENCES

Acharya, D., & Shrivastava, A. (2008). *Indigenous herbal medicines: Tribal formulations and traditional herbal practices.* Jaipur, India: Aavishkar.

American Academy of Family Physicians, American Academy of Pediatrics, American College of Physicians, & American Osteopathic Association. (2010). Joint principles for medical education of physicians as preparation for practice in the patient-centered medical home. Retrieved from http://www.acponline.org/running_practice /delivery_and_payment_models/pcmh/under-standing/educ-joint-principles.pdf

American Academy of Nurse Practitioners Certification Program. (2012). *Candidate and renewal handbook 2012–2013.* Retrieved from http: //www.aanpcertification.org/ptistore/resource /documents/Candidate_Handbook.pdf

American Association of Colleges of Nursing. (2006). *The essentials of doctoral education for advanced nursing practice*. Retrieved from http://www.aacn.nche.edu/DNP/pdf/Essentials.pdf

American Association of Colleges of Nursing. (2009). Frequently asked questions: Question 6. Retrieved from http://www.aacn.nche.edu/dnp/dnpfaq.htm

American Association of Colleges of Nursing. (2012). 2012 data on doctoral programs. Retrieved from http://www.aacn.nche.edu/dnp

American Holistic Nurses Association. (n.d.). Who we are. Retrieved from http://www.ahna.org/Aboutus/tabid/1158/Default.aspx

American Holistic Nurses' Credentialing Corporation. (2012). Certification criteria. Retrieved from http://ahncc.org/certificationprocess.html

American Nurses Association. (2001). *Scope and standards of nursing informatics practice*. Washington, DC: Author.

American Nurses Association. (2007). *Public health nursing: Scope and standards of practice*. Silver Spring, MD: Nursesbooks.org.

American Nurses Credentialing Center. (2012). Advanced public health nursing certification requirements. Retrieved from http://www.nursecredentialing.org/Certification/NurseSpecialties/AdvPublicHealth.html

American Nurses Credentialing Center. (2014). 2014 certification renewal requirements. Retrieved from http://www.nursecredentialing.org/RenewalRequirements.aspx

American Public Health Association. (1996). A statement of APHA public health nursing. Retrieved from http://www.apha.org/policies-and-advocacy/public-health-policy-statements

American Society of Registered Nurses. (2008). Nurse practitioners as entrepreneurs: Constrained or liberated? *Journal of Advanced Practice Nursing*. Retrieved from http://www.asrn.org/journal-advanced-practice-nursing/february-2008.html

Association of State and Territorial Directors of Nursing. (2008). *Report on a public health nurse to population ratio*. Washington, DC: Author.

Association of State and Territorial Directors of Nursing, Centers for Disease Control and Prevention, & Partners' Cooperative Agreement. (2009). *State public health nursing executive leadership functions*. Washington, DC: Author.

Barnes, P., Bloom, B., & Nahin, R. (2007). Complementary and alternative medicine use among adults and children. United States, 2007. *CDC National Health Statistics Report #12*. DHHS Publication No. (PHS) 2009-1250.

Baron, R. (2010). Meaningful use of health information technology is managing information. *Journal of the American Medical Association, 304*(1), 89–90.

Bayer, R., Gostin, L., Jennings, S., & Steinbock, B. (2007). *Public health ethics: Theory, policy and practice*. New York, NY: Oxford University Press.

Bersin, J. (2008). *The training measurement book: Best practices, proven methodologies, and practical approaches*. San Francisco, CA: Pfeiffer.

Blair, K. A., Dennehy, P., & White, P. (2005). *Nurse practitioner faculty practice: An expectation of professionalism* (National Organization of Nurse Practitioner Faculties position paper). Retrieved from http://c.ymcdn.com/sites/www.nonpf.org/resource/resmgr/imported/FPStatement2005Final.pdf

Borycki, E., Lemieux-Charles, L., Nagle, L., & Eysenbach, G. (2009). Evaluating the impact of hybrid electronic–paper environments upon novice nurse information seeking. *Methods of Information in Medicine, 28*(2), 137–143.

Boyd, M., Luetje, V., & Eckert, A. (1992). Creating organizational change in an inpatient long-term care facility. *Psychosocial Rehabilitation Journal, 15*(3), 47–54.

Boyer, E. (1990). *Scholarship reconsidered: Priorities of the professorate*. Princeton, NJ: Carnegie Foundation for the Advancement of Teaching.

Burnes, B. (2004). Kurt Lewin and complexity theories: Back to the future? *Journal of Change Management, 4*(4), 309–325.

Center for Spirituality and Healing. (2008). About. Retrieved from http://www.csh.umn.edu/about/home.html

Centers for Disease Control and Prevention. (n.d.). *Local public health system performance assessment*. Washington, DC: Department of Health and Human Services.

Centers for Disease Control and Prevention. (2011, May 20). Ten great public health achievements—United States 2001-2010. *Morbidity and Mortality Weekly Report, 60*(19), 619–623. Retrieved from http://www.cdc.gov/mmwr/preview/mmwrhtml/mm6019a5.htm

Centers for Medicare and Medicaid Services. (2012). Medicare and Medicaid programs electronic health record incentive program. *Federal Register, 75*(8), 1844–2011. Retrieved from http://www.cms.hhs.gov/Recovery/Downloads/CMS-2009-0117-0002.pdf

Cherry, K. (2011). Lewin's leadership styles. Retrieved from http://psychology.about.com/od/leadership/a/leadstyles.htm

Commission on Collegiate Nursing Education. (2008). *Criteria for evaluation of nurse practitioner programs*. Retrieved from http://www.aacn.nche.edu/leading-initiatives/education-resources/evalcriteria2008.pdf

D'Amour, D., Ferrada-Videla, M., San Martin-Rodriquez, L., & Beaulieu, M. D. (2005). The conceptual basis for interprofessional collaboration: Core concepts and theoretical frameworks. *Journal of Interprofessional Care, 19*(Suppl. 1), 116–131.

Dayhoff, N., & Moore, P. (2003). Entrepreneurship: Start-up questions. *Clinical Nurse Specialist, 17*, 86–87.

Dennis, A., & Wixom, B. (2003). *System analysis and design* (2nd ed.). New York, NY: Wiley.

Diers, D. (1995). Clinical scholarship. *Journal of Professional Nursing, 11*(1), 24–30.

Dilts, R., Grinder, J., Delozier, J., & Bandler, R. (1980). *Neuro-linguistic programming. Volume I: The study of the structure of subjective experience*. Cupertino, CA: Meta.

Dimick, C. (2008). Record limbo: Hybrid systems add burden and risk to data reporting. *Journal of AHIMA, 79*(11), 28–32.

Dossey, B., Selanders, L., Beck, D. M., & Attewell, A. (2005). *Florence Nightingale today: Healing, leadership, global action*. Washington, DC: Nursesbooks.org.

Failla, K. (2008). Manager and staff perceptions of the manager's leadership style. *Journal of Nursing Administration, 38*(11), 480–487.

Guyatt, G., & Rennie, D. (2002). *Users' guides to the medical literature: A manual for evidence-based clinical practice*. Chicago, IL: American Medical Association.

Hall, T. (2008). Minimizing hybrid records. Tips for reducing paper documentation as new systems come online. *Journal of AHIMA, 79*(11), 42–45.

Hamilton, W., Round, A., Sharp, D., & Peters, T. (2003, December). The quality of record keeping in primary care: A comparison of computerized paper and hybrid systems. *British Journal of General Practice, 53*(497), 929–933.

Hanson, C., & Bennett, S. (2005). Business planning and reimbursement mechanisms. In A. Hamric, J. Spross, & C. Hanson (Eds.), *Advanced practice nursing: An integrative approach* (4th ed., pp. 543–574). St. Louis, MO: Saunders-Elsevier.

Hasnain-Wynia, R. (2006). Is evidence-based medicine patient-centered and is patient-centered care evidence-based? *Health Services Research, 41*(1), 1–8. Retrieved from http://www.ncbi.nlm.nih.gov/pmc/articles/PMC1681528/

Health Resources and Services Administration. (2010). HRSA study finds nursing workforce is growing. Retrieved from http://www.hrsa.gov/about/news/pressreleases/2010/100922nursingworkforce.html

Institute of Medicine. (1988). *The future of public health*. Washington, DC: National Academy Press.

Institute of Medicine. (1999). *To err is human: Building a safer health system*. Washington, DC: National Academy Press.

Institute of Medicine. (2003). *Keeping patients safe: Transforming the work environment of nurses*. Washington, DC: National Academies of Medicine.

Institute of Medicine. (2010). *The future of nursing: Leading change, advancing health*. Washington, DC: National Academies of Medicine.

Jewish Women's Archive. (n.d.). Lillian Wald. Retrieved from http://jwa.org/womenofvalor/wald

Keller, L., & Strohschein, S. (2012). Population-based public health nursing practice: The intervention wheel. In M. Stanhope & J. Lancaster (Eds.), *Public health nursing: Population-centered health care in the community* (pp. 186–215). Philadelphia, PA: Elsevier.

Kelly, K. (2010). Is the DNP the answer to the nursing faculty shortage? Not likely! *Nursing Forum, 45*(4), 266–270.

Kotter, J. (1996). *Leading change*. Boston, MA: Harvard Business School Press.

Leven, R., Keefe, J., & Marren, J. (2010). Evidence-based practice improvement: Merging 2 paradigms. *Journal of Nursing Care Quality, 25*(2), 117–126.

Lieberman, J. (1993). *Light: Medicine of the future—how we can use it to heal ourselves now*. Santa Fe, NM: Inner Traditions/Bear & Company.

Love, J. (2005). *The visionary entrepreneur*. Retrieved from http://www.advancingwomen.com/entrepreneurialism/35341.php

Luecke, R. (2004). *Managing projects large and small*. Boston, MA: Harvard Business School Press.

Manchester, G., Raia, T., Scott, J., Emery, L., & Russo, A. (1992). Primary care health information system: A hybrid electronic–paper medical record system. *Journal of Ambulatory Care Management, 15*(3), 13–29.

Mann, J. D. (2009, January–February). Practicing presence through Breema. *Spirituality and Health*, 1–2.

Melnyk, B., & Fineout-Overholt, E. (2011). *Evidence-based practice in nursing and healthcare: A guide to best practice*. Philadelphia, PA: Lippincott Williams & Wilkins.

Minnesota Department of Health. (2007). *Cornerstones of public health nursing*. Retrieved from http://www.health.state.mn.us/divs/opi/cd/phn/docs/0710phn_cornerstones.pdf

Monsen, K. (2005). Use of the Omaha System in practice. In K. Martin (Ed.), *The Omaha System: A key to practice, documentation, and information management* (pp. 58–83). St. Louis, MO: Elsevier.

National Association of County Health Officials. (1994). *Blueprint for a healthy community: A guide for local health departments*. Washington, DC: Author.

National Center for Complementary and Alternative Medicine. (2007). What is CAM? Retrieved from http://nccam.nih.gov/sites/nccam.nih.gov/files/D347_05-25-2012.pdf

National Center for Complementary and Alternative Medicine. (2012). Homeopathy: An introduction. Retrieved from http://nccam.nih.gov/health/homeopathy

National Center for Health Statistics. (2010). *Health, United States, 2010—with special feature on death and dying*. National Center for Health Statistics. Hyattsville, MD: Centers for Disease Control.

National League for Nursing (NLN). (2002). *The preparation of nurse educators* (NLN position paper). Retrieved from http://www.nln.org/aboutnln/PositionStatements/preparation051802.pdf

National League for Nursing. (2008). *Preparing the next generation of nurses to practice in a technology-rich environment: An informatics agenda*. Retrieved from http://www.nln.org/aboutnln/positionstatements/informatics_052808.pdf

National Organization of Nurse Practitioner Faculties Faculty Practice Committee. (2000). *Faculty practice and promotion and tenure*. Retrieved from http://c.ymcdn.com/sites/www.nonpf.org/resource/resmgr/imported/FPguide1100.pdf

New York State Education Department, Office of the Professions. (2014). License requirements: Nurse practitioner. Retrieved from http://www.op.nysed.gov/prof/nurse/np.htm

Nicholes, R., & Dyer, J. (2012). Is eligibility for tenure possible for the Doctor of Nursing Practice–prepared faculty? *Journal of Professional Nursing, 28*(1), 13–17.

Nightingale, F. (1946). *Notes on nursing: What it is, and what it is not*. Philadelphia, PA: Lippincott. (Original work published 1859)

Olds, D., Eckenrode, J., Henderson, C., Kitzman, H., Powers, J., Cole, R., . . . Luckey D. (1997). Long-term effects of home visitation on maternal life course and child abuse and neglect: Fifteen-year follow-up of a randomized trial. *Journal of the American Medical Association, 278*(8), 637–643.

Otto, H. A., & Knight, J. W. (1979). *Dimensions in wholistic healing: New frontiers in the treatment of the whole person*. Chicago, IL: Burnham.

Peraino, R. (2011). *Dedicated to change in the delivery of healthcare: Why patient centered care?* Retrieved from http://www.patientcenteredcare.net

Public Health Accreditation Board. (2011). *Standards and measures*. Retrieved from http://www.phaboard.org/wp-content/uploads/PHAB-Standards-and-Measures-Version-1.0.pdf

Public Health Functions Steering Committee. (1998). Public health in America. Retrieved from http://www.health.gov/phfunctions/public.htm

Quad Council of Public Health Nursing Organizations. (2005). *Scope and standards of public health nursing practice*. Washington, DC: American Nurses Association.

Quad Council of Public Health Nursing Organizations. (2007). *Scope and standards of public health nursing*. Washington, DC: American Nurses Association.

Quad Council of Public Health Nursing Organizations. (2009). *Competencies for public health nursing practice*. Washington, DC: Association of State and Territorial Directors of Nursing.

Regal, P. H. (1990). The language of proof. In *The anatomy of judgment* (pp. 255–293). Minneapolis, MN: University of Minnesota Press.

Robert Wood Johnson Foundation. (2011). APRNs: A "big part of the solution" to the primary care provider shortage. Retrieved from http://www.rwjf.org/humancapital/product.jsp?id=72775&print=true&referer=http%3A//w

Rollet, J., & Lebo, S. (2007). 2007 salary survey results: A decade of growth. Results of the 2007 National Salary and Workplace Survey of Nurse Practitioners. *Advance for Nurse Practitioners*. Retrieved from http://nurse-practitioners.advanceweb.com/Article/2007-Salary-Survey-Results-A-Decade-of-Growth-3.aspx

Rush University. (n.d.). Doctor of Nursing Practice leadership tracks. Retrieved from http://www.rushu.rush.edu/servlet/Satellite?c=RushUnivLevel4Page&cid=1320160314993&pagename=Rush%2FRushUnivLevel4Page%2FLevel_4_College_GME_CME_Page

Sackett, D., Straus, S., & Richardson, W. (2000). *Evidence-based medicine: How to practice and teach EBM*. London, England: Livingstone.

Scherger, J. (2010). Meaningful use of HIT saves lives. *Modern Medicine, 87*(9), 8–9.

Shane, S. (2004). *A general theory of entrepreneurship: The individual opportunity nexus*. New Horizons in Entrepreneurship Series. Northampton, MA: Edward Elgar.

Smith, M. (2001). *Kurt Lewin: Groups, experiential learning and action research*. Retrieved from http://infed.org/mobi/kurt-lewin-groups-experiential-learning-and-action-research

Sperhac, A., & Clinton, P. (2008). Doctorate of Nursing Practice: Blueprint for excellence. *Journal of Pediatric Health Care, 22*(3), 146–151.

Stanhope, M., & Lancaster, J. (2012). *Public health nursing: Population-centered care in the community*. Philadelphia, PA: Elsevier.

Stefl, M. (2008). Common competencies for all healthcare managers: The healthcare leadership alliance model. *Journal of Health Care Management, 53*(6), 360–373.

Taylor, J. (2006). *A survival guide for project managers* (2nd ed.). New York, NY: American Management Association.

Tracy, M. (2005). Direct clinical practice. In A. Hamric, J. Spross, & C. Hanson (Eds.), *Advanced practice nursing: An integrative approach* (4th ed., pp. 123–158). St. Louis, MO: Saunders-Elsevier.

Trivieri, L., & Anderson, J. W. (2002). *Alternative medicine: The definitive guide*. Berkeley, CA: Celestial Arts.

United Nations. (2002). *End poverty 2015 Millennium Development Goals*. Retrieved from http://www.un.org/millenniumgoals/reports.shtml

University of Minnesota. (n.d.). School of Nursing: Doctor of Nursing Practice: Integrative health and healing. Retrieved from http://www.nursing.umn.edu/DNP/specialties/integrative-health-and-healing/

U.S. Department of Health and Human Services, Health Resources and Services Administration, Bureau of Health Professionals, Division of Nursing. (1984). *Consensus conference on the essentials of public health nursing practice and education*. Rockville, MD: Author.

U.S. Department of Health and Human Services, Secretary's Advisory Committee on National Health Promotion and Disease Prevention Objectives for 2020. (2008). *Phase I report: Recommendations for the framework and format of Healthy People 2020*. Retrieved from http://healthypeople.gov/2020/about/advisory/PhaseI.pdf

Watson, G. (2011). Definition of entrepreneurship. Retrieved from http://www.gregwatson.com/entrepreneurship-definition

Wisconsin Nurses Association. (2011). *Advanced practice nurses*. Retrieved from http://www.wisconsinnurses.org/APN.php

Wood, D. (2009). *Why have nurses left the profession?* Retrieved from http://www.nursezone.com/nursing-news-events/more-news/Why-Have-Nurses-Left-the-Profession_29118.aspx

Influencing and Leading Change in the Complex Healthcare Environment: The Role of the Advanced Practice Nurse

Anne M. Barker

CHAPTER OBJECTIVES

1. Use a contemporary model to lead and influence practice changes in healthcare organizations.

2. Apply concepts from complexity science to better understand how to realize successful, sustained organizational change.

3. Apply the concepts of transformational leadership theory to the role of the advanced practice nurse as a leader and influencer of change.

4. Reflect on one's leadership skills and plans for professional development.

This chapter provides a foundation from which advanced practice nurses can recognize and embrace their role as leaders and influencers of practice changes in healthcare organizations. There are a myriad of opportunities for the advanced practice nurse to partner with members of the interprofessional team to increase the efficiency and effectiveness of health care, improve quality and safety, and reduce costs. This chapter focuses on changes at the level at which most advanced practice nurses function (the microsystem) versus major organizational changes.

The first part of this chapter presents an eight-step change model that is informed by both a traditional understanding of organizational change coupled with a basic understanding of complexity science. In this model, change happens by appealing to the vision and values of others rather than by coaxing and manipulation. The second part of the chapter presents transformational leadership as a theory and strategy advanced practice nurses can apply to be leaders and influencers of change in healthcare systems. A model of leadership is presented to assist the reader in actualizing the characteristics of effective leadership, whether in a formal managerial role or a staff position.

THE EVOLUTION OF THEORIES OF ORGANIZATIONAL CHANGE

Theories and models of organizational change have evolved over the last 70 years. One of the earliest change theories was introduced in 1947 by Kurt Lewin. He proposed a three-step model for managing change that still can be applied today:

1. *Unfreezing:* Challenging the status quo to gain support that a change is needed
2. *Freezing:* Making a change
3. *Refreezing:* Solidifying the change into the culture

Over time, other models (Barker, Sullivan, & Emery, 2005; Kanter, 1983; Kotter, 2012) have proposed a varying number of steps to implement change. However, all basically have four distinct phases: assessing the problem/need for change, setting change objectives, implementing change, and evaluating the outcomes of the change.

COMPLEXITY SCIENCE: A NEW PARADIGM FOR UNDERSTANDING ORGANIZATIONAL CHANGE

Despite these traditional models and theories of change, Kotter (2012) suggested that more than 70% of all major change initiatives in organizations fail because managers do not see the change holistically and follow it through.

This author suggests that the reason organizational changes fail to be sustainable is that, compounding Kotter's findings, change leaders fail to recognize how people behave and engage in contemporary, complex environments. A new view of how the world works—complexity science—can shed light on why organizational change initiatives often fail.

Before considering complexity science, it is first important to understand its predecessor, the modern worldview. Based on neoclassical thought arising from the work of scientists such as Newton and Galileo, the underlying view of how the world functions is that it is mechanistic, assuming cause and effect, linear relationships, and predictability. Over the centuries, this worldview revolutionized the understanding of how the world works and has been responsible for many scientific advancements. Applied to organizations, the modern worldview has led to the establishment of organizational hierarchies with well-defined systems of control (policies, procedures, complex planning algorithms, and so forth) with the intent to regulate processes, systems, and people in the organization to achieve predictable outcomes.

However, this modern worldview is now being replaced by a postmodern worldview as scientists, leaders, and individuals discover that the world, organizations, events, and people are not controllable and predictable. Understanding is growing that we do not know many things about how the world and humans work. In concert with the postmodern worldview, an emerging school of organizational thought suggests that leaders need to abandon the old ways of thinking about organizations and embrace new ones that use complexity science as a framework.

Complexity science, a broad term that embraces theories and concepts from the natural sciences, including chaos, complexity, and quantum theories, provides a new understanding. The basic element of complexity science is the *complex adaptive system*. *Complex* denotes that the world is composed of a diverse and vast number of elements that are multidimensional, interconnected, and interactive. These elements form *systems*, which are sets of related parts that are connected, work together, and self-regulate. *Adaptive* suggests these systems can process information and adapt to changes in order to learn from experiences so as to survive and thrive.

By definition, complex adaptive systems do not significantly differ from the traditional definition of organizational systems. However, the concept of complexity reformulates thinking to view systems as messy, disorganized, and unpredictable versus mechanistic, controllable, and predictable. Complexity science views systems holistically, recognizing that the elements in the systems cannot be separated and pulled apart. Complexity science focuses on the interconnection of the elements and recognizes that elements can change and grow based on these connections.

Traditional systems theory places a system in an environment in which it interacts. Complexity science emphasizes that this environment is also a complex adaptive system. This principle is called embeddedness and offers further understanding of why organizations are unpredictable and people and events are not controllable. To illustrate, the department in which the advanced practice nurse works is a complex adaptive system composed of a large number of individuals representing different professions, levels of expertise, educational backgrounds, religions, genders, ages, races, and so forth. These individuals interact with each other and depend on one another to complete the work of the department. Further, the department is embedded in other complex adaptive systems such as the healthcare organization, the community, the healthcare industry, society, and so forth.

A CHANGE MODEL INFORMED BY COMPLEXITY SCIENCE

The model (**Table 5-1**) presented in this chapter is an eight-step model that combines lessons from traditional theories of change with those of complexity science. As with all models, each step

is an iterative process, where moving through one step multiple times may inform the previous step or a later step. For example, a change implementation should not be decided on before the stakeholders are analyzed. However, once the implementation is decided on, new stakeholders may be identified and added to the analysis.

In this section the author suggests a general approach to change. Change is very complex, thus the guidance provided should be modified based on many factors, including the following:

- The source of change, which can be proposed by top management, direct care providers, and those in midlevel positions
- The magnitude of the change, which can be small changes affecting one to several people at the departmental level to large transformational changes affecting the entire organization
- How many disciplines/staff are affected by the change
- If multiple change projects occur at the same time
- The urgency for making the change

TABLE 5-1	Eight Steps of the Change Process
Step 1	Making Sense/Unfreezing
Step 2	Leading or Serving on an Interprofessional Change Team
Step 3	Developing a Team Vision and Charge
Step 4	Identifying and Analyzing Forces of Change
Step 5	Developing a Work Plan for Change Implementation
Step 6	Implementing Change
Step 7	Evaluating Outcomes and Refining as Needed
Step 8	Incorporating Changes into the Culture/Refreezing

Step 1: Making Sense/Unfreezing

This first step has been referred to as unfreezing, creating dissatisfaction, creating a sense of urgency, and sense making, but all have the same intent: people need to understand the internal and external environments that are driving the need for change. The advanced practice nurse first undertakes to develop a personal understanding and acceptance that a practice change is called for, whether initiating the change or not. This understanding can emerge from personal observations and concerns about a practice, internal data suggesting a problem, and new knowledge attained externally.

Next is to help others to answer the following question: Why is a specific practice change needed based on what is happening in the external and internal environments? By virtue of their education and specialization, advanced practice nurses are well suited to influence others on the interprofessional team to consider and make a practice change by helping them understand why the status quo is ineffective and why new ways of acting are called for. Complexity science suggests that people change based on interconnections and relations. Thus, widespread discussion is suggested versus limiting the discussion to just a few.

Strategies to help make sense of a need for change include the following:

■ Provide data and information about the department's performance as compared to competitors' performance, evidence, and clinical practice guidelines. This is one of the most important strategies for several reasons. Having data preimplementation of a change is important in order to measure results postimplementation. Further, top management, whose support is needed to be successful, use data to make decisions. Projects that save money, improve access, generate revenue, improve outcomes, improve satisfaction, and improve safety are more likely be supported than are projects that appeal to softer outcomes such as improved resilience, better leadership, improved quality of life, and so forth. In other words, the advanced practice nurse makes a business case for the change.

■ Help others on the team understand the issues and trends in the external environment and the impact on their work.

■ Bring back information from educational experiences, the literature, and conferences.

■ Encourage others to engage in external activities and to bring back to the department what they learned.

■ Role-model high expectations related to system processes and client outcomes.

■ Discuss vision and values for the outcomes of the proposed change.

■ Demonstrate why the change is worth the time and effort.

Step 2: Leading or Serving on an Interprofessional Change Team

Complexity science proposes that relationships and the connections between people in organizations are the most important elements for successful functioning of the system and for making sustained, positive change. Thus, changes should be planned and implemented by a change team, not by one or two people imposing their ideas and processes on others. The best change outcomes involve the ideas and expertise of many people, and the contributions of many can lead to the most successful, sustained change.

A diverse representation of all key stakeholders, including staff members, clinical disciplines, shifts, levels of personnel, and informal leaders, should be included on a change team. Further, people with expertise in budgeting and program evaluation could be very valuable in some instances. Members of the change team need to be credible and able to build trust among themselves, and they need to be seen as trustworthy by those affected by the change.

Step 3: Developing a Team Vision and Charge

One of the first activities in which the team engages is to develop a team vision and charter. A vision for the change project, similar to a departmental or organizational vision, helps the team appreciate the meaning and purpose of the work of the team, aligns the team toward a common goal, and commits the team to a desirable future.

To develop a vision, a simple visioning exercise can be used. Each member of the team should close their eyes and envision the desirable end result. Each person writes the vision on paper and then reads the statement to the group. After each member contributes, the team begins to identify themes, clarify what is being discussed, and identify areas of agreement and disagreement. One person should record themes. To avoid wasting time, one or two people should be asked to draft the vision statement and bring it back to the group for final revisions and approval. A sample team vision can be found in **Figure 5-1**.

Next, the team develops a team charter. Charters can range from simple one-page documents such as the one shown in Figure 5-1 to more complex documents that might also include how the team communicates outside meetings, the strengths of the team, each member's developmental needs, details on the roles of each person, and so forth. In Figure 5-1, the team charter documents the team purpose, vision, team processes, team expectations, and deliverables.

Step 4: Identifying and Analyzing Forces of Change

The next step is to identify the forces (people, values, technology, and structures) that facilitate change and those that resist change. This strategy, called a force field analysis, was first introduced by Kurt Lewin (1947) and still has applicability today. During this step, the team assesses these forces and considers strategies to strengthen the facilitating forces and to decrease the resisting forces.

The team can conduct this analysis by using poster paper or a whiteboard. No matter the media, someone should be assigned to capture this analysis on paper, which can be referred to as the process progresses. **Figure 5-2** is an example of a force field analysis for the team presented in the previous step. In the middle of the figure, the team has provided a brief description of the proposed change. On the left-hand side of the figure, the forces that drive a change are listed, and on the right side, those forces that resist the change are listed.

To identify the source of change, ask the following questions:

- What data are available that either support or refute the need for the change?
- Who are the individuals and groups affected by the change? Of these, who might be supportive of the change? Who might resist the change? Who has influence and who does not? (This is called a stakeholder analysis.)
- Is the change congruent with the mission, vision, values, and strategic plans of the parent organization and the department?
- Is the organizational culture one that supports risk taking and learning or is it rigid and resistant to change?
- Is there enough time to plan and implement the change?
- Are there enough resources (space, money, human resources) to support the change?
- What are the costs of the change? Are these driving or resisting forces?
- Is the change easy to implement or complex?
- Will there be a need to develop the people affected by the change?

Once the forces of change are analyzed, the team next assigns each force a relative number to signify its strength. In the example, the driving forces scored x points and the restraining forces also scored x points. This then suggests to the team that the restraining forces should be considered and that steps to reduce these forces should be taken. For instance, the new faculty members without curriculum expertise can be developed. This action can be part of the objectives of the next step.

FIGURE 5-1 Sample team charter.

Purpose

The purpose of the team is to review the current specialization track in nursing administration to ensure that appropriate content is presented, that there is no duplication of content or assignments among the courses, and that the content is consistent with professional standards.

Vision

At the completion of the project, the nursing administration specialty track will prepare students to be prominent transformational leaders in their healthcare organizations. The curriculum will be contemporary, reflecting professional standards in nursing administration and the application of best practice in teaching and learning. Potential students will seek admission to our School of Nursing based on its reputation for preparing nurse leaders. Employers will prefer to employ our students with the firm knowledge that graduates are ready to assume leadership in the healthcare organization.

Team Members

- Linda Morality, Team Leader
- Anita Baxter
- Anna Maria Sarvonovich
- Joan Pettie

Team Process

- The leader will prepare a written agenda.
- The team will meet monthly on the third Monday of the month from 11 a.m. to 1 p.m.
- A written work plan will be developed and reviewed each meeting to note the status of each step.
- Meetings will start and end on time.
- If someone is unable to attend a meeting, that person must notify the team leader and is responsible for implementing what decisions and assignments were made.
- The recorder will rotate for each meeting.

Team Expectations

- Meeting will begin and end on time
- Everyone is expected to contribute and no one person should monopolize the discussion.
- Members will come to each meeting fully prepared with any assignments completed.
- Cell phones will be on vibrate, face down. Should members need to text or take a call, they should leave the room.
- No sidebars.
- One person speaks at a time.

Deliverables

The courses will be revised and implemented by September 2015.

FIGURE 5-2	Force field analysis.

Driving Forces		Restraining Forces
Faculty content experts	The purpose of the team is to review the current specialization track in nursing administration to ensure that appropriate content is presented, that there is no duplication of content or assignments among the courses, and that the content is consistent with professional standards.	Members are located at different sites
Current courses		
		Complex implementation
No costs except time		
Past experience		Time commitments of team

Step 5: Developing a Work Plan for Change Implementation

After completing the team charter and the force field analysis, the change team is prepared to develop an implementation plan. If there are no preimplementation data to support the change, the team can consider whether it is feasible or practical to collect data prior to the implementation. For instance, in the practice setting this may be accomplished by a retrospective review of medical records. Another approach might be to make the change in one area and not in another, and then to compare differences. (The reader will be introduced to these and other methods in research courses.)

The team can use **Table 5-2** as a template for documenting objectives, plans, timelines,

TABLE 5-2	Work Plan for Implementation of a Change

Objective	Plan	Responsible Person	Timeline	Evaluation/ Outcomes

Source: Barker, A., Sullivan, D., & Emery, M. (2006). *Leadership competencies for clinical managers: The renaissance of transformational leadership*. Sudbury, MA: Jones and Bartlett.

responsible parties, and evaluation. As the team develops the implementation plan, several considerations can help make the change successful and sustainable:

- Consider plans that are flexible with a few simple specifications as guidelines. This allows for better strategies and ways of doing things to emerge from many individuals during the implementation phase. It also allows for small successes to happen that can build confidence, energize people for more change, and calm the doubters. Paradoxically, it also allows for failures to happen, but when they do they are small moments of learning rather than large setbacks. New actions and ideas emerge from the failures as well as from the successes.

- Consider taking multiple actions for one or more objectives. Although this can be at times confusing, and perhaps resource intensive, it also allows for the best solutions to emerge through trial and error. For example, the advanced practice nurse in a primary care clinic may want to set up a system to get information from clients about their satisfaction with services. Several initiatives can be taken at the same time, such as focus groups, written surveys, and informal conversations with patients and family.

- Consider pilot tests of the change to assess its practicality and to iron out problems.

- Consider evaluations of structures, processes, and outcomes. Determining how the change will be evaluated before its actual implementation is important.

- Do not overlook the need for people to learn new behaviors and ways of doing the work. Although often this means offering workshops and seminars of varying lengths to introduce the change, learning while doing is a more effective approach.

Step 6: Implementing Change

Next, the team rolls out the implementation plan. The responsibility of the change team during this phase is to be visible, seek feedback, provide encouragement, communicate, and resolve problems as they occur. The key to success is to listen to those involved in and affected by the change and to take their ideas and concerns seriously. These are the individuals with whom the change will succeed or fail. Further, they are the individuals who can best express successes and failures. For example, if the change project is to decrease noise, only the patient and family can assess if the change has been successful or not.

Step 7: Evaluating Outcomes and Refining as Needed

The purpose of this step is to ask whether the objectives of the change project, as set out in the work plan, have been met. The decisions about what is to be evaluated, who is evaluating, and how to evaluate have already been made during step 5. At the predetermined time, data are collected to determine what has been successful and what has not been successful and why. Adjustments are made based on the findings of the evaluation and new actions taken. Once these actions are taken, evaluations are done again until the expected results are achieved.

Step 8: Incorporating Changes into the Culture/Refreezing

During this phase, providing positive feedback is the most powerful tool to sustain change. This feedback happens on two fronts: showing appreciation for the people who implemented the change and sharing widely the successes attained. The evaluation data from the previous step are also shared.

THE CALL FOR ACTION: TRANSFORMATIONAL LEADERSHIP

Advanced practice nurses are being called on and challenged to lead changes in healthcare organizations to improve quality, decrease adverse events, reduce costs, and enhance patient satisfaction. Transformational leadership is widely accepted in the healthcare industry and nursing is the preferred leadership style to accomplish this goal. In 2004, the Institute of Medicine (IOM) devoted an entire chapter in the landmark report *Keeping Patients Safe: Transforming the Work Environment of Nurses* to the theory and evidence of transformational leadership. The report cited studies that suggest that transformational leadership is associated with better patient outcomes, fewer medical errors, and greater staff satisfaction. In a subsequent report (IOM 2010), the IOM recommends that no matter their formal positions in organizations, "all nurses must be leaders in the design, implementation, and evaluation of, as well as advocacy for, the ongoing reforms to the system that will be needed" (p. 221).

Additionally, the Magnet Recognition Program model has five components, one of which is transformational leadership. The rationale for recommending transformational leadership is that the goal of leadership is not to keep organizations stable but rather to transform values, beliefs, and behaviors to meet the demands of healthcare reform (American Nurses Credentialing Center, 2014).

THE EVOLUTION OF LEADERSHIP THEORIES

Ancient scholars and philosophers such as Plato and Confucius observed and wrote about leadership, but it was not until the 1930s and the onset of World War II that one can find formal theories and empirical studies of organizational leadership. During the first half of the 20th century, several important themes emerged that still have relevance in today's organizations. First, most theories purported that a democratic, participatory style with positive, supportive relationships between the manager and followers is generally more effective than are autocratic styles of leadership (Fielder, 1957; Likert, 1957; White & Lippit, 1950). Second, the leader must pay attention to organizational goals (Blake & Mouton, 1985; House, 1971).

And last, the theories maintained and research studies further supported, the behaviors and attitudes of the leader affect follower satisfaction and group performance (Fielder, 1957; White & Lippit, 1950). During the 1980s, the view of leadership theory underwent a major paradigm shift from a focus on tasks and systems of controls to one of building the organizational culture to provide an environment in which people are successful and organizational outcomes are positive.

In 1978 James McGregor Burns proposed a new leadership theory that he called transformational leadership. In his seminal work, *Leadership*, Burns described the leadership style and strategies of famous political leaders such as Mahatma Gandhi, Franklin Roosevelt, and John Kennedy. This work resonated with organizational scholars and practitioners, forming the basis for most of the contemporary writing about leadership. Burns (1978) defines transformational leadership as occurring "when two or more persons engage with others in such a way that the leader and followers raise one another to higher levels of motivation and morality" (p. 20). In other words, both the leader and follower find meaning and purpose in their work, growing and developing as a result of the relationship.

A CONTEMPORARY LEADERSHIP MODEL FOR ADVANCED PRACTICE NURSES

Although transformational leadership has been an enduring and often preferred leadership style since the 1980s, it is still evolving. **Figure 5-3** displays a model developed by the author as a result of working with advanced practice nursing students who lead, influence, and participate in practice changes in healthcare organizations. The foundation of the model is transformational leadership and trust. The four pillars of leadership are supported by this foundation, ultimately resulting in a desirable healthcare system as defined by the Institute of Medicine (2004).

FIGURE 5-3   Leadership model.

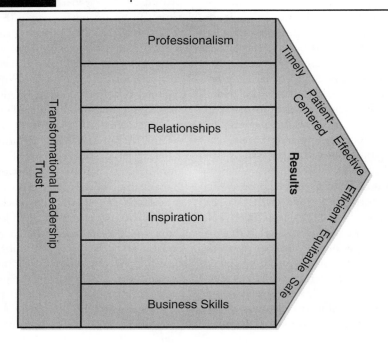

The Foundation

People can be influenced by leaders in whom they believe and trust. A desirable vision of where the team is headed provides meaning and purpose to the work and aligns the team toward common goals. To best accomplish this the advanced practice nurse can adopt strategies of transformational leadership and trust.

Transformational Leadership

To summarize, the important concepts of transformational leadership theory are as follows:

- The relationships between leaders and their colleagues are characterized by engagement versus passivity.
- Transformational leaders bring out the best in the team and performance beyond expectations.

- Transformational leadership is based on empowering the team to work together toward a common vision versus power over others and imposing one's ideas and will.
- Transformational leadership is ethical and focuses on the goals of the organization and development of all the team versus self-aggrandizement and personal gain at the expense of others (Barker et al., 2005).

Trust

Trust was identified, based on Burns's work, as a basic ingredient for successful transformational leadership (Bennis & Nanus, 1985). Recently, there has been a renewed interest and appreciation for the importance of trust as the foundation for leadership and team effectiveness. The importance of organizational trust cannot be overstated. In the literature on this topic, the following positive organizational outcomes have been associated with high levels of organizational trust:

- Enhanced employee performance
- Improved organizational effectiveness
- Greater commitment to the organization
- Good communications and information sharing
- Less resistance to organizational change
- Improved team functioning
- Improved job satisfaction/retention
- Greater participation in decision making and problem solving (Barker et al., 2005)

An important characteristic about trust is that trust begets trust, and mistrust begets mistrust. In other words, trusting behaviors can lead to increased trust, and, in contrast, distrusting behaviors can decrease mutual trust (Zand, 1972). For example, open, honest communication is one of several trusting behaviors. If the advanced practice nurse communicates with another person openly and honestly, the other person will come to trust her; in turn, the other person will likewise communicate openly and honestly, leading to a cycle of trust.

Covey (n.d.), who is currently the top expert in organizational trust, defines trust as "both character (who you are) and competence (your strengths and the results you produce)." Character is one's integrity and intent. These are actualized in such behaviors as follows (Covey, 2005):

- Walking the talk—the congruency between what one says and does
- Looking out for the good of others as well as of oneself
- Doing the right thing even if it is unpopular or difficult
- Keeping commitments to others
- Being consistent and dependable in what one does
- Engaging in honest, transparent communications

- Listening actively
- Being candid
- Displaying basic honesty and moral character
- Acting ethically and with good intentions and motives
- Fulfilling one's fiduciary obligations by placing the concern of others above one's own

Competence is one's talents, skills, knowledge to work with others, and proven ability to deliver results. Simply stated, leaders have no credibility if they do not produce deliverables that contribute to organizational success. Competence is demonstrated by the following behaviors (Covey, 2005):

- Influencing others by setting mutual goals and directions together versus control
- Empowering others by giving people the opportunity to take action, providing them the resources to be successful, supporting their efforts, and providing the necessary information to get the work done
- Demonstrating good decision-making skills so that others develop a trust in the decisions that are made and changes that occur

Pillars of Leadership

The model includes four pillars of leadership that are supported by the foundation of transformational leadership and trust:

I. Professionalism
II. Inspirational motivation
III. Interpersonal relationships
IV. Business skills

Each of these pillars is briefly discussed, and each topic deserves further understanding by the novice advanced practice nurse.

Pillar I: Professionalism

At the core of being professional is being self-aware by reflecting on one's experiences, skills, knowledge, values and attitudes, and feedback from others. To be self-aware, advanced practice nurses reflect on personal thoughts and actions to gain an understanding of their leadership skills, values, and knowledge and identify their strengths and areas in need of further development as a leader.

There are a number of models of self-reflection, but for the purpose of this chapter, two models specific to nursing and health care have been combined to assist advanced practice nurses to engage in self-reflection—Gibb's (1988) classic model and Johns's (1994) model. Despite their age, these models are still widely used in nursing and provide a concrete framework for self-reflection. **Figure 5-4** provides a framework and questions to consider for self-reflection on leadership skills.

Pillar II: Inspiration

Transformational leaders motivate and inspire followers, generating excitement and sustaining a positive belief about the work to be accomplished, by doing the following:

- Articulating a credible vision for others
- Providing a work environment in which people find meaning and purpose in their work
- Setting realistic and achievable, yet high expectations for themselves and others. This is known as the Pygmalion effect. Simply put, expectations drive behaviors, and on a subconscious level people will live up to the standards set. For instance, when a team believes they are the "best team," have the best patient outcomes, and relate to one another better than similar teams do, the team members will act to maintain and confirm this expectation.
- Demonstrating to others that their contributions to the work of the organization have meaning and purpose that result in positive outcomes for clients, their families, and the community

---

FIGURE 5-4   Reflection on leadership skills.

Think about a recent situation in which you assumed a leadership role, whether it was formal or informal.

Describe the situation, including the who, what, where, when, and how. Describe your role as leader. Be objective and factual.

Write down how you **felt** about the situation. Include both your positive and negative feelings. How do you think others felt in the situation?

Using the model in Figure 5-3, **evaluate** how effective you were as the leader. Consider each of the following elements:

- Did you engage the other individuals in the situation to move toward a desired goal?
- What was the level of trust among the involved individuals?
- How well did you manage conflict, communication, and collaboration?
- What professional skills did you exhibit? Which might have been better employed?
- What business skills were needed? Did you use them effectively?

Overall, what can you **conclude** and what did you learn? What were the results? What would you do differently the next time? What would you do the same?

Write down one or two self-development goals for **actions** to take next time you confront a similar situation.

- Being optimistic and passionate
- Encouraging questioning, the challenging of assumptions, out-of-the-box thinking, and by fostering creativity, innovation, and risk taking
- Engaging with and treating each person as unique

Pillar III: Interpersonal Relationships

Transformational leaders build positive interpersonal relationships by engaging with individuals and groups in a way that is characterized by open and honest communication. Communication has two elements: knowing what, when, how, and to whom to communicate and, equally important, how to listen. Communications need to be open, accurate, and candid. At the same time, the advanced practice nurse needs to know when to keep information confidential and when to be discreet, avoiding gossip and harmful rumor spreading.

In both the practice and educational settings, evidence is growing that quality patient-centered care requires the collaboration of the clinical disciplines. Collaboration is defined by these underlying concepts sharing, partnership, power, and interdependency (D'Amour, Ferrad-Videla, Rodriquez, & Beaulieu, 2005, pp.119–120):

- Sharing includes shared responsibilities, decision making, values, data, planning, and intervention.
- Partnerships are two or more people of different disciplines working together for mutual patient outcomes. The relationship is characterized by trust and respect. These types of partnerships emerge through understanding and appreciating the roles of each discipline and their unique contributions to patient-centered care. Understanding begins in the educational setting in the preparation of health professionals.
- Power is shared among the group rather than one person being viewed as the most powerful team member. In other words,

all team members are empowered to work toward the outcomes.
- Interdependency means that the team works together versus autonomously

Pillar IV: Business Competency

At the end of the day, the measure of competent leadership is whether healthcare practices were improved by working with others and employing their skills and competence. Throughout their education and practice, advanced practice nurses are exposed to and can achieve a further depth of understanding of many of the following business competencies:

- Understanding the healthcare delivery system
  - Policy
  - Healthcare economics
  - Healthcare delivery system
  - Current and future trends
- Understanding the organization
  - Mission and vision
  - Strategic plan
  - Finance
  - Quality
  - Information systems
  - Care delivery system
  - Relationships with the community
  - Marketing

Results

The third part of the model, the roof, is the results. As stated previously, leaders have no credibility if they do not produce results that contribute to the organization's success. In this model, the results are organized by the IOM's (2001) recommendations for quality health care:

- *Safe:* Avoiding injuries to patients from the care that is intended to help them
- *Effective:* Providing services based on scientific knowledge to all who can benefit, and

refraining from providing services to those not likely to benefit

- *Patient-centered:* Providing care that is respectful of and responsive to individual patient preferences, needs, and values, and ensuring that patient values guide all clinical decisions
- *Timely:* Reducing waits and sometimes harmful delays for both those who receive and those who give care
- *Efficient:* Avoiding waste, including waste of equipment, supplies, ideas, and energy
- *Equitable:* Providing care that does not vary in quality because of personal characteristics such as gender, ethnicity, geographic location, and socioeconomic status

DISCUSSION QUESTIONS ———

1. Describe a change you have either participated in or observed in your organization. Using the eight-step model of change, analyze which suggested strategies were employed and which were not. Was the change sustained successfully? If yes, why? If no, why not? What could have been done differently?

2. Complete the visioning exercise described in the text for yourself. Share this with other students in your class.

3. Using Figure 5-4, reflect on your leadership skills. Develop an action plan for leadership development.

REFERENCES ———

American Nurses Credentialing Center. (2014). Magnet Recognition Program model. Retrieved from http://www.nursecredentialing.org/Magnet /ProgramOverview/New-Magnet-Model

Barker, A. M., Sullivan, D. T., & Emery, M. J. (2005). *Leadership competencies: The renaissance of transformational leadership.* Sudbury, MA: Jones and Bartlett.

Bennis, W. G., & Nanus, B. (1985). *Leaders: The strategies for taking charge.* New York, NY: Harper & Row.

Blake, R. R., & Mouton, J. S. (1985). *The managerial grid III.* Houston, TX: Gulf.

Burns, J. M. (1978). *Leadership.* New York, NY: Harper & Row.

Covey, S. (n.d.). How we define trust. Retrieved from http://www.coveylink.com/about-coveylink/how -we-define-trust.php

Covey, S. (2005). *The speed of trust: The one thing that changes everything.* New York, NY: Simon and Schuster.

D'Amour, D., Ferrad-Videla, M., & Rodriquez, L., & Beaulieu, M. D. (2005). The conceptual basis for interprofessional collaboration: Core concepts and theoretical frameworks. *Journal of Interprofessional Care, 19*(1), 115–131.

Fielder, F. E. (1957). *A theory of leadership effectiveness.* New York, NY: McGraw-Hill.

Gibbs, G. (1988). *Learning by doing: A guide to teaching and learning methods.* Oxford, England: Further Education Unit.

House, R. J. (1971). A path goal theory of leadership effectiveness. *Administrative Science Quarterly, 15,* 321–338.

Institute of Medicine. (2001). *Crossing the quality chasm: A new health system for the 21st century.* Retrieved from http://www.iom.edu/Reports/2001 /Crossing-the-Quality-Chasm-A-New-Health -System-for-the-21st-Century.aspx

Institute of Medicine. (2004). Keeping patients safe: Transforming the work environment of nurses. Retrieved from http://www.iom.edu/Reports/2003 /Keeping-Patients-Safe-Transforming-the-Work -Environment-of-Nurses.aspx

Institute of Medicine. (2010). *The future of nursing: Leading change, advancing health.* Retrieved from http://www.iom.edu/Reports/2010/the-future -of-nursing-leading-change-advancing-health.aspx

Johns, C. (1994). Nuances of reflection. *Journal of Clinical Nursing, 3,* 71–75.

Kanter, R. M. (1983). *The change masters.* New York, NY: Simon and Schuster.

Kotter, J. (2012). *Leading change.* Cambridge, MA: Harvard Business Review Press.

Lewin, K. (1947). Frontiers in group dynamics: Concepts, method, and reality in social science, social equilibrium, and social change. *Human Relations, 1*(1), 5–41.

Likert, R. (1957). *The human organization: Its management and values.* New York, NY: McGraw-Hill.

White, R. K., & Lippit, R. (1950). *Autocracy and democracy: An experimental inquiry.* New York, NY: Harper and Brothers.

Zand, D. E. (1972). Trust and managerial problem solving. *Administrative Science Quarterly, 17*(2), 229–239.

CHAPTER 6

© A-R-T/Shutterstock

Interprofessional Collaboration for Improving Patient and Population Health

Laurel Ash and Catherine Miller

CHAPTER OBJECTIVES

1. Identify workforce and regulatory issues that affect interprofessional collaboration in the clinical setting.

2. Discuss barriers to and drivers of effective collaboration among inter-professional healthcare teams.

3. Discuss stages of effective team development.

4. Analyze components of a work culture that supports collaboration.

5. Review leadership theories and consider the roles that leaders play in improving population health.

BACKGROUND

The *Consensus Model for APRN Regulation*, prepared by the APRN Consensus Work Group and the National Council of State Boards of Nursing APRN Advisory Committee (2008) and endorsed by numerous nursing organizations, defined advanced practice registered nurse (APRN) practice as practice in one of four recognized roles: certified nurse practitioner, certified nurse-midwife, clinical nurse specialist,

and certified registered nurse anesthetist. The primary focus of an APRN's practice includes provision of direct patient or population care. Conventionally, APRNs are prepared in accredited programs, sit for national certification, and meet regulatory requirements authorizing license to practice as an APRN. A number of nurses with advanced graduate preparation function in specialties that do not fall into these categories yet advance the health of an organization, population, or aggregate or provide indirect patient care. Such roles may work in the areas of administration, informatics, education, and public health. Discussions are ongoing as to how these specialty practices fit into the traditional definition of APRN practice and subsequently the Doctor of Nursing Practice (DNP) role. This chapter uses the term *APRN* to reflect all advanced roles of nursing practice.

Numerous research has documented well the impact that APRNs have on health outcomes, including the ability to deliver excellent quality, cost-effective care with high levels of patient satisfaction (Cunningham, 2004; Dailey, 2005; Horrocks, Anderson, & Salisbury, 2002; Ingersoll, McIntosh, & Williams, 2000; Lambing, Adams, Fox, & Devine, 2004; Laurant et al., 2004; Miller, Snyder, & Lindeke, 2005; Mundinger et al., 2000). The world is changing, and APRNs must position themselves to be at the table with other disciplines and professionals in order to emphasize the influence of nursing care on the health of individuals or populations. The complexity of the current healthcare delivery system, trends in patient demographics, epidemiological changes of disease and chronic conditions, economic challenges, the need for improved patient safety, and the call for a redesign or reform of the healthcare delivery system will challenge all professionals to envision health care in new ways.

Healthcare reform is a prominent issue for health professionals, policymakers, and the public. During the 2008 presidential campaign, president-elect Obama announced a comprehensive healthcare reform proposal (Kaiser Family Foundation [KFF], 2008). This proposal outlined key points regarding restructuring our present system. As a foundation, all individuals and communities must be guaranteed a set of essential preventive care services. Reform must include measures to improve health outcomes and safeguard patients from preventable

medical error. Obama's platform supported programs that use collaborative teams as a means to deliver comprehensive, cost-effective, and safe care to persons with chronic conditions (KFF, 2008). Access to safe, effective, and affordable health care is a concern shared by the American public and rated of significant importance in a national poll, conducted by researchers from the Kaiser Family Foundation and the Harvard School of Public Health and released in January 2009.

Healthcare reform, formally known as the Patient Protection and Affordable Care Act (Public Law 111-148), was signed into law March 23, 2010, by President Barack Obama. This comprehensive set of enactments aims to control healthcare expenditures, enhance access to care, and improve patient care delivery and quality of health care (KFF, 2011; Patient Protection and Affordable Care Act [PPACA], 2010). Nursing is highlighted throughout the Act as playing a key role in addressing multiple reforms. Shortages of primary care physicians, particularly in certain geographic and underserved areas, contribute to access problems. Because the Act intends to extend health coverage to many more millions of Americans, further burdens are placed on an already stressed system. This legislation recognizes advanced practice nurses, particularly nurse practitioners, as part of the solution to raise numbers of primary care providers and expands funding for nurse practitioner training and education. Additionally, a number of provisions specifically identify nurses as interprofessional team leaders and members. The Medical/HealthCare Home provision (KFF, 2011; PPACA, 2010, Section 3502) explicitly identified interdisciplinary teams—to include nurses, nurse practitioners, physicians, pharmacists, social workers, and other allied health professionals—to provide coordinated, integrated, and evidence-based care to patients and families, particularly those with complex healthcare needs. The Public Health Services Act of PPACA was amended to support nurse-managed health centers (KFF, 2011; PPACA, 2010, Section 5208). The grant appropriates funds and authorizes advanced practice nurses to coordinate and deliver comprehensive primary and wellness care to underserved, vulnerable populations. Nurses must be the major providers of services in a team led by an advanced practice nurse. Demonstration projects, such as Independence at Home (KFF, 2011; PPACA, 2010, Section 3024), clearly designate nurse practitioners as leaders of and participants in healthcare teams aimed at improving health outcomes and reducing costs to home-bound Medicare beneficiaries. DNP-prepared nurses, at the highest level of clinical nursing practice, must fully participate as team leaders and members in innovative models of care delivery and document improved healthcare outcomes because of such collaboration and leadership.

The professions of nursing and medicine agree on the need to create organizational environments that promote interprofessional collaboration. The American Nurses Association (ANA, 2008) report *ANA's Health System Reform Agenda* places particular emphasis on the role of collaboration in chronic disease management and patient safety. The American College of Physicians (ACP, 2009) also acknowledges that the future of healthcare delivery requires interprofessional teams that are prepared to meet the diverse, multifaceted health issues of the population. Providers, policy leaders, and health systems will need to shift their mindset from traditional models of linear, disease-focused care to new delivery approaches. In a redesigned model, each discipline brings specialized skills and abilities, practices at the highest level of the individual provider's ability, assumes new roles, and participates in a collaborative manner with other professionals to provide high-quality, safe, cost-effective, patient-focused care. This call to action demands that APRNs perform at the highest level of clinical expertise, the Doctor of Nursing Practice, and collaborate

interprofessionally to improve patient and population health outcomes.

In 2008, the Institute of Medicine (IOM), in partnership with the Robert Wood Johnson Foundation (RWJF), convened an 18-member panel of physicians, nurses, educators, policymakers, economists, and public health experts to examine, debate, and problem-solve critical healthcare issues and, in particular, the role that nurses play in transforming the healthcare system. In October 2010, the panel released its findings in an evidence-based report, *The Future of Nursing: Leading Change, Advancing Health* (IOM, 2011). This 500-plus-page document highlighted nursing's reputation for safe, high-quality care and provided specific recommendations to further advance skills and expertise of nurses to lead change. The report proposed that nurses attain higher educational levels to address increasingly complex health issues; that outdated organizational and regulatory barriers be removed to allow nurses to practice to the full extent of their education and training; and that nurses be provided opportunities to assume leadership positions and be full collaborative partners with physicians and other healthcare professionals in redesigning health care in the United States (IOM, 2011).

To improve quality, maximize resources, and coordinate care, an interdisciplinary approach to care for patients with complex health needs is best. To foster positive collaborative behaviors between professionals, reduce biases of other disciplines, and ultimately improve patient outcomes, nursing education needs to expand to include competencies in interprofessional teamwork and collaboration in clinical environments (IOM, 2011). All nurses will benefit from enhanced leadership, political suaveness, advocacy, and health policy development skills, all of which are components of DNP programs.

Although the IOM is a highly regarded institution, not all health professions embrace the *Future of Nursing* report. Mistrust between disciplines persists. The American Medical Association issued a response to the report that challenged nursing's role, iterated that a "physician-led team approach to care helps ensure high quality patient care and value for health care spending," and emphasized the differences in physician and nurse practitioner education, suggesting that nurses are less prepared to deliver primary care (American Medical Association, 2010). Full partnership is a work in progress; DNP-prepared nurses must embrace these challenges and practice to the highest level to design, collaborate, lead, and document results of innovative models of care and resultant improved healthcare outcomes.

Merriam-Webster's Collegiate Dictionary defines *collaborate* as "to labor together, to work jointly with others." Leaders in the business world further describe collaboration as a concept involving "strategic alliances" or "interpersonal networks" in an effort to accomplish a project (Ring, 2005). As healthcare professionals, we can learn from successful business and management practices and use the collaboration processes of communicating, cooperating, transferring knowledge, coordinating, problem solving, and negotiating to more effectively reach a healthcare goal or outcome. The ACP (2009) suggested that collaboration involves mutual acknowledgment, understanding, and respect for the complementary roles, skills, and abilities of the interprofessional team. Effective collaborative partnerships promote quality and cost-effective care through an intentional process that allows members to exchange pertinent knowledge and ideas and subsequently engage in a practice of shared decision making. The purpose of this chapter is to generate a better understanding of interprofessional collaboration, distinguish which elements DNPs must possess to successfully collaborate with other professionals to improve the health status of persons or groups, and provide an overview of models of interprofessional collaboration in the real world.

IMPROVING HEALTH OUTCOMES

The IOM's 2001 report, *Crossing the Quality Chasm: A New Health System for the 21st Century*, identified four key issues contributing to poor quality of care and undesirable health outcomes: the complexity of the knowledge, skills, interventions, and treatments required to deliver care; the increase in chronic conditions; inefficient, disorganized delivery systems; and challenges to greater implementation of information technology. The report went on to outline 10 recommendations intended to improve health outcomes, one of which focuses on interprofessional collaboration. It emphasized the need for providers and institutions to actively collaborate, exchange information, and make provisions for care coordination because the needs of any persons or population are beyond the expertise of any single health profession (IOM, 2001; Yeager, 2005). An earlier IOM report (1999), *To Err Is Human: Building a Safer Health System*, addressed issues related to patient safety and errors in health care. This report articulated interprofessional communication and collaboration as primary measures to improve quality and reduce errors.

Accrediting and regulatory bodies such as The Joint Commission (2008) recognize interprofessional collaboration as an essential component of the prevention of medical error. This organization's mission is to continuously improve the safety and quality of care through the measure and evaluation of outcomes data. It has targeted improved communication and collaboration among providers, staff, and patients as a means to better protect patients from harm. Improved patient safety outcomes can be additionally facilitated through collaborative efforts such as development of interdisciplinary clinical guidelines and interprofessional curricula that incorporate proven strategies of team management and collaboration processes. Doctorally prepared APRNs are well positioned to participate in and lead interprofessional collaborative teams in efforts to improve health outcomes of the individual patient or target population (American Association of Colleges of Nursing [AACN], 2006b).

INTERPROFESSIONAL COLLABORATION

The terms *interdisciplinary* and *interprofessional* are often used interchangeably in the literature about collaborative teams, but each has a slightly different connotation. Interprofessional collaboration describes the interactions among individual professionals who may represent a particular discipline or branch of knowledge but who additionally bring their unique educational backgrounds, experiences, values, roles, and identities to the process. Each professional may possess some shared or overlapping knowledge, skills, abilities, and roles with other professionals with whom he or she collaborates. Hence, the term *interprofessional* offers a broader definition than *interdisciplinary*, which is more specific to the knowledge ascribed to a particular discipline. DNP-prepared nurses are suited to serve as effective collaborative team leaders and participants not only because of the scientific knowledge, skills, and abilities related to their distinctive advanced nursing practice disciplines but also because of their comprehension of organizational and systems improvements, outcome evaluation processes, healthcare policy, and leadership. This new skill set will be critical for DNP-prepared nurses leading teams in the complex and ever changing health arena. The AACN's (2006b) *Essentials of Doctoral Education for Advanced Nursing Practice* added that collaborative teams must remain "fluid depending upon the needs of the patient (population) . . . and [DNP-prepared nurses] must be prepared to play a central role in establishing interprofessional teams, participating in the work of the team and assuming leadership of the team when appropriate" (p. 14).

The concept of interprofessional collaborations to improve health outcomes is not new; it has been and continues to be the cornerstone of public health practice. Effective public health system collaborations are critical to protect populations from disease and injury and to promote health. Public health collaborations have involved not only vested professionals but also systems of communities, governmental agencies, nonprofit organizations, and private-sector groups to address a common goal or complex health outcome (Wilson & Bekemeir, 2004). DNP-prepared nurses can benefit from the experiences of public health colleagues and expand the definition of interprofessional panel collaboration. This is particularly relevant when considering potential stakeholders and in assembling the team. Successful implementation of a system or organizational improvement may require collaborations outside the typical healthcare team. The purpose or outcome of the project may dictate the need to include patient or family representation in accordance with their ability and willingness to participate, as well as professionals from information and technology, health policy, administration, governing boards, and library science.

INTERPROFESSIONAL HEALTHCARE TEAMS

Many healthcare practitioners indicate that they practice within an interprofessional team. Often, this involves each professional addressing a particular portion of patient or population care, working *independently of* and in parallel or in sequence with one another, with the physician frequently assuming the role of team leader (Robert Wood Johnson Foundation [RWJF], 2008). Drinka and Clark (2000) reinforced the need to function *interdependently* and engage in collaborative problem solving. All too often, competition exists between roles, with each discipline holding to the belief that it is the most qualified to manage the patient or problem, thus negatively influencing the functioning of the team. In effective interprofessional teams, members recognize and value dissimilar professional perspectives and overlapping roles, and they share decision making and leadership to best meet the needs of the patient or problem at hand (Drinka & Clark, 2000). To achieve optimal health outcomes, it is essential for DNP-prepared nurses and other health professionals to engage in true collaborative interprofessional practices. These types of collaborative practices are most successful when (1) the complexity of the problem is high, (2) the team shares a common goal or vision for the outcome, (3) members have distinct roles, (4) members recognize the value of each other's positions, and (5) each offers unique contributions toward the improved patient or population outcome (ACP, 2009; Drinka & Clark, 2000; RWJF, 2008). This model for interprofessional healthcare teams will require DNP-prepared nurses to have a thorough understanding of effective collaboration—in addition to a firm grounding in effective communication, team processes, and leadership—to bring forth innovative strategies to improve health and health care.

Benefits of Collaboration

The literature of the past two decades documents well the numerous benefits of collaborative practices, including reduced error, decreased lengths of stay, improved health, better pain management, improved quality of life, and higher patient satisfaction (Brita-Rossi et al., 1996; Chung & Nguyen, 2005; Cowan et al., 2006; D'Amour & Oandasan, 2005; Drinka & Clark, 2000; Grady & Wojner, 1996; IOM, 1999; The Joint Commission, 2008; Yeager, 2005). Nelson et al. (2002) and Sierchio (2003) noted the additional benefits to healthcare systems of cost savings and healthy work environments. High-performing collaborative teams promote job satisfaction (D'Amour & Oandasan, 2005; Hall, Weaver, Gravelle, & Thibault, 2007; Sierchio, 2003), support a positive workplace atmosphere, and provide a sense of accomplishment while valuing the unique work and contributions of team members. These issues

are particularly relevant to nursing practice. Addressing concerns of nursing shortages, improving working environments, and promoting measures to increase job satisfaction all have been found to correlate with lower rates of nurse burnout (Vahey, Aiken, Sloane, Clarke, & Vargas, 2004) and in turn indirectly influence nurse retention and recruitment.

The concept of "value added" has been discussed as an indirect benefit of effective collaboration (Dunevitz, 1997; Kleinpell et al., 2002). The term *value added* indicates the growth or improvement experienced in a group, project, or organization over a period, which yields an indirect "value" gained by a patient or population. Such value-added contributions may be the improvement to patient care delivery over time resulting from the rich professional interactions and exchanges that occur within an interprofessional team meeting. This enhanced communication would be more beneficial than is the communication required from professionals working independently of one another. Value-added benefits may additionally be evident from the process itself, such as the creative problem solving that occurs during a brainstorming session designed to address a community health problem.

Barriers to and Drivers of Effective Collaboration in Interprofessional Healthcare Teams

Barriers

In spite of the mandates or recommendations by the IOM, RWJF, ANA, and The Joint Commission, effective interprofessional collaboration has yet to be adopted in any widespread form in the United States to improve patient or population outcomes. Literature from both Canada and Britain also makes recommendations for interprofessional collaboration to improve care (Oandasan et al., 2004), along with current thinking as to why healthcare systems have not adopted interprofessional healthcare teams. Some of the barriers to interprofessional collaboration include (1) gender, power, socialization, education, status, and cultural differences between professions (Hall, 2005; Whitehead, 2007); (2) lack of a payment system and structures that reward interprofessional collaboration; (3) the misunderstanding of the scope and contribution of each profession; and (4) turf protection (Patterson, Grenny, McMillan, & Switzler, 2002). The DNP-prepared nurse needs a comprehensive understanding of these barriers to provide fresh, creative thinking and leadership for the healthy development and sustainment of collaboration.

Nursing and medicine were and are often considered central players in healthcare teams; an examination of the issues related to these two professions is prudent. Nurse and physician role differences are easier to understand in light of the historical roles of gender. In the 19th century, nurses cared for patients in hospitals, whereas physicians cared for patients in their offices or patients' homes. According to Lynnaugh and Reverby's (1990) *Ordered to Care: The Dilemma of American Nursing 1850–1945*, whereas physicians were "welcome visitors," hospitals were run by lay boards and often staffed by "live in" nurses (p. 26). That changed when medicine became more science oriented and doctors realized that hospitals were full of sick patients to whom they could apply their newly developed knowledge of science. Medicine soon controlled hospitals and defended this control with the argument that it owned "special knowledge" to diagnose and treat. Physicians were able to convince the public that nurses were not trustworthy enough to manage medications or capable of obtaining the "special knowledge" that physicians had (often because of the menstrual cycle). Nurses soon became handmaidens to physicians; they needed to be "self-less, knowledgeless and virtuous" (Gordon, 2005, p. 63).

Nursing education in the 20th century was designed to provide cheap labor for hospitals while educating its new workforce. Nurses came to view themselves as working for doctors, not patients. Nurses were valued for their virtue, not for their knowledge (Buresh & Gordon, 2006). Most nurse leaders either accepted this subjugated role or were unable to change it. As nursing lost power, medicine increased its social status by high-tech innovations in acute care (along with reimbursement for them). Healthcare delivery became fragmented based on physician specialty care for patients with acute care needs. Indeed, medicine dominated health care in the 20th century.

It can be argued that this physician-dominant, fragmented care has driven up healthcare costs, promoted polypharmacy, and encouraged "silo" practices. Wheatley (2005) compared organizations to the biological natural world. In the biological world, if a species becomes too dominant and loses its ability to work when the environment shifts, the entire system can collapse. According to *Healthy People 2020* (U.S. Department of Health and Human Services, 2010), the nation's healthcare system will be challenged to provide effective chronic disease prevention and treatment. The current system, which is based on episodic care, will not serve the needs of the population. To meet the needs of the early 21st century, DNP-prepared nurses will need to bring a full nursing perspective into the healthcare environment, along with the empowerment of other members of the team to improve the viability and strength of the healthcare system.

Physicians have also been closely aligned with the financial success of healthcare organizations (often hospitals) and therefore have often been designated leaders for any clinically based team. Even today, the ACP (2009) concluded that the "patient is best served by a multidisciplinary team where the clinical team is led by the physician" (p. 2). Although physicians may have the most training in diagnosis and treatment of disease, they may not always be the best choice to lead teams. Haas (1977) discussed the "cloak of competence" that is expected of physicians by society. Medical students are socialized to adopt this "cloak" or image of confidence and perceived competence to meet societal expectations and may bring this "decisiveness" to the interprofessional arena. This may lead the physician to believe that he or she must always make the final decision in the team, which may result in a professional power imbalance whereby physicians have more power than other members of the team do.

The issue of "disruptive behavior" in the workplace has been studied recently in light of the connection between poor communication and adverse events (The Joint Commission, 2008). Rosenstein's (2002) qualitative study of physician–nurse relations found that almost all nurses in the study experienced some sort of "disruptive physician behavior," including verbal abuse. Rosenstein and O'Daniel (2008) repeated this work, expanded to include disruptive behavior by both nurses and physicians. This second report concluded that whereas "physician disruptive behavior is usually more direct and overt, nurse disruptive behaviors more frequently take the form of back-door undermining, clique formation, and other types of passive-aggressive behavior" (Rosenstein & O'Daniel, 2008, p. 467).

In its *Essentials of Doctoral Education for Advanced Nursing Practice*, the AACN (2006b) discussed the need for interprofessional healthcare teams to function as high-performance teams. High-performance teams are those that emphasize the skills, abilities, and unique perspective of each team member. If the nurses (or other team members) remain invisible, the overall effectiveness of the team will be impaired.

To work on interprofessional teams, nurses need to articulate the role they play in improving patient care. The work that nurses perform is often not recognized by other healthcare professionals and reimbursement systems or found within the nomenclature of electronic health records. Many tasks that nurses perform are difficult to quantify, such as supporting a family

through a crisis. A vital responsibility of the DNP-prepared nurse (likely collaborating with other nursing PhD colleagues) is to articulate to the public, insurers, and policymakers the role that nurses play in promoting positive patient and family outcomes.

Another key factor in empowering nurses in interprofessional collaboration is the importance of role identification and clarity. In the United States, there is confusion about the education and titling of nurses. Although many states protect the title of "nurse," the public (including other healthcare professionals) continues to be confused about just who nurses are. Nurses in administration may not identify themselves as nurses, whereas some medical assistants may call themselves "nurses." Although the work that medical assistants do with patients is valuable, it is not nursing. The first step to getting our voices heard is to identify who we are and to call ourselves "nurses" at all levels. It is important that as nurses work to gain visibility and voice, they remain open to listening to other voices on the team.

Drivers

Successful Team Development What are the stages of development that transform groups of disparate professionals into high-performance teams? Tuckman and Jensen (1977) and many others believe that teams go through stages, including forming, storming, norming, performing, and adjourning. Amos, Hu, and Herrick (2005) recommended that nurses understand these developmental stages in order to promote the development of a successful team.

Forming is the stage when the team first comes together to serve a specific purpose. Team members come into the group as individuals and get to know each other while determining the mission of the team, along with their roles and responsibilities. The development of trust is key in this stage. Davoli and Fine (2004) suggested incorporating activities that are designed to show the human side of each team member, such as "icebreakers" or "member check-in" (p. 269).

In an interdisciplinary team, it is likely there are members from diverse professions, each with its own culture and language. An important first task of an interdisciplinary team is to discuss and understand the scope of each profession represented (Hall, 2005). It is likely there will be both overlap and diversity of function and skills among the professions. It is also important to develop a sense of shared language by reducing the use of professional jargon. Although it may be unintentional, jargon can prevent knowledge sharing, hinder communication, and promote power imbalances. Standardized tools such as SBAR (situation, background, assessment, and recommendation), developed and used by Kaiser Permanente, can be used by interprofessional teams for discussion and problem solving regarding patient situations (Leonard, Graham, & Bonacum, 2004).

In the *storming* stage, team members have not fully developed trust, and conflict inevitably arises. Within interprofessional teams, members come from diverse disciplines and worldviews. It is highly likely that there will be a wide range of opinions and thoughts related to the issues and work of the team. It is important to face this conflict directly, however, to move on to the next stage. During the storming stage, it is vital that members learn to listen to one another with tolerance and patience (Lee, 2008). If the team does not go through this stage successfully, differences between individuals will not be brought into the team process and outcome. Conflict resolution is discussed at length later in this chapter.

Norming is the stage in which team members begin to develop a team identity. It is still important for the team to elicit differences of opinion in order to prevent "groupthink."

In the *performing* stage, team members work together to achieve team goals. Individual and professional turf needs are set aside in order for the team to be effective in its mission. In this stage, the team members also learn to be flexible in tasks and roles in order to achieve the team's goals.

Finally, the stage of *adjourning* concludes the formation of a team. The team evaluates its performance and progress by reviewing whether outcomes were met.

The following factors assist teams to progress through the stages of team development:

- Shared purpose, goal, and buy-in of members
- Reciprocal trust in team members
- Recognition and value of the unique role or skills each brings
- Functioning at the highest level of skill, ability, or practice
- Clear understanding of roles and the responsibilities of team members to meet goals
- Work culture and environment that embrace the collaborative process
- Collective cognitive responsibility and shared decision making

Shared Purpose For a team to be effective, there must be a shared purpose or vision (Kouzes & Pozner, 2007). The purpose of the interprofessional healthcare team is based on improving some aspect of patient or population health outcomes. Competing needs of team members must be tabled in favor of the greater purpose. Turf wars and politicized thinking have no place in an effective interprofessional healthcare team. The leader must inspire this shared vision and elicit buy-in from each member. As Wheatley (2005) suggested, creativity is unleashed in people when they find "meaning" or purpose in "real" work. Meaningful teamwork can create synergistic solutions from members when the team has shared meaning or vision. Patterson et al. (2002) described how free-flowing dialogue helps "fill the pool" of shared meaning. By allowing dialogue to be safe, more people can add their meaning to the "shared pool," giving the group a higher IQ. Learning to make dialogue safe is a skill that drives trust.

Team Members and Reciprocal Trust An effective team must include the development of reciprocal trust between members. According to Kouzes and Pozner (2007), members of a high-trust team must continue to work to maintain interpersonal relationships with one another. In addition to the group mission and goals, the work of the group must also include getting to know one another. The leader or facilitator who is willing to trust others in the group enough to show vulnerability and give up control often creates a culture of trust. The leader must have enough self-confidence to be willing to be the first to be transparent; because trust is contagious, others will likely follow. Team members and leaders need to listen intently and value the unique viewpoints of others in the group. If the group fails to develop trust or to listen to and value each other, it is likely that group members will resist and sabotage the group's efforts (Wheatley, 2005). Many authors describe this aspect of team leadership as leading with the heart: looking at how the heart can help shape dialogue and goals (Kouzes & Pozner, 2007; Patterson et al., 2002).

Because of growth in global businesses, along with economic and time constraints, many teams now meet in virtual formats. Virtual formats can unite team members from different cultural groups and social constructs. The question many have is, What components are necessary to build trust in virtual teams? Kouzes and Pozner (2007) proposed that a group can only become a team when members have met face to face four to five times. These authors suggested that "virtual trust, like virtual reality, is one step removed from the real thing" (Kouzes & Pozner, 2007, p. 241). Other sources discussed the very real possibility of developing trust via virtual means (Grabowski & Roberts, 1999; Greenberg, Greenberg, & Antonucci, 2007; Kirkman, Rosen, Gibson, Tesluk, & McPherson, 2002). Mayer, Davis, and Schoorman (1995) proposed that trust consists of three dimensions: ability, benevolence, and integrity. There is some

evidence that when teams meet face to face, they form trust based on benevolence, whereas virtual teams rely more on ability. For example, in teams that meet in person, benevolence or interpersonal trust is enhanced by informal personal meetings that occur at lunch or in the copy room. Virtual groups tend to develop trust based on performance and ability of team members.

Because of the lack of eye contact and body language in virtual interactions, communication patterns should be more deliberate. Greenberg et al. (2007) proposed that trust building in virtual teams intentionally includes activities that promote both cognitive and affective trust. Cognitive trust is implicated in the formation of "swift, but fragile trust" during the early development of the team (Greenberg et al., 2007, p. 325). For cognitive trust to develop, individual team members need to believe that group members have both ability (competence) and integrity. One action to promote a sense of competence in individual team members is to have the team leader introduce members and endorse their abilities and why they were chosen for the team. Another important asset for building the sense of integrity is for team members to keep deadlines and stay engaged in the process (no freeloading). Affective trust is essential during later stages of the team's development and is vital to the functioning of team members in order to complete the task. Development of affective trust is based on benevolence and relies on team members seeing the humanity in one another, with development of true caring and concern.

Holton (2001) recommended that virtual teams include time in "caring talk," which she defined as "personal conversations and story-telling" (p. 36). G. Boehlhower (personal communication, April 10, 2009) recommended that virtual teams begin their meeting time with "check in, story-telling, deep questioning and dialogue, and affirmation." He went on to state that he "sees the level of trust develop regularly" in online groups when the human side of individuals is shared. As discussed earlier in this chapter, this type of sharing may be started with icebreakers, check-ins, and checkouts.

DNPs will likely gain experience with online relationship building during their education and can continue to experiment with team building in face-to-face and virtual formats based on the current evidence. The use of video conferencing (which includes visual and nonverbal cues) enhances the richness of communication and thus decreases ambiguity and increases trust. It may be that the communication channel (face to face, video or audio conferencing, group chat, text, email, etc.) should be matched to the purpose of the communication (Clark, Clark, & Crossley, 2010).

Recognition and Value of Each Team Member According to Burkhardt and Alvita (2008), "Each person is a moral agent and must be recognized as worthy of dignity and respect" (p. 219). Without respect, the work of the group cannot move forward; dialogue is halted. Respect among team members is vital because, as Patterson et al. (2002) noted, "Respect is like air. If it goes away, it is all people can think about" (p. 71). Each member's voice must be heard and respected whether he or she is the highest educated member or not. To do this, team members must recognize, often on the basis of an individual's professional skill set, the moral agency of each member and his or her unique skills and abilities.

Using structure in interprofessional team dialogue may be called for as a result of the entrenched perceived power and authority of individual members and the professions they represent. Such methods as the Indian talking stick and Johari window can be used proactively to be sure that all team members feel they have a voice, are understood, and are free to share their thoughts and feelings. The concept behind the talking stick is that only the person who is holding the stick may speak. When the person finishes speaking, the stick is passed to the next speaker. That next person may not argue or disagree with the former speaker, but is to restate what has been said. This process allows for all team members to be and feel understood (Covey, 2004).

The Johari window is a tool developed in 1955 by Joseph Luft and Harry Ingham (Chapman, 2008). It is used to help build trust among group members by encouraging appropriate self-disclosure. The Johari window has four quadrants: the open area, the blind area, the hidden area, and the unknown area. The goal is to increase the open area so that team members can be more productive because communication is not hampered by "distractions, mistrust, confusion, conflict and misunderstanding" (Chapman, 2008, p. 4). One team member (the subject) is given a list of 55 adjectives and is told to pick 5 or 6 that describe himself or herself. Another team member is given the same list and also picks out 5 or 6 words that describe the subject. The adjectives are then placed in the four quadrants (Chapman, 2008):

1. Both team members know the open area.
2. Only the subject, not the other team member, knows the hidden area.
3. Only the team member, not the subject, knows the blind spot.
4. The unknown area includes adjectives picked by neither subject nor team member and may or may not be applicable to the subject.

The Johari tool can assist team members to learn about themselves and each other. Appropriate and sensitive increases in the open area can be promoted by the use of team-building exercises and games, along with teams engaging in nonworktime activities.

Functioning at the Highest Level American health care is expensive, but not always effective. There is pressure for innovative models of care that are cost effective and that improve outcomes for patients. Many clinical systems have begun to use episodic treatment groups (ETGs) to measure patient outcomes and provider performance (Fortham, Dove, & Wooster, 2000). Examples of ETGs are those for chronic diseases such as diabetes, asthma, depression, and hypertension. Guideline development by such groups as the Institute for Clinical Systems Integration (ICSI) can provide evidence-based pathways of care for the various ETGs.

In the past, physicians have felt the need to perform all the primary care tasks for patients. Given the current complexity and expense of health care, it is not possible for one group to do it all. This realization has led to the concept of having all healthcare providers work to the top of their licenses. This involves a shifting of tasks, often with each discipline giving up some tasks that can be done by another care provider more cost effectively. An example of working to the top of one's license is for advanced practice nurses to take more responsibility for routine chronic and acute care and health maintenance, while physicians perform the diagnosing and treatment of more complex unstable patients, and registered nurses (RNs) assume the roles of care coordinator (including pre- and postvisit planning), coach, and educator. In this example, all disciplines may need to give up some tasks in order to be cost effective. An exemplar of a program that utilizes healthcare providers at the top of their licenses is the DIAMOND (Depression Improvement Across Minnesota—Offering a New Direction) project (Institute for Clinical Systems Integration [ICSI], 2007). At the center of the DIAMOND project is a case manager (typically an RN) who has 150 to 200 patients with depression in an outpatient setting. The case manager works with a consulting psychiatrist to review patients on a weekly basis (typically 2 hours per week). This has proven to be a cost-effective model that provides better depression outcomes than standard care does. The challenge is to provide a payment structure that rewards this type of innovative care.

Clear Understanding of Roles and Responsibilities During the forming stage of the team (and beyond), it is vital that each team member understand his or her role and responsibilities. Role uncertainty can lead to conflict among team members and decrease team functioning (Baker, Baker, & Campbell, 2003). The leader should be certain that each team member has a clear understanding of his or her role by having the members restate their role to the team. This type of candid discussion can occur only if the team feels that open communication is safe. A clear understanding of each team member's role helps to prevent role overlap as well as tasks falling through the cracks (Lewis, 2007).

Work Culture That Embraces Collaboration Some of the components of a work culture that embraces collaboration are (1) providing psychological safety, (2) a flattened power differential (hierarchy), (3) administrative support and resultant resources allocated for collaboration (Kelly, 2008), and (4) physical space design that promotes collaboration, such as rooms for interdisciplinary interaction (Lindeke & Sieckert, 2005).

According to Edmonson (2006), organizations that support "upward voice" promote a culture of psychological safety. She went on to state that "upward voice is communication directed to someone higher in the organizational hierarchy with perceived power or authority to take action on the problem or suggestion" (p. 1). Some tangible evidence of this is leaders who walk around the organization and initiate conversation, suggestion boxes placed around the organization, and an open door policy. Individuals must have the sense that they can readily ask questions, try out new ideas and innovations, and ask for support from others.

Another way to promote psychological safety within an organization is by inspiring employee confidence in the fact that there will not be a penalty for admitting to mistakes. Safety culture research is shifting from focusing on only the role of individuals in errors to the role of systems. Healthcare leaders have had to explore other industry successes that promote safety, such as in aviation, where the focus of safety improvement is on the systems in which individuals operate (Feldman, 2008). Authors such as Snijders, Kollen, Van Lingen, Fetter, and Molendijik (2009) have recommended a nonpunitive incident-reporting system to improve safety standards. A nonpunitive incident-reporting system helps ensure that issues are brought to the forefront so that improvements can be made. The Agency for Healthcare Research and Quality (2009) has developed evaluation tools for primary care offices, nursing homes, and hospitals with questions related to psychological safety and communication. DNPs are required to provide leadership and recommend resources to champion the culture of both psychological and systems safety within the organizations they serve.

Collective Cognitive Responsibility and Shared Decision Making As fundamental as it is for each team member to have a clear understanding of individual roles and responsibilities, it is also essential for high-performance teams to have a culture of shared decision making or collective cognitive responsibility. Scardamalia (2002) described collective cognitive responsibility in terms of team members having responsibility not only for the outcome of the group but also for staying cognitively involved in the process as things unfold. She described the functioning of a surgical team, in which members not only perform their assigned tasks but also stay involved in the entire process. The responsibility for the outcome lies not just with the leader of the surgical team but with the entire team as a whole.

A key component of shared decision making is that it usually occurs at the point of service (Golanowski, Beaudry, Kurz, Laffey, & Hook, 2007; Porter-O'Grady, 1997). Porter-O'Grady stated that "the point of decision making in the clinical delivery system is the place where patients and providers meet" (p. 41), which has implications for including patients as collaborators on the interprofessional team.

Healthcare systems, as complex adaptive systems, require flexibility and continuous participation, learning, and sharing (Begun, Zimmerman, & Dooley, 2003). All the interprofessional healthcare team members must stay engaged in the process at the point of service for the outcome of care to be successful.

STRONG LEADERSHIP

There is no dispute that redesigning health care will require strong leadership. As opposed to "management," which seeks to control and manage, leaders seek to create and inspire change (Kotter, 1990). Leadership theories generally fall under the classifications of behavioral, contingency, contemporary, and Wheatley's "new leadership" approaches (Kelly, 2008). Behavioral theories posit that leadership style or behavior is the most important factor in the outcome desired. Behavioral approaches include autocratic, democratic, and laissez-faire, based on where the power or decision making occurs and the type of worker or task involved. Contingency theories recognize that there is more to leadership than the leader's behavior. One type of contingency theory is situational leadership, developed by Hershey and Blanchard (Blanchard, 2008), in which follower maturity is evaluated and determines the amount of direction, support, or delegation from the leader to the follower. Contemporary theories include transformational leadership, which the IOM (2003) deemed vital to the achievement of the transformation of health care.

Transformational Leadership

The IOM (2003) report recommended transformational leadership to make the necessary changes to improve patient safety. Transformational leadership, developed first by Burns (1978), is based on the concept of empowering all team members (including the leader) to work together to achieve a shared goal. This fits with Covey's (2004) definition of leadership: "Leadership is communicating to people their worth and potential so clearly that they come to see it in themselves" (p. 98).

The transformational leader need not be in a formal position of administration, but can lead from any position within the organization and operates through an ethical and moral perspective. Transformational leaders lead with a clear vision and use coaching, inspiring, and mentoring to transform themselves, followers, and organizations (Burns, 1978; Kelly, 2008).

Complexity Leadership or "New Leadership"

Complexity leadership is the name given to the new paradigm of thinking about leadership that unites science and management to solve problems. Complexity has contributions from chaos theory and similarities to the thinking of such nurse theorists as Rogers, Newman, and Watson (Crowell, 2011). Margaret Wheatley (2005) described this "new way" of leadership, which is contrary to the Western style of linear, hierarchical organizations. She bases her view of organizations on biology, which is self-organizing and complex. Instead of seeing change as negative, Wheatley views change as life itself. She stated, "Nothing alive, including us, resists creative motions. However, all of life resists control. All of life reacts to any process that inhibits its freedom to create itself" (p. 28). She recommended that teams self-organize to build communities that are no longer ruled by "command and control" (p. 68). Wheatley suggested that instead of viewing organizations and workers as machines, organizations model themselves after living systems, which are adaptive, creative, and depend on one another for growth and sustainability.

Leadership Versus Management

Whereas management is the coordination of resources to meet organizational goals,

leadership is built on relationships. Kouzes and Pozner (2007), in their seminal book *The Leadership Challenge*, examined leaders over 25 years and determined that leadership is a relationship in which leaders do five things:

1. *Model the way.* The leader must be aware of his or her own values and live a life that expresses those values.
2. *Inspire a shared vision.* The leader must be able to imagine the future and inspire others to share that vision.
3. *Challenge the process.* Leaders are engaged in the processes of the team and continually looking for innovations. They are willing to take risks and learn from experiences.
4. *Enable others to act.* Leaders help to build trust in relationships through collaboration and competence.
5. *Encourage the heart.* Leaders identify the contributions of each individual team member and encourage celebration when victories occur.

Anyone can be a leader; a formal title is not necessary.

EFFECTIVE COMMUNICATION

> Remember not only to say the right thing in the right place, but far more difficult still, to leave unsaid the wrong thing at the tempting moment.
>
> —Benjamin Franklin

All the work of interprofessional collaborations involves communication. Success or failure of the team is dependent on the effectiveness of the communication processes. Communication is a complex process of transmitting a message from a sender to a receiver. The sender must effectively deliver the content, and the receiver must in turn correctly interpret or decipher the message. Many errors can occur within this exchange, and skilled communicators must make a concerted effort to deliver clear, consistent messages to prevent misinterpretation and loss of meaning.

Communication is more than the exchange of verbal information; in fact, the majority of communication is nonverbal. The DNP must be accomplished not only in the art of verbal and written communication but also in the interpretation and effective use of nonverbal communiqués such as silence, gestures, facial expressions, body language, tone of voice, and space (Sullivan, 2004).

In addition to sending congruent verbal and nonverbal messages, it is vital for DNPs to employ strategies that enhance communication within the interprofessional team setting. Determining the timing and best medium for what, how, and when to deliver a message is a necessary skill (Sullivan, 2004). Appropriate timing of key messages increases the likelihood that the message will have the desired impact on the recipient. The message may be phrased well but rejected if the intended audience is not receptive. Consider the availability and state of mind of the recipient. Is there adequate time for the discussion? Is the recipient distracted, emotionally or physically? Are other issues more pressing now? Such factors may contribute to misinterpretation or lack of objectivity regarding the communication. DNPs must reflect on whether an alternate time, venue, or medium may provide a more appropriate means by which to deliver the message. For instance, if the message is of a sensitive, confidential matter, face-to-face communication would be preferable to an email message, voicemail correspondence, or team discussion (Sullivan, 2004). In group settings, it is imperative to allow participants enough time to provide objective information and express thoughts, viewpoints, and opinions about the situation in order for meaningful collaboration to occur.

Buresh and Gordon (2006), in their book *From Silence to Voice: What Nurses Know and Must Communicate to the Public*, suggest the use of the "voice of agency" when communicating the role of nursing to others. Within the collaborative team, it is imperative that DNP members

clearly communicate nursing's involvement in a patient care scenario or clinical project and, more important, articulate the level of clinical judgment and rationale required for such actions. It is important and necessary to embrace the opportunity to communicate to the team the role of the DNP in enhanced care delivery. This voice of agency is not boastful nor an attempt to be superior, but rather an accurate acknowledgment of the unique contributions, value added, and improved patient outcomes resulting from expert nursing care. Conversely, it may reflect the negative consequences or potential for error averted as a result of the expertise, skills, and knowledge of doctorally prepared nurses. Davoli and Fine (2004) offered a similar perspective and noted, "Collaboration gives providers an opportunity to be introspective and solidify their role through the contributions they make. A successful collaborative process will enhance one's professional identity" (p. 268). Draye, Acker, and Zimmer (2006), in their article on the practice doctorate in nursing, proposed that the educational preparation of DNPs include opportunity for the student to convene an interprofessional team. This experience allows the student to incorporate strategies to promote effective team functioning while communicating the unique contributions of nursing required for the improved health outcome.

Buresh and Gordon (2006) went on to discuss the role that self-presentation plays in communicating information regarding the competency and credibility of the DNP to team members, patients, or the public. Attire and manner of address influence the perceptions of others. What does dress communicate if Mary wears teddy bear scrubs rather than street clothes and a lab coat to a committee meeting? How might the DNP's role be valued if she were introduced as Mary from pediatrics versus Dr. Mary Jones, pediatric nurse practitioner? How are physician colleagues addressed in similar workplace encounters? Introductions using one's full name and credentials convey professionalism, respect, and credibility on par with other healthcare professional colleagues (Buresh & Gordon, 2006).

Ineffective communication is a major obstacle in interprofessional collaboration, is directly related to quality of patient care, and contributes to adverse health outcomes (Clarin, 2007; IOM, 1999). Some barriers that lead to communication breakdowns are specific to interactions between the sender and receiver, whereas others relate to the organizational system. Defensiveness on the part of either participant can hamper communications (Sullivan, 2004). These behaviors may result from lack of self-confidence, a fear of rejection, or perceived threat to self-image or status. Defensiveness impedes communication by displacing anger via verbal aggression or conflict avoidance. Awareness of this mechanism and developing an approach to manage it in the context of the collaborative team are necessary attributes of an effective DNP leader.

As healthcare teams become more global and virtual, the potential for language and cultural communication barriers increases. Misreading body language or misinterpretation of the spoken or written message often results from a lack of understanding regarding language (especially in translation) and cultural differences (Sullivan, 2004). What one group finds acceptable another may consider offensive, such as eye contact, physical touch, or the use of space. Room for misinterpretation exists in translation. Language used by Western cultures typically is direct and explicit, in which the background is not necessarily required to interpret the meaning of the message. This may differ from cultures that use indirect communication, in which the intent of the message often relies on the context in which it is used (Brett, Behfar, & Kern, 2006). DNPs and interprofessional colleagues have an obligation to increase their cultural competence and understanding of health issues and healthcare disparities to dispel any misconceptions, particularly if the team is composed of persons from diverse cultures.

Jargon is another "language" that can pose a barrier to understanding (Davoli & Fine, 2004; Sullivan, 2004). Unfamiliar terms can lead to confusion and error and should be avoided to prevent unfavorable outcomes. Although professional jargon may serve as a type of verbal shorthand among some group members, it can also be a form of intimidation or exclusion and contribute to an imbalance of knowledge or power within the team (Davoli & Fine, 2004). Lindeke and Block (2001) stressed that collaborative teams communicate with a shared, inclusive (i.e., "we," "our") language to prevent this imbalance and promote participation of all members. Effective communication involves the use of a common, shared language that is understood by all members of the team.

Preconceived assumptions and biases prevent the listener from tuning in and focusing on the content (Sullivan, 2004). This hinders the communication process because the receiver has formulated a predetermined judgment or drawn a conclusion before all the information is shared or facts validated. Effective communicators need to suspend judgments until all viewpoints are shared.

Gender differences in style and approach to communication can also pose obstacles (Sullivan, 2004). Subtle differences exist in how men and women perceive the same message. In collaborative teams, women may strive for consensus, whereas men may place emphasis on hierarchy and "leading the team." Differences exist in the use of questions and interruptions in communications. An appreciation and understanding of these dissimilarities can prepare the DNP to function more effectively in teams of mixed gender.

Organizations and systems may pose additional obstacles to effective interprofessional communications. Outdated, limited, or unavailable technologies, such as video

TABLE 6-1	Measures to Improve Communication

- Maintain eye contact: Convey interest, attentiveness. (United States/Canada)
- Speak concisely: Avoid jargon.
- Use questions wisely: Clarify or elicit further information.
- Avoid qualifiers or tags (e.g., "sort of," "kind of," "I don't know if you would be interested"): These reduce the effectiveness of one's message.
- Be aware of gestures, facial expressions, posture: Send positive nonverbal signals (e.g., smiling conveys warmth, leaning forward indicates receptivity, and open-palm gestures suggest accessibility).
- Avoid defensiveness.
- Avoid responding emotionally: Never raise your voice, yell, or cry.

conferencing, messaging, or paging systems, or lack of electronic health record interoperability between systems can significantly impair the ability of members to communicate on a timely basis. This can be of vital importance to patient safety when attempting to communicate critical changes in patient status, medications, or lab values. The system further contributes to communication problems when the roles and responsibilities of team members are unclear. Participants may be hesitant or resistant to engage in exchanges or knowledge sharing. Clear designation of roles is of particular importance in virtual organizations and teams (i.e., electronically linked providers). In these collaborative environments, risks can be mitigated if members have a clear understanding of what is expected of each other and have a preestablished path of communication (Grabowski & Roberts, 1999) (see **Table 6-1**).

CONFLICT RESOLUTION

As both leaders and members of interprofessional teams, DNPs need to develop and continue to refine skills related to conflict resolution. Conflicts are inevitable and are even vital for interprofessional team effectiveness. *Conflict* is defined in many ways but generally includes disagreement, interference, and negative emotion (Barki & Hartwick, 2001). If conflict is disruptive or dysfunctional, team efforts can decrease communication and thus team functioning. On the other hand, conflict that is constructive leads to superior results by including the "shared pool of meaning" of all team members. According to Patterson et al. (2002), the "larger the shared pool, the smarter the decisions" (p. 21).

As stated earlier, nurses over the last century have often used passive-aggressive methods to resolve conflict, such as avoidance, withholding, smoothing over, and compromising (Feldman, 2008). These methods do not promote dialogue, the most central means to attain the shared pool of meaning of the entire team. DNPs need to lead nurses and other professionals in techniques that promote dialogue and thus collaboration between professionals. The purposes of collaborative conflict management are to promote win-win versus win-lose solutions. The skills for conflict resolution and improving dialogue can be learned. According to Patterson et al. (2002) in their book *Crucial Conversations*, conflict resolution includes such methods as starting with the heart, making conversation safe, staying in dialogue when emotions are high, using persuasion, and promoting positive actions. Most of the skills related to collaborative conflict management are intertwined with effective communication skills and the development of emotional intelligence.

Chinn (2008) offered suggestions that are foundational for the transformation of conflict into solidarity and diversity. These recommendations begin before there is any conflict in a group or team and include rotating leadership, practicing critical reflection, and adopting customs to value diversity. By rotating leadership, the team members all have a stake in the outcome of the team goals and processes. When a conflict arises, involved parties can step back while other members rise up to help lead the team. Critical reflection can be accomplished by incorporating a closing time at which all team members can share their thoughts and feelings about the team process. By practicing ways to value diversity, such as developing team processes during meetings that show appreciation and value for each individual, conflict can move from violence to peaceful recognition of the diversity of alternative views.

EMOTIONAL INTELLIGENCE

Emotional intelligence (EI) is yet another valuable attribute of successful interprofessional leadership. EI is the awareness of the role that emotion plays in personal relationships and the purposeful use of emotion to communicate, build rapport, and motivate self and others. These characteristics have been found to play a far greater role than cognitive abilities in the success or failure of a leader (Goleman, Boyzatsis, & McKee, 2002).

Goleman et al. (2002) outlined five realms of EI: self-awareness, self-regulation, motivation, empathy, and social skills. Self-awareness involves recognizing your own emotions and the effect your mood and confidence level have on persons. Maintaining your composure in high-emotion meetings or challenging clinical situations is an example of effectual

self-regulation. Conflict is a natural process of interprofessional teamwork, which can lead to positive or negative group functioning, depending on leadership style. Emotionally intelligent leaders have the ability to adapt, withhold judgment, and exhibit self-control in emotionally charged situations. An optimistic attitude, passion, and commitment to pursuing the goals of the group and desire for excellence help provide the motivation factor of EI. Leaders who are sensitive and empathetic to the needs and perspectives of others encourage the group to carry on and perform to its best ability.

Drinka and Clark (2000) talked about the role of "reflective practice" in interprofessional team practice. This concept builds on the self-awareness and empathy qualities of EI: the understanding of how our professional cultures, preparations, and experiences shape how we function in teams, as well as the ability to appreciate the similar and dissimilar perspectives of other interprofessional team members.

A fifth element is that of social skill: the ability to build rapport, network, communicate, and facilitate change. As an effective leader, it is imperative to foster a system of open, timely communication—whether by face-to-face communication, phone, or electronic means—to meet the desired outcomes for the project, patient, or population successfully. Regularly practicing relaxation techniques and rehearsing responses prior to anticipated stressful encounters allow one to manage reactions in an emotionally intelligent manner. DNPs can develop these skills with regular practice, self-reflection, coaching, and feedback from colleagues and can use "EQ" (emotional intelligence quotient) as a tool to gauge their performance as leaders.

McCallin and Bamford (2007) suggested that EI is integral to effective interdisciplinary team functioning. Healthcare providers may be highly skilled in practicing emotionally intelligent interactions with their patients and families but may receive little preparation in promoting emotionally intelligent, healthy communication and functioning between professionals. Miller et al. (2008) specifically explored the role of EI in nursing practice as it relates to interprofessional team functioning. In this qualitative study, the ability of the nurse to effectively collaborate on interprofessional teams was influenced by his or her degree of EI. Nurses who engaged in *esprit de corps* (significant role embracing to the exclusion of other professionals) were considerably less able to function successfully on the team, less able to have other members appreciate nursing's contribution to patient care, and generally less engaged in team processes. These researchers support the need to address not only the cognitive aspects of interprofessional teamwork but also the emotional aspects of optimal team functioning. DNP leaders versed in EI work are well suited to recognize individual and personality differences among team members and can build on them, mentor colleagues, and use EI to influence the effectiveness of the team and improve patient outcomes and satisfaction among interprofessional team members.

NECESSITIES FOR COLLABORATION

Change Agent: Lewin's Model

The objective of interprofessional collaboration is, of course, to generate a practice or systems enhancement to improve the health of an individual or population. Whether implementing an evidence-based practice effort or a quality improvement initiative, some sort of change is required. Even what many group members view as a desirable change will inevitably encounter some reluctance or resistance. The ability to facilitate change or serve as an agent of change is a key function required for successful collaboration. DNPs must be versed in one or more theories of change to effectively motivate and move the collaborative team to the optimal goal.

Lewin's (1951) force field analysis model is a classic framework for understanding the process of change within a group, system, or health initiative. Lewin's theory recognizes change as a constant factor of life ensuing from a dynamic balance of driving and opposing forces. The desired change results from the addition of driving forces or the diminishing of opposing forces and progresses over a series of three stages: unfreezing, moving, and refreezing. Unfreezing necessitates assessing the need and preparing members to move from the status quo to an improved level of practice, whereas the movement phase involves the addition of driving forces to motivate and empower members to adopt the improved perspective while simultaneously minimizing restraining forces that pose barriers to the desired change (Lewin, 1951; Miller, 2008). Driving forces must outweigh opposing forces to shift the equilibrium in the direction of the desired change. The improvements must then be secured, or allowed to refreeze, in order to maintain the desired change (Lewin, 1951; Miller, 2008).

Continuous Reflective Learning

The drivers of effective interprofessional teams discussed in this chapter evolve in teams over time. Knowing the drivers is the first step in the development of both personal and team skills, but individual team members and the team as a whole need continuous reflection. Each leader and follower should develop habits that build in time for personal reflection and growth. Many find that reading sacred texts or poetry, listening to music, practicing yoga, praying, meditating, exercising, connecting with spiritual leaders, or being in nature allow for deep, reflective thinking and learning. Covey (1991) called this "sharpening the saw" (p. 38) and recommended that people proactively plan for daily time to renew themselves. The wholeness of each team member is vital for the best functioning of the entire team.

Teams within healthcare organizations in the 21st century will need to practice continuous reflective learning (developed by Senge, 1990) to adapt to the rapid changes taking place. Interprofessional teams can utilize the vast organizational behavior research on the significance of continuous reflective learning. Edmonson (1999) defined team learning as "the activities carried out by team members through which a team obtains and processes data that allow it to adapt and change" (p. 352). Spending some time on reflection regarding team functioning is vital to learning. Structural practices that foster team learning include providing time during each meeting for reflection, leaving the worksite for retreats, conducting "critical incident" evaluations, discussing errors and failures, using patient satisfaction surveys and interviews, and celebrating successes.

The Patient and Family as Interprofessional Team Members

As health care reorganizes into interprofessional teams in which primary care is the hub of the system, central team members will be patients and their families. Patients and their families will need to be invited into and supported in the interprofessional collaboration process through actions that promote meaningful dialogue, patient empowerment, self-efficacy, and activation (Hibbard, Stockard, Mahoney, & Tusler, 2004). Some tools the DNP may want to recommend include patient or family focus groups, satisfaction surveys, personal health records, decisional guides such as the *Ottawa Personal Decision Guide* (O'Connor, 2006), and advance directives, along with ongoing patient education regarding the patients' and families' role in health care.

MODELS FOR IMPLEMENTATION: FROM PROJECT TO PRACTICE

Value of Incorporating Collaborative Work into Educational Preparation Curricula

Although there is a growing body of evidence regarding the benefits of collaboration between disciplines in the delivery of optimal patient care, few healthcare professionals have received any formal training in this concept during their educational preparation. Students in health professional programs often are taught in both the classroom and clinical setting by faculty from the same professional background. They have little opportunity to learn about the work of other disciplines or participate in any shared learning experience. Brewer (2005) described this pattern of education as "silo" preparation, in which each discipline believes it is best qualified to care for the patient. Without a formal structure and support for learning and practicing a team approach to care delivery in the educational setting, negative attitudes, prejudices, and misunderstanding of roles can occur. These contribute to an inability to collaborate effectively and to consult with other providers as practicing professionals and may lead to discipline overlap and competition rather than collaboration for delivery of care.

A Cochrane systematic review of interprofessional education interventions (Reeves et al., 2008) examined six studies—four randomized controlled and two controlled before-and-after designs in a variety of settings. Interprofessional education was defined as any type of educational experience or learning opportunity in which interactive learning occurred between two or more health-related disciplines. Although a number of positive outcomes were noted, further rigorous studies are needed to draw conclusive evidence supporting core elements of interprofessional education and the subsequent impact of interprofessional collaborative education on health outcomes.

In an effort to increase the ability of health professional teams to deliver optimal patient care, RWJF funded educational programs (Partnerships for Quality Education [PQE]) designed to improve interprofessional collaboration, chronic disease management, systems-based care, and quality (RWJF, 2008). These initiatives were developed to provide nurse practitioners, physicians, and other allied healthcare providers with educational experiences, skills, and attitudes to deliver better quality care than could be provided by any single discipline. One funded model was Collaborative Interprofessional Team Education (CITE); the objective of this program was to design collaborative clinical and educational interventions for health professional students from medicine, nursing, social work, and pharmacy (RWJF, 2008). The program did make some strides toward improvement in participants' understanding of and attitudes toward other professions.

Whitehead (2007) offered some insight into the challenges of engaging medical students in interprofessional educational programs. Real and perceived power, high degree of status, professional socialization, and decision-making responsibility can limit the ability of physicians to collaborate with other members of the healthcare team unless efforts to change the culture, flatten hierarchy, and share responsibility are promoted. A number of additional obstacles prevented full implementation of the CITE initiative, including differing academic schedules and a lack of faculty practicing in teams to effectively mentor and model for students (RWJF, 2008).

The primary objective of Achieving Competence Today (ACT), another PQE initiative, was to promote interprofessional collaboration and quality improvement in the curriculum of healthcare professionals within two academic health centers (Ladden, Bednash, Stevens, & Moore, 2006; RWJF, 2008). Four disciplines worked jointly to plan and implement a quality improvement project. As a result, core competencies necessary for successful interprofessional teams were identified, and researchers suggested measures for incorporating these competencies into the educational preparation of future students as a means to improve quality and safety in health care.

DNP programs can build on concepts of interprofessional education by allowing and encouraging programs to use faculty from a variety of disciplines to prepare DNP students. Interprofessional faculty can add a depth and richness to the DNP curriculum by bringing and sharing skills, knowledge, and the highest level of expertise in areas of clinical practice—whether it be business and management, pharmacy, public policy, psychology, medicine, or informatics (AACN, 2006a). Educational experience related to interprofessional collaboration as a means to improve quality or promote safety should be highly visible within the scholarly DNP project.

Role of the Scholarly Project: Real Interdisciplinary Collaboration

The Essentials of Doctoral Education for Advanced Nursing Practice (AACN, 2006b) refers to the final DNP scholarly project or capstone as a culminating immersion experience that affords the opportunity to integrate and synthesize all elements of doctoral education competencies within an interprofessional work environment. DNP-led scholarly projects provide a venue for students to assume leadership roles for effective interprofessional collaboration to improve health care, patient outcomes, and healthcare systems.

The DNP project "Optimal Use of Individualized Asthma Action Plans in an Electronic Health Record" (Miller, 2008) involved a number of opportunities for interprofessional collaboration. This process improvement project involved a systems change designed to improve pediatric asthma care delivery in a regional health system. An asthma action plan tool built into the electronic health record of a multispecialty regional health system served as a vehicle for the delivery of evidence-based practice. Distinct DNP-led interprofessional teams collaborated during various stages of program planning, implementation, and evaluation. Collaboration with nursing professionals and professionals in the fields of informatics, information technology, statisticians, and management was active throughout the project, particularly during tool development and in the implementation phase. Key to ensuring effective communication within this group was using a common language and developing a clear understanding of each other's roles and contributions. A second opportunity for interprofessional collaboration occurred during the implementation phase. Each member of the pediatric asthma team—the DNP, clinical nurse specialist, and physician—came to the project with his or her own agenda and perspective. Frequent revisiting of desired project outcomes, goals, and objectives was necessary early on to develop a cohesive, unified collaboration.

A third DNP-led collaboration took place at the pilot project site, a regional primary care clinic. This collaboration, which initially presented many challenges, involved physicians, nursing, administrative management, and administrative support. This site had recently been acquired by the parent organization. Previous quality improvement initiatives had been attempted and, because of a variety of factors, were not successfully implemented. A number of barriers to collaboration were anticipated at this site, including a sense of mistrust and resistance to change. Building trusting, nonthreatening relationships with staff and providers was a much needed starting point. Issues of power were foreseeable between the physicians and the project manager. Initially, this group expressed hesitancy with the concept of anyone other than the physician being responsible for the optimal delivery of pediatric asthma care. It is important to acknowledge that providers might experience competing loyalties as they struggle to prioritize and balance the additional time needed to implement a project along with time required to see other patients or perform other duties. Avoiding these barriers requires mutual respect for each other's role, purpose, and workload. It is vital to continually clarify and communicate the shared vision of the collaborative project—in this case, improved asthma care for children. Building relationships, seeking team

member input, and developing a shared vision play critical roles in negotiating hurdles for interprofessional collaboration and for effective project implementation and evaluation.

In the DNP project "Developing a Population-Focused Student Health Service" (Ash, 2005), interprofessional collaboration morphed from providers within the student health services (SHS) to a broad range of professionals. The ecological approach (NASPA, 2004) was used in the final stages of the student DNP project, which broadened the stakeholders and thus the collaborating professionals. The ecological perspective views the connections between health and learning within the campus setting (Sacher et al., 2005). The initial task force led by the DNP student included a project mentor who was an expert in group work as a result of his education and experience as a master of social work. His skills in the so-called softer side of team development molded the experience by bringing all the team members into the process. He was also continually willing to try new approaches and then evaluate the outcomes. He had direct access to the vice president of student affairs, who was also known to be innovative and skilled in human relationships because of his background in counseling. A current DNP student project, which is an offshoot of the former project, is preventing chronic disease through screening, nonpharmacologic and pharmacologic interventions, and healthcare coaching. This project will include nonhealthcare team members (coaches) to facilitate the attainment of healthcare goals.

Unlike many healthcare-related projects, there were no physicians on the interprofessional team. This may have changed the leadership and political issues that have plagued nurse–physician relationships in the past. The DNP student may have struggled to lead a team that included a physician. If, however, a physician was part of the team, increased efforts could have been made to develop reciprocal trust and to recognize and value each profession. Having a physician from outside the college may have afforded an opportunity for increased networking of the interprofessional team within the community in which the college is situated.

Some of the drivers of interprofessional team functioning, such as trust, recognition and value of team members, and a shared purpose, were already present on this team at some level. Team members knew each other and had passion for the team purpose: developing a culture that embraces health and well-being. The team members work within a college that espouses "Benedictine values" (College of St. Scholastica, 2009), which include community, hospitality, and stewardship. This emphasis on Benedictine values provided a work culture that embraced collaboration, which is a driver of interprofessional teams.

One of the barriers that plagued the team was that there was no clear understanding of roles and responsibilities. The team met and formed ideas that the team leader and mentor needed to follow through on. This team structure has changed since the end of the DNP project and now comprises four separate working groups focused on student health, faculty and staff health, marketing, and academic integration. The project, now entitled Well U, has been in full swing for more than 4 years.

The use of Wheatley's (2005) "new leadership" approach helps account for the success of this project. The college campus, in relationship to health, could be seen as chaotic; once the relationships were formed between team members, however, information and ideas flowed. The team came to understand that all connections were vital to the development of a college-wide culture that embraced health and well-being. A long-term approach to building cultural change continues in this project. **Table 6-2** shows interprofessional team members in the DNP project.

Interprofessional collaboration is not limited to efforts in the United States. In two reports to the Minister of Health in Canada, the Health Professions Regulatory Advisory Council (2008, 2009) reviewed the scope of practice of nurse

TABLE 6-2 Interprofessional Team Members

Initial Task Force	Final Multi-Interprofessional Team
DNP student	DNP student
MSW mentor	MSW mentor
RN from SHS	RN from SHS
Student	Student
	Director of Institutional Research and Assessment
	VP for Enrollment Management
	Registrar
	Manager, Wellness Center
	International student advisor
	Department chair, Physical Therapy

practitioners and the need for interprofessional collaboration as a means to address primary care provider shortages and comprehensive, quality care. As a result, the Minister of Health supported initiatives for innovative practice models to improve access and quality of care for underserved Canadian residents. In the DNP-led project, "A Nurse Practitioner-Led Clinic in Thunder Bay" (Thibeault, 2011), a team of nurse practitioners, registered nurses, social worker, dietitian, pharmacist, administrator, and community representative designed and implemented a comprehensive primary care clinic that opened its doors to Thunder Bay residents in November 2010. The clinic's primary focus is comprehensive care across the life span, with a focus on health promotion, disease prevention, and chronic care delivery. The clinic has exceeded initial goals of increasing access for unattached patients and reducing costly emergency room visits.

SUMMARY

Given their advanced preparation, DNPs are well positioned to participate and lead interprofessional teams. Recognizing obstacles and developing strategies to reduce such barriers are key functions of interprofessional team leadership. All members of the interprofessional team need to have preparation and opportunities to rehearse this new approach to patient care delivery. Incorporating shared interdisciplinary learning experiences into the educational preparation of healthcare professionals provides the foundation for forming partnerships rather than competition for patient care delivery. Further study is needed to demonstrate the most effective educational interventions to prepare healthcare providers for successful collaborative work.

Workforce and regulatory issues may present both challenges and opportunities for interprofessional collaborations. Shortages of physician primary care providers, particularly in rural settings, are likely to influence both the configuration and function of the interprofessional team (ACP, 2009; Minnesota

Department of Health [MDH], 2009). DNP-prepared primary care providers can help to fill this gap but must be allowed (regulatory wise) to practice at the top of their education and scope; this will necessitate that physician colleagues reexamine and relinquish some of the responsibilities and tasks traditionally "owned" by medicine. Nursing and medicine will need to work together to devise a vision for this new collaborative practice model to most efficiently and effectively address the needs of the population and improve the quality of care provided.

The American Academy of Pediatrics' concept of a "medical home" suggests that all individuals, particularly those with complex or chronic health conditions, should receive a comprehensive, coordinated approach to health care and social services (MDH, 2009). The proposed Health Care Home initiatives expand the definition of primary care provider to include physicians, APRNs, and physician assistants (MDH, 2009). The primary care provider will lead and coordinate the efforts of the interprofessional team to best meet the needs of the patient. Nurse practice acts, regulations, and reimbursement issues must be reviewed and revised to support the ability of APRNs to assume this role and deliver comprehensive care. Continued research is needed to identify the full impact of workforce and regulatory issues on these collaborations as well as strategies to address these concerns. DNPs in both direct (certified nurse practitioner [CNP], clinical nurse specialist [CNS], certified registered nurse anesthetist [CRNA], certified nurse-midwife [CNM]) and indirect provider roles (health policymakers, administrators, informatics specialists, public health experts) must continue to effectively work with other members of the healthcare team to deliver comprehensive, patient-centered care. Interprofessional collaborations are an important facet of a reformed healthcare delivery system and a vital step toward improving health outcomes and reducing medical error.

DISCUSSION QUESTIONS _____

1. What is the difference between shared decision making and collective cognitive responsibility?

2. How does leadership differ from management?

3. Consider a conflict in your clinical practice setting. As an advanced practice nurse, what is your role in assisting the team to resolve the issue(s)?

4. What is your vision of the ideal interdisciplinary team?

REFERENCES _____

Agency for Healthcare Research and Quality. (2009). *Surveys on patient safety culture*. Retrieved from http://www.ahrq.gov/qual/patientsafetyculture/

American Association of Colleges of Nursing. (2006a). *DNP roadmap task force report, October 20, 2006*. Retrieved from http://www.aacn.nche.edu/dnp/roadmapreport.pdf

American Association of Colleges of Nursing. (2006b). *The essentials of doctoral education for advanced nursing practice*. Washington, DC: Author.

American College of Physicians. (2009). *Nurse practitioners in primary care* [Policy monograph]. Philadelphia, PA: Author.

American Medical Association. (2010, October 5). *AMA responds to IOM report on future of nursing*. Retrieved from http://www.ama-assn.org/ama/pub/news/news/nursing-future-workforce.page

American Nurses Association. (2008, February). *ANA's health system reform agenda*. Silver Spring, MD: Author. Retrieved from http://www.nursingworld.org/Content/HealthcareandPolicyIssues/Agenda/ANAsHealthSystemReformAgenda.pdf

Amos, M., Hu, J., & Herrick, C. (2005). The impact of team building on communication and job satisfaction of nursing staff. *Journal for Nurses in Staff Development, 21*(1), 10–16.

APRN Consensus Work Group & National Council of State Boards of Nursing APRN Advisory Committee. (2008, July). *Consensus model for APRN regulation: Licensure, accreditation, certification and education*. APRN Joint Dialogue Group Report. Retrieved from http://www.aacn.nche.edu/education-resources/APRNReport.pdf

Ash, L. (2005). *Developing a population-focused student health service* (Unpublished doctoral dissertation). Rush University, Chicago, IL.

Baker, S., Baker, K., & Campbell, M. (2003). *Complete idiot's guide to project management*. Indianapolis, IN: Alpha.

Barki, H., & Hartwick, J. (2001). Interpersonal conflict and its management in information system development. *MIS Quarterly, 25*(2), 195–228.

Begun, J., Zimmerman, B., & Dooley, K. (2003). Health care organizations as complex adaptive systems. In S. M. Mick & M. Wyttenbach (Eds.), *Advances in health care organization theory* (pp. 253–288). San Francisco, CA: Jossey-Bass. Retrieved from http://www.change-ability.ca/Complex_Adaptive.pdf

Blanchard, K. (2008). Situational leadership. *Leadership Excellence, 25*(5), 19.

Brett, J., Behfar, K., & Kern, M. (2006, November). Managing multicultural teams. *Harvard Business Review, 84*(11), 84–91. Retrieved from Business Source Premier database.

Brewer, C. (2005). The health care workforce. In A. Kovner & J. Knickman (Eds.), *Health care delivery in the United States* (pp. 320–326). New York, NY: Springer.

Brita-Rossi, P., Adduci, D., Kaufman, J., Lipson, S. J., Totte, C., & Wasserman, K. (1996). Improving the process of care: The cost-quality value of interdisciplinary collaboration. *Journal of Nursing Care Quality, 10*(2), 10–16.

Buresh, B., & Gordon, S. (2006). *From silence to voice: What nurses know and must communicate to the public*. Ithaca, NY: Cornell University Press.

Burkhardt, M., & Alvita, K. (2008). *Ethics and issues in contemporary nursing*. Clifton Park, NY: Thomson Delmar Learning.

Burns, J. (1978). *Leadership*. New York, NY: Harper and Row.

Chapman, A. (2008). Johari window: Ingham and Luft's Johari window model diagrams and examples—for self-awareness, personal development, group development and understanding relationships. Retrieved from http://www.businessballs.com/johariwindowmodel.htm

Chinn, P. (2008). *Peace and power*. Sudbury, MA: Jones and Bartlett.

Chung, H., & Nguyen, P. H. (2005). Changing unit culture: An interdisciplinary commitment to improve pain outcomes. *Journal for Healthcare Quality: Official Publication of the National Association for Healthcare Quality, 27*(2), 12–19.

Clarin, O. A. (2007). Strategies to overcome barriers to effective nurse practitioner and physician collaboration. *Journal for Nurse Practitioners, 3*(8), 538–548.

Clark, W., Clark, L., & Crossley, K. (2010). Developing multidimensional trust without touch in virtual teams. *Marketing Management Journal, 20*(1), 177–193.

College of St. Scholastica. (2009). Guiding documents. Retrieved from http://www.css.edu /About/Leadership/Guiding-Documents.html

Covey, S. (1991). *Principle-centered leadership*. New York, NY: Summit Books.

Covey, S. (2004). *The eighth habit: From effectiveness to greatness*. New York, NY: Free Press.

Cowan, M. J., Shapiro, M., Hays, R. D., Afifi, A., Vazirani, S., Ward, C. R., & Ettner, S. L. (2006). The effect of a multidisciplinary hospitalist/physician and advanced practice nurse collaboration on hospital costs. *Journal of Nursing Administration, 36*(2), 79–85.

Crowell, D. (2011). *Complexity leadership*. Philadelphia, PA: F. A. Davis.

Cunningham, R. (2004, March). Advanced practice nursing outcomes: A review of selected empirical literature. *Oncology Nursing Forum, 31*(2), 219–232. Retrieved from CINAHL Plus with Full Text database.

Dailey, M. (2005, April). Interdisciplinary collaboration: Essential for improved wound care outcomes and wound prevention in home care. *Home Health Care Management and Practice, 17*(3), 213–221. Retrieved from CINAHL Plus with Full Text database.

D'Amour, D., & Oandasan, I. (2005). Interprofessionality as the field of interprofessional practice and interprofessional education: An emerging concept. *Journal of Interprofessional Care, 19*, 8–20.

Davoli, G. W., & Fine, L. J. (2004). Stacking the deck for success in interprofessional collaboration. *Health Promotion Practice, 5*(3), 266–270.

Draye, M. A., Acker, M., & Zimmer, P. A. (2006). The practice doctorate in nursing: Approaches to transform nurse practitioner education and practice. *Nursing Outlook, 54*(3), 123–129.

Drinka, T., & Clark, P. (2000). *Health care teamwork: Interdisciplinary practice and teaching*. Westport, CT: Auburn House.

Dunevitz, B. (1997). Perspectives in ambulatory care. Collaboration—in a variety of ways—creates health care value. *Nursing Economics, 15*(4), 218–219.

Edmonson, A. (1999). Psychological safety and learning behavior in work teams. *Administrative Science Quarterly, 44*(2), 350–383.

Feldman, H. (2008). *Nursing leadership: A concise encyclopedia*. New York, NY: Springer.

Fortham, M., Dove, H., & Wooster, L. (2000). Episodic treatment groups (ETGs): A patient classification system for measuring outcomes performance by episode of care. *Topics in Healthcare Information Management, 21*(2), 51–61.

Golanowski, M., Beaudry, D., Kurz, L., Laffey, W., & Hook, M. (2007). Inter-disciplinary shared decision-making: Taking shared governance to the next level. *Nursing Administration Quarterly, 31*(4), 341–353.

Goleman, D., Boyzatsis, R., & McKee, A. (2002). *Primal leadership: Realizing the power of emotional intelligence*. Boston, MA: Harvard Business School Press.

Gordon, S. (2005). *Nursing against the odds*. Ithaca, NY: Cornell University Press.

Grabowski, M., & Roberts, K. (1999, November). Risk mitigation in virtual organizations. *Organization Science, 10*(6), 704–721. Retrieved from Business Source Premier database.

Grady, G. F., & Wojner, A. W. (1996). Collaborative practice teams: The infrastructure of outcomes management. *AACN Clinical Issues: Advanced Practice in Acute & Critical Care, 7*(1), 153–158.

Greenberg, P., Greenberg, R., & Antonucci, Y. (2007). Creating and sustaining trust in virtual teams. *Business Horizons, 50*(4), 325–333.

Haas, J. (1977). The professionalism of medical students: Developing a cloak of confidence. *Symbolic Interaction, 1*(1), 71–88.

Hall, P. (2005). Interprofessional teamwork: Professional cultures as barriers. *Journal of Interprofessional Care, 19*(Suppl. 1), 188–196.

Hall, P., Weaver, L., Gravelle, D., & Thibault, H. (2007). Developing collaborative person-centred practice: A pilot project on a palliative care unit. *Journal of Interprofessional Care, 21*(1), 69–81.

Health Professions Regulatory Advisory Council. (2008). *A report to the Minister of Health and Long-Term Care on the review of the scope of practice for registered nurses in the extended class (nurse practitioners)*. Toronto, Ontario, Canada: Author.

Health Professions Regulatory Advisory Council. (2009). *Critical links: Transforming and supporting patient care: A report to the Minister of Health and Long Term Care on mechanisms to facilitate and support interprofessional collaboration and a new framework*

for the prescribing and use of drugs by non-physician regulated health professions. Toronto, Ontario, Canada: Author.

Hibbard, J. H., Stockard, J., Mahoney, E. R., & Tusler, M. (2004). Development of the patient activation measure (PAM): Conceptualizing and measuring activation in patient and consumers. *Health Services Research, 39*(4), 1005–1026.

Holton, J. A. (2001). Building trust and collaboration in a virtual team. *Team Performance Management, 7*(3), 36–47.

Horrocks, S., Anderson, E., & Salisbury, C. (2002, April 6). Systematic review of whether nurse practitioners working in primary care can provide equivalent care to doctors. *British Medical Journal, 324*(7341), 819–823. Retrieved from CINAHL Plus with Full Text database.

Ingersoll, G. L., McIntosh, E., & Williams, M. (2000). Nurse sensitive outcomes of advanced practice. *Journal of Advanced Nursing, 32*(5), 1272–1281.

Institute for Clinical Systems Integration. (2007). *DIAMOND: Depression improvement across Minnesota—offering a new direction.* Retrieved from http://www.health.state.mn.us/healthreform/homes/payment/archives/paymentsteering090624_DIAMOND.pdf

Institute of Medicine. (1999). *To err is human: Building a safer health system.* Washington, DC: National Academies Press.

Institute of Medicine. (2001). *Crossing the quality chasm: A new health system for the 21st century.* Washington, DC: National Academies Press.

Institute of Medicine. (2003). *Health professions education: A bridge to quality.* Washington, DC: National Academies Press.

Institute of Medicine. (2011). *The future of nursing: Leading change, advancing health.* Washington, DC: National Academies Press.

The Joint Commission. (2008). *Accreditation program: Ambulatory health care national patient safety goals.* Retrieved from http://www.jointcommission.org/standards_information/jcfaq.aspx?ProgramId=39

Kaiser Family Foundation. (2008). *President-elect Barack Obama's health care reform proposal.* Retrieved from http://kaiserfamilyfoundation.files.wordpress.com/2013/01/obama_health_care_reform_proposal.pdf

Kaiser Family Foundation. (2011, April 15). *Summary of the Affordable Care Act.* Retrieved from http://www.kff.org/healthreform/upload/8061.pdf

Kaiser Family Foundation/Harvard School of Public Health Survey. (2009). *Toplines: The public's health care agenda for the new president and Congress* (Publication No. 7853). Retrieved from http://www.kff.org/kaiserpolls/upload/7853.pdf

Kelly, P. (2008). *Nursing leadership and management.* Clifton Park, NY: Delmar.

Kirkman, B., Rosen, L., Gibson, C. B., Tesluk, P., & McPherson, S. (2002). Five challenges to virtual team success: Lessons from Sabre, Inc. *Academy of Management Executive, 16*(3), 67–79.

Kleinpell, R. M., Faut-Callahan, M. M., Lauer, K., Kremer, M. J., Murphy, M., & Sperhac, A. (2002). Collaborative practice in advanced practice nursing in acute care. *Critical Care Nursing Clinics of North America, 14*(3), 307–313.

Kotter, J. (1990). What leaders really do. *Harvard Business Review, 68*, 104.

Kouzes, J., & Pozner, B. (2007). *The leadership challenge.* San Francisco, CA: Wiley.

Ladden, M., Bednash, G., Stevens, D., & Moore, G. (2006). Educating interprofessional learners for quality, safety and systems improvement. *Journal of Inter-professional Care, 20*(5), 497–509.

Lambing, A., Adams, D., Fox, D., & Divine, G. (2004, August). Nurse practitioners' and physicians' care activities and clinical outcomes with an inpatient geriatric population. *Journal of the American Academy of Nurse Practitioners, 16*(8), 343–352. Retrieved from CINAHL Plus with Full Text database.

Laurant, M., Reeves, D., Hermens, R., Braspenning, J., Grol, R., & Sibbald, B. (2004, December). Substitution of doctors by nurses in primary care. *Cochrane Database of Systematic Reviews.* Retrieved from CINAHL Plus with Full Text database.

Lee, S. (2008). *The five stages of team development.* Retrieved from http://ezinearticles.com/?The-Five-Stages-of-Team-Development&id=1254894

Leonard, M., Graham, S., & Bonacum, D. (2004). The human factor: The critical importance of effective teamwork and communication in providing safe care. *Quality and Safety in Health Care, 13*(Supp. 1), 85–90.

Lewin, K. (1951). Frontiers in group dynamics. In D. Cartwright (Ed.), *Field theory in social science* (pp. 188–237). New York, NY: Harper.

Lewis, J. (2007). *Fundamentals of project management.* New York, NY: AMACOM.

Lindeke, L. L., & Block, D. E. (2001). Interdisciplinary collaboration in the 21st century. *Minnesota Medicine, 84*(6), 42–45.

Lindeke, L. L., & Sieckert, A. M. (2005). Nurse–physician workplace collaboration. *Online Journal of Issues in Nursing, 10*(1). Retrieved from http://www.nursingworld.org/MainMenuCategories/ANAMarketplace/ANAPeriodicals/OJIN/TableofContents/Volume102005/No1Jan05/tpc26_416011.aspx

Lynnaugh, J., & Reverby, S. (1990). *Ordered to care: The dilemma of American nursing 1850–1945.* New York, NY: Cambridge University Press.

Mayer, R. C., Davis, J. H., & Schoorman, F. D. (1995). An integrative model of organizational trust. *Academy of Management Review, 20,* 709-734.

McCallin, A., & Bamford, A. (2007). Interdisciplinary teamwork: Is the influence of emotional intelligence fully appreciated? *Journal of Nursing Management, 15*(4), 386-391.

Miller, C. (2008). *Optimal use of individualized asthma action plans in an electronic health record* (Unpublished doctoral dissertation). University of Minnesota, Minneapolis.

Miller, K. L., Reeves, S., Zwarenstein, M., Beales, J. D., Kenaszchuk, C., & Gotlib Conn, L. (2008). Nursing emotion work and interprofessional collaboration in general medicine wards: A qualitative study. *Journal of Advanced Nursing, 64*(4), 332-343.

Miller, M., Snyder, M., & Lindeke, L. (2005, September). Forces of change. Nurse practitioners: Current status and future challenges. *Clinical Excellence for Nurse Practitioners, 9*(3), 162-169. Retrieved from CINAHL Plus with Full Text database.

Minnesota Department of Health. (2009). *Health workforce shortage study report: Report to the Minnesota legislature 2009.* St. Paul, MN: Author.

Mundinger, M., Kane, R., Lenz, E., Totten, A., Tsai, W., Cleary, P., . . . Shelanski, M. L. (2000). Primary care outcomes in patients treated by nurse practitioners or physicians: A randomized trial. *Journal of the American Medical Association, 283*(1), 59-68. Retrieved from CINAHL Plus with Full Text database.

NASPA. (2004). *Leadership for a healthy campus: An ecological approach for student success.* Retrieved from http://www.naspa.org/constituent-groups/kcs/wellness-and-health-promotion/resources

Nelson, E. C., Batalden, P. B., Huber, T. P., Mohr, J. J., Godfrey, M. M., Headrick, L. A., . . . Wasson, J. H. (2002). Microsystems in health care: Part 1. Learning from high-performing front-line clinical units. *The Joint Commission Journal on Quality Improvement, 28*(9), 472-493.

Oandasan, I., D'Amour, D., Zwarenstein, M., Barker, K., Purden, M., Beaulieu, M. D., . . . Tregunno, D. (2004). *Interprofessional education for collaborative patient-centred practice: An evolving framework* [Executive summary]. Retrieved from http://www.ferasi.umontreal.ca/eng/07_info/IECPCP_Final_Report.pdf

O'Connor, A. (2006). *Ottawa personal decision guide* [Pamphlet]. University of Ottawa, Ontario, Canada: Ottawa Health Research Institute.

Patient Protection and Affordable Care Act (PPACA), Pub. L. No. 111-148, §2702, 124 Stat. *119,* 318-319 (2010).

Patterson, K., Grenny, J., McMillan, R., & Switzler, A. (2002). *Crucial conversations: Tools for talking when stakes are high.* New York, NY: McGraw-Hill.

Porter-O'Grady, T. (1997). *Whole systems shared governance.* Gaithersburg, MD: Aspen.

Reeves, S., Zwarenstein, M., Goldman, J., Barr, H., Freeth, D., Hammick, M., & Koppel, I. (2008). Interprofessional education: Effects on professional practice and health care outcomes [Review]. *Cochrane Database of Systematic Reviews, 1,* CD002213. doi:10.1002/14651858.CD002213.pub2

Ring, P. (2005, January). Collaboration. In *Blackwell encyclopedic dictionary of organizational behavior.* Retrieved from Blackwell Encyclopedia of Management Library database.

Robert Wood Johnson Foundation. (2008, April). Partnerships for quality education (Robert Wood Johnson Grant Results Reports). Retrieved from http://www.rwjf.org/pr/product.jsp?id=17748

Rosenstein, A. (2002). The impact of nurse–physician relationships on nurse satisfaction and retention. *American Journal of Nursing, 102*(6), 26-34.

Rosenstein, A., & O'Daniel, M. (2008). A survey of the impacts of disruptive behaviors and communication defects on public safety. *The Joint Commission Journal on Quality and Patient Safety, 34*(8), 464-471.

Sacher, L., Moses, K., Fabiano, P., Haubenreiser, J., Grizzel, J., & Mart, S. (2005, March). *College health: Stretch your definitions of the core concepts, assumptions and practices.* American College Health Association. PowerPoint presentation at NASPA (Student Affairs Administration in Higher Education) session, Washington, DC.

Scardamalia, M. (2002). Collective cognitive responsibility for the advancement of knowledge. In B. Smith (Ed.), *Liberal education in a knowledge society* (pp. 67-98). Chicago, IL: Open Court.

Senge, P. (1990). *The art and discipline of the learning organization.* New York, NY: Doubleday.

Sierchio, G. P. (2003). A multidisciplinary approach for improving outcomes. *Journal of Infusion Nursing, 26*(1), 34–43.

Snijders, C., Kollen, B., Van Lingen, R., Fetter, W., & Molendijk, H. (2009). Which aspects of safety culture predict incident reporting behavior in neonatal intensive care units? A multilevel analysis. *Critical Care Medicine, 37*(1), 61–67.

Sullivan, E. J. (2004). *Becoming influential: A guide for nurses.* Upper Saddle River, NJ: Pearson Prentice Hall.

Thibeault, L. (2011). *A nurse practitioner led clinic in Thunder Bay* (Unpublished doctoral dissertation). College of St. Scholastica, Duluth, MN.

Tuckman, B. W., & Jensen, M. A. C. (1977). Stages of small-group development revisited. *Group & Organization Management, 2*(4), 419–427. doi:10.1177/105960117700200404

U.S. Department of Health and Human Services. (2010). *About Healthy People 2020.* Retrieved from http://www.healthypeople.gov/2020/about/default.aspx

Vahey, D. C., Aiken, L. H., Sloane, D. M., Clarke, S. P., & Vargas, D. (2004). Nurse burnout and patient satisfaction. *Medical Care, 42*(Suppl. 2), 1157–1166.

Wheatley, M. (2005). *Finding our way: Leadership for an uncertain time.* San Francisco, CA: Berrett-Koehler.

Whitehead, C. (2007). The doctor dilemma in interprofessional education and care: How and why will physicians collaborate? *Medical Education, 41*(10), 1010–1016.

Wilson, J., & Bekemeir, B. (2004). Public health. In *Encyclopedia of leadership* (Vol. 3, pp. 1271–1274). Thousand Oaks, CA: Sage.

Yeager, S. (2005). Interdisciplinary collaboration: The heart and soul of healthcare. *Critical Care Nursing Clinics of North America, 17*(2), 143–148.

PART 2

Healthcare Delivery and Health Policy for Advanced Practice: Core Knowledge

For the advanced practice nurse, understanding the system in which one works is an essential foundation for successful practice. In acting simultaneously as an advocate for the consumer and as a provider and manager of care, nurses in advanced practice need basic knowledge of the following topics:

- The structure, operations, scope, and characteristics of the healthcare delivery system

- The means by which the healthcare delivery system is financed, including national healthcare expenditures and sources of payment

- The trends that will influence the future of the system

- Ways in which nurses can influence healthcare policy and, conversely, the ways in which policy influences practice

The information provided in Part 2 can help the reader move beyond the perspective of the nursing profession to a broader understanding of the healthcare organization, relationships with other members of the interdisciplinary team, and the forces that affect current and future practices. The ultimate goal is to prepare the reader as an advanced practice nurse to provide high-quality, cost-effective care, to participate in the design and implementation of programs in a variety of systems, and to assume leadership for practice changes.

In reviewing the information provided in this part, it is helpful to think of the issues as constituting a triad of cost, quality, and access. Any change to correct an issue in one component will have a significant and possibly negative effect on the other two. For instance, with the implementation of the Affordable Care Act, millions more citizens are insured and have access to health care, so costs may increase as a result of increased demands on the system, and these cost increases may, in turn, affect quality if healthcare organizations are not funded properly.

The chapters in Part 2 were selected from several books. Chapters 7 and 8 are the introductory chapters in *Delivering Health Care in America: A Systems Approach*, by Shi and Singh (Jones & Bartlett Learning, 2015). These chapters provide a foundation for understanding the healthcare delivery system. In Chapter 7, Shi and Singh paint a realistic—albeit gloomy—portrait of a complex, massive healthcare "system" in the United States. Because of the diversity of stakeholders in the U.S. healthcare system, including multiple providers, multiple payers, and the government, they suggest revolutionary changes in health care will be difficult, if not impossible, to achieve in this country. In Chapter 8, the same authors discuss issues of beliefs, values, and health. Although much of the content is not new to nursing—whose theorists and writers have focused on health as a metaparadigm for the profession for more than 60 years (see Part 4)—this chapter explores in depth the concept of holistic health and values from the perspective of policy and leadership.

Chapter 9 provides a discussion of clinical microsystems, which are defined as the combination of a small group of people who work together in a defined setting on a regular basis—or as needed—to provide care and the individuals who receive that care (who also can be recognized as part of a discrete subpopulation of patients). The majority of advanced practice nurses and readers of this book work in microsystems, as defined here, where direct care to patients is provided. Viewing the organization in which one works and interacts with the interprofessional team is empowering.

In Chapter 10, Schulz introduces the reader to microeconomics. This is not an easy read, as much of the information and language is new to most advanced practice nurses. However, the information provided will assist the reader is viewing health care from an economic perspective. Although the discussion uses hospitals as an example, the basic principles of competition, regulation, and the profit motive apply to any healthcare organization and, for nurse educators, institutions of higher education.

Chapter 11 was selected to give an overview of the major concepts of the regulation of health professionals, with emphasis on the oversight of advanced practice nurses who provide direct patient care. Understanding the process of licensure and credentialing and their effects on the practice of advanced practice nursing is fundamental to practicing as a competent practitioner. In this chapter, Loversidge reviews the historical roots of the regulation of advanced practice nursing at state and federal levels and provides the reader with the tools to navigate the regulatory process and become a confident spokesperson for issues critical to all advanced practice nurses.

CHAPTER 7

An Overview of U.S. Healthcare Delivery

Leiyu Shi and Douglas A. Singh

© A-R-T/Shutterstock

CHAPTER OBJECTIVES

1. Understand the basic nature of the U.S. healthcare system.
2. Outline the key functional components of a healthcare delivery system.
3. Understand healthcare reform and the Affordable Care Act.
4. Discuss the primary characteristics of the U.S. healthcare system.
5. Describe why it is important for advanced practice nurses to understand the intricacies of the healthcare delivery system.
6. Understand healthcare delivery systems in selected countries.
7. Point out global health challenges and reform efforts.
8. Describe the systems model as a framework for studying the health services system in the United States. The U.S. healthcare delivery system is a behemoth that is almost impossible for any single entity to manage and control.

INTRODUCTION

The United States has a unique system of healthcare delivery unlike any other healthcare system in the world. Most developed countries have national health insurance programs run by the government and financed through general taxes. Almost all citizens in such countries are entitled to receive healthcare services. Such is not yet the case in the United States, where not all Americans are automatically covered by health insurance.

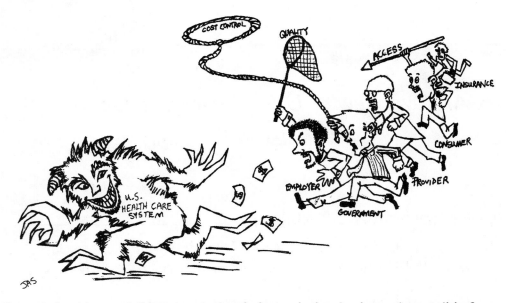

The U.S. healthcare delivery system is a behemoth that is almost impossible for any single entity to manage and control.
Source: Shi, L., & Singh, D. (2015). Delivering health care in America: A systems approach (6th ed.). Burlington, MA: Jones & Bartlett.

The U.S. healthcare delivery system is really not a system in its true sense, even though it is called a system when reference is made to its various features, components, and services. Hence, it may be somewhat misleading to talk about the American healthcare delivery "system" because a true system does not exist (Wolinsky, 1988). One main feature of the U.S. healthcare system is that it is fragmented because different people obtain health care through different means. The system has continued to undergo periodic changes, mainly in response to concerns regarding cost, access, and quality.

Describing healthcare delivery in the United States can be a daunting task. To facilitate an understanding of the structural and conceptual basis for the delivery of health services, a systems framework is presented at the end of the chapter, and, for the sake of simplicity, the mechanisms of health services delivery in the United States are collectively referred to as a system.

AN OVERVIEW OF THE SCOPE AND SIZE OF THE SYSTEM

Table 7-1 demonstrates the complexity of healthcare delivery in the United States. Many organizations and individuals are involved in health care, ranging from educational and research institutions, medical suppliers, insurers, payers, and claims processors to healthcare providers. Multitudes of providers are involved in the delivery of preventive, primary, subacute, acute, auxiliary, rehabilitative, and continuing care. An increasing number of managed care organizations (MCOs) and integrated networks now provide a continuum of care, covering many of the service components.

The U.S. healthcare delivery system is massive, with total employment that reached over 16.4 million in 2010 in various health delivery settings. This included more than 838,000 professionally active doctors of medicine (MDs), 70,480 osteopathic physicians (DOs), and

| TABLE 7-1 | The Complexity of Healthcare Delivery |

Education/ Research	Suppliers	Insurers	Providers	Payers	Government
Medical schools	Pharmaceutical companies	Managed care plans	*Preventive Care*	Blue Cross/ Blue Shield plans	Public insurance financing
Dental schools	Multipurpose suppliers	Blue Cross/ Blue Shield plans	Health departments		Health regulations
Nursing programs	Biotechnology companies		*Primary Care*	Commercial insurers	Health policy
Physician assistant programs		Commercial insurers	Physician offices	Employers	Research funding
Nurse practitioner programs		Self-insured employers	Community health centers	Third-party administrators	Public health
Physical therapy, occupational therapy, speech therapy programs		Medicare	Dentists	State agencies	
		Medicaid	Nonphysician providers		
		VA	*Subacute Care*		
		Tricare	Subacute care facilities		
Research organizations			Ambulatory surgery centers		
Private foundations			*Acute Care*		
U.S. Public Health Service (AHRQ, ATSDR, CDC, FDA, HRSA, IHS, NIH, SAMHSA)			Hospitals		
			Auxiliary Services		
			Pharmacists		
			Diagnostic clinics		
			X-ray units		
			Suppliers of medical equipment		
			Rehabilitative Services		
			Home health agencies		
			Rehabilitation centers		
			Skilled nursing facilities		
			Continuing Care		
			Nursing homes		
			End-of-Life Care		
			Hospices		
			Integrated		
Professional associations			Managed care organizations		

(continues)

TABLE 7-1	The Complexity of Healthcare Deliver *(continued)*
Trade associations	Integrated networks

Note: AHRQ, Agency for Healthcare Research and Quality; ATSDR, Agency for Toxic Substances and Disease Registry; CDC, Centers for Disease Control and Prevention; FDA, Food and Drug Administration; HRSA, Health Resources and Services Administration; IHS, Indian Health Service; NIH, National Institutes of Health; SAMHSA, Substance Abuse and Mental Health Services Administration; VA, Veterans Administration.

Source: Shi, L., & Singh, D. (2015). *Delivering health care in America: A systems approach* (6th ed.). Burlington, MA: Jones & Bartlett.

2.6 million active nurses (U.S. Census Bureau, 2012). The vast number of healthcare and health services professionals (5.98 million) work in ambulatory health service settings, such as the offices of physicians, dentists; and other health practitioners; medical and diagnostic laboratories; and home healthcare service locations. This is followed by hospitals (4.7 million) and nursing and residential care facilities (3.13 million). The vast array of healthcare institutions includes approximately 5,795 hospitals, 15,700 nursing homes, and 13,337 substance abuse treatment facilities (U.S. Census Bureau, 2012).

In 2011, 1,128 federally qualified health center grantees, with 138,403 full-time employees, provided preventive and primary care services to approximately 20.2 million people living in medically underserved rural and urban areas (Health Resources and Services Administration, 2013). Various types of healthcare professionals are trained in 159 medical and osteopathic schools, 61 dental schools, more than 100 schools of pharmacy, and more than 1,500 nursing programs located throughout the country (U.S. Bureau of Labor Statistics, 2011). Multitudes of government agencies are involved with the financing of health care, medical research, and regulatory oversight of the various aspects of the healthcare delivery system.

A Broad Description of the System

U.S. healthcare delivery does not function as a rational and integrated network of components designed to work together coherently. To the contrary, it is a kaleidoscope of financing, insurance, delivery, and payment mechanisms that remain loosely coordinated. Each of these basic functional components—financing, insurance, delivery, and payment—represents an amalgam of public (government) and private sources. Thus, government-run programs finance and insure health care for select groups of people who meet each program's prescribed criteria for eligibility. To a lesser degree, government programs also deliver certain healthcare services directly to certain recipients, such as veterans, military personnel, American Indians/Alaska Natives, and some of the uninsured. However, the financing, insurance, payment, and delivery functions are largely in private hands.

The market-oriented economy in the United States attracts a variety of private entrepreneurs driven by the pursuit of profits obtained by carrying out the key functions of healthcare delivery. Employers purchase health insurance for their employees through private sources, and employees receive healthcare services delivered by the private sector. The government finances public insurance through Medicare, Medicaid, and the Children's Health Insurance Program (CHIP) for a significant portion of the low-income, elderly, disabled, and pediatric populations. However, insurance arrangements for many publicly insured people are made through private entities, such as health maintenance organizations (HMOs), and healthcare services are rendered by private physicians and hospitals. The blend of public and private involvement in the delivery of health care has had several reults:

- A multiplicity of financial arrangements that enable individuals to pay for healthcare services

- Numerous insurance agencies or MCOs that employ varied mechanisms for insuring against risk

- Multiple payers that make their own determinations regarding how much to pay for each type of service

- A large array of settings where medical services are delivered

- Numerous consulting firms offering expertise in planning, cost containment, electronic systems, quality, and restructuring of resources

There is little standardization in a system that is functionally fragmented, and the various system components fit together only loosely. Such a system is not subject to overall planning, direction, and coordination from a central agency, such as the government. Duplication, overlap, inadequacy, inconsistency, and waste exist, leading to complexity and inefficiency, due to the missing dimension of system-wide planning, direction, and coordination. The system as a whole does not lend itself to standard budgetary methods of cost control. Each individual and corporate entity within a predominantly private entrepreneurial system seeks to manipulate financial incentives to its own advantage, without regard to its impact on the system as a whole. Hence, cost containment remains an elusive goal. In short, the U.S. healthcare delivery system is like a behemoth or an economic megalith that is almost impossible for any single entity to manage or control. The U.S. economy is the largest in the world, and, compared to other nations, consumption of healthcare services in the United States

represents a greater proportion of the country's total economic output. Although the system can be credited for delivering some of the best clinical care in the world, it falls short of delivering equitable services to every American.

An acceptable healthcare delivery system should have two primary objectives: (1) it must enable all citizens to obtain needed healthcare services, and (2) the services must be cost effective and meet certain established standards of quality. The U.S. healthcare delivery system falls short of both these ideals. On the other hand, certain features of U.S. health care are the envy of the world. The United States leads the world in the latest and the best in medical technology, training, and research. It offers some of the most sophisticated institutions, products, and processes of healthcare delivery.

Basic Components of a Health Services Delivery System

Figure 7-1 illustrates that a healthcare delivery system incorporates four functional components—financing, insurance, delivery, and payment—also known as the *quad-function model*. Healthcare delivery systems differ depending on the arrangement of these components. The four functions generally overlap, but the degree of overlap varies between a private and a government-run system and between a traditional health insurance and managed care–based system. In a government-run system, the functions are more closely integrated and may be indistinguishable. Managed care arrangements also integrate the four functions to varying degrees.

Financing

Financing is necessary to obtain health insurance or to pay for healthcare services. For most privately insured Americans, health insurance is employment based; that is, the employers finance health care as a fringe benefit. A dependent spouse or children may also be covered by the working spouse's or working parent's employer.

FIGURE 7-1   Basic healthcare delivery functions.

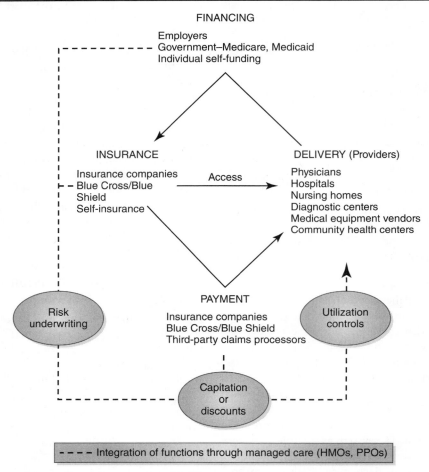

Source: Shi, L., & Singh, D. (2015). *Delivering health care in America: A systems approach* (6th ed.). Burlington, MA: Jones & Bartlett.

Most employers purchase health insurance for their employees through an MCO or an insurance company selected by the employer. Small employers may or may not be in a position to afford health insurance coverage for their employees. In public programs, the government functions as the financier; the insurance function may be carved out to an HMO.

Insurance

Insurance protects the insured against catastrophic risks when needing expensive healthcare services. The insurance function also determines the package of health services the insured individual is entitled to receive. It specifies how and where healthcare services may be received. The MCO or insurance company also functions as a claims processor and manages the disbursement of funds to the healthcare providers.

Delivery

The term *delivery* refers to the provision of healthcare services by various providers. The term *provider* refers to any entity that delivers healthcare services and either can independently bill for those services or is tax supported. Common examples of providers include physicians, nurse practitioners in some states, dentists, optometrists, and therapists in private practices, hospitals, and diagnostic and imaging clinics, and suppliers of medical equipment (e.g., wheelchairs, walkers, ostomy supplies, oxygen). With few exceptions, most providers render services to people who have health insurance. With a few exceptions, even those covered under public insurance programs receive healthcare services from private providers.

Payment

The payment function deals with reimbursement to providers for services delivered. The insurer determines how much is paid for a certain service. Funds for actual disbursement come from the premiums paid to the MCO or insurance company. The patient is usually required, at the time of service, to pay an out-of-pocket amount, such as $25 or $30, to see a physician. The remainder is covered by the MCO or insurance company. In government insurance plans, such as Medicare and Medicaid, tax revenues are used to pay providers.

INSURANCE AND HEALTHCARE REFORM

In 2009, there were 194.5 million Americans with private health insurance coverage (U.S. Census Bureau, 2012). The U.S. government finances health benefits for certain special populations, including government employees, the elderly (people age 65 and older), people with disabilities, some people with very low incomes, and children from low-income families. The program for the elderly and certain disabled individuals is called Medicare. The program for the indigent, jointly administered by the federal government and state governments, is named Medicaid. The program for children from low-income families, another federal/state partnership, is called the Children's Health Insurance Program (CHIP). In 2009, there were 43.4 million Medicare beneficiaries and 47.8 million Medicaid recipients, but 50.7 million people (16.7%) remained without any health insurance (U.S. Census Bureau, 2012).

Even the predominant employment-based financing system in the United States has left some employed individuals uninsured for two main reasons: (1) In many states, employers are not mandated to offer health insurance to their employees; therefore, some employers, due to economic constraints, do not offer it. Some small businesses simply cannot get group insurance at affordable rates and, therefore, are not able to offer health insurance as a benefit to their employees. (2) In many work settings, participation in health insurance programs is voluntary and does not require employees to join. Some employees choose not to sign up, mainly because they cannot afford the cost of health insurance premiums. Employers rarely pay 100% of the insurance premium; most require their employees to pay a portion of the cost, called premium cost sharing. People such as those who are self-employed have to obtain health insurance on their own. Individual rates are typically higher than group rates available to employers. In the United States, working people earning low wages have been the most likely to be uninsured because most cannot afford premium cost sharing and are not eligible for public benefits.

In the U.S. context, *healthcare reform* refers to the expansion of health insurance to cover the uninsured—those without private or public health insurance coverage. The Affordable Care Act (ACA) of 2010 is the most sweeping healthcare reform in recent U.S. history. One of the main objectives of the ACA is to reduce the number of uninsured. This section provides a brief overview of how the ACA plans to accomplish this.

The ACA was rolled out gradually starting in 2010 when insurance companies were mandated to start covering children and young adults younger than the age of 26 under their parents' health insurance plans. Most other insurance provisions went into effect on January 1, 2014, except for a mandate for employers to provide health insurance, which is postponed until 2015. The ACA requires that all U.S. citizens and legal residents must be covered by either public or private insurance. The law also relaxed standards to qualify additional numbers of people for Medicaid, although many states have chosen not to implement it based on the U.S. Supreme Court's ruling in 2012. Individuals without private or public insurance must obtain health insurance from participating insurance companies through Web-based, government-run exchanges; failing do so, they must pay a tax. The main function of the exchanges—also referred to as health insurance marketplaces—is to first determine whether an applicant qualifies for Medicaid or CHIP programs. If an applicant does not qualify for a public program, the exchange enables the individual to compare health plans offered by private insurers and to purchase a suitable health plan. Federal subsidies have been made available to people with incomes up to 400% of the federal poverty level to partially offset the cost of health insurance. Small employers can also obtain health coverage for their employees through the exchanges. The law mandates insurance plans to cover a variety of services referred to as "essential health benefits."

The open enrollment period for the exchanges closed on April 30, 2014. A total of 8,019,763 people selected a marketplace plan (CNN Health, 2014). A predictive model developed by Parente and Feldman (2013) estimated that, at best, full implementation of the ACA will reduce the number of uninsured by more than 20 million. If achieved, this would be the largest coverage expansion in recent U.S. history. Nevertheless, by its own design, the ACA will fail to achieve universal coverage that would enable all citizens and legal residents to have health insurance.

ROLE OF MANAGED CARE

Under traditional insurance, the four basic health delivery functions have been fragmented; that is, the financiers, insurers, providers, and payers have often been different entities, with a few exceptions. During the 1990s, however, healthcare delivery in the United States underwent a fundamental change involving a tighter integration of the basic functions through managed care.

Previously, fragmentation of the functions meant a lack of control over utilization and payments. The quantity of health care consumed refers to utilization of health services. Traditionally, determination of the utilization of health services and the price charged for each service have been left up to the insured individuals and the providers of health care. As a result of rising healthcare costs, however, current delivery mechanisms have instituted some controls over both utilization and price.

Managed care is a system of healthcare delivery that (1) seeks to achieve efficiencies by integrating the four functions of healthcare delivery discussed earlier, (2) employs mechanisms to control (manage) utilization of medical services, and (3) determines the price at which the services are purchased and, consequently, how much the providers get paid. The primary financier is still the employer or the government, as the case may be. Instead of purchasing health insurance through a traditional insurance company, the employer contracts with an MCO, such as an HMO or a preferred provider organization (PPO), to offer a selected health plan to its employees. In this case, the MCO functions like an insurance company and promises to provide healthcare services contracted under the health plan to the enrollees of the plan. The term *enrollee* (member) refers to the individual covered under the plan. The contractual arrangement between the MCO and the enrollee—including the collective array of covered health services that the enrollee is entitled to—is referred to as the *health plan* (or "plan," for short). The health plan uses selected providers from whom the enrollees can choose to receive services.

Compared with health services delivery under fee-for-service, managed care was successful in accomplishing cost control and greater integration of healthcare delivery. By ensuring access to needed health services, emphasizing preventive care, and maintaining a broad provider network, effective cost-saving measures can be implemented by managed care without compromising access and quality, thus providing healthcare budget predictability unattainable by other kinds of healthcare deliveries.

MAJOR CHARACTERISTICS OF THE U.S. HEALTHCARE SYSTEM

In any country, certain external influences shape the basic character of the health services delivery system. These forces consist of the political climate of a nation; economic development; technological progress; social and cultural values; physical environment; population characteristics, such as demographic and health trends; and global influences (**Figure 7-2**). The combined interaction of these environmental forces influences the course of healthcare delivery.

FIGURE 7-2 External forces affecting healthcare delivery.

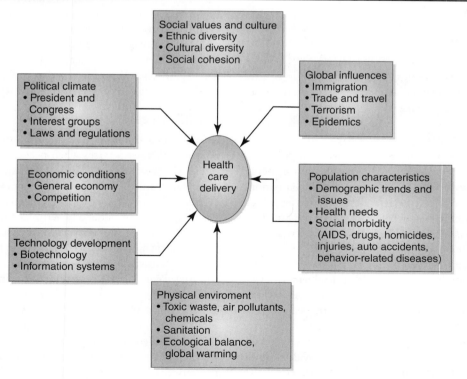

Source: Shi, L., & Singh, D. (2015). *Delivering health care in America: A systems approach* (6th ed.). Burlington, MA: Jones & Bartlett.

Ten basic characteristics differentiate the U.S. healthcare delivery system from that of most other countries:

1. No central agency governs the system.
2. Access to healthcare services is selectively based on insurance coverage.
3. Health care is delivered under imperfect market conditions.
4. Third-party insurers act as intermediaries between the financing and delivery functions.
5. The existence of multiple payers makes the system cumbersome.
6. The balance of power among various players prevents any single entity from dominating the system.
7. Legal risks influence practice behavior of providers.
8. Development of new technology creates an automatic demand for its use.
9. New service settings have evolved along a continuum.
10. Quality is no longer accepted as an unachievable goal.

No Central Agency

The U.S. healthcare system is not administratively controlled by a department or an agency of the government. Most other developed nations have national healthcare programs in which every citizen is entitled to receive a defined set of healthcare services. To control costs, these systems use global budgets to determine total healthcare expenditures on a national scale and to allocate resources within budgetary limits. Availability of services, as well as payments to providers, is subject to such budgetary constraints. The governments of these nations also control the proliferation of healthcare services, especially costly medical technology. System-wide controls over the allocation of resources determine to what extent government-sponsored healthcare services are available to citizens. For instance, the availability of specialized services is restricted.

By contrast, the United States has mainly a private system of financing and delivery. Private financing, predominantly through employers, accounts for approximately 53% of total healthcare expenditures; the government finances the remaining 47%. Private delivery of health care means that the majority of hospitals and physician clinics are private businesses, independent of the government. No central agency monitors total expenditures through global budgets or controls the availability and utilization of services. Nevertheless, the federal and state governments play an important role in healthcare delivery. They determine public-sector expenditures and reimbursement rates for services provided to Medicare, Medicaid, and CHIP beneficiaries. The government also formulates standards of participation through health policy and regulation, meaning providers must comply with the standards established by the government to be certified to provide services to Medicare, Medicaid, and CHIP beneficiaries. Certification standards are also regarded as minimum standards of quality in most sectors of the healthcare industry.

Partial Access

Access means the ability of an individual to obtain healthcare services when needed, which is not the same as having health insurance. Americans can access healthcare services if they (1) have health insurance through their employers, (2) are covered under a government healthcare program, (3) can afford to buy insurance with their own private funds, (4) are able to pay for services privately, or (5) can obtain charity or subsidized care. Health insurance is the primary means for ensuring access. Although the uninsured can access certain types of services, they often encounter barriers to obtaining needed health care. Federally supported health centers, for example, provide physician/nurse practitioner services to anyone regardless of ability to pay. Such centers and other types of free clinics, however, are located only in certain geographic areas and provide limited specialized services. Under U.S. law, hospital emergency departments are required to evaluate a patient's condition and render medically needed services for which the hospital does not receive any direct payments unless the patient is able to pay. Uninsured Americans, therefore, are able to obtain medical care for acute illness. Hence, one can say that the United States does have a form of universal catastrophic health insurance even for the uninsured (Altman & Reinhardt, 1996). On the other hand, the uninsured generally have to forgo continual basic and routine care, commonly referred to as *primary care.*

Countries with national healthcare programs provide universal coverage. However, access to services when needed may be restricted because no healthcare system has the capacity to deliver on demand every type of service for its citizens. Hence, universal access—the ability of all citizens to obtain health care when needed—remains mostly a theoretical concept.

The main goal of the ACA is to increase access and make it more affordable. As just mentioned, having coverage does not necessarily equate to access. Cost of insurance, cost of care, availability of services, and a relatively large number of uninsured still cast some doubts on whether the ACA will successfully achieve access for a large segment of the U.S. population.

Imperfect Market

In the United States, even though the delivery of services is largely in private hands, health care is only partially governed by free market forces. The delivery and consumption of health care in the United States does not quite pass the basic test of a free market, as subsequently described. Hence, the system is best described as a quasi-market or an imperfect market.

Under free-market conditions, there is an inverse relationship between the quantity of medical services demanded and the price of medical services. That is, quantity demanded goes up when the prices go down and vice versa. On the other hand, there is a direct relationship between price and the quantity supplied by the providers

of care. In other words, providers are willing to supply higher quantities at higher prices and vice versa. In a free market, the quantity of medical care that patients are willing to purchase, the quantity of medical care that providers are willing to supply, and the price reach a state of equilibrium. The equilibrium is achieved without the interference of any nonmarket forces. It is important to keep in mind that these conditions exist only under free-market conditions, which are not characteristic of the healthcare market.

In a free market, multiple patients (buyers) and providers (sellers) act independently, and patients can choose to receive services from any provider. Providers do not collude to fix prices, nor are prices fixed by an external agency. Rather, prices are governed by the free and unencumbered interaction of the forces of supply and demand (**Figure 7-3**). Demand—that is, the quantity of health care purchased—in turn, is driven by the prices prevailing in the free market. Under free-market conditions, the quantity demanded will increase as the price is lowered for a given product or service. Conversely, the quantity demanded will decrease as the price increases.

Under casual observation, it may appear that multiple patients and providers do exist. Most patients, however, are now enrolled in either a private health plan or a government-sponsored program or programs. These plans act as intermediaries for the patients, and the consolidation of patients into health plans has the effect of shifting the power from the patients to the administrators of the plans. The result is that the health plans, not the patients, are the real buyers in the healthcare services market. Private health plans, in many instances, offer their enrollees a limited choice of providers rather than an open choice.

Theoretically, prices are negotiated between the payers and providers. In practice, however, prices are determined by the payers, such as MCOs, Medicare, and Medicaid. Because prices are set by agencies external to the market, they are not governed by the unencumbered forces of supply and demand.

FIGURE 7-3 Relationship among price, supply, and demand under free-market conditions.

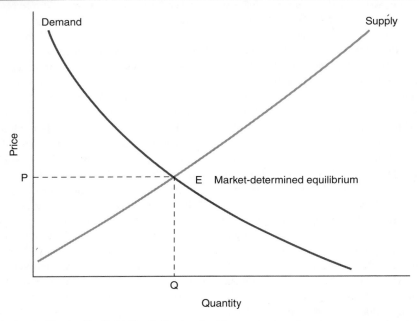

Source: Shi, L., & Singh, D. (2015). *Delivering health care in America: A systems approach* (6th ed.). Burlington, MA: Jones & Bartlett.

For the healthcare market to be free, unrestrained competition must occur among providers based on price and quality. The consolidation of buying power in the hands of private health plans, however, has been forcing providers to form alliances and integrated delivery systems on the supply side. In certain geographic sectors of the country, a single giant medical system has taken over as the sole provider of major healthcare services, restricting competition. As the healthcare system continues to move in this direction, it appears that only in large metropolitan areas will there be more than one large integrated system competing to get the business of the health plans.

A free market requires that patients have information about the appropriateness of various services. Such information is difficult to obtain because technology-driven medical care has become highly sophisticated. New diagnostic methods, intervention techniques, and more effective drugs fall in the domain of the professional physician. Also, medical interventions are commonly required in a state of urgency. Hence, patients have neither the skills nor the time and resources to obtain accurate information when needed. Channeling all healthcare needs through a primary care provider can reduce this information gap when the primary care provider acts as the patient's advocate or agent. Conversely, the Internet is becoming a prominent source of medical information, and medical advertising is having an impact on consumer expectations.

In a free market, patients must directly bear the cost of services received. The purpose of insurance is to protect against the risk of unforeseen catastrophic events. Because the fundamental purpose of insurance is to meet major expenses when unlikely events occur, having insurance for basic and routine health care undermines the principle of insurance. When you buy home insurance to protect your property against the unlikely event of a fire, you do not anticipate the occurrence of a loss. The probability that you will suffer a loss by fire is very small. If a fire does occur and cause major damage, insurance will cover the loss, but insurance does not cover routine wear and tear on the house, such as chipped paint or a leaky faucet. Health insurance, however, generally covers basic and routine services that are predictable. Health insurance coverage for minor services, such as colds and coughs, earaches, and so forth, amounts to prepayment for such services. Health insurance has the effect of insulating patients from the full cost of health care. There is a moral hazard that, once enrollees have purchased health insurance, they will use healthcare services to a greater extent than if they were to pay for these services out-of-pocket.

At least two additional factors limit the ability of patients to make decisions. First, decisions about the utilization of health care are often determined by need rather than by price-based demand. *Need* has been defined as the amount of medical care that medical experts believe a person should have to remain or become healthy (Feldstein, 1993). Second, the delivery of health care can result in demand creation. This follows from self-assessed need, which, coupled with moral hazard, leads to greater utilization, creating an artificial demand because prices are not taken into consideration. Practitioners who have a financial interest in additional treatments also create artificial demand (Hemenway & Fallon, 1985), referred to as provider-induced demand or supplier-induced demand. Functioning as patients' agents, physicians

exert enormous influence on the demand for healthcare services (Altman & Wallack, 1996). Demand creation occurs when physicians prescribe medical care beyond what is clinically necessary. This can include practices such as making more frequent follow-up appointments than necessary, prescribing excessive medical tests, or performing unnecessary surgery (Santerre & Neun, 1996).

In a free market, patients have information on price and quality for each provider. The current system has other drawbacks that obstruct information-seeking efforts. Item-based pricing is one such hurdle. Surgery is a good example to illustrate item-based pricing, also referred to as "fee for service." Patients can generally obtain the fees the surgeon would charge for a particular operation. But the final bill, after the surgery has been performed, is likely to include charges for supplies, use of the hospital's facilities, and services performed by providers such as anesthesiologists, nurse anesthetists, and pathologists. These providers, sometimes referred to as phantom providers, who function in an adjunct capacity, bill for their services separately. Item billing for such additional services, which sometimes cannot be anticipated, makes it extremely difficult to ascertain the total price before services have actually been received. Package pricing can help overcome these drawbacks, but it has made relatively little headway for pricing medical procedures. *Package pricing* refers to a bundled fee for a package of related services. In the surgery example, this would mean one all-inclusive price for the surgeon's fees, hospital facilities, supplies, diagnostics, pathology, anesthesia, and postsurgical follow-up.

Third-Party Insurers and Payers

Insurance often functions as the intermediary among those who finance, deliver, and receive health care. The insurance intermediary does not have the incentive to be the patient's advocate on either price or quality. At best, employees can air their dissatisfactions with the plan to their employer, who has the power to discontinue the current plan and choose another company. In reality, however, employers may be reluctant to change plans if the current plan offers lower premiums compared to a different plan.

Multiple Payers

A national healthcare system is sometimes also referred to as a *single-payer system* because there is one primary payer, the government. When delivering services, providers send the bill to an agency of the government that subsequently sends payment to each provider. In contrast, the United States has a multiplicity of health plans. Multiple payers often represent a billing and collection nightmare for the providers of services. Multiple payers make the system more cumbersome in several ways:

- It is extremely difficult for providers to keep tabs on the numerous health plans. For example, it is difficult to keep up with which services are covered under each plan and how much each plan will pay for those services.

- Providers must hire claims processors to bill for services and monitor receipt of payments. Billing practices are not standardized, and each payer establishes its own format.

- Payments can be denied for not precisely following the requirements set by each payer.

- Denied claims necessitate rebilling.

- When only partial payment is received, some health plans may allow the provider to balance bill the patient for the amount the health plan did not pay. Other plans prohibit balance billing. Even when the balance-billing option is available to the provider, it triggers a new cycle of billings and collection efforts.

- Providers must sometimes engage in lengthy collection efforts, including writing collection letters, turning delinquent accounts over to collection agencies, and finally writing off as bad debt amounts that cannot be collected.

- Government programs have complex regulations for determining whether payment is made for services actually delivered. Medicare, for example, requires that each provider maintain lengthy documentation on services provided. Medicaid is known for lengthy delays in paying providers.

It is generally believed that the United States spends far more on administrative costs—costs associated with billing, collections, bad debts, and maintaining medical records—than do the national healthcare systems in other countries.

Power Balancing

The U.S. health services system involves multiple players, not just multiple payers. The key players in the system have been physicians, administrators of health service institutions, insurance companies, large employers, and the government. Big business, labor, insurance companies, physicians, and hospitals make up the powerful and politically active special interest groups represented before lawmakers by high-priced lobbyists. Each set of players has its own economic interests to protect. Physicians, for instance, want to maintain their incomes and have minimum interference with the way they practice medicine; institutional administrators seek to maximize reimbursement from private and public insurers. Insurance companies and MCOs are interested in maintaining their share of the health insurance market; large employers want to contain the costs they incur providing health insurance as a benefit to their employees. The government tries to maintain or enhance existing benefits for those covered under public insurance programs and simultaneously contain the cost of providing these benefits. The problem is that self-interests of different players are often at odds. For example, providers seek to increase government reimbursement for services delivered to Medicare, Medicaid, and CHIP beneficiaries, but the government wants to contain cost increases. Employers dislike rising health insurance premiums. Health plans, under pressure from the employers, may constrain fees for the providers, who then resent these cuts.

The fragmented self-interests of the various players produce countervailing forces within the system. In an environment that is rife with motivations to protect conflicting self-interests, achieving comprehensive system-wide reforms has been next to impossible, and cost containment has remained a major challenge. Consequently, the approach to healthcare reform in the United States has been characterized as incremental or piecemeal, and the focus of reform initiatives has been confined to health insurance coverage and payment cuts to providers rather than how care can be better provided.

Litigation Risks

America is a litigious society. Motivated by the prospects of enormous jury awards, Americans are quick to drag an alleged offender into a courtroom at the slightest perception of incurred harm. Private healthcare providers have become increasingly susceptible to litigation. Hence, in the United States, the risk of malpractice lawsuits is a real consideration in the practice of medicine. To protect themselves against the possibility of litigation, it is not uncommon for practitioners to engage in what is referred to as *defensive medicine* by prescribing additional diagnostic tests, scheduling return checkup visits, and maintaining copious documentation. Many of these additional efforts may be unnecessary; hence, they are costly and inefficient.

High Technology

The United States has been the hotbed of research and innovation in new medical technology. Growth in science and technology often creates demand for new services despite shrinking resources to finance sophisticated care. People generally equate high-tech care to high-quality care. They want "the latest and the best," especially when health insurance will pay for new treatments. Physicians and technicians want to try the latest gadgets. Hospitals compete on the basis of having the most modern equipment and facilities. Once capital investments are made, costs must be recouped through utilization. Legal risks for providers and health plans alike may also play a role in discouraging denial of new technology. Thus, several factors promote the use of costly new technology once it is developed.

Continuum of Services

Medical care services are classified into three broad categories: curative (e.g., drugs, treatments, and surgeries), restorative (e.g., physical, occupational, and speech therapies), and preventive (e.g., prenatal care, mammograms, and immunizations). Healthcare settings are no longer confined to the hospital and the physician's office, where many of the aforementioned services were once delivered. Additional settings, such as home health, subacute care units, and outpatient surgery centers, have emerged in response to the changing configuration of economic incentives. **Table 7-2** depicts the continuum of healthcare services. The healthcare continuum in the United States remains lopsided, with a heavier emphasis on specialized services than on preventive services, primary care, and management of chronic conditions.

Quest for Quality

Even though the definition and measurement of quality in health care are not as clear-cut as they are in other industries, the delivery sector of health care has come under increased pressure to develop quality standards and demonstrate compliance with those standards. There are higher expectations for improved health outcomes at the individual and broader community levels. The concept of continual quality improvement has also received much emphasis in managing healthcare institutions.

TABLE 7-2 The Continuum of Healthcare Services

Types of Health Services	Delivery Settings
Preventive care	Public health programs
	Community programs
	Personal lifestyles
	Primary care settings
Primary care	Physician's office or clinic
	Community health centers
	Self-care
	Alternative medicine
	Medical homes
Specialized care	Specialist provider clinics
Chronic care	Primary care settings
	Specialist provider clinics
	Home health
	Long-term care facilities
	Self-care
	Alternative medicine
Long-term care	Long-term care facilities
	Home health
Subacute care	Special subacute units (hospitals, long-term care facilities)
	Home health
	Outpatient surgical centers
Acute care	Hospitals
Rehabilitative care	Rehabilitation departments (hospitals, long-term care facilities)
	Home health
	Outpatient rehabilitation centers
End-of-life care	Hospice services provided in a variety of settings

Source: Shi, L., & Singh, D. (2015). *Delivering health care in America: A systems approach* (6th ed.). Burlington, MA: Jones & Bartlett.

TRENDS AND DIRECTIONS

Since the final 2 decades of the 20th century, the U.S. healthcare delivery system has continued to undergo certain fundamental shifts in emphasis These transformations are summarized in **Figure 7-4**.

Promotion of health while reducing costs has been the driving force behind these trends.

| FIGURE 7-4 | Trends and directions in healthcare delivery. |

◊ Illness ⟶ Wellness

◊ Acute care ⟶ Primary care

◊ Inpatient ⟶ Outpatient

◊ Individual health ⟶ Community well-being

◊ Fragmented care ⟶ Managed care

◊ Independent institutions ⟶ Integrated systems

◊ Service duplication ⟶ Continuum of services

Source: Shi, L., & Singh, D. (2015). *Delivering health care in America: A systems approach* (6th ed.). Burlington, MA: Jones & Bartlett.

An example of a shift in emphasis is the concept of health itself: The focus is changing from illness to wellness. Such a change requires new methods and settings for wellness promotion, although the treatment of illness continues to be the primary goal of the health services delivery system. The ACA is moving in that direction, partly by shifting focus from disease treatment to disease prevention, better health outcomes for individuals and communities, and lower healthcare costs.

Significance for Healthcare Practitioners

An understanding of the intricacies within the health services system would be beneficial to all those who come in contact with the system. In their respective training programs, health professionals, such as physicians, nurses, technicians, therapists, dietitians, and pharmacists, as well as others, may understand their own individual roles but remain ignorant of the forces outside their profession that could significantly affect current and future practices. An understanding of the healthcare delivery system can attune advanced practice nurses to their relationship with the rest of the healthcare environment. It can help them understand changes and the impact of those changes on their own practice. Adaptation and relearning are strategies that can prepare health professionals to cope with an environment that will see ongoing change long into the future. For example, many of the ACA's requirements present both opportunities and challenges for healthcare practitioners. For example, besides increasing the number of the insured who will flock to providers to receive services, the ACA places additional responsibilities on providers to deliver services in a more coordinated manner while also improving the quality of care. However, healthcare practitioners are concerned that changes in the ACA regarding healthcare financing may affect the availability of adequate and sustainable funding as they make adjustments to cope with the influx of recently insured consumers who are likely to have greater healthcare needs than the general population does.

Significance for Healthcare Managers

An understanding of the healthcare system has specific implications for health services managers, who must understand the macroenvironment in which they make critical decisions in planning and strategic management, regardless of whether they manage a private institution or a public service agency.

Such decisions and actions, eventually, affect the efficiency and quality of services delivered. The interactions among the system's key components and the implications of those interactions must be well understood because the operations of healthcare institutions are strongly influenced, either directly or indirectly, by the financing of health services, reimbursement rates, insurance mechanisms, delivery modes, new statutes and legal opinions, and government regulations.

The environment of healthcare delivery will continue to remain fluid and dynamic. The viability of delivery settings, and, thus, the success of healthcare managers, often depends on how the managers react to the system dynamics. Timeliness of action is often a critical factor that can make the difference between failure and success. Following are some more specific reasons why understanding the healthcare delivery system is indispensable for healthcare managers.

Positioning the Organization

Managers need to understand their own organizational position within the macroenvironment of the healthcare system. Senior managers, such as chief executive officers, must constantly gauge the nature and impact of the fundamental shifts illustrated in Figure 7-4. Managers need to consider which changes in the current configuration of financing, insurance, payment, and delivery might affect their organization's long-term stability. Middle and first-line managers also need to understand their role in the current configuration and how that role might change in the future. How should resources be realigned to effectively respond to those changes? For example, these managers need to evaluate whether certain functions in their departments will have to be eliminated, modified, or added. Would the changes involve further training? What processes are likely to change and how? What do the managers need to do to maintain the integrity of their institution's mission, the goodwill of the patients they

serve, and the quality of care? Well-thought-out and appropriately planned change is likely to cause less turbulence for the providers as well as for the recipients of care.

Handling Threats and Opportunities

Changes in any of the functions of financing, insurance, payment, and delivery can present new threats or opportunities in the healthcare market. Healthcare managers are more effective if they proactively deal with any threats to their institution's profitability and viability. Managers need to find ways to transform certain threats into new opportunities.

Evaluating Implications

Managers are better able to evaluate the implications of health policy and new reform proposals when they understand the relevant issues and how such issues link to the delivery of health services in the establishments they manage. The expansion of health insurance coverage under the ACA brings more individuals into the healthcare system, creating further demand for health services. Planning and staffing for the right mix of healthcare workforce to meet this anticipated surge in demand are critical.

Planning

Senior managers are often responsible for strategic planning regarding which services should be added or discontinued, which resources should be committed to facility expansion, or what should be done with excess capacity. Any long-range planning must take into consideration the current makeup of health services delivery, the evolving trends, and the potential impact of these trends.

Capturing New Markets

Healthcare managers are in a better position to capture new health services markets if they understand emerging trends in the financing, insurance, payment, and delivery functions. New opportunities must be explored before any newly evolving segments of the market get overcrowded. An understanding of the dynamics within the system is essential to forging new marketing strategies to stay ahead of the competition and often to finding a service niche.

Complying with Regulations

Delivery of healthcare services is heavily regulated. Healthcare managers must comply with government regulations, such as standards of participation in government programs, licensing rules, and security and privacy laws regarding patient information, and must operate within the constraints of reimbursement rates. The Medicare and Medicaid programs have, periodically, made drastic changes to their reimbursement methodologies that have triggered the need for operational changes in the way services are organized and delivered. Private agencies, such as The Joint Commission, also play an indirect regulatory role, mainly in the monitoring of quality of services. Healthcare managers have no choice but to play by the rules set by the various public and private agencies. Hence, it is paramount that healthcare managers acquaint themselves with the rules and regulations governing their areas of operation.

Following the Organizational Mission

Knowledge of the healthcare system and its development is essential for effective management of healthcare organizations. By keeping up to date on community needs, technological progress, consumer demand, and economic prospects, managers can be in a better position to fulfill their organizational missions to enhance access, improve service quality, and achieve efficiency in the delivery of services.

Significance for Educational Settings

Nurse educators should teach students at all levels about how the healthcare system is organized and the impact on their practice. Helping students to recognize why certain decisions and actions are taken in different healthcare settings prepares them for the reality of the constraints that may influence their practice once they enter the market.

There is a recent recognition of the importance of interprofessional teams for delivering quality, safe care. Working with and appreciating other disciplines begins in educational settings with two or more disciplines learning together, appreciating each other's roles and contributions, and making decisions together about patient outcomes.

HEALTHCARE SYSTEMS OF OTHER COUNTRIES

By 2012, the 25 wealthiest nations all had some form of universal coverage (Rodin & de Ferranti, 2012). Canada and western European nations have used three basic models for structuring their national healthcare systems:

1. In a system under national health insurance (NHI), such as in Canada, the government finances health care through general taxes, but the actual care is delivered by private providers. In the context of the quad-function model, NHI requires a tighter consolidation of the financing, insurance, and payment functions coordinated by the government. Delivery is characterized by detached private arrangements.

2. In a national health system (NHS), such as in Great Britain, in addition to financing a tax-supported NHI program, the government manages the infrastructure for the delivery of medical care. Under such a system, the government operates most of the medical institutions. Most healthcare providers, such as physicians, are either government employees or are tightly organized in a publicly managed infrastructure. In the context of the quad-function model, NHS requires a tighter consolidation of all four functions.

3. In a socialized health insurance (SHI) system, such as in Germany, government-mandated

contributions by employers and employees finance health care. Private providers deliver healthcare services. Private not-for-profit insurance companies, called sickness funds, are responsible for collecting the contributions and paying physicians and hospitals (Santerre & Neun, 1996). In a socialized health insurance system, insurance and payment functions are closely integrated, and the financing function is better coordinated with the insurance and payment functions than in the United States. Delivery is characterized by independent private arrangements. The government exercises overall control.

GLOBAL HEALTH CHALLENGES AND REFORM

Developing countries, containing almost 85% of the world's population, claim only 11% of the world's health spending. Yet, these countries account for 93% of the worldwide burden of disease. The six developing regions of the world are East Asia and the Pacific, Europe (mainly eastern Europe) and Central Asia, Latin America and the Caribbean, the Middle East and North Africa, South Asia, and sub-Saharan Africa. Of these, the latter two have the least resources and the greatest health burden. On a per capita basis, industrialized countries have six times as many hospital beds and three times as many physicians as developing countries. People with private financial means can find reasonably good health care in many parts of the developing world. However, the majority of the populations have to depend on limited government services that are often of questionable quality, as evaluated by Western standards. As a general observation, government financing for health services increases in countries with higher per capita incomes (Schieber & Maeda, 1999).

There is a huge gap in health care and health status between developing and developed countries. For example, in 2009, the global life expectancy at birth was 68 years of age, while life expectancy in the African region was only

54. Infant mortality rates varied between 2 per 1,000 live births and 114 per 1,000 live births. There were also wide variations in health care for pregnant women, availability of skilled health personnel for childbirth, and access to medicine (World Health Organization, 2012).

The poor quality and low efficiency of healthcare services in many countries, especially services provided by the public sector, which is often the main source of care for poor people, have become serious issues for decision makers in these countries (Sachs, 2012). These factors combined with the rising out-of-pocket costs and high numbers of uninsured forced many governments to launch healthcare reform efforts. Many low- and middle-income countries are moving toward universal health coverage (Lagomarsino, Garabrant, Adyas, Muga, & Otoo, 2012). On the other hand, international health assistance plays a significant role in health care in many developing countries. Global aid increased from $10 billion in 2000 to $27 billion in 2010 (Sachs, 2012). However, the total international aid started to fall in 2011 because of a global recession (Organisation for Economic Co-operation and Development, 2012).

THE SYSTEMS FRAMEWORK

A system consists of a set of interrelated and interdependent, logically coordinated components designed to achieve common goals. Even though the various functional components of the health services delivery structure in the United States are, at best, only loosely coordinated, the main components can be identified using a systems model. The systems framework used here helps one understand that the structure of healthcare services in the United States is based on some foundations, provides a logical arrangement of the various components, and demonstrates a progression from inputs to outputs. The main elements of this arrangement are system inputs (resources), system structure, system processes, and system outputs (outcomes). In addition, system outlook (future directions) is a necessary feature of a dynamic system (see **Figure 7-5**).

System Foundations

The current healthcare system is not an accident. Historical, cultural, social, and economic factors explain its current structure. These factors also affect forces that shape new trends and developments, as well as those that impede change.

System Resources

No mechanism for health services delivery can fulfill its primary objective without deploying the necessary human and nonhuman resources. Human resources consist of the various types and categories of workers directly engaged in the delivery of health services to patients. Such personnel—physicians, nurses, dentists, pharmacists, other doctorally trained professionals,

---

FIGURE 7-5　The systems model.

ENVIRONMENT

I. SYSTEM FOUNDATIONS
Cultural Beliefs and Values and Historical Developments
"Beliefs, Values, and Health"
"The Evolution of Health Services in the United States"

↓

System Features

II. SYSTEM RESOURCES
Human Resources
"Health Services Professionals"

Nonhuman Resources
"Medical Technology"

"Health Services Financing"

III. SYSTEM PROCESSES
The Continuum of Care
"Outpatient and Primary Care Services"

"Inpatient Facilities and Services"

"Managed Care and Integrated Organizations"

Special Populations
"Long-Term Care"

"Health Services for Special Populations"

IV. SYSTEM OUTCOMES
Issues and Concerns
"Cost, Access, and Quality"

Change and Reform
"Health Policy"

↓

FUTURE TRENDS

V. SYSTEM OUTLOOK
"The Future of Health Services Delivery"

Source: Shi, L., & Singh, D. (2015). *Delivering health care in America: A systems approach* (6th ed.). Burlington, MA: Jones & Bartlett.

and numerous categories of allied health professionals—usually have direct contact with patients. Numerous ancillary workers—billing and collection agents, marketing and public relations personnel, and building maintenance employees—often play an important, but indirect, supportive role in the delivery of health care.

Resources are closely intertwined with access to health care. For instance, in certain rural areas of the United States, access is restricted because of a shortage of health professionals within certain categories. Development and diffusion of technology also determine the caliber of health care to which people may have access. Financing for health insurance and reimbursement to providers affect access indirectly.

System Processes

System resources influence the development and change in the physical infrastructure—such as hospitals, clinics, and nursing homes—essential for the different processes of healthcare delivery. Most healthcare services are delivered in noninstitutional settings, mainly associated with processes referred to as outpatient care. Institutional health services provided in hospitals, nursing homes, and rehabilitation institutions, for example, are predominantly inpatient services . Managed care and integrated systems represent a fundamental change in the financing (including payment and insurance) and delivery of health care. Special institutional and community-based settings have been developed for long-term care. Delivery of services should be tailored to meet the special needs of certain vulnerable population groups.

System Outcomes

System outcomes refers to the critical issues and concerns surrounding what the health services system has been able to accomplish, or not accomplish, in relation to its primary objective: to provide to an entire nation cost-effective health services that meet certain established standards of quality. The previous three elements of the systems model play a critical role in fulfilling this objective. Access, cost, and quality are the main outcome criteria to evaluate the success of a healthcare delivery system. Issues and concerns regarding these criteria trigger broad initiatives for reforming the system through health policy.

System Outlook

A dynamic healthcare system must be forward looking. In essence, it must project into the future the accomplishment of desired system outcomes in view of anticipated social, economic, political, technological, informational, ecological, anthro-cultural, and global forces of change.

SUMMARY

The United States has a unique system of healthcare delivery. Its basic features characterize it as a patchwork of subsystems. Health care is delivered through an amalgam of private and public financing, through private health insurance and public insurance programs; the latter programs are for special groups. Contrary to popular opinion, healthcare delivery in the United States is not governed by free-market principles; at best, it is an imperfect market. Yet the system is not dominated or controlled by a single entity as would be the case in national healthcare systems.

No country in the world has a perfect system, and most nations with a national healthcare program also have a private sector that varies in size. Because of resource limitations, universal access remains a theoretical concept even in countries that offer universal health insurance coverage. The developing countries of the world also face serious challenges due to scarce resources and strong underlying needs for services.

Healthcare managers must understand how the healthcare delivery system works and evolves. Such an understanding can help them maintain a strategic position within the macroenvironment of the healthcare system. The systems framework provides an organized approach to understanding the various components of the U.S. healthcare delivery system.

ACA TAKEAWAY

- The main goal of the ACA is to increase access to health care and make it more affordable, mainly for those who were previously uninsured.

- All U.S. citizens and legal residents are required to have health insurance or pay a fine.

- Two main avenues for covering the uninsured are expansion of Medicaid and purchase of subsidized private health insurance through government-run exchanges.

- Insurance companies are required to include coverage for a variety of healthcare services.

- The ACA fails to achieve universal coverage; it also may not successfully achieve access for a large segment of the U.S. population.

- The ACA promises to shift focus from disease treatment to disease prevention and improved health outcomes.

- Additional responsibilities are placed on providers to deliver services in a more coordinated manner while also improving the quality of care.

DISCUSSION QUESTIONS

1. Using the principles of complexity science, why does cost containment remain an elusive goal in U.S. health services delivery?

2. Why is it that, despite public and private health insurance programs, some U.S. citizens are without healthcare coverage? How will the ACA change this?

3. How does the intermediary role of insurance affect your practice setting and the care you provide?

4. Who are the major players in the U.S. health services system? What are the positive and negative effects of the often conflicting self-interests of these players? How can organizations at the local level begin to connect the players to improve safety and quality while at the same time reduce costs?

5. Why is it important for advanced practice nurses to understand the intricacies of the healthcare delivery system?

6. Provide a general overview of the Affordable Care Act. How has the implementation of the ACA affected your organization and your practice?

REFERENCES

Altman, S. H., & Reinhardt, U. E. (1996). Introduction: Where does health care reform go from here? An uncharted odyssey. In S. H. Altman & U. E. Reinhardt (Eds.), *Strategic choices for a changing health care system* (pp. xxi–xxxii). Chicago, IL: Health Administration Press.

Altman, S. H., & Wallack, S. S. (1996). Health care spending: Can the United States control it? In S. H. Altman & U. E. Reinhardt (Eds.), *Strategic choices for a changing health care system* (pp. 1–32). Chicago, IL: Health Administration Press.

Canadian Institute for Health Information. (2012). *National health expenditure trends, 1975 to 2012.* Ottawa, ON: The Institute. Retrieved from https://secure.cihi.ca/free_products/NHEXTrendsReport2012EN.pdf

Church, J., & Barker, P. (1998). Regionalization of health services in Canada: A critical perspective. *International Journal of Health Services, 28*(3), 467–486.

CNN Health. (2014, May 5). Obamacare: Enrollment statistics and Medicaid expansion. Retrieved from http://www.cnn.com/interactive/2013/09/health/map-obamacare

Feldstein, P. J. (1993). *Health care economics* (4th ed.). New York, NY: Delmar.

Health Resources and Services Administration. (2013). Health center snapshot 2011. Retrieved from http://www.hrsa.gov/data-statistics/health-center-data/index.html

Hemenway, D., & Fallon, D. (1985). Testing for physician-induced demand with hypothetical cases. *Medical Care, 23*(4), 344–349.

Lagomarsino, G., Garabrant, A., Adyas, A., Muga, R., & Otoo, N. (2012). Moving towards universal health coverage: Health insurance reforms in nine developing countries in Africa and Asia. *Lancet, 380*(9845), 933–943.

Organisation for Economic Co-operation and Development. (2012). Development: Aid to developing countries falls because of global recession. Retrieved from http://www.oecd.org/development /developmentaidtodevelopingcountriesfallsbe causeofglobalrecession.htm

Parente, S. T., & Feldman, R. (2013). Microsimulation of private health insurance and Medicaid take-up following the U.S. Supreme Court decision upholding the Affordable Care Act. *Health Services Research, 48*(2 Pt. 2), 826–849.

Rodin, J., & de Ferranti, D. (2012). Universal health coverage: The third global health transition? *Lancet, 380*(9845), 861–862.

Sachs, J. D. (2012). Achieving universal health coverage in low-income settings. *Lancet, 380*(9845), 944–947.

Santerre, R. E., & Neun, S. P. (1996). *Health economics: Theories, insights, and industry studies.* Chicago, IL: Irwin.

Schieber, G., & Maeda, A. (1999). Health care financing and delivery in developing countries. *Health Affairs, 18*(3), 193–205.

Shi, L., & Singh, D. (2015). *Delivering health care in America: A systems approach* (6th ed.). Burlington, MA: Jones & Bartlett.

U.S. Bureau of Labor Statistics. (2011). *Occupational outlook handbook, 2010–2011.* Retrieved from http://www.bls.gov/ooh/home.htm

U.S. Census Bureau. (2012). The 2012 statistical abstract. Retrieved from http://www.census.gov /compendia/statab/cats/health_nutrition /health_care_resources.html

U.S. Department of Health and Human Services. (2013). About the law. Retrieved from http://www .hhs.gov/healthcare/rights/index.html

Wolinsky, F. D. (1988). *The sociology of health: Principles, practitioners, and issues* (2nd ed.) Belmont, CA: Wadsworth.

World Health Organization. (2012). *World health statistics 2012.* Retrieved from http://www.who.int /gho/publications/world_health_statistics /2012/en

CHAPTER 8

Beliefs, Values, and Health

Leiyu Shi and Douglas A. Singh

CHAPTER OBJECTIVES

1. Understand the concepts of health and disease, risk factors, and the role of health promotion and disease prevention.

2. Summarize the disease prevention requisites under the Affordable Care Act.

3. Understand public health and appreciate its expanding role in health protection both in the United States and globally.

4. Explore the determinants of health and measures related to health.

5. Understand the American anthro-cultural values and their implications for healthcare delivery.

6. Evaluate justice and equity in health care according to contrasting theories.

7. Explore the integration of individual and population health.

INTRODUCTION

From an economic perspective, curative medicine appears to produce decreasing returns in health improvement while increasing healthcare expenditures (Saward & Sorensen, 1980). There has also been a growing recognition of the benefits to society from the promotion of health and prevention of disease, disability, and premature death. However, progress in this direction has been slow because of the prevailing social values and beliefs that still focus on curing

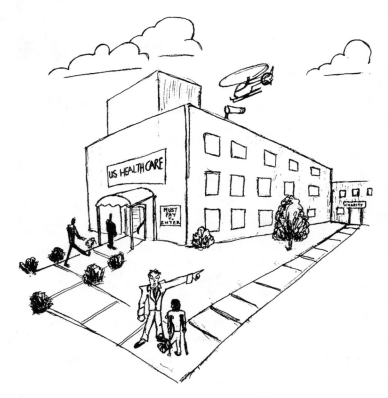

"This is the market justice system. Social justice is over there."

diseases rather than promoting health. The common definitions of health, as well as measures for evaluating health status, reflect similar inclinations. This chapter proposes a balanced approach to health, although fully achieving such an ideal is not without difficult challenges. The 10-year Healthy People initiatives, undertaken by the U.S. Department of Health and Human Services (U.S. DHHS) since 1980, illustrate steps taken in this direction, even though these initiatives have been typically strong in rhetoric but weak in actionable strategies and sustainable funding.

Anthro-cultural factors reflected in the beliefs and values ingrained in the American culture have been influential in laying the foundations of a system that has remained predominantly private, as opposed to a tax-financed national healthcare program.

This chapter further explores the issue of equity in the distribution of health services, using the contrasting theories of market justice and social justice. U.S. healthcare delivery incorporates both principles, which are complementary in some ways and which create conflicts in other areas. The Affordable Care Act (ACA) tilts the system more toward a social justice orientation, places a greater emphasis on preventive services, but does not quite promise to achieve equitable access to health care for all Americans.

SIGNIFICANCE FOR ADVANCED PRACTICE NURSES

Materials covered in this chapter have several implications for nurses in administration, practice, and education: (1) The health status of a population has tremendous bearing on the utilization of health services, assuming the services are readily available. Planning of health services and practice changes must be governed by demographic and health trends and initiatives toward reducing disease and disability. (2) The basic meanings of health, determinants of health, and health risk appraisal should be used to design appropriate educational, preventive, and therapeutic initiatives. (3) There is a growing emphasis on evaluating the effectiveness of healthcare organizations based on the contributions they make to community and population health. The concepts discussed in this chapter can guide advanced practice nurses in implementing programs of most value to their communities. (4) Quantified measures of health status and utilization can be used to evaluate the adequacy and effectiveness of existing programs, plan new strategies, measure progress, and discontinue ineffective services.

BASIC CONCEPTS OF HEALTH

Health

In the United States, the concepts of health and health care have largely been governed by the medical model, more specifically referred to as the biomedical model. The *medical model* defines health as the absence of illness or disease. This definition implies that optimum health exists when a person is free of symptoms and does not require medical treatment. However, it is not a definition of health in the true sense. This prevailing view of health emphasizes clinical diagnosis and medical interventions to treat disease or symptoms of disease, while prevention of disease and health promotion are not included. Therefore, when the term *healthcare delivery* is used, in reality it refers to medical care delivery.

Medical sociologists have gone a step further in defining health as the state of optimum capacity of an individual to perform his or her expected social roles and tasks, such as work, school, and doing household chores (Parsons, 1972). A person who is unable (as opposed to unwilling) to perform his or her social roles in society is considered sick. However, this concept also seems inadequate because many people continue to engage in their social obligations despite suffering from pain, cough, colds, and other types of temporary disabilities, including mental distress. Then, there are those who shirk from their social responsibilities even when they may be in good health. In other words, optimal health is not necessarily reflected in a person's engagement in social roles and responsibilities.

An emphasis on both physical and mental dimensions of health is found in the definition of health proposed by the Society for Academic Emergency Medicine, according to which health is "a state of physical and mental well-being that facilitates the achievement of individual and societal goals" (Ethics Committee, Society for Academic Emergency Medicine, 1992). This view of health recognizes the importance of achieving harmony between the physiological and emotional dimensions.

The World Health Organization (WHO) definition of health is most often cited as the ideal for healthcare delivery systems; it recognizes that optimal health is more than a mere absence of disease or infirmity. WHO defines health as "a state of complete physical, mental and social well-being and not merely the absence of disease or infirmity" (WHO, 1948). As a biopsychosocial model, WHO's definition specifically identifies social well-being as a third dimension of health. For example, having a social support network is positively associated with life stresses, self-esteem, and social relations. Conversely, many studies show that social isolation is associated with a higher risk for poor health and mortality (Pantell et al., 2013).

WHO has also defined a healthcare system as all the activities whose primary purpose is to promote, restore, or maintain health (McKee, 2001). As this chapter points out, health care should include much more than medical care. Thus, *health care* can be defined as a variety of services believed to improve a person's health and well-being.

There has been a growing interest in holistic health, which emphasizes the well-being of every aspect of what makes a person whole and complete. Thus, holistic medicine seeks to treat the individual as a whole person (Ward, 1995). For example, diagnosis and treatment should take into account the mental, emotional, spiritual, nutritional, environmental, and other factors surrounding the origin of disease (Cohen, 2003).

Holistic health incorporates the spiritual dimension as a fourth element—in addition to the physical, mental, and social aspects—necessary for optimal health (**Figure 8-1**). A growing volume of medical literature, both in the United States and abroad, points to the healing effects of a person's religion and spirituality on

morbidity and mortality. The importance of spirituality as an aspect of health care is also reflected in a number of policy documents produced by the WHO (2003) and other bodies.

From an extensive review of literature, Chida, Steptoe, and Powell (2009) concluded that religious practice/spirituality was associated with reductions in death from all causes and death from cardiovascular diseases. Heart patients who attended regular religious services were found to have a significant survival advantage (Oman, Kurata, Strawbridge, & Cohen, 2002). Religious and spiritual beliefs and practices have shown a positive impact on a person's physical, mental, and social well-being. Many studies have shown positive relations between religious practice and protective health behaviors (Chida et al., 2009). Several religious communities promote healthy lifestyles associated with reduced tobacco use and alcohol consumption, as well as healthy diet. An examination of literature found a reduced risk for cancer in these communities (Hoff, Johannessen-Henry, Ross, Hvidt, & Johansen, 2008). Spiritual well-being has also been recognized as an important

FIGURE 8-1   The four dimensions of holistic health.

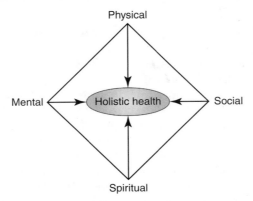

Source: Shi, L., & Singh, D. (2015). *Delivering health care in America: A systems approach* (6th ed.). Burlington, MA: Jones & Bartlett.

internal resource for helping people cope with illness. For instance, a study conducted at the University of Michigan found that 93% of the women undergoing cancer treatment indicated that their religious lives helped them sustain their hope (Roberts, Brown, Elkins, & Larson, 1997). Studies have found that a large percentage of patients want their physicians to consider their spiritual needs, and almost half expressed a desire for the physicians to pray with them if they could (Post, Puchalski, & Larson, 2000).

The spiritual dimension is frequently tied to one's religious beliefs, values, morals, and practices. Broadly, it is described as meaning, purpose, and fulfillment in life; hope and will to live; faith; and a person's relationship with God (Marwick, 1995; Ross, 1995; Swanson, 1995). A clinically tested scale to measure spiritual well-being included categories such as belief in a power greater than oneself, purpose in life, faith, trust in providence, prayer, meditation, group worship, ability to forgive, and gratitude for life (Hatch, Burg, Naberhaus, & Hellmich, 1998).

The Committee on Religion and Psychiatry of the American Psychiatric Association has issued a position statement to emphasize the importance of maintaining respect for a patient's religious and spiritual beliefs. For the first time, "religious or spiritual problem" was included as a diagnostic category in *Diagnostic and Statistical Manual of Mental Disorders, Fifth Edition* (*DSM-5*). The holistic approach to health also alludes to the need for incorporating alternative therapies into the predominant medical model.

Quality of Life

The term *quality of life* is used to capture the essence of overall satisfaction with life during and following a person's encounter with the healthcare delivery system. Thus, the term is employed in two ways. First, it is an indicator of how satisfied a person is with the experiences while receiving health care. Specific life domains, such as comfort factors, respect, privacy, security, degree of independence, decision-making autonomy, and attention to personal preferences, are significant to most people. These factors are now regarded as rights that patients can demand during any type of healthcare encounter. Second, quality of life can refer to a person's overall satisfaction with life and with self-perceptions of health, particularly after some medical intervention. The implication is that desirable processes during medical treatment and successful outcomes would, subsequently, have a positive effect on an individual's ability to function, carry out social roles and obligations, and have a sense of fulfillment and self-worth.

Risk Factors and Disease

The occurrence of disease involves more than just a single factor. For example, the mere presence of tubercle bacillus does not mean the infected person will develop tuberculosis. Other factors, such as poverty, overcrowding, and malnutrition, may be essential for development of the disease (Friedman, 1980). Hence, tracing *risk factors*—attributes that increase the likelihood of developing a particular disease or negative health condition in the future—requires a broad approach. One useful explanation of disease occurrence (for communicable diseases, in particular) is provided by the tripartite model, sometimes referred to as the epidemiology triangle (**Figure 8-2**). Of the three entities in this model, the *host* is the organism—generally, a human—that becomes sick. Factors associated with the host include genetic makeup, level of immunity, fitness, and personal habits and behaviors. However, for the host to become sick, an *agent* must be present, although presence of an agent does not ensure that disease will occur. In the previous example, tubercle bacillus is the agent for tuberculosis. Other examples are chemical agents, radiation, tobacco smoke, dietary indiscretions, and nutritional deficiencies. The third entity, *environment*,

FIGURE 8-2 The epidemiology triangle.

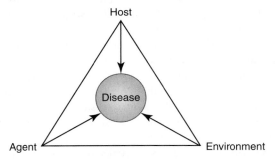

Source: Shi, L., & Singh, D. (2015). *Delivering health care in America: A systems approach* (6th ed.). Burlington, MA: Jones & Bartlett.

is external to the host and includes the physical, social, cultural, and economic aspects of the environment. Examples include sanitation, air pollution, anthro-cultural beliefs, social equity, social norms, and economic status. The environmental factors play a moderating role that can either enhance or reduce susceptibility to disease. Because the three entities often interact to produce disease, disease prevention efforts should focus on a broad approach to mitigate or eliminate risk factors associated with all three entities.

Behavioral Risk Factors

Certain individual behaviors and personal lifestyle choices represent important risk factors for illness and disease. For example, smoking has been identified as the leading cause of preventable disease and death in the United States, because it significantly increases the risk of heart disease, stroke, lung cancer, and chronic lung disease (U.S. DHHS, 2004). Substance abuse, inadequate physical exercise, a high-fat diet, irresponsible use of motor vehicles, and unsafe sex are additional examples of behavioral risk factors. (**Table 8-1** presents the percentage of the U.S. population with selected behavioral risks.)

Acute, Subacute, and Chronic Conditions

Disease can be classified as acute, subacute, or chronic. An *acute condition* is relatively severe, episodic (of short duration), and often treatable and subject to recovery. Treatments are generally provided in a hospital. Examples of acute conditions are a sudden interruption of kidney function or a myocardial infarction (heart attack). A *subacute condition* is a less severe phase of an acute illness. It can be a postacute condition, requiring continuity of treatment after discharge from a hospital. Examples include ventilator and head trauma care. A *chronic condition* is one that persists over time, is not severe, but is generally irreversible. A chronic condition may be kept under control through appropriate medical treatment, but if left untreated, the condition may lead to severe and life-threatening health problems. Examples of chronic conditions are hypertension, asthma, arthritis, heart disease, and diabetes. Contributors to chronic disease include ethnic, cultural, and behavioral factors and the social and physical environment, discussed later in this chapter.

In the United States, chronic diseases have become the leading cause of death and

TABLE 8-1	Percentage of U.S. Population with Behavioral Risks	

Behavioral Risks	Percentage of Population	Year
Alcohol (12 years and older)	51.8	2010
Marijuana (12 years and older)	6.9	2010
Cocaine use (12th graders)	1.1	2011
Cocaine use (10th graders)	0.7	2011
Cocaine use (8th graders)	0.8	2011
Cigarette smoking (18 years and older)	19.0	2011
Hypertension (20 years and older)	31.9	2009–2010
Overweight (20–74 years)	68.5	2007–2010
Serum cholesterol (20 years and older)	13.6	2009–2010

Nore: Data are based on household interviews of a sample of the civilian.

Source: Data from National Center for Health Statistics. (2012). *Health, United States, 2009*. Hyattsville, MD: U.S. Department of Health and Human Services, pp. 276, 281, 283, 292, 293, 301.

disability. Almost 50% of Americans have at least one chronic illness (Robert Wood Johnson Foundation [RWJF], 2010), and 8.7 out of every 10 deaths are attributable to chronic disease (WHO, 2011). Among both the younger and older age groups (ages 18 and up), hypertension was ranked the most common chronic condition, followed by cholesterol disorders. Among children up to age 17, respiratory diseases and asthma were the most common chronic conditions (Agency for Healthcare Research and Quality, 2006). The incidence of childhood chronic diseases has almost quadrupled over the past four decades, mostly the result of a threefold increase in childhood obesity (Partnership to Fight Chronic Disease [PFCD], 2009). Moreover, 26% of adults aged 18 or older had multiple chronic conditions in 2010. The combination of arthritis and hypertension was the most common dyad, and the combination of arthritis, hypertension, and diabetes was the most common triad (Ward & Schiller, 2010).

It is estimated that 75% of total health expenditures in the United States are attributable to the treatment of chronic conditions (PFCD, 2009). In 2011, total healthcare costs associated with the treatment of chronic diseases were approximately $1.7 trillion (PFCD, 2009). In addition, health disparities continue to be a serious threat to the health and well-being of some population groups. For example, African American, Hispanic, American Indian, and Alaskan Native adults are twice as likely as white adults to have diabetes (Centers for Disease Control and Prevention [CDC], 2010a).

There are three main reasons behind the rise of chronic conditions in the U.S. population: (1) New diagnostic methods, medical procedures, and pharmaceuticals have significantly improved the treatment of acute illnesses, survival rates, and longevity, but these achievements have come with the consequence of a larger number of people living with chronic conditions. The prevalence of chronic disease is expected to continue to rise with an aging population and longer life expectancy. (2) Screening and diagnosis have expanded in scope, frequency, and accuracy (RWJF, 2010). (3) Lifestyle choices, such as high-salt and high-fat diets and sedentary lifestyles, are risk factors that contribute to the development of chronic conditions. To address these issues, the U.S. Department of Health and Human Services (DHHS) launched a comprehensive initiative with the aid of $650 million allocated under the American Recovery and Reinvestment Act of 2009. The goal of this initiative—Communities Putting Prevention to Work—is to "reduce risk factors, prevent/delay chronic disease, promote wellness in children and adults, and provide positive, sustainable health change in communities" (U.S. DHHS 2010b).

Health Promotion and Disease Prevention

A program of health promotion and disease prevention is built on three main principles: (1) An understanding of risk factors associated with host, agent, and/or environment. Risk factors and their health consequences are evaluated through a process called *health risk appraisal*. Only when the risk factors and their health consequences are known can interventions be developed to help individuals adopt healthier lifestyles. (2) Interventions for counteracting the key risk factors include two main approaches: (a) behavior modification geared toward the goal of adopting healthier lifestyles and (b) therapeutic interventions. Both are discussed in the next paragraphs. (3) Adequate public health and social services, as discussed later in this chapter, include all health-related services designed to minimize risk factors and their negative effects in order to prevent disease, control disease outbreaks, and contain the spread of infectious agents.

Various avenues can be used for motivating individuals to alter behaviors that may contribute to disease, disability, or death. Behavior

can be modified through educational programs and incentives directed at specific high-risk populations. In the case of cigarette smoking, for example, health promotion aims at building people's knowledge, attitudes, and skills to avoid or quit smoking. It also involves reducing advertisements and other environmental enticements that promote nicotine addiction. Financial incentives/disincentives, such as a higher cigarette tax, have been used to discourage purchase of cigarettes.

Therapeutic interventions fall into three areas of preventive effort: primary prevention, secondary prevention, and tertiary prevention. *Primary prevention* refers to activities undertaken to reduce the probability that a disease will develop in the future (Kane, 1988). Its objective is to restrain the development of a disease or negative health condition before it occurs. Therapeutic intervention would include community health efforts to assist patients in smoking cessation and exercise programs to prevent conditions such as lung cancer and heart disease. Safety training and practices at the workplace can reduce serious work-related injuries. Prenatal care is known to lower infant mortality rates. Immunization has had a greater impact on prevention against childhood diseases and mortality reduction than any other public health intervention besides clean water (Plotkin & Plotkin, 1999). Hand washing, refrigeration of foods, garbage collection, sewage treatment, and protection of the water supply are also examples of primary prevention (Timmreck, 1994). There have been numerous incidents where emphasis on food safety and proper cooking could have prevented outbreaks of potentially deadly episodes, such as those caused by *E. coli*.

Secondary prevention refers to early detection and treatment of disease. Health screenings and periodic health examinations are just two examples. Screening for hypertension, cancers, and diabetes, for example, has been instrumental in prescribing early treatment. The main

| TABLE 8-2 | Annual Percent Decline in U.S. Cancer Mortality, 1991–2010 | | | |

Type of Cancer	1991–1995	1994–2003	1998–2007	2001–2010
All cancers	3.0	1.1	1.4	1.5
Breast cancer	6.3	2.5	2.2	2.2
Cervical cancer	9.7	3.6	2.6	1.5
Ovarian cancer	4.8	0.5	0.8	2.0
Prostate cancer	6.3	3.5	3.1	2.7

Source: Data from National Center for Health Statistics of the Centers for Disease Control and Prevention, National Cancer Institute, SEER Cancer Statistics Review, 1975–2010.

objective of secondary prevention is to block the progression of a disease or an injury from developing into an impairment or disability (Timmreck, 1994).

Tertiary prevention refers to interventions that could prevent complications from chronic conditions and prevent further illness, injury, or disability. For example, regular turning of bed-bound patients prevents pressure sores; rehabilitation therapies can prevent permanent disability; and infection control practices in hospitals and nursing homes are designed to prevent iatrogenic illnesses, that is, illnesses or injuries caused by the process of health care.

As shown in **Table 8-2**, prevention, early detection, and treatment efforts helped reduce cancer mortality quite significantly between 1991 and 2010. This decrease was the first sustained decline since record keeping was instituted in the 1930s.

Disease Prevention Under Healthcare Reform

Prevention and wellness have received a great deal of emphasis in the health reform law. The ACA requires Medicare and private health insurance plans to provide a range of preventive services with no out-of-pocket costs. As a result, in 2011 and 2012, an estimated 71 million Americans with private insurance gained access to preventive services (U.S. DHHS, 2013).

The ACA established the Prevention and Public Health Fund (PPHF), which has distributed almost $3.2 billion toward national preventive efforts and toward improving health outcomes and enhancing quality of health care (American Public Health Association, 2013). Grants have been issued to reduce chronic diseases. The Office of the Surgeon General has developed a National Prevention Strategy that encourages partnerships among federal, state, tribal, local, and territorial governments; business, industry, and other private sector partners; philanthropic organizations; community and faith-based organizations; and everyday Americans to improve health through prevention (National Prevention Council, 2011). The Centers for Disease Control and Prevention established a National Diabetes Prevention Program. In 2012, six organizations received $6.75 million to develop partnerships that reach a large numbers of individuals with pre-diabetes (CDC, 2013a, 2013b).

In 2011, $10 million was made available to establish and evaluate comprehensive workplace wellness programs (U.S. DHHS, 2011a). Beginning in 2014, $200 million in wellness grant funding will be available to small businesses to encourage the formation of wellness programs and employee incentivizing (Anderko et al., 2012).

PUBLIC HEALTH

Public health remains poorly understood by its prime beneficiaries, the public. For some people, public health evokes images of a massive social enterprise or welfare system. To others, the term means healthcare services for everyone. Still another image of public health is that of a body of knowledge and techniques that can be applied to health-related problems (Turnock, 1997). However, none of these ideas adequately reflects what public health is.

The Institute of Medicine (IOM) proposed that the mission of public health is to fulfill "society's interest in assuring conditions in which people can be healthy" (IOM, 1988, p. 7). Public health deals with broad societal concerns about ensuring conditions that promote optimum health for the society as a whole. It involves the application of scientific knowledge to counteract any threats that may jeopardize health and safety of the general population. Because of its extensive scope, the vast majority of public health efforts are carried out by government agencies, such as the CDC in the United States.

Three main distinctions can be seen between the practices of medicine and public health: (1) Medicine focuses on the individual patient— diagnosing symptoms, treating and preventing disease, relieving pain and suffering, and maintaining or restoring normal function. Public health, conversely, focuses on populations (Shi & Johnson, 2014). (2) The emphases in modern medicine are on the biological causes of disease and developing treatments and therapies. Public health focuses on (a) identifying the environmental, social, and behavioral risk factors as well as emerging or potential risks that may threaten people's health and safety, and (b) implementing population-wide interventions to minimize those risk factors (Peters, Drabant, Elster, Tierney, & Hatcher, 2001). (3) Medicine focuses on the treatment of disease and recovery of health. Public health deals with various efforts to prevent disease and counteract threats that may negatively affect people's health.

Public health activities can range from providing education on nutrition to passing laws that enhance automobile safety. For example, public health includes dissemination to the public and to health professionals timely information about important health issues, particularly when communicable diseases pose potential threats to large segments of a population.

Compared to the delivery of medical services, public health involves a broader range of professionals. The medical sector encompasses physicians, nurses, dentists, therapists, social workers, psychologists, nutritionists, health educators, pharmacists, laboratory technicians, health services administrators, and so forth. In addition to these professionals, public health also involves professionals such as sanitarians, epidemiologists, statisticians, industrial hygienists, environmental health specialists, food and drug inspectors, toxicologists, and economists (Lasker, 1997).

Health Protection and Environmental Health

Health protection is one of the main public health functions. In the 1850s, John Snow successfully traced the risk of cholera outbreaks in London to the Broad Street water pump (Rosen, 1993). Since then, *environmental health* has specifically dealt with preventing the spread of disease through water, air, and food (Schneider, 2000). Environmental health science, along with other public health measures, was instrumental in reducing the risk of infectious diseases during the 1900s. For example, in 1900, pneumonia, tuberculosis, and diarrhea, along with enteritis, were the top three killers in the United States (CDC, 1999);

TABLE 8-3	Leading Causes of Death, 2010	

Cause of Death	Deaths	Percentage
All causes	2,468,435	100.0
Diseases of the heart	597,689	24.2
Malignant neoplasms	574,743	23.3
Chronic lower respiratory diseases	138,080	5.6
Cerebrovascular diseases	129,476	5.2
Unintentional injuries	120,859	4.9
Alzheimer's disease	83,494	3.4
Diabetes mellitus	69,071	2.8
Nephritis, nephrotic syndrome, and nephrosis	50,476	2.0
Influenza and pneumonia	50,097	2.0
Suicide	38,364	1.6

Source: Data from National Center for Health Statistics. (2013). *Health, United States, 2012.* Hyattsville, MD: U.S. Department of Health and Human Services, p. 88.

that is no longer the case today (see **Table 8-3**). With the rapid industrialization during the 20th century, environmental health faced new challenges due to serious health hazards from chemicals, industrial waste, infectious waste, radiation, asbestos, and other toxic substances. In the 21st century, chemical, biological, and nuclear agents in the hands of terrorists and rogue nations has emerged as a new environmental threat.

Health Protection During Global Pandemics

Over time, public health has become a complex global undertaking. Its main goal of protecting the health and safety of populations from a variety of old and new threats cannot be achieved without global cooperation. In 2003, severe acute respiratory syndrome (SARS)—a contagious disease that is accompanied by fever and symptoms of pneumonia or other respiratory illness—spread from China to Canada. Worldwide, more than 8,000 people were affected (CDC, 2012).

The global threat of avian influenza has also elicited a public health response. The CDC launched a website dedicated to educating the public about avian influenza, how it is spread, and past and current outbreaks. The website contains specific information for health professionals, travelers, the poultry industry, state departments of health, and people with possible exposures to avian influenza (CDC, 2007).

After a novel H1N1 influenza virus emerged from Mexico in April 2009, U.S. health officials anticipated and prepared for an influenza pandemic, and it stretched the response capabilities of the public health system. The virus affected every U.S. state, and Americans were left unprotected because of the unavailability of antiviral medications. Since then, a global effort has been undertaken to establish collaborative networks to exchange information and contain global pandemics (WHO, 2013).

Health Protection and Preparedness in the United States

Since the horrific events of what is commonly referred to as 9/11 (September 11, 2001), the United States has opened a new chapter in health protection. The efforts to protect the health and safety of Americans began in June 2002 when President Bush signed into law the Public Health Security and Bioterrorism Preparedness Response Act of 2002. Subsequently, the Homeland Security Act of 2002 created the Department of Homeland Security (DHS) and called for a major restructuring of the nation's resources with the primary mission of helping prevent, protect against, and respond to any acts of terrorism in the United States. It also provided better tools to contain attacks on the food and water supplies; protect the nation's vital infrastructures, such as nuclear facilities; and track biological materials anywhere in the United States. The term *bioterrorism* encompasses the use of chemical, biological, and nuclear agents to cause harm to relatively large civilian populations.

Now, health protection and preparedness involves a massive operation to deal with any natural or man-made threats. Dealing with such threats requires large-scale preparations, which include appropriate tools and training for workers in medical care, public health, emergency care, and civil defense agencies at the federal, state, and local levels. It requires national initiatives to develop countermeasures, such as new vaccines, a robust public health infrastructure, and coordination among numerous agencies. It requires an infrastructure to handle large numbers of casualties and isolation facilities for contagious patients. Hospitals, public health agencies, and civil defense must be linked together through information systems. Containment of infectious agents, such as smallpox, necessitates quick detection, treatment, isolation, and organized efforts to protect the unaffected population. Rapid cleanup, evacuation of the affected population, and transfer of victims to medical care facilities require detailed plans and logistics.

The United States has confronted major natural disasters, such as Hurricane Katrina in 2005, Hurricane Sandy in 2012, and tornadoes in Oklahoma in 2013, as well as man-made mass casualties such as the Boston Marathon Bombing on April 15, 2013. Health protection and preparedness have become ongoing efforts through revitalized initiatives such as the Pandemic and All-Hazards Preparedness Act (PAHPA) of 2006, which also authorized a new Assistant Secretary for Preparedness and Response (ASPR) within the DHHS and called for the establishment of a quadrennial National Health Security Strategy (NHSS). The CDC has developed the National Biosurveillance Strategy for Human Health, which covers six priority areas: electronic health information exchange, electronic laboratory information exchange, unstructured data, integrated biosurveillance information, global disease detection and collaboration, and biosurveillance workforce. Based on the National Health Security Strategy developed by the DHHS in 2009, *Healthy People 2020* focused on four areas of reinforcement under an overarching goal to "improve the Nation's ability to prevent, prepare for, respond to, and recover from a major health incident": time to release official information about a public health emergency, time for designated personnel to respond to an emergency, Laboratory Response Network (LRN) laboratories, and time to develop after-action reports and improvement plans in states (U.S. DHHS, 2010a). A progress report shows that most states and localities have strong biological laboratory capabilities and capacities, with nearly 90% of laboratories in the LRN reachable around the clock (CDC, 2010b).

In 2011, the Health Alert Network (HAN) was established, which is a nationwide program designed to facilitate communication, information, and distance learning related to health threats, including bioterrorism (U.S. DHHS, 2011b). When fully established, the network will link the various local health departments as well as other components of bioterrorism preparedness and response, such as laboratories and state health departments.

One of the key concepts of preparedness is *surge capacity*, defined as "the ability of a healthcare facility or system to expand its operations to safely treat an abnormally large influx of patients" (Bonnett & Peery, 2007). The initial response is conducted at a local healthcare facility, such as a hospital. Strategies for expanding the surge capacity of a hospital include early discharge of stable patients, cancellation of elective procedures and admissions, conversion of private rooms to double rooms, reopening of closed areas, revision of staff work hours to a 12-hour disaster shift, callback of off-duty personnel, and establishment of temporary external shelters for patient holding (Hick et al., 2004).

If the local-level response becomes overloaded or incapacitated, it requires activation of a second tier of disaster response—community-level surge capacity. Cooperative regional planning necessitates sharing of staff and supplies across a network of regional healthcare facilities (Hick et al., 2004). An important aspect of disaster planning at the community level focuses on the transportation logistics of the region. The quantity of ambulances in the area and the means of accessing these resources during an event could be crucial to delivering proper care to critical patients (Kearns, Hubble, Holmes, & Cairns, 2013). The final tier of disaster response involves federal aid under the National Disaster Medical System (NDMS), which actually dates back to the 1980s and was designed to accommodate large numbers of military casualties. Disaster Medical Assistance Teams (DMATs) are a vital component of the NDMS that directly respond to the needs of an overwhelmed community. DMATs deploy with trained personnel (in both medical and ancillary services), equipped with tents, water filtration, generators, and medical supplies (Stopford, 2005).

Despite the progress made, disaster preparedness efforts in the United States remain fragmented and underfunded. For example, review, rotation, replacement, and upgrade of equipment and supplies in the system on a regular basis have remained a challenge (Cohen & Mulvaney, 2005).

DETERMINANTS OF HEALTH

Health determinants are major factors that, over time, affect the health and well-being of individuals and populations. An understanding of health determinants is required for any positive interventions necessary to improve health and longevity.

Blum's Model of Health Determinants

In 1974, Blum (1981) proposed an "Environment of Health" model, later called the "Force Field and Well-Being Paradigms of Health" (**Figure 8-3**). Blum proposed four major inputs that contributed to health and well-being. These main influences (called "force fields") are environment, lifestyle, heredity, and medical care, all of which must be considered simultaneously when addressing the health status of an individual or a population. In other words, there is no single pathway to better health, because health determinants interact in complex ways. Consequently, improvement in health requires a multipronged approach.

The four wedges in Figure 8-3 represent the four major force fields. The size of each wedge signifies its relative importance. Thus, the most important force field is environment, followed by lifestyles and heredity. Medical care has the least impact on health and well-being.

FIGURE 8-3 The Force Field and Well-Being Paradigms of Health.

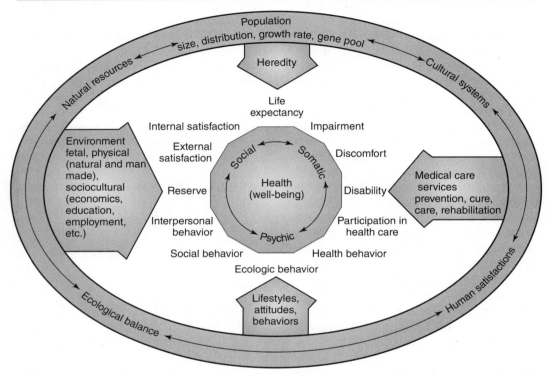

Source: Reproduced from H. L. Blum, Planning for Health, © 1981, Human Sciences Press, with kind permission of Lynda L. Brothers.

Blum's model also explains that the four main forces operate within a much broader context and are affected by broad national and international factors, such as a nation's population characteristics, natural resources, ecological balance, human satisfactions, and cultural systems. Among these factors, type of healthcare delivery system can also be included. In the United States, the preponderance of healthcare expenditures is devoted to the treatment of medical conditions rather than to the prevention and control of factors that produce those medical conditions in the first place. This misdirection can be traced to the conflicts that often result from the beliefs and values ingrained in the American culture.

Environment

Environmental factors encompass the physical, socioeconomic, sociopolitical, and sociocultural dimensions. Among physical environmental factors are air pollution, food and water contaminants, radiation, toxic chemicals, wastes, disease vectors, safety hazards, and habitat alterations.

The relationship of socioeconomic status (SES) to health and well-being may be explained by the general likelihood that people who have better education also have higher incomes. The greater the economic gap between the rich and the poor in a given geographic area, the worse the health status of the population in that area is likely to be. It has been suggested that wide income gaps produce less social cohesion, greater psychosocial stress, and, consequently, poorer health (Wilkinson, 1997). For example, social cohesion—characterized by a hospitable social environment in which people trust each other and participate in communal activities—is linked to lower overall mortality and better self-rated health (Kawachi, Kennedy, & Glass, 1999; Kawachi, Kennedy, Lochner, & Prothrow-Stith, 1997). Even countries with national health insurance programs, such as Britain, Australia, Denmark, and Sweden, experience persistent and widening disparities in health according to socioeconomic status (Pincus, Esther, DeWalt, & Callahan, 1998). The joint relationship of income inequality and availability of primary care has also been found to be significantly associated with individuals' self-rated health status (Shi, Starfield, Politzer, & Regan, 2002).

Lifestyle

Lifestyle, or behavioral risk factors, were previously discussed. This section provides some illustrations of how lifestyle factors are related to health. Studies have shown that diet and foods, for example, play a major role in most of the significant health problems of today. Heart disease, diabetes, stroke, and cancer are but some of the diseases with direct links to dietary choices. Throughout the world, incidence and mortality rates for many forms of cancer are rising. Yet research has clearly indicated that a significant portion of cancer is preventable. Researchers estimated that 40% to 60% of all cancers, and as many as 35% of cancer deaths, are linked to diet (American Institute for Cancer Research, 1996). Current research also shows that a diet rich in fruits, vegetables, and low-fat dairy foods, and with reduced saturated and total fat, can substantially lower blood pressure (see, for example, the DASH Eating Plan recommended by U.S. DHHS [2006]). The role of exercise and physical activity as a potentially useful, effective, and acceptable method is significant in reducing the risk of colon cancer (Macfarlane & Lowenfels, 1994) as well as many other health problems.

Heredity

Genetic factors predispose individuals to certain diseases. For example, cancer occurs when the body's healthy genes lose their ability to suppress malignant growth or when other genetic processes stop working properly, although this does not mean that cancer is entirely a disease of the genes (Davis & Webster, 2002). A person can do little about the genetic makeup he or she has inherited. However, lifestyles and behaviors that a person may currently engage in can have significant influences on future progeny. Advances in gene therapy hold the promise of treating a variety of inherited or acquired diseases.

Medical Care

Even though the other three factors are more important in the determination of health, medical care is, nevertheless, a key determinant of health. Both individual and population health are closely related to having access to adequate preventive and curative healthcare services. Despite the fact that medical care, compared to the other three factors, has the least impact on health and well-being, Americans' attitudes toward health improvement focus on more medical research, development of new medical technology, and spending more on high-tech medical care. Yet, significant declines in mortality rates were achieved well before the modernization of Western medicine and the escalation in medical care expenditures.

The availability of primary care may be one alternative pathway through which income inequality influences population-level health outcomes. Research by Shi and colleagues (1999, 2001) suggests that access to primary care, in addition to income inequality, significantly correlates with reduced mortality, increased life expectancy, and improved birth outcomes. In the United States, individuals living in states with a higher primary care physician-to-population ratio are more likely to report good health than are those living in states with a lower ratio (Shi et al., 2002).

Contemporary Models of Health Determinants

More recent models have built upon Blum's framework of health determinants. For example, the model proposed by Dahlgren and Whitehead (2006) states that age, sex, and genetic makeup are fixed factors, but other factors in the surrounding layers can be modified to positively influence population health. Individual lifestyle factors have the potential to promote or damage health, and social interactions can sustain people's health; but living and working conditions; food supplies; access to essential goods and services; and the overall economic, cultural, and environmental conditions have wider influences on individual and population health.

Ansari and colleagues (2003) proposed a public health model of the social determinants of health in which the determinants are categorized into four major groups: social determinants, healthcare system attributes, disease-inducing behaviors, and health outcomes.

The WHO Commission on Social Determinants of Health (2007) concluded that "the social conditions in which people are born, live, and work are the single most important determinant of one's health status." The WHO model provides a conceptual framework for understanding the socioeconomic and political contexts, structural determinants, intermediary determinants (including material circumstances, social-environmental circumstances, behavioral and biological factors, social cohesion, and the healthcare system), and the impact on health equity and well-being measured as health outcomes.

U.S. government agencies, such as the CDC and DHHS, have recognized the need to address health inequities. The CDC's National Center for HIV/AIDS, Viral Hepatitis, STD, and TB Prevention adopted the WHO framework on social determinants of health to use as a guide for its activities (see **Figure 8-4**).

ANTHRO-CULTURAL BELIEFS AND VALUES

A value system orients the members of a society toward defining what is desirable for that society. It has been observed that even a society as complex and highly differentiated as in the United States can be said to have a relatively well-integrated system of institutionalized common values at the societal level (Parsons, 1972). Although such a view may still prevail, American society now has several different subcultures that have grown in size as a result of a steady influx of immigrants from different parts of the world.

The current system of health services delivery traces its roots to the traditional beliefs and values espoused by the American people. The value and belief system governs the training and general orientation of healthcare providers, type of health delivery settings, financing and allocation of resources, and access to health care.

Some of the main beliefs and values prevalent in the American culture are outlined as follows:

1. A strong belief in the advancement of science and the application of scientific methods to medicine were instrumental in creating the medical model that primarily governs healthcare delivery in the United States.

| **FIGURE 8-4** | WHO Commission on Social Determinants of Health conceptual framework. |

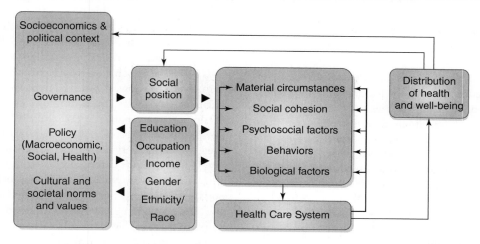

Source: Centers for Disease Control and Prevention. (2010). *Establishing a holistic framework to reduce inequities in HIV, viral hepatitis, STDs, and tuberculosis in the United States.* Retrieved from http://www.cdc.gov/socialdeterminants/docs/SDH-White-Paper-2010.pdf

In turn, the medical model has fueled the tremendous growth in medical science and technological innovation. As a result, the United States has been leading the world in medical breakthroughs. These developments have had numerous implications for health services delivery:

a. They increase the demand for the latest treatments and raise patients' expectations for finding cures.

b. Medical professionals have been preoccupied with clinical interventions, whereas the holistic aspects of health and use of alternative therapies have not received adequate emphasis.

c. Healthcare professionals have been trained to focus on physical symptoms rather than the underlying causes of disease.

d. Integration of diagnosis and treatment with disease prevention has been lagging behind.

e. Most research efforts have focused on the development of medical technology. Commitment of resources to the preservation and enhancement of health and well-being has lagged behind.

f. Medical specialists, using the latest technology, are held in higher esteem and earn higher incomes than general practitioners do.

g. The desirability of healthcare delivery institutions, such as hospitals, is often evaluated by their acquisition of advanced technology.

h. Whereas biomedicine has taken central stage, diagnosis and treatment of mental health have been relegated to a lesser status.

i. The biomedical model has neglected the social and spiritual elements of health.

2. America has been a champion of capitalism. Due to a strong belief in capitalism, health care has largely been viewed as an economic good (or service), not as a public resource.

3. A culture of capitalism promotes entrepreneurial spirit and self-determination. Hence, individual capabilities to obtain health services have largely determined the production and consumption of health care—which services will be produced, where and in what quantity, and who will have access to those services. Some key implications are:

   a. Upper-tier access to healthcare services is available mainly through private health insurance. Those with public insurance fall in a second tier. The uninsured make up a third tier.

   b. A clear distinction exists between the types of services provided for poor and for affluent communities and between those in rural and inner-city locations.

   c. The culture of individualism emphasizes individual health rather than population health. Medical practice, therefore, has been directed at keeping the individual healthy rather than keeping the entire community healthy.

   d. A concern for the most underprivileged classes in society—the poor, the elderly, the disabled, and children—led to the creation of the public programs Medicaid, Medicare, and the Children's Health Insurance Program (CHIP).

4. Principles of free enterprise and a general distrust of big government have kept the delivery of health care largely in private hands. Hence, a separation also exists between public health functions and the private practice of medicine.

EQUITABLE DISTRIBUTION OF HEALTH CARE

Scarcity of economic resources is a central economic concept. From this perspective, health care can be viewed as an economic good. Two fundamental questions arise with regard to how scarce healthcare resources ought to be used: (1) How much health care should be produced? (2) How should health care be distributed? The first question concerns the appropriate combination in which health services ought to be produced in relation to all other goods and services in the overall economy. If more health care is produced, a society may have to do with less of some other goods, such as food, clothing, and transportation. The second question affects individuals at a more personal level. It deals with who can receive which type of medical service, and how access to services will be restricted.

The production, distribution, and subsequent consumption of health care must be perceived as equitable by a society. No society has found a perfectly equitable method to distribute limited economic resources. In fact, any method of resource distribution leaves some inequalities. Societies, therefore, try to allocate resources according to some guiding principles acceptable to each society. Such principles are ingrained in a society's value and belief system. It is recognized that not everyone can receive everything medical science has to offer.

A just and fair allocation of health care poses conceptual and practical difficulties; hence, a theory of justice needs to resolve the problem of healthcare allocation (Jonsen, 1986). Even though various ethical principles can be used to guide decisions pertaining to just and fair allocation of health care in individual circumstances, the broad concern about equitable access to health services is addressed by two contrasting theories referred to as market justice and social justice.

Market Justice

The principle of market justice ascribes the fair distribution of health care to the market forces in a free economy. Medical care and its benefits are distributed based on people's willingness and ability to pay (Santerre & Neun, 1996). In other words, people are entitled to purchase a share of the available goods and services that they value. They are to purchase these valued goods and services by means of wealth acquired through their own legitimate efforts. This is how most goods and services are distributed in a free market. The free market implies that giving people something they have not earned would be morally and economically wrong.

The characteristics of a free market are preconditions to the distribution of healthcare services according to market justice principles. It should be added that health care in the United States is not delivered in a free market; rather, it is delivered in a quasi-market. Hence, market justice principles are only partially applicable to the U.S. healthcare delivery system. Distribution of health care according to market justice is based on the following key assumptions:

- Health care is like any other economic good or service, the distribution and consumption of which are determined by free-market forces of supply and demand.

- Individuals are responsible for their own achievements. From the rewards of their achievements, people are free to obtain various economic goods and services, including health care. When individuals pursue their own best interests, the interests of society as a whole are best served (Ferguson & Maurice, 1970).

- People make rational choices in their decisions to purchase healthcare products and services. Grossman (1972) proposed that health is also an investment commodity. People consider the purchase of health services as an investment. For example, the

investment has a monetary payoff when it reduces the number of sick days, making extra time available for productive activities, such as earning a living. Or it can have a utility payoff—a payoff in terms of satisfaction—when it makes life more enjoyable and fulfilling.

- People, in consultation with their physicians, know what is best for them. This assumption implies that people place a certain degree of trust in their physicians and that the physician–patient relationship is ongoing.

- The marketplace works best with minimum interference from the government. In other words, the market, rather than the government, can allocate healthcare resources in the most efficient and equitable manner.

Under market justice, the production of health care is determined by how much the consumers are willing and able to purchase at the prevailing market prices. Thus, prices and ability to pay ration the quantity and type of healthcare services people consume. The uninsured and those who lack sufficient income to pay privately face barriers to obtaining health care. Such limitations to obtaining health care are referred to as "rationing by ability to pay" (Feldstein, 1994), demand-side rationing, or price rationing. To an extent, barriers faced by the uninsured would be overcome through charitable services.

The key characteristics and their implications under the system of market justice are summarized in **Table 8-4**. Market justice emphasizes individual, rather than collective, responsibility for health. It proposes private, rather than government, solutions to social problems of health.

Social Justice

The idea of social justice is at odds with the principles of capitalism and market justice.

TABLE 8-4	Comparison of Market Justice and Social Justice

Market Justice	Social Justice
Characteristics	
• Views health care as an ecwonomic good	• Views health care as a social resource
• Assumes free-market conditions for health services delivery	• Requires active government involvement in health services delivery
• Assumes that markets are more efficient in allocating health resources equitably	• Assumes that the government is more efficient in allocating health resources equitably
• Production and distribution of health care determined by market-based demand	• Medical resource allocation determined by central planning
• Medical care distribution based on people's ability to pay	• Ability to pay inconsequential for receiving medical care
• Access to medical care viewed as an economic reward of personal effort and achievement	• Equal access to medical services viewed as a basic right
Implications	
• Individual responsibility for health	• Collective responsibility for health
• based on individual purchasing power	• Everyone is entitled to a basic package of benefits
• Limited obligation to the collective good	• Strong obligation to the collective good
• Emphasis on individual well-being	• Community well-being supersedes that of the individual
• Private solutions to social problems	• Public solutions to social problems
• Rationing based on ability to pay	• Planned rationing of health care

Source: Shi, L., & Singh, D. (2015). *Delivering health care in America: A systems approach* (6th ed.). Burlington, MA: Jones & Bartlett.

The term *social justice* was invented in the 19th century by the critics of capitalism to describe the "good society" (Kristol, 1978). According to the principle of social justice, the equitable distribution of health care is a societal responsibility, which is best achieved by letting the government take over the production and distribution of health care. Social justice regards health care as a social good—as opposed to an economic good—that should be collectively financed and available to all citizens regardless

of the individual recipient's ability to pay. The main characteristics and implications of social justice are summarized in Table 8-4.

Canadians and Europeans long ago reached a broad consensus that health care is a social good (Reinhardt, 1994). Public health also has a social justice orientation (Turnock, 1997). Under the social justice system, inability to obtain medical services because of a lack of financial resources is considered inequitable. Accordingly, a just distribution of health care must be based on need, not simply on one's ability to purchase in the marketplace (demand). Need for health care is determined either by the patient or by a health professional.

The principle of social justice is also based on certain assumptions:

- Health care is different from most other goods and services. Health-seeking behavior is governed primarily by need rather than by ability to pay.

- Responsibility for health is shared. Individuals are not held completely responsible for their condition because factors outside their control may have brought on the condition. Society is held responsible because individuals cannot control certain environmental factors, such as economic inequalities, unemployment, or unsanitary conditions.

- Society has an obligation to the collective good. The well-being of the community is superior to that of the individual. An unhealthy individual is a burden on society. A person carrying a deadly infection, for example, is a threat to society. Society, therefore, is obligated to cure the problem by providing health care to the individual, because, by doing so, the whole society would benefit.

- The government rather than the market can better decide through central planning how much health care to produce and how to distribute it among all citizens.

Just like true market justice does not exist in health care, true social justice also does not exist. This is because no society can afford to provide unlimited amounts of health care to all its citizens (Feldstein, 1994). The government may offer insurance coverage to all, but subsequently has to find ways to limit the availability of certain healthcare services. For example, under social justice, the government decides how technology will be dispersed and who will be allowed access to certain types of costly high-tech services, even though basic services may be available to all. The government engages in supply-side rationing, which is also referred to as planned rationing or nonprice rationing. In social justice systems, the government uses the term *health planning* to limit the supply of healthcare services, although the limited resources are often more equally dispersed throughout the country than is generally the case under a market justice system. It is because of the necessity of rationing health care that citizens of a country can be given universal coverage, but not universal access. Even when a covered individual has a medical need, depending on the nature of health services required, he or she may have to wait until services become available.

Justice in the U.S. Health Delivery System

In a quasi- or imperfect market, which characterizes healthcare delivery in the United States, elements of both market and social justice exist. In some areas, the principles of market and social justice complement each other. In other areas, the two present conflicts.

The two contrasting principles complement each other with employer-based health insurance for most middle-class working Americans (market justice) and publicly financed Medicare, Medicaid, and CHIP coverage for certain disadvantaged groups (social justice). Insured populations access healthcare services delivered mainly by private practitioners and private institutions (market justice). Tax-supported county and city hospitals, public health clinics, and community health centers can be accessed by the uninsured in areas where such services are available (social justice).

Market and social justice principles create conflicts when healthcare resources are not uniformly distributed throughout the United States, and there is a general shortage of primary care physicians. Consequently, in spite of having public insurance, many Medicaid-covered patients have difficulty obtaining timely access, particularly in rural and inner-city areas.

In part, this conflict is created by artificially low reimbursement from public programs, whereas reimbursement from private payers is more generous.

In the past, market justice principles have been dominant in the United States, but the ACA promises to change that and swing the pendulum more toward social justice. Massive new government subsidies are available to many people who can purchase private insurance through government-run exchanges. Medicaid is being expanded significantly for low-income families. These expansions will be paid through a number of new taxes provided for in the ACA. However, the ACA is not designed to achieve universal coverage; it may also not successfully achieve access for a large segment of the U.S. population, particularly if the providers are unable to meet the law's demands within reimbursement constraints.

Limitations of Market Justice

The principles of market justice work well in the allocation of economic goods when the unequal distribution of the goods does not affect the larger society. For example, people live in different sizes and styles of homes, drive different types of automobiles, and spend their money on a variety of things based on individual success, but the allocation of certain resources has wider repercussions for society. In these areas, market justice has severe limitations:

1. Market justice principles fail to rectify critical human concerns. Pervasive social problems, such as crime, illiteracy, and homelessness, can significantly weaken the fabric of a society. Indeed, the United States has recognized such issues and instituted programs based on social justice to combat the problems through added police protection, publicly supported education, and subsidized housing for many of the poor and elderly. Health care is an important social issue because it not only affects human productivity and achievement but also provides basic human dignity.

2. Market justice does not always protect a society. Individual health issues can have negative consequences for society because ill health is not always confined to the individual. The AIDS epidemic is an example in which society can be put at serious risk. Initial spread of the SARS epidemic in Beijing, China, was largely due to patients with SARS symptoms being turned away by hospitals because they were not able to pay in advance for the cost of the treatment. Similar to clean air and water, health care is a social concern that, in the long run, protects against the burden of preventable disease and disability, a burden that is ultimately borne by society.

3. Market justice does not work well in healthcare delivery. A growing national economy and prosperity in the past did not materially reduce the number of uninsured Americans. On the other hand, the number of uninsured increases during economic downturns. For example, during the 2007–2009 recession, 5 million Americans lost employment-based health insurance (Holahan, 2011).

INTEGRATION OF INDIVIDUAL AND POPULATION HEALTH

It has been recognized that typical emphasis on the treatment of acute illness in hospitals, biomedical research, and high technology has not significantly improved the population's health. Consequently, the medical model should be integrated with a disease-prevention, health-promotion, primary care–based model. Society will always need the benefits of modern science and technology for the treatment of disease, but disease prevention, health promotion, and primary care can prevent certain health problems, delay the onset of disease, and prevent disability and premature death. An integrated approach will improve the overall health of the population, enhance people's quality of life, and conserve healthcare resources.

The real challenge for the healthcare delivery system is to incorporate the medical and wellness models within the holistic context of health. The Ottawa Charter for Health Promotion, for instance, mentions caring, holism, and ecology as essential issues in developing strategies for health promotion (de Leeuw, 1989). *Holism* and *ecology* refer to the complex relationships that exist among the individual, the healthcare delivery system, and the physical, social, cultural, and economic environmental factors. In addition, as the increasing body of research points out, the spiritual dimension must be incorporated into the integrated model.

Another equally important challenge for the healthcare delivery system is to focus on both individual and population health outcomes. The nature of health is complex, and the interrelationships among the physical, mental, social, and spiritual dimensions are not well understood. How to translate this multidimensional framework of health into specific actions that are efficiently configured to achieve better individual and community health is one of the greatest challenges healthcare systems face.

For an integrated approach to become reality, resource limitations make it necessary to deploy the best American ingenuity toward health-spending reduction, elimination of wasteful care, promotion of individual responsibility and accountability for one's health, and improved access to basic services. In a broad sense, these services include medical care, preventive services, health promotion, and social policy to improve education, lifestyle, employment, and housing (**Figure 8-5**). The Ottawa Charter has proposed achieving health objectives through social public policy and community action. An integrated approach also necessitates creation of a new model for training healthcare professionals by forming partnerships with the community (Henry, 1993). The subsequent paragraphs describe examples

---

FIGURE 8-5   Integrated model for holistic health.

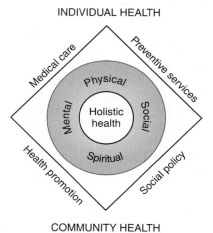

Source: Shi, L., & Singh, D. (2015). *Delivering health care in America: A systems approach* (6th ed.). Burlington, MA: Jones & Bartlett.

of community partnership reflected in community health assessment and Healthy People initiatives.

Community Health Assessment

Community health assessment is a method used to conduct broad assessments of populations at a local or state level. For integrating individual and community health, the assessment is best conducted by collaboration among public health agencies, hospitals, and other healthcare providers. Community hospitals, in particular, are increasingly held accountable for the health status of the communities in which they are located. To fulfill this mission, hospitals must first conduct a health assessment of their communities. Such assessments provide broad perspectives of the populations' health and point to specific needs that healthcare providers can address. These assessments can help pinpoint interventions that should be given priority to improve the populations' health status or address critical issues pertaining to certain groups within the populations.

Healthy People Initiatives

Since 1980, the United States has undertaken 10-year plans outlining certain key national health objectives to be accomplished during each of the 10-year periods. The objectives are developed by a consortium of national and state organizations under the leadership of the U.S. Surgeon General. The first of these programs, with objectives for 1990, provided national goals for reducing premature deaths among all age groups and for reducing the average number of days of illness among those older than age 65. A final review of this program concluded that positive changes in premature death had been achieved for all age categories except adolescents, and illness among the elderly had not been reduced. However, the review set the stage for development and modification of goals and objectives for the subsequent 10-year program (Chrvala & Bulger, 1999).

Healthy People 2000: National Health Promotion and Disease Prevention Objectives identified three main goals to be reached by the year 2000: increase the span of healthy life for Americans, reduce health disparities, and achieve access to preventive services by all Americans (U.S. DHHS, 1992). According to the final review, the major accomplishments included surpassing the targets for reducing deaths from coronary heart disease and cancer; meeting the targets for incidence rates for AIDS and syphilis, mammography exams, violent deaths, and tobacco-related deaths; nearly meeting the targets for infant mortality and number of children with elevated levels of lead in the blood; and making some progress toward reducing health disparities among special populations.

Healthy People 2010: Healthy People in Healthy Communities continued in the earlier traditions as an instrument to improve the health of the American people in the first decade of the 21st century. It focused on two broad goals: (1) to increase quality and years of healthy life and (2) to eliminate health disparities. It went a step beyond the previous initiatives by emphasizing the role of community partners—businesses, local governments, and civic, professional, and religious organizations—as effective agents for improving health in their local communities (U.S. DHHS, 1998). The final report revealed that 23% of the targets were met or exceeded and the nation had made progress in 48% of the targets. Specifically, life expectancy at birth, expected years in good or better health, and expected years free of activity limitations all improved, while expected years free of selected chronic diseases decreased. However, the goal of reducing health disparities has not been achieved. Health disparities in about 80% of the objectives have not changed and even increased in another 13% of the objectives (National Center for Health Statistics, 2012b). Hence, challenges remain in the reduction of chronic conditions and health disparities among population groups.

Launched in 2010, *Healthy People 2020* (U.S. DHHS, 2010a) has a fivefold mission: (1) Identify nationwide health improvement priorities. (2) Increase public awareness and understanding of the determinants of health, disease, and disability and the opportunities for progress. (3) Provide measurable objectives and goals that can be used at the national, state, and local levels. (4) Engage multiple sectors to take actions that are driven by the best available evidence and knowledge. (5) Identify critical research and data collection needs. Its four overarching goals are to

1. Attain high-quality, longer lives free of preventable disease, disability, injury, and premature death.

2. Achieve health equity, eliminate disparities, and improve the health of all groups.

3. Create social and physical environments that promote good health for all.

4. Promote quality of life, healthy development, and healthy behaviors across all life stages.

The overarching goals are in line with the tradition of earlier Healthy People initiatives but place particular emphasis on the determinants of health. **Figure 8-6** illustrates the Action Model to Achieve Healthy People 2020 Overarching Goals. This model illustrates that interventions (i.e., policies, programs, information) influence

FIGURE 8-6 Action Model to Achieve U.S. *Healthy People 2020* Overarching Goals.

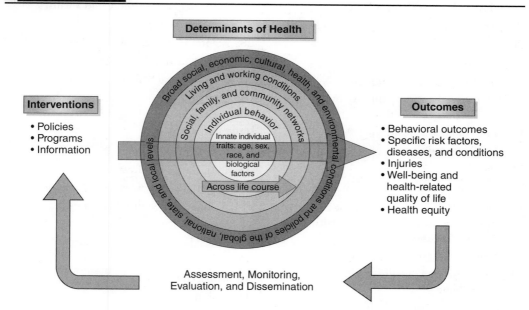

Source: U.S. Department of Health and Human Services. Office of Disease Prevention and Health Promotion. Healthy People 2020. Washington, DC. Available at https://www.healthypeople.gov /sites/default/files/Phasel_0.pdf. Accessed December 15th, 2014.

the determinants of health at four levels: (1) individual; (2) social, family, and community; (3) living and working conditions; and (4) broad social, economic, cultural, health, and environmental conditions, leading to improvement in outcomes. Results are to be demonstrated through assessment, monitoring, and evaluation, and the dissemination of findings would provide feedback for future interventions.

Healthy People 2020 is differentiated from previous Healthy People initiatives by including multiple new topic areas in its objective list, such as adolescent health, genomics, global health, health communication and health information technology, and social determinants of health. *Healthy People 2020* has 42 topic areas, with 13 new areas (underlined in **Table 8-5**).

TABLE 8-5	List of *Healthy People 2020* Topic Areas

1. Access to Health Services
2. Adolescent Health
3. Arthritis, Osteoporosis, and Chronic Back Conditions
4. Blood Disorders and Blood Safety
5. Cancer
6. Chronic Kidney Disease
7. Dementias, Including Alzheimer's Disease
8. Diabetes
9. Disability and Health
10. Early and Middle Childhood
11. Educational and Community-Based Programs
12. Environmental Health
13. Family Planning
14. Food Safety
15. Genomics
16. Global Health
17. Health Communication and Health Information Technology
18. Healthcare-Associated Infections
19. Health-Related Quality of Life and Well-Being
20. Hearing and Other Sensory or Communication Disorders
21. Heart Disease and Stroke
22. HIV
23. Immunization and Infectious Diseases
24. Injury and Violence Prevention
25. Lesbian, Gay, Bisexual, and Transgender Health
26. Maternal, Infant, and Child Health
27. Medical Product Safety
28. Mental Health and Mental Disorders
29. Nutrition and Weight Status
30. Occupational Safety and Health
31. Older Adults
32. Oral Health
33. Physical Activity
34. Preparedness
35. Public Health Infrastructure
36. Respiratory Diseases
37. Sexually Transmitted Diseases
38. Sleep Health
39. Social Determinants of Health
40. Substance Abuse
41. Tobacco Use
42. Vision

Source: Shi, L., & Singh, D. (2015). *Delivering health care in America: A systems approach* (6th ed.). Burlington, MA: Jones & Bartlett.

Measurement of *Healthy People 2020*

Healthy People 2020 establishes four foundational health measures to monitor progress toward achieving its goals. The foundational health measures include general health status, health-related quality of life and well-being, determinants of health, and disparities. Measures of general health status include life expectancy, healthy life expectancy, years of potential life lost, physically and mentally unhealthy days, self-assessed health status, limitation of activity, and chronic disease prevalence. Measures of health-related quality of life and well-being include physical, mental, and social health-related quality of life; well-being/satisfaction; and participation in common activities. *Healthy People 2020* defines determinants of health as "a range of personal, social, economic, and environmental factors that influence health status. Determinants of health include such things as biology, genetics, individual behavior, access to health services, and the environment in which people are born, live, learn, play, work, and age." Measures of disparities and inequity include differences in health status based on race/ethnicity, gender, physical and mental ability, and geography (U.S. DHHS, 2010a).

There has been ongoing review of how well the healthcare system is working toward achievement of the delineated goals. The findings of these ongoing studies are compared to the baseline data from the beginning of the 10-year period to determine whether adequate progress has occurred.

Global health is also an important topic area in *Healthy People 2020*. The measurement of global health focuses on two aspects. The first is to measure the reduction of global diseases in the United States, including malaria and tuberculosis (TB). The second is to measure "global capacity in support of the International Health Regulations to detect and contain emerging health threats" (U.S. DHHS, 2010a). The indicators include the number of Global Disease Detection (GDD) Regional Centers worldwide, the number of public health professionals trained by GDD programs worldwide, and the number of diagnostic tests established or improved by GDD programs (U.S. DHHS, 2010a).

SUMMARY

The delivery of health care is primarily driven by the medical model, which emphasizes illness rather than wellness. Holistic concepts of health, along with the integration of medical care with preventive and health promotional efforts, need to be adopted to significantly improve the health of Americans. Such an approach would also require individual responsibility for one's own health-oriented behaviors, as well as community partnerships to improve both personal and community health. An understanding of the determinants of health, health education, community health assessment, and national initiatives, such as Healthy People, are essential to accomplishing these goals. *Healthy People 2020*, launched in 2010, continues its goals of improving health and eliminating disparities. Public health has gained increased importance because of a growing recognition of its role in health protection, environmental health, and preparedness for natural disasters and bioterrorism. Public health has now become global in its scope.

The various facets of health and its determinants, and ongoing initiatives in the areas of prevention, health promotion, health protection, and equality are complex undertakings and require substantial financial resources. Objective measures play a critical role in evaluating the success of various programs, as well as for directing future planning activities.

The broad concern about equitable access to health services is addressed by the contrasting theories of market justice and social justice. Countries offering universal coverage have adopted the principles of social justice under which the government finances healthcare services and decides on the distribution of those services. However, because no country can afford to provide unlimited amounts of health care to all citizens, supply-side rationing becomes inevitable. Many of the characteristics of the U.S. healthcare system trace back to the beliefs and values underlying the American culture. The principles of market justice have been dominant, but social justice is also apparent in publicly financed programs and in the health reform initiatives under the ACA. Under market justice, not all citizens have health insurance coverage, a phenomenon called demand-side rationing.

ACA TAKEAWAY

■ Medicare and private health plans are required to cover a range of recommended preventive services with no out-of-pocket costs.

■ The ACA has provided funds to expand preventive national efforts.

■ Wellness grants are made available to small businesses to encourage wellness programs.

■ The ACA will move U.S. health care toward social justice. Yet it is unlikely to achieve justice and equity in providing access to health care for all Americans.

DISCUSSION QUESTIONS

1. How can you use the health risk appraisal for health promotion and disease prevention in your practice?

2. Discuss the definitions of health, health promotion, and disease prevention presented in this chapter in terms of their implications for your practice.

3. Since the tragic events of 9/11, what "preparedness"-related measures have been taken in your setting to cope with potential natural and man-made disasters? Assess their effectiveness.

4. The Blum model points to four key determinants of health. Discuss their implications for your practice.

5. Discuss the main cultural beliefs and values in American society that have influenced you, your practice, and your organization.

6. Discuss how the concepts of market justice and social justice are evident in your practice. In what way do the two principles complement each other and in what way are they in conflict?

7. Reflect on how the integration of individual and population health could inform practice changes.

8. How can the objectives set forth in *Healthy People 2020* guide your practice changes?

REFERENCES

Agency for Healthcare Research and Quality. (2006). The Medical Expenditure Panel Survey (MEPS). Retrieved from http://www.ahrq.gov/research /data/meps/index.html

American Institute for Cancer Research. (1996). *Food, nutrition and the prevention of cancer: A global perspective*. Washington, DC. Retrieved from http://www .aicr.org/site/PageServer

American Public Health Association. (2013). Prevention and Public Health Fund. Updated chart of Prevention and Public Health Fund allocations, FY 2010 enacted through FY 2014 request. Retrieved from http://www.apha.org /NR/rdonlyres/A448A5CD-6BFE-4AA5-B25D-DF59C195484E/0/PPH2010201441613.pdf

Anderko, L., Roffenbender, J. S., Goetzel, R. Z., Millard, F., Wildenhaus, K., DeSantis, C., & Novelli, W. (2012). Promoting prevention through the Affordable Care Act: Workplace wellness. *Preventing Chronic Disease, 9*, E175. doi: http://dx.doi. org/10.5888/pcd9.120092

Ansari, Z., Carson, N. J., Ackland, M. J., Vaughan, L., & Serraglio, A. (2003). A public health model of the social determinants of health. *Sozial und Präventivmedizin/Social and Preventive Medicine, 48*(4), 242–251.

Blum, H. L. (1981). *Planning for health* (2nd ed.). New York, NY: Human Sciences Press.

Bonnett, C., & Peery, B. C. (2007). Surge capacity: A proposed conceptual framework. *American Journal of Emergency Medicine, 25*, 297–306.

Centers for Disease Control and Prevention. (1999). Control of infectious diseases. *Morbidity and Mortality Weekly Report, 48*(29), 621.

Centers for Disease Control and Prevention. (2007). Avian influenza (bird flu). Retrieved from http://www.cdc.gov/flu/avian/

Centers for Disease Control and Prevention. (2010a). *Establishing a holistic framework to reduce inequities in HIV, viral hepatitis, STDs, and tuberculosis in the United States.* Retrieved from http://www.cdc.gov/social determinants/docs/SDH-White-Paper-2010.pdf

Centers for Disease Control and Prevention. (2010b). *Public health preparedness: Strengthening the nation's emergency response state by state.* Retrieved from http://www.bt.cdc.gov/publications/2010phprep

Centers for Disease Control and Prevention. (2012). SARS basics fact sheet. Retrieved from http://www.cdc.gov/sars/about/fs-SARS.html

Centers for Disease Control and Prevention. (2013a). National Diabetes Prevention Program. Retrieved from http://www.cdc.gov/diabetes/prevention/about.htm

Centers for Disease Control and Prevention. (2013b). National Diabetes Prevention Program: Funded organizations. Retrieved from http://www.cdc.gov/diabetes/prevention/about.htm

Chida, Y., Steptoe, A., & Powell, L. H. (2009). Religiosity/spirituality and mortality. *Psychotherapy and Psychosomatics, 78,* 81–90.

Chrvala, C. A., & Bulger, R. J. (Eds.). (1999). *Leading health indicators for Healthy People 2010: Final report.* Washington, DC: National Academy of Sciences.

Cohen, M. H. (2003). *Future medicine.* Ann Arbor: University of Michigan Press.

Cohen, S., & Mulvaney, K. (2005). Field observations: Disaster medical assistance team response for Hurricane Charley, Punta Gorda, Florida, 2004. *Disaster Management and Response,* 22–27.

Dahlgren, G., & Whitehead, M. (2006). *European strategies for tackling social inequities in health: Concepts and principles for tackling social inequities in health: Levelling up (part 2).* Studies on Social and Economic Determinants of Population Health no. 3. Denmark: World Health Organization. Retrieved from http://www.euro.who.int/—data/assets/pdf_file/0018/103824/E89384.pdf

Davis, D. L., & Webster, P. S. (2002, November). The social context of science: Cancer and the environment. *Annals of the American Academy of Political and Social Science, 584,* 13–34.

de Leeuw, E. (1989). Concepts in health promotion: The notion of relativism. *Social Science and Medicine, 29*(11), 1281–1288.

Ethics Committee, Society for Academic Emergency Medicine. (1992). An ethical foundation for

health care: An emergency medicine perspective. *Annals of Emergency Medicine, 21*(11), 1381–1387.

Feldstein, P. J. (1994). *Health policy issues: An economic perspective on health reform.* Ann Arbor, MI: AUPHA/HAP.

Ferguson, C. E., & Maurice, S. C. (1970). *Economic analysis.* Homewood, IL: Richard D. Irwin.

Friedman, G. D. (1980). *Primer of epidemiology.* New York, NY: McGraw-Hill.

Grossman, M. (1972). On the concept of health capital and the demand for health. *Journal of Political Economy, 80*(2), 223–255.

Hatch, R. L., Burg, M. A., Naberhaus, D. S., & Hellmich, L. K. (1998). The Spiritual Involvement and Beliefs Scale: Development and testing of a new instrument. *Journal of Family Practice, 46,* 476–486.

Henry, R. C. (1993). Community partnership model for health professions education. *Journal of the American Podiatric Medical Association, 83*(6), 328–331.

Hick, J., Hanfling, D., Burstein, J. L., DeAtley, C., Barbisch, D., Bogdan, G. M., & Cantrill, S. (2004). Health care facility and community strategies for patient care surge capacity. *Annals of Emergency Medicine, 44,* 253–261.

Hoff, A., Johannessen-Henry, C. T., Ross, L., Hvidt, N. C., & Johansen, C. (2008). Religion and reduced cancer risk—what is the explanation? A review. *European Journal of Cancer, 44*(17), 2573–2579.

Holahan, J. (2011). The 2007–09 recession and health insurance coverage. *Health Affairs, 30*(1), 145–152.

Institute of Medicine. (1988). *The future of public health.* Washington, DC: National Academies Press.

Jonsen, A. R. (1986). Bentham in a box: Technology assessment and health care allocation. *Law, Medicine, and Health Care, 14*(3–4), 172–174.

Kane, R. L. (1988). Empiric approaches to prevention in the elderly: Are we promoting too much? In R. Chernoff & D. A. Lipschitz (Eds.), *Health promotion and disease prevention in the elderly* (pp. 127–141). New York, NY: Raven Press.

Kawachi, I., Kennedy, B. P., & Glass, R. (1999). Social capital and self-rated health: A contextual analysis. *American Journal of Public Health, 89,* 1187–1193.

Kawachi, I., Kennedy, B. P., Lochner, K., & Prothrow-Stith, D. (1997). Social capital, income inequality, and mortality. *American Journal of Public Health, 87,* 1491–1498.

Kearns, R., Hubble, M. W., Holmes, J. H., IV, & Cairns, B. A. (2013). Disaster planning: Transportation resources and considerations for managing a burn disaster. *Journal of Burn Care and Research*, 1–12.

Kristol, I. (1978). A capitalist conception of justice. In R. T. De George & J. A. Pichler (Eds.), *Ethics, free enterprise, and public policy: Original essays on moral issues in business* (pp. 57–69). New York, NY: Oxford University Press.

Lasker, R. D. (1997). *Medicine and public health: The power of collaboration*. New York, NY: New York Academy of Medicine.

Macfarlane, G. J., & Lowenfels, A. B. (1994). Physical activity and colon cancer. *European Journal of Cancer Prevention, 3*(5), 393–398.

Marwick, C. (1995). Should physicians prescribe prayer for health? Spiritual aspects of well-being considered. *Journal of the American Medical Association, 273*(20), 1561–1562.

McKee, M. (2001). Measuring the efficiency of health systems. *British Medical Journal, 323*(7308), 295–296.

National Center for Health Statistics. (2012a). *Health, United States, 2009.* Hyattsville, MD: U.S. Department of Health and Human Services.

National Center for Health Statistics. (2012b). *Healthy People 2010 final review.* Retrieved from http://www.cdc.gov/nchs/healthy_people/hp2010/hp2010_final_review.htm

National Center for Health Statistics. (2013). *Health, United States, 2012.* Hyattsville, MD: U.S. Department of Health and Human Services.

National Prevention Council. (2011). *Nation prevention strategy: America's plan for better health and wellness.* Washington, DC: U.S. Department of Health and Human Services.

Oman, D., Kurata, J. H., Strawbridge, W. J., & Cohen, R. D. (2002). Religious attendance and cause of death over 31 years. *International Journal of Psychiatry and Medicine, 32*, 69–89.

Pantell, M., Rehkopf, D., Jutte, D., Syme, S. L., Balmes, J., & Adler, N. (2013). Social isolation: A predictor of mortality comparable to traditional clinical risk factors. *American Journal of Public Health, 103*(11), 2056–2062.

Parsons, T. (1972). Definitions of health and illness in the light of American values and social structure. In E. G. Jaco (Ed.), *Patients, physicians and illness: A sourcebook in behavioral science and health* (2nd ed.). New York, NY: Free Press.

Partnership to Fight Chronic Disease. (2009). *Almanac of chronic disease*. Retrieved from http://www.fightchronicdisease.org/sites/fightchronicdisease.org/files/docs/2009AlmanacofChronicDisease_updated81009.pdf

Peters, K. E., Drabant, E., Elster, A. B., Tierney, M., & Hatcher, B. (2001). *Cooperative actions for health programs: Lessons learned in medicine and public health collaboration.* Chicago, IL: American Medical Association.

Pincus, T., Esther, R., DeWalt, D. A., & Callahan, L. F. (1998). Social conditions and self-management are more powerful determinants of health than access to care. *Annals of Internal Medicine, 129*(5), 406–411.

Plotkin, S. L., & Plotkin, S. A. (1999). A short history of vaccination. In S. A. Plotkin & W. A. Orenstein (Eds.), *Vaccines* (3rd ed.). Philadelphia, PA: Saunders.

Post, S. G., Puchalski, C. M., & Larson, D. B. (2000). Physicians and patient spirituality: Professional boundaries, competency, and ethics. *Annals of Internal Medicine, 132*(7), 578–583.

Reinhardt, U. E. (1994). Providing access to health care and controlling costs: The universal dilemma. In P. R. Lee & C. L. Estes (Eds.), *The nation's health* (4th ed., pp. 263–278). Boston, MA: Jones & Bartlett.

Robert Wood Johnson Foundation. (2010). Chronic care: Making the case for ongoing care. Retrieved from http://www.rwjf.org/pr/product.jsp?id=50968

Roberts, J. A., Brown, D., Elkins, T., & Larson, D. B. (1997). Factors influencing views of patients with gynecologic cancer about end-of-life decisions. *American Journal of Obstetrics and Gynecology, 176*, 166–172.

Rosen, G. (1993). *A history of public health.* Baltimore, MD: Johns Hopkins University Press.

Ross, L. (1995). The spiritual dimension: Its importance to patients' health, well-being and quality of life and its implications for nursing practice. *International Journal of Nursing Studies, 32*(5), 457–468.

Santerre, R. E., & Neun, S. P. (1996). *Health economics: Theories, insights, and industry studies.* Chicago, IL: Irwin.

Saward, E., & Sorensen, A. (1980). The current emphasis on preventive medicine. In S. J. Williams (Ed.), *Issues in health services* (pp. 17–29). New York, NY: Wiley.

Schneider, M. J. (2000). *Introduction to public health.* Gaithersburg, MD: Aspen.

Shi, L., & Johnson, J. (Eds.). (2014). *Public health administration: Principles for population-based management* (3rd ed.). Burlington, MA: Jones & Bartlett.

Shi, L., & Singh, D. (2015). *Delivering health care in America: A systems approach* (6th ed.). Burlington, MA: Jones & Bartlett.

Shi, L., & Starfield, B. (2001). Primary care physician supply, income inequality, and racial mortality in

US metropolitan areas. *American Journal of Public Health, 91*(8), 1246–1250.

Shi, L., Starfield, B., Kennedy, B., & Kawachi, I. (1999). Income inequality, primary care, and health indicators. *Journal of Family Practice, 48*(4), 275–284.

Shi, L., Starfield, B., Politzer, R., & Regan, J. (2002). Primary care, self-rated health, and reduction in social disparities in health. *Health Services Research, 37*(3), 529–550.

Stopford, B. (2005). The National Disaster Medical System—America's medical readiness force. *Disaster Management and Response*, 53–56.

Swanson, C. S. (1995). A spirit-focused conceptual model of nursing for the advanced practice nurse. *Issues in Comprehensive Pediatric Nursing, 18*(4), 267–275.

Timmreck, T. C. (1994). *An introduction to epidemiology.* Boston, MA: Jones & Bartlett.

Turnock, B. J. (1997). *Public health: What it is and how it works.* Gaithersburg, MD: Aspen Publishers.

U.S. Department of Health and Human Services. (1992). *Healthy People 2000: National health promotion and disease prevention objectives.* Boston, MA: Jones & Bartlett.

U.S. Department of Health and Human Services. (1998). *Healthy People 2010 objectives: Draft for public comment.* Washington, DC: U.S. Government Printing Office.

U.S. Department of Health and Human Services. (2004). *The health consequences of smoking: A report of the Surgeon General.* Retrieved from http://www.surgeongeneral.gov/library /reports/50-years-of-progress/

U.S. Department of Health and Human Services. (2006). *Your guide to lowering blood pressure.* Retrieved from http://www.nhlbi.nih.gov/health /public/heart/hbp/dash/new_dash.pdf

U.S. Department of Health and Human Services. (2010a). *Healthy People 2020.* Retrieved from http://healthypeople.gov/2020

U.S. Department of Health and Human Services. (2010b). *Summary of the prevention and wellness initiative—community component.* Retrieved from http://www.cdc.gov/chronicdisease/recovery /docs/PW_Community_fact_sheet_final.pdf

U.S. Department of Health and Human Services. (2011a, June 23). $10 million in Affordable Care Act funds to help create workplace health programs [News release]. Retrieved from http://www. businesswire.com/news/home/20110623005954 /en/10-Million-Affordable-Care-Act-funds -create#.VBMMf2OaViY

U.S. Department of Health and Human Services. (2011b). *National Health Security Strategy 2009.* Retrieved from http://www.phe.gov/Preparedness /planning/authority/nhss/Pages/default.aspx

U.S. Department of Health and Human Services. (2012). Medicare preventive services. Retrieved from http://www.hhs.gov/healthcare/prevention /seniors/medicare-preventive-services.html

U.S. Department of Health and Human Services. (2013). Affordable Care Act rules on expanding access to preventive services for women. Retrieved from http://www.hhs.gov/healthcare/facts/fact sheets/2011/08/womensprevention08012011a .html

U.S. Department of Health and Human Services, the Secretary's Advisory Committee on National Health Promotion and Disease Prevention Objectives for 2020. (2008). *Phase I report: Recommendations for the framework and format of Healthy People 2020.* Retrieved from http://healthypeople. gov/2020/about/advisory/PhaseI.pdf

Ward, B. (1995). Holistic medicine. *Australian Family Physician, 24*(5), 761–762, 765.

Ward, B. W., & Schiller, J. S. (2010). Prevalence of multiple chronic conditions among US adults: Estimates from the National Health Interview Survey. *Preventing Chronic Diseases, 10*, 120203.

WHO Commission on Social Determinants of Health. (2007). *A conceptual framework for action on the social determinants of health.* Geneva, Switzerland: World Health Organization. Retrieved from http://www.who.int/social_determinants /resources/csdh_framework_action_05_07.pdf

Wilkinson, R. G. (1997). Comment: Income, inequality, and social cohesion. *American Journal of Public Health, 87*, 1504–1506.

World Health Organization. (1948). *Preamble to the constitution.* Geneva, Switzerland: Author.

World Health Organization. (2003). *WHO definition of palliative care.* Geneva, Switzerland: Author.

World Health Organization. (2011). *Noncommunicable diseases country profiles.* Retrieved from http://www.who.int/nmh/publications /ncd_profiles2011/en

World Health Organization. (2013). *Pandemic influenza preparedness framework.* Retrieved from http://www.who.int/influenza/resources /pip_framework/en

CHAPTER 9

The Healthcare Interdisciplinary Context: A Focus on the Microsystem Concept

Julie K. Johnson

© A-R-T/Shutterstock

LEARNING OBJECTIVES

1. Apply the concepts of the microsystem to understand one's practice environment.
2. Understand the theoretical underpinnings of the microsystem.
3. Define the essential elements of a microsystem.
4. Describe research that has identified high-performing microsystems.
5. Describe one method for assessing the functioning of a microsystem.
6. Explore the potential link between microsystems and patient safety.

INTRODUCTION

Health care is provided in complex environments with intricate webs of relationships. These relationships represent the multiple interactions with people, information, technology, culture, and the physical environment in which patient care is provided. The organization of health care can be described in many different ways, for example, a clinic, a clinical department within a hospital, an inpatient unit, or a primary care setting, among others. Of course, all these are accurate organizational descriptions and provide some insight into the types of care processes and providers in each area. Another framework to describe how health care is organized is the clinical microsystem. The clinical microsystem, as an organizational construct, is a systems approach for providing clinical care that is based on theories from organizational development, leadership, and quality improvement.

A clinical microsystem can be defined as the combination of a small group of people who work together in a defined setting on a regular basis—or as needed—to provide care and the individuals who receive that care (who also can be recognized as part of a discrete subpopulation of patients). Based on this definition, the essential elements of the microsystem include a designated group of specific patients, clinicians and support staff, information and information technology specialists, and care processes. The clinical purpose and its setting define the essential components of the microsystem. For example, a microsystem that provides pediatric cardiovascular surgical care has a very specific purpose that outlines the required components to accomplish the purpose. The purpose of the microsystem also identifies the patient population eligible to receive care (e.g., pediatric patients with cardiovascular problems that need surgical repair) as well as the clinicians (surgeons, anesthesiologists, cardiologists, and nurses) and other service providers. This type of microsystem looks quite different from a microsystem that has the mission of providing outpatient care. Microsystems evolve over time as they respond to the needs of their patients and providers as well as to external pressures such as regulatory and accreditation requirements.

A clinical microsystem (as an example of a complex adaptive system) is often embedded in a larger organizational context. For example, several microsystems may exist within an outpatient clinic and hundreds of microsystems may exist within a hospital.

Microsystems exist everywhere, but their levels of functioning vary. One contributing factor is the ability of individual caregivers to recognize their efforts as part of a microsystem. Previous research on clinical microsystems (described later in this chapter) has identified 10 success factors, as summarized in **Table 9-1** (Mohr, 2000). Every clinical microsystem possesses each of these factors in varying degrees. A high-performing microsystem (i.e., a microsystem that consistently and reliably achieves the best outcomes for its patients) would rate the highest on each of these factors.

As a functioning unit, the microsystem has clinical as well as business aims, linked processes, and a shared information and technology environment. It produces services and care that can be measured as performance outcomes. The microsystem construct explicitly demonstrates the caregiving system. It builds on systems theory by recognizing that "important systems' characteristics include the system-environment boundary, input, output, process, goal-directedness, and interaction of the elements of the system" (Bertalanffy, 1968).

Systems, in general, often bring up images of "well-oiled machines." However, healthcare systems are often cumbersome, unwieldy, unfriendly, and opaque to their users, who are the patients, physicians, nurses, and staff who frequent the microsystem. Healthcare systems are best described as complex adaptive systems. As such, they are a collection of individuals who are free to act in ways that are not totally predictable. Their organizational boundaries are "fuzzy"; their membership changes, and their members simultaneously can be members of other systems. Furthermore, given the complexity of these systems, the actions of individuals are interconnected so that the action of one changes the context for all the others (Plsek & Greenhalgh, 2001). The clinical microsystem is a complex adaptive system, and as such it must: (a) do the work, (b) meet member needs, and (c) maintain itself as a functioning clinical unit.

In its *Crossing the Quality Chasm* report, the Institute of Medicine identified multiple layers of the healthcare system that influence the ability to improve care (Berwick, 2002):

- the patients' experience;
- the functioning of the microsystem;
- the functioning of the organizations that house or otherwise support microsystems; and
- the environment (e.g., policy, payment, and regulation) that shapes the behavior, interests, and opportunities of the organizations.

TABLE 9-1	Characteristics of High-Performing Microsystems

Microsystem Characteristic	Definition
Leadership	The role of leaders is to maintain balance while reaching collective goals, and to empower individual autonomy and accountability through building knowledge, respectful action, reviewing, and reflecting.
Organizational support	The larger organization looks for ways to support the work of the microsystem and coordinate the hand-offs between microsystems.
Staff focus	There is selective hiring of the best qualified employees. An orientation process is designed and implemented to fully integrate new staff into an organization's culture and work roles. Expectations of staff are high regarding performance, continuing education, professional growth, collaboration, and networking.
Education and training	All clinical microsystems are responsible for the ongoing education and training of staff and for aligning daily work roles with training competencies. Academic clinical microsystems have the additional responsibility of training students.
Interdependence	The interaction of staff is characterized by trust, collaboration, a willingness to help each other, appreciation of complementary roles, respect, and recognition that each staffer contributes individually to a shared purpose.
Patient focus	The primary concern is to meet all patient needs: caring, listening, educating, responding to special requests, innovating to meet patient needs, and smooth service flow.
Community and market focus	The microsystem is a resource for the community and the community is a resource for the microsystem. The microsystem establishes excellent and innovative relationships with the community.
Performance results	Performance focuses on improving patient outcomes, avoiding unnecessary costs, streamlining delivery, using data feedback, promoting positive competition, and engaging in frank discussions about performance.
Process improvement	An atmosphere for learning and redesign is supported by the continuous monitoring of care, use of benchmarking, frequent tests of change, and a staff that has been empowered to innovate
Information and information technology	Information is the key connector for staff to patients, staff to staff, and needs with actions to meet those needs. Technology facilitates effective communication. Multiple formal and informal channels are used to keep all system members fully informed, provide a forum for member input, and ensure that everyone is in the loop on important topics.

Source: Freshman, B., Rubino, L., & Chassiakos, Y. (2010). *Collaboration across the disciplines in health care*. Sudbury, MA: Jones and Bartlett.

| FIGURE 9-1 | The chain effect in improving healthcare quality and patient safety. |

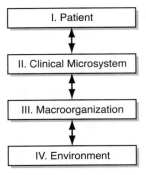

Source: Freshman, B., Rubino, L., & Chassiakos, Y. (2010). *Collaboration across the disciplines in health care.* Sudbury, MA: Jones and Bartlett.

Efforts at each of the different levels of the healthcare system—patient, microsystem, macroorganization, environment—and the interactions between them can positively influence the ability to achieve patient safety and quality of care objectives. **Figure 9-1** illustrates the interactions of these elements.

ROOTS OF THE CLINICAL MICROSYSTEM CONCEPT

The conceptual underpinnings of the clinical microsystem are based on ideas developed by Deming (1986), Senge (1990), Wheatley (1992), and others who have applied systems thinking to organizational development, leadership, and quality improvement.

Bertalanffy (1968), founder of the mathematical Theory of Systems, defined a system as a set of interacting, interrelated, or interdependent elements that work together in a particular environment to perform the functions that are required to achieve the system's aim. The importance of understanding systems as interrelated parts of a whole cannot be overstated.

Comprehending the assembly of the system as a whole can inform the work of those who are trying to create successful, interdependent systems (Batalden & Mohr, 1997). Learning to see interrelationships rather than linear cause-and-effect chains as well as grasping the phenomenon of change as a process, rather than a snapshot, are essential for understanding systems (Senge, 1990). Systems have certain rules (or principles) that help us predict how they will behave (Ackoff, 1974, 1994).

- The whole has one or more defining functions.
- Each part can affect the behavior or properties of the whole.
- Each part is necessary but alone is insufficient to carry out the defining function of the whole.
- Behavior and properties of one part of the system depend on the behavior and properties of at least one other part of the system.

Systems thinking is the cornerstone of how "learning organizations" view their world

(Senge, 1990). Learning organizations are those that measure outcomes and strive for improvement. Many fields outside health care, including education, telecommunications, and aviation, use systems theory to better serve their clients, understand applicable research, improve outcomes, and ensure quality and safety. Recognizing feedback from the system and then using that feedback for design and redesign of services is an inherent element of systems thinking.

The seminal idea for the clinical microsystem stems from the work of James Brian Quinn (Quinn, 1992). Quinn analyzed the world's best-of-best service organizations, such as FedEx, Mary Kay Cosmetics, McDonald's, Scandinavian Airlines, and Nordstrom's. He focused on determining what these extraordinary organizations were doing to achieve high quality, explosive growth, high margins, and wonderful reputations with customers. He found that these leading service organizations organized around, and continually engineered, the frontline relationships that connected the needs of customers with the organization's core competency. Quinn termed this frontline activity that embedded the service delivery process the "smallest replicable unit" or the "minimum replicable unit." This smallest replicable unit, what we call the microsystem, is the key to implementing effective strategy, information technology, and other critically important aspects of intelligent enterprise.

STUDY OF HIGH-PERFORMING MICROSYSTEMS

Qualitative research methods have been used to understand processes and outcomes of care in designing and redesigning care around the clinical microsystem (Barach & Johnson, 2006; Galvan, Bacha, Mohr, & Barach, 2005). In the late 1990s, under the aegis of the Institute of Medicine (IOM) and with funding by the Robert Wood Johnson Foundation, Mohr (2000) and Donaldson

and Mohr (2000) investigated high-performing clinical microsystems. This research was based on a national search for the highest-quality clinical microsystems. Forty-three clinical units were identified using theoretical sampling, and their leaders were interviewed using a semistructured interview protocol. The results of the interviews were analyzed to determine the characteristics that seemed to be most responsible for enabling these microsystems to be effective. The results suggested that eight dimensions were associated with high quality of care:

1. integration of information;
2. measurement;
3. interdependence of the care team;
4. supportiveness of the larger system;
5. constancy of purpose;
6. connection to community;
7. investment in improvement; and
8. alignment of role and training.

These eight factors became a framework for evaluating clinical microsystems. Each dimension can be thought of on a continuum that represents the presence of the characteristic in the microsystem.

The Dartmouth study (funded by the Robert Wood Johnson Foundation to continue and build on the IOM study) was based on 20 case studies of high-performing clinical microsystems and included on-site interviews with every member of each microsystem, plus analysis of individual microsystem performance data (Batalden, Nelson, Edwards, Godfrey, & Mohr, 2003; Batalden, Nelson, Mohr, et al., 2003; Godfrey, Nelson, Wasson, Mohr, & Batalden, 2003; Huber et al., 2003; Kosnik & Espinosa, 2003; Mohr et al., 2003; Nelson et al., 2002; Nelson et al., 2003; Wasson, Godfrey, Nelson, Mohr, & Batalden, 2003). As a result of this work, the dimensions of high-performing microsystems have been further refined and expanded to include two additional categories. Table 9-1 lists the dimensions of high-performing microsystems and provides an operational definition of each. For example, increased awareness of the small frontline work unit as a microsystem also means recognizing the characteristics that contribute to the unit's identity and being mindful of the reliability of these characteristics.

ASSESSING PERFORMANCE OF THE MICROSYSTEM

Several tools and techniques are available for microsystems that wish to engage in self-assessment based on microsystem characteristics. The success characteristics emerged from the analysis of the coded interview transcripts; they reflect how members of high-performing microsystems describe their work and how it was done. Consequently, they provided the framework for a microsystem-specific analysis of performance, which is the basis of the Microsystem Assessment Tool (MAT). The MAT (**Appendix 9-1**) is designed to help understand microsystems and how those functioning within them can improve their performance (Mohr & Batalden, 2002; Mohr, Batalden, & Barach, 2004). It addresses the nature of the interaction between the microsystem and the parent organization, and offers considerable insight into the functioning of a microsystem. The MAT is designed to be used quickly and easily by microsystem members to evaluate their own frontline units.

Additionally, there is a series of "toolkits" and "workbooks" to provide a path forward for assessing one's microsystem. Workbooks are available for different types of clinical microsystems, including the following:

- Primary care practices
- Specialty practices
- Cystic fibrosis programs
- Brain trauma programs
- Inpatient care units
- Emergency departments

Each workbook uses a standard approach to conduct a full assessment of a microsystem based on the "5 P" method, which includes assessments of the different aspects of a clinical microsystem: purpose, patients, professionals and staff, processes, and patterns of performance (outcomes, values, beliefs, and practices). The workbooks, which are available electronically at http://www.clinicalmicrosystem.org, include a variety of methods and tools to evaluate each respective aspect of a microsystem.

LEADERSHIP FOR PATIENT SAFETY IN THE MICROSYSTEM

The clinical microsystem—as a unit of research, analysis, and practice—is an important level at which to focus patient safety and quality improvement interventions. It is at this system level that most patients and caregivers meet, and it is at this level that real changes in patient care can be made.

Safety is a property of the clinical microsystem that can be achieved only through a systematic application of a broad array of process, equipment, organization, supervision, training, simulation, and teamwork changes. **Table 9-2** builds on the research of high-performing microsystems and provides specific actions that can be further explored. This list provides an organizing framework and a place to start applying patient safety concepts to microsystems.

CONCLUSION

The microsystem concepts have evolved from systems theory and primary research on characteristics of high-performing clinical units. Specific interventions can be implemented to embed quality and safety into a microsystem. Table 9-2 offers several suggestions related to each of the microsystem characteristics that might serve as a guiding framework to be adapted and used by individual microsystems. Leaders should promote safety as a priority for the organization, but they should allow individual microsystems to create innovative strategies for improvement.

TABLE 9-2	Linkage of Microsystem Characteristics to Patient Safety

Microsystem Characteristic	Steps Linked to Improved Patient Safety
Leadership	■ Define the quality and safety vision of the organization ■ Identify the existing constraints within the organization ■ Allocate resources for plan development, implementation, and ongoing monitoring and evaluation ■ Build in microsystems participation and input to plan development ■ Align organizational quality and safety goals ■ Engage the Board of Trustees in ongoing conversations about the organizational progress toward achieving safety goals ■ Promote and recognize prompt truth-telling about errors or hazards ■ Certify helpful changes to improve safety
Organizational support	■ Work with clinical microsystems to identify patient safety issues and make relevant local changes ■ Put the necessary resources and tools into the hands of individuals
Staff focus	■ Assess current safety culture ■ Identify the gap between current culture and safety vision ■ Plan cultural interventions ■ Conduct periodic assessments of culture ■ Celebrate examples of desired behavior (e.g., acknowledgment of an error)
Education and training	■ Develop patient safety curriculum ■ Provide training and education of key clinical and management leadership ■ Develop a core of staff with patient safety skills who can work across microsystems as a resource
Interdependence of the care team	■ Build PDSA* into debriefings ■ Use daily huddles to debrief and to celebrate identifying errors
Patient focus	■ Establish patient and family partnerships ■ Support disclosure and truth around medical error
Community and market focus	■ Analyze safety issues in community and partner with external groups to reduce risk to population
Performance results	■ Develop key safety measures ■ Create feedback mechanisms to share results with Microsystems
Process improvement	■ Identify patient safety priorities based on assessment of key safety measures ■ Address the work that will be required at the microsystem level
Information and information technology	■ Enhance error reporting systems ■ Build safety concepts into information flow (e.g., checklists, reminder systems)

*PDSA (Plan-Do-Study-Act)

Source: Freshman, B., Rubino, L., & Chassiakos, Y. (2010). *Collaboration across the disciplines in health care.* Sudbury, MA: Jones and Bartlett.

Simply bringing individuals together to perform a specified task does not automatically ensure that they will function as a team. Effective teamwork depends on the willingness of clinicians from diverse backgrounds to cooperate toward a shared goal, to communicate, to work together effectively, and to improve. Each team member must be able to: (a) anticipate the needs of the others, (b) adjust to each other's actions and to the changing environment, (c) monitor each other's activities and distribute workload dynamically, and (d) have a shared understanding of accepted processes and how events and actions should proceed. Microsystems with clear goals and effective communication strategies can adjust to new information with speed and effectiveness to enhance real-time problem solving. Individual behaviors change more readily on a team because team identity is less threatened by change than are individuals. Behavioral attributes of effective teamwork, including enhanced interpersonal skills, can extend positively to other clinical arenas.

Turning a clinical unit into an effective microsystem requires substantial planning and practice. There is a natural resistance among many to moving beyond individual roles and accountability toward a team mindset. One can promote and facilitate this commitment by using the following guidelines:

1. Foster a shared awareness of each member's tasks and role on the team through cross-training and other team training modalities.

2. Train members in specific teamwork skills such as communication, situation awareness, leadership, follower-ship, resource allocation, and adaptability.

3. Conduct team training in simulated scenarios with a focus on both team behaviors and technical skills.

4. Train team leaders in the necessary leadership competencies to build and maintain effective teams.

5. Establish and consistently utilize reliable methods of team performance evaluation and rapid feedback.

As we continue to move beyond conceptual theory and research to the application of new understandings and concepts in clinical settings, the emerging fields of chaos theory, complexity science, complex adaptive systems, and lean production have influenced how these concepts have been applied to improving microsystems (Arrow, McGrath, & Berdahl, 2000; Peters, 1987; Plsek & Greenhalgh, 2001; Plsek & Wilson, 2001). The result is an ongoing process of continuous quality improvement that is enhanced by collaboration among microsystems and their researchers to share information, successes, and best practices. (Updates on these efforts are available at http://clinicalmicrosystem.org [Trustees of Dartmouth College, 2008].)

DISCUSSION QUESTIONS

1. Describe a clinical microsystem with which you are familiar. What is the aim of the microsystem, and what are its core elements?

2. Use the Microsystem Assessment Tool (Appendix 9-1) to assess the microsystem in which you work.

3. What are the types of strategies you might use to help a clinical microsystem move toward a higher level of functioning?

4. Access the workbook for your specific setting at http://www.clinicalmicrosystem.org. These workbooks are quite extensive. At this point you may want to browse the main features and save the workbook for later reference.

REFERENCES

Ackoff, R. (1974). *Redesigning the future*. New York, NY: Wiley.

Ackoff, R. (1994). *The Democratic corporation*. New York, NY: Oxford University Press.

Arrow, H., McGrath, J., & Berdahl, J. (2000). *Small groups as complex systems.* Thousand Oaks, CA: Sage.

Barach, P., & Johnson, J. K. (2006). Understanding the complexity of redesigning care around the clinical microsystem. *Quality and Safety in Health Care, 15*(Suppl. 1), i10–i16.

Batalden, P., & Mohr, J. (1997). Building knowledge of health care as a system. *Quality Management in Health Care, 5,* 1-12.

Batalden, P. B., Mohr, J. K., Nelson, E. C., Plume, S. K., Baker, G. R., Wasson, J. H., . . . Wisniewski, J. J. (1997). Continually improving the health and value of health care for a population of patients: The panel management process. *Quality Management in Health Care, 5,* 41-51.

Batalden, P., Nelson, E., Edwards, W., Godfrey, M., & Mohr, J. (2003). Microsystems in health care: Part 9. Developing small clinical units to attain peak performance. *The Joint Commission Journal on Quality and Safety, 29,* 575-585.

Batalden, P. B, Nelson, E. C., Mohr, J. K., Godfrey, M. M., Huber, T., Kosnik C., & Ashling, K. (2003). Microsystems in health care: Part 5. How leaders are leading. *The Joint Commission Journal on Quality and Safety, 29,* 297-308.

Bertalanffy, L. V. (1968). *General system theory: Foundations, development, applications.* New York, NY: George Braziller.

Berwick, D. (2002). A user's manual for the IOM's "Quality Chasm" report. *Health Affairs, 21,* 80-90.

Deming, W. E. (1986). *Out of the crisis.* Cambridge: Massachusetts Institute of Technology Center for Advanced Engineering Study.

Donaldson, M. S., & Mohr, J. K. (2000). *Improvement and innovation in health care microsystems.* A technical report for the Institute of Medicine Committee on the Quality of Health Care in America. Princeton, NJ: Robert Wood Johnson Foundation.

Freshman, B., Rubino, L., & Chassiakos, Y. (2010). *Collaboration across the disciplines in health care.* Sudbury, MA: Jones and Bartlett.

Galvan, C., Bacha, E., Mohr, J., & Barach, P. (2005). A human factors approach to understanding patient safety during pediatric cardiac surgery. *Progress in Pediatric Cardiology, 20,*13-20.

Godfrey, M. M., Nelson, E. C., Wasson, J. H., Mohr, J. J., & Batalden, P. B. (2003). Microsystems in health care: Part 3. Planning patient-centered services. *The Joint Commission Journal on Quality and Safety, 29,* 159-170.

Huber, T., Godfrey, M., Nelson, E., Mohr, J., Campbell, C., & Batalden P. (2003). Microsystems in health care: Part 8. Developing people and improving worklife: What front-line staff told us. *The Joint Commission Journal on Quality and Safety, 29,* 512-522.

Kosnik, L., & Espinosa, J. (2003). Microsystems in health care: Part 7. The microsystem as a platform for merging strategic planning and operations. *The Joint Commission Journal on Quality and Safety, 29,* 452-459.

Mohr, J. (2000). *Forming, operating, and improving microsystems of care.* Hanover, NH: Center for the Evaluative Clinical Sciences, Dartmouth College.

Mohr, J. J., Barach, P., Cravero, J. P., Blike, G. T., Godfrey, M. M., Batalden, P. B., & Nelson, E. C. (2003). Microsystems in health care: Part 6. Designing patient safety into the microsystem. *The Joint Commission Journal on Quality and Safety, 29,* 401-408.

Mohr, J., & Batalden, P. (2002). Improving safety at the front lines: The role of clinical microsystems. *Quality and Safety in Health Care, 11,* 45-50.

Mohr, J., Batalden, P., & Barach, P. (2004). Integrating patient safety into the clinical microsystem. *Quality and Safety in Health Care, 13*(Suppl. 2), ii34-ii38.

Nelson, E. C., Batalden, P. B., Homa, K., Godfrey, M. M., Campbell, C., Headrick, L. A., . . . Wasson, J. H. (2003). Microsystems in health care: Part 2. Creating a rich information environment. *The Joint Commission Journal on Quality and Safety, 29,* 5-15.

Nelson, E., Batalden, P., Huber, T., Mohr, J. J., Campbell, C., Headrick, L. A., & Wasson, J. H. (2002). Microsystems in health care: Part 1. Learning from high-performing front-line clinical units. *The Joint Commission Journal on Quality and Safety, 28,* 472-493.

Nelson, E. C., Batalden, P. B., Mohr, J. J., & Plume, S. K. (1998). Building a quality future. *Frontiers of Health Services Management, 15,* 3-32.

Peters, T. (1987). *Thriving on chaos: Handbook for a management revolution.* New York, NY: Harper & Row.

Plsek, P. E., & Greenhalgh, T. (2001). Complexity science: The challenge of complexity in health care. *British Medical Journal, 323,* 625-628.

Plsek, P. E., & Wilson, T. (2001). Complexity, leadership, and management in health care organisations. *BMJ, 523*(7315), 746-749.

Quinn, J. B. (1992). *The intelligent enterprise.* New York, NY: Free Press.

Senge, P. (1990). *The fifth discipline.* New York, NY: Doubleday.

Trustees of Dartmouth College. (2008). Clinical microsystems. Retrieved from http://clinicalmicrosystem.org/

Wasson, J. H., Godfrey, M. M., Nelson, E. C., Mohr, J. J., & Batalden, P. B. (2003). Microsystems in health care: Part 4. Planning patient-centered care. *The Joint Commission Journal on Quality and Safety, 29*, 227–237.

Wheatley, M. (1992). *Leadership and the new science: Learning about organization from an orderly universe.* San Francisco, CA: Berrett-Koehler.

APPENDIX 9-1

Microsystem Assessment Tool

Characteristics and Definition	Description			
Leadership				
1. Leadership: The role of leaders is to balance setting and reach collective goals, and to empower individual autonomy and accountability through building knowledge, respectful action, reviewing, and reflecting.	■ Leaders often tell me how to do my job and leave little room for innovation and autonomy. Overall, they don't foster a positive culture.	■ Leaders struggle to find the right balance between reaching performance goals and supporting and empowering the staff.	■ Leaders maintain constancy of purpose, establish clear goals and expectations, and foster a respectful positive culture. Leaders take time to build knowledge, review and reflect, and take action about microsystems and the larger organization.	■ Can't rate
2. Organizational support: The larger organization looks for ways to support the work of the microsystem and coordinate the hand-offs between microsystems.	■ The larger organization isn't supportive in a way that provides recognition, information, and resources to enhance my work.	■ The larger organization is inconsistent and unpredictable in providing the recognition, information, and resources needed to enhance my work.	■ The larger organization provides recognition, information, and resources that enhance my work and makes it easier for me to meet the needs of patients.	■ Can't rate
Staff				
3. Staff focus: There is selective hiring of the right kind of people. The orientation process is designed to fully integrate new staff into culture and work roles.	■ I am not made to feel like a valued member of the microsystem. My orientation was incomplete.	■ I feel like I am a valued member of the microsystem, but I don't think the microsystem is doing all that it could to support education	■ I am a valued member of the microsystem and what I say matters. This is evident through staffing, education and training,	■ Can't rate

(continues)

Characteristics and Definition	Description			
Expectations of staff are high regarding performance, continuing education, professional growth, and networking.	My continuing education and professional growth needs are not being met.	and training of staff, workload, and professional growth.	workload, and professional growth.	
4. Education and training: All clinical microsystems have responsibility for the ongoing education and training of staff and for aligning daily work roles with training competencies. Academic clinical microsystems have the additional responsibility of training students.	■ Training is accomplished in disciplinary silos (e.g., nurses train nurses, physicians train residents, etc.). The educational efforts are not aligned with the flow of patient care, so that education becomes an "add-on" to what we do.	■ We recognize that our training could be different to reflect the needs of our microsystem, but we haven't made many changes yet. Some continuing education is available to everyone.	■ There is a team approach to training, whether we are training staff, nurses, or students. Education and patient care are integrated into the flow of work in a way that benefits both from the available resources. Continuing education for all staff is recognized as vital to our continued success.	■ Can't rate
5. Interdependence: The interaction of staff is characterized by trust, collaboration, willingness to help each other, appreciation of complementary roles, respect, and recognition that all contribute individually to a shared purpose.	■ I work independently and I am responsible for my own part of the work.	■ The care approach is interdisciplinary, but we are not always able to work together as an effective team.	■ Care is provided by an interdisciplinary team characterized by trust, collaboration, appreciation of complementary roles, and a recognition that all contribute individually to a shared purpose.	■ Can't rate

Characteristics and Definition	Description			
Patient				
6. Patient focus: The primary concern is to meet all patient needs: caring, listening, educating, and responding to special requests, innovating to meet patient needs, and smooth service flow.	▪ Most of us, including our patients, would agree that we do not always provide patient-centered care. We are not always clear about what patients want and need.	▪ We are actively working to provide patient-centered care and we are making progress toward more effectively and consistently learning about and meeting patient needs.	▪ We are effective in learning about and meeting patient needs: caring, listening, educating, responding to special requests, and smooth service flow.	▪ Can't rate
7. Community and market focus: The microsystem is a resource for the community; the community is a resource to the microsystem; the microsystem establishes excellent and innovative relationships with the community.	▪ We focus on the patients who come to our unit. We haven't implemented any outreach programs in our community. Patients and their families often make their own connections to the community resources they need.	▪ We have tried a few outreach programs and have had some success, but it is not the norm for us to go out into the community or actively connect patients to the community resources that are available to them.	▪ We are doing everything we can to understand our community. We actively employ resources to help us work with the community. We add to the community and draw on resources from the community meet patient needs.	▪ Can't rate
Performance				
8. Performance results: Performance focuses on patient outcomes, avoidable costs, streamlining	▪ We don't routinely collect data on the process or outcomes of the care we provide.	▪ We often collect data on the outcomes of the care we provide and on	▪ Outcomes (clinical, satisfaction, financial, technical, and safety) are routinely measured; we	▪ Can't rate

(continues)

Characteristics and Definition	Description			
delivery, using data feedback, promoting positive competition, and frank discussions about performance.		some processes of care.	feed data back to staff and we make changes based on data.	
9. Process improvement: An atmosphere for learning and redesign is supported by the continuous monitoring of care, use of benchmarking, frequent tests of change, and staff members who have been empowered to innovate.	■ The resources required (in the form of training, financial support, and time) are rarely available to support improvement work. Any improvement activities we do are in addition to our daily work.	■ Some resources are available to support improvement work, but we don't use them as often as we could. Change ideas are implemented without much discipline.	■ There are ample resources to support continual improvement work. Studying, measuring, and improving care in a scientific way are essential parts of our daily work.	■ Can't rate

Information and Information Technology

10. Information and information technology: Information is *the* connector: (a) staff to patients, (b) staff to staff, (c) needs with actions to meet needs. Technology facilitates effective communication and multiple formal and informal channels are used to keep everyone informed all of the time, to listen to everyone's ideas, and to ensure that everyone is connected on important topics.

Given the complexity of information and the use of technology in the microsystem, assess your microsystem on the following three characteristics: (1) integration of information with patients, (2) integration of information with providers and staff, and (3) integration of information with technology.

A. Integration of information with patients	■ Patients have access to some standard information that is available to all patients.	■ Patients have access to standard information that is available to all patients. We've started to think about how to improve the	■ Patients have a variety of ways to get the information they need, and it can be customized to meet their individual learning styles. We routinely ask	■ Can't rate

Characteristics and Definition	Description			
		■ information they are given to better meet their needs.	■ patients for feedback about how to improve the information we give them.	
B. Integration of information with providers and staff	■ I am always tracking down the information I need to do my work.	■ Most of the time I have the information I need, but sometimes essential information is missing and I have to track it down.	■ The information I need to do my work is available when I need it.	■ Can't rate
C. Integration of information with technology	■ The technology I need to facilitate and enhance my work is either not available to me, or it is available but not effective. The technology we currently have does not make my job easier.	■ I have access to technology that will enhance my work, but it is not easy to use and seems to be cumbersome and time-consuming.	■ Technology facilitates a smooth linkage between information and patient care by providing timely and effective access to a rich information environment. The information environment has been designed to support the work of the clinical unit.	■ Can't rate

Instructions: Each of the "success" characteristics (e.g., leadership) is followed by a series of three descriptions. For each characteristic, please check [√] the description that best describes your current microsystem and the care it delivers or use the microsystem with which you are most familiar.

Source: © Julie K. Johnson, MSPH, PhD

Microeconomics in the Hospital Firm: Competition, Regulation, the Profit Motive, and Patient Care

Mary Anne Schultz

CHAPTER OBJECTIVES

1. Provide a broad view of the economics involved in the hospital environment that includes competition, regulation, and patient care.

2. Understand the impact of regulation in the U.S. healthcare system and costs associated with it.

3. Demonstrate the impact of electronic medical records and how this affects the healthcare industry.

INTRODUCTION

Since the introduction of a prospective payment system (PPS) for health care 25 years ago, hospital services have become increasingly driven by the market forces of price and quality. Rooted in a tradition of caring, hospitals were once seen as places where people could be healed and have their physical needs met—all through the professionalism and trust of healthcare providers. This was the hospital's mission. Today, hospitals are businesses, big and small, where patient care is but one service and patients are no longer the only constituent. The processes are now high technology, caring, curing in some cases, research based, and financially driven, serving a number of stakeholders such as physicians, investors, patients and families, and employees such as nurses, to name a few.

Balancing the goals of the players and supporting the many purposes of a hospital require identification of the pressures shaping its operation. Chiefly, these are (1) competition, (2) regulation,

(3) the profit motive, and (4) quality patient care. This chapter examines these key forces from the standpoint of theory and practices in both microeconomics and cost accounting. Health care once derived its processes almost solely from mission, but now a hospital's margin is first because without a (profit) margin the organization, like all businesses, ceases to exist, and hence there is no mission. This chapter in no way provides a comprehensive survey of these interrelated forces but instead offers an explanatory primer, with examples, for a hospital's economic and business behavior. An overview of the disciplines of both microeconomics and cost accounting is provided to acquaint the reader with what is probably an entirely new way of thinking (and talking) about the institution called a hospital. This way, the profession, through the nurse managers and other nurse administrators, communicates with key non-provider hospital decision makers, such as the chief executive officer or chief financial officer, with the same language and thus on a level playing field.

MICROECONOMICS, COST ACCOUNTING, AND NURSING

This section addresses the question, "What is microeconomics (and, in turn, cost accounting) and what has it to do with nursing?" Economics, the study of how society allocates scarce resources, can be divided into two categories, macroeconomics and microeconomics. Macroeconomics (the prefix *macro* meaning large) is the study of the market system on a large scale. Macroeconomics considers the aggregate performance of all markets (so, the performance or outcomes of all companies or firms in all industries) and gives us indices or measures (indicators) of a nation's economy such as stock prices, interest rates, jobless claims, and housing starts. For purposes of this chapter, macroeconomics might serve as a context within which we describe the typical hospital (hospital firm)

behavior with respect to (1) revenue optimization, (2) expense reduction, and (3) production of patient outcomes at an acceptable (not maximal) level of quality. Microeconomics, the study of individual consumers in relationship to their markets, is concerned with the choices made by smaller economic units such as consumers or individual (hospital) firms. A key topic in this chapter, microeconomics gives us concepts such as profit, profit maximization, price strategy, and non-price competition to consider.

Cost accounting is an element of financial management that generates information about the costs of an organization and its components. As such, it is a subset of accounting in general and encompasses the development and provision of a wide range of financial management that is useful to managers in their organizational roles. Keep in mind that the goal in generating this information is to provide a basis for decision making. A quintessential question in our field is this: What should the nurse-to-patient ratio be and on what basis is this decided? The field of cost accounting, borrowing from financial accounting (information generated by firms largely for external purposes, e.g., the Internal Revenue Service) while encompassing managerial accounting (information generated by firms for their own internal use), affords us tools to address the tough staffing questions such as break-even analysis, profitability analysis, make-versus-buy decision making, marginal cost calculations, and cost–quality trade-off analysis. The relationship of the accounting disciplines is depicted in **Figure 10-1**. It is the considered opinion of the author that these domains, economics and accounting, were once considered mutually exclusive from the field of nursing. Only as the number of nurses undertaking formal study of these quantitative disciplines, such as in Master of Business Administration (MBA) or Master of Public Health (MPH) programs, increased did our field place itself on equal footing with lay administrators at the top of the hospital hierarchy.

FIGURE 10-1 Relationship of the accounting disciplines.

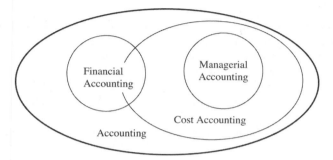

Source: Dunham-Taylor, J., & Pinczuk, J. (2015). *Financial management for nurse managers: Merging the heart with the dollar* (3rd ed.). Burlington, MA: Jones & Bartlett.

The nurse at the top of the administrative hierarchy, the nurse executive, may have trained with advanced preparation in all three disciplines discussed here, microeconomics, cost accounting, and nursing. The American Organization of Nurse Executives (2005) published its view of the core competencies that the nurse executive should have. Among these are analyses of supply and demand data, analysis of financial statements, and articulation of business models based on economics, strategic and business planning, and the development of future business skill sets in leadership team members, all of which are listed under the Business Skills subsection of the document. This is brought to the attention of the reader to dramatize how important it is for current and future nurse leaders to maintain their own skill set in business and financial matters and to message this process with key leaders in their organizations such as nurse managers. The deployment of nurse resources at the unit level could quite possibly be the most important decision made in hospital care because it is through the provision of quality nursing care that quality patient outcomes are realized.

Today, baccalaureate nursing schools traditionally require one course in leadership, often at the senior level. This course may not include financial content. Some schools are beginning to offer a separate course in nursing management that does address lower-level financial decision making, for example, the use of budgeting and marketing tools for nurse managers on the unit level. All, or nearly all, baccalaureate programs offer a course in health systems that analyzes healthcare organizations on the macrolevel, but the core quantitative courses and tools needed to place nursing on equal footing with lay decision makers reside in MBA or MPH programs and only some Master of Science in Nursing (MS or MSN) programs, including the new DNP programs (Doctor of Nursing Practice), in which the volume and type of financial preparation for these future leaders vary.

This does not mean that every nurse prepared at the baccalaureate or higher level must be a manager per se. It also does not mean that the nurse administrator must be a junior chief financial officer. Rather, a nurse executive must possess the financial knowledge necessary to make system-focused decisions that integrate the clinical and business aspects of health care (Lemire, 2000).

Nursing administration, one form of advanced practice (Harris, Huber, Jones, Manojlovich, & Reineck, 2006), is an at-risk specialty given numerous reports of dropping enrollment in graduate nursing administration programs (Herrin, Jones, Krepper, Sherman, & Reineck, 2006); a perceived lack of attractiveness of nursing administration as a viable graduate program choice (Rudan, 2002); widespread nurse executive burnout (Rollins, 2008); and the dire situation of the aging nurse faculty workforce (Berlin & Sechrist, 2002). Without this vital specialty, nursing could lose its scientific basis for practice, nurse managers at the unit level might lose recently acquired gains in real autonomy and decision making, and, most of all, research done by nurses on the effectiveness of their measures will continue to be invisible in healthcare quality, health services research, health policy, and healthcare finance initiatives (Lang, 2003). This discussion is an appeal to the reader regarding the uniqueness of the nursing administration specialty as well as the special challenges afforded the profession if our critical mass of economic and systems thinkers continues to deteriorate.

COMPETITION

Theory of the firm, the theory of supply and demand, explains and predicts price, quantity of products, and the likelihood of survival of firms in a competitive industry. Before the PPS was introduced into the healthcare market, hospital firms operated on a cost-plus basis, billing insurers for the total consumption of resources by an individual patient. After 1983, hospitals were switched to a diagnosis-related group (DRG) basis for reimbursement, receiving compensation for what a typical patient within a medical diagnosis and selected other medical conditions would consume. This departure from the cost-plus reimbursement scheme ended the era of price competition in health care, and hospitals began to compete

on a nonprice, or quality, basis, which is when patient outcomes magnified in importance.

For centuries, the relationship of the demand for a product or service to its supply has been thought to be largely the result of the intervening variable of price. In the fictional "market for widgets," supply of a product consistently meets the demand for it, given a set of assumptions about the market for widgets. This theory, theory of the firm, explains a lot about the way the world works pending the strength of these assumptions: a large numbers of buyers and sellers, perfect information about the product, absence of barriers to entry and exit as a business entity in the industry, and homogeneity of the product. Note that a full description of all four assumptions as they pertain to markets for health care is beyond the scope of this text, yet a focus on two of the assumptions—a large number of healthcare buyers and sellers and the existence of good information—is key.

In health care, the four assumptions are less clearly visible than in the fictitious market for widgets for a variety of reasons. Among them are the fact that relatively little is known to the buyer of hospital care (the insurance company) about the quality of care purchased from the seller (in our case, the hospital), and the demand for hospital care is a derived demand. This is to say that it comes from health insurance companies as the intermediary between hospital care providers such as hospitals and the individual consumer–patient. When health care entered the competitive arena, decision makers became highly sensitized to the customary business practices of restricting expenses and maximizing revenue while producing a service of measurable quality whenever possible. (Note that the language "an acceptable level of quality" should not be confused with something time-honored verbalized by nursing such as "the highest possible level of quality.")

The change from a system loosely concerned with quality of care, through the professionalism and trust of providers, to a system that prices services strategically while competing on quality has resulted in a cost-conscious era unlike that ever seen before. It is widely recognized that as hospitals compete to provide services, they attempt to (1) optimize profit through pricing strategies, (2) reduce expenses through decisions about personnel and equipment, and (3) achieve reimbursable patient outcomes by satisfying recipients of care through both high-technology and caring approaches. This means that hospitals seek to strike a vital balance between cost reduction and quality of care to adapt successfully to external competitive threats to their survival. For example, the ratio of nurses or operating expenses to patient days is a resource input that may influence the output of the system in the provision of quality care.

Better care provision (a result of wise resource allocation) may result in better patient outcomes (output) that results in better reimbursement and is alleged to be a benefit of an openly competitive, deregulated hospital market. Hospitals that can demonstrate higher quality of care, or even adequacy of care, will win higher reimbursement, or bids, for reimbursement plans, more patients, and better-qualified care providers. Over time, "good" hospitals will survive because they have established a pattern of good outcomes. The higher the hospital's performance or improvement, the higher the value-based incentive payments.

Additional evidence that this theory, theory of the firm, which explains a lot of how the world works, explains at least some things about how the world of hospital care works can be found through such organizations as HealthGrades, a leading independent health-care ranking company (see www.healthgrades .com), and *U.S. News and World Report*'s ranking system (see http://health.usnews.com/sections /health/best-hospitals). Both report such measures as risk-adjusted mortality rates and complication rates as patient-population-specific measures of comparative quality.

Also, hospitals can be designated as Magnet hospitals by the American Nurses Credentialing Center (ANCC; see www.nursecredentialing .org/Magnet/ProgramOverview.aspx), which means they meet process and structural criteria validated by a site visit from the ANCC. Only those hospitals known to be a good place to practice nursing are ranked as such, and the term originally meant that the hospital "attracted" nurses and patients.

The inner workings of these organizations cited in the previous two paragraphs and detailed descriptions of their methodologies, too complex to be reported here, can be found at their respective websites. Also, a primer on what risk-adjusted mortality rates means, as an overall general measure of quality or at least adequacy of any one hospital, is discussed in a later section. In summary, the importance of these hospital ranking systems, or stamps of approval as the public might see them, is this: The information about the quality of the product or service of a hospital is accurate enough to be used for comparison ratings used by payers as well as by others interested in these data. Hence, the information qualifies as perfect information (not to be taken literally).

What microeconomic theory states regarding the eventual number of hospital firms within an industry under long-run equilibrium (hospitals that rival or compete over a long time) is this: Those hospital firms with better products or services will survive, and those with inferior products and services will not. This is the result of the achievement of quality held by payers and consumers, which, in part, drives the industry's (derived) demand. Unfortunately, relatively little is known about the tenets of competition in health care. More will be known as variations in the quality of patient outcomes based on reimbursement in hospitals become available in the future. So, the usefulness of this theory for the explanation and prediction of future activities in health care remains challenged. This is not to say that "Supply and demand—it just doesn't work in health care!" is an emotionally charged statement devoid of reason. It is, instead, appropriate to say that predictive power of the theory in health care is limited more than its explanatory power interpreting the how and why of a hospital firm's behavior. Stated another way, all hospitals seek to maximize patient outcomes/reimbursement and thus maximize performance ratings.

In the world of competitive hospital management, decision makers continually forecast, or second guess, what their rivals will do when they introduce such novelties as courting new profitable patient populations or programs such as breast centers, cancer centers, symptom-management clinics, and addiction rehabilitation. In short, hospitals must innovate with new programs, new patient populations, or quality initiatives to survive and better achieve the continuum of care in the value-based environment. New sources of (perfect or symmetric) information on hospital care continually become available in both print and electronic media, so decision makers must be savvy regarding patient outcome comparisons. Just as automobiles are rated for gas consumption and airlines for on-time arrivals, payers and consumers contract for hospital care based on price and quality through managed care negotiations.

REGULATION AND MANAGED CARE

The soaring cost of health care has been one of the most pressing domestic issues for decades. Politicians and pundits speak of how changes in laws could affect this crisis, sometimes provoking a discussion of socialized medicine and cross-country comparison of U.S. versus "other" healthcare expenditures and outcomes. With no clear answer to this type of healthcare bill emerging soon, most would agree that although our healthcare system is among the most market oriented (competitively driven) in the world, it remains the most heavily regulated sector of the U.S. economy (Conover, 2004). This author states that the costs of regulation are the benefits

we would derive with alternative uses of those resources. After reviewing the literature on 47 different kinds of healthcare regulations, it was estimated that the net burden of health services regulation on society was $169.1 billion annually. For the novice in economic thinking, let's examine what some of the costs of regulation are said to be. In lay terms, it is the sum total of all expenditures by federal or state regulators that oversee, inspect, supervise, monitor, or award privileges to healthcare providers such as physicians, nurses, and hospitals. In just a quick survey of hospital and nursing regulation costs alone, consider these:

- The Centers for Medicare and Medicaid Services (CMS) utilization reviews of appropriateness
- Occupational Safety and Health Administration (OSHA) inspection of workplace safety
- The National Labor Relations Board monitoring of nurse unions
- National Council of State Boards of Nursing licensing exam requirements
- Every state board of nursing, medicine, pharmacy, respiratory therapy, and physical therapy
- American Association of Colleges of Nursing and National League for Nursing accreditation of nursing schools
- National Practitioner Data Bank housing information on practitioners
- Limitations on medical resident or registered nurse (RN) working hours
- Fraud and abuse protections

Each one of these organizations or protections has staff, overhead, a place of business to run, and extensive reporting requirements to yet another governmental or quasi-governmental organization. The author makes a convincing case that if health care were deregulated, the cost savings from this could realize gains in health promotion and prevention.

Although in our discussion of rivalry and what hospital firms must do to survive, indeed thrive, a convincing case is made about the benefits of the competitive, or market-driven, environment for hospital care, this is not diametrically opposed to regulatory efforts. This needs to be said because, in essence, a highly competitive market-driven industry is a bit like the polar opposite of one that is highly or completely regulated as is the case in countries with a national single-payer health system. In short, the market for hospitals is not what is known as "purely competitive" as is the market for widgets; far from it. It holds, instead, a complicated mixture of free-market principles, huge regulatory demands, a demand for sick-care services that is derived and not direct, and the most complicated reimbursement scheme known in modern times in any industry.

Managed care, a concept and term invented by Alain Enthoven (1986), was originally intended to reduce healthcare costs to society through the restriction of resource allocation and to improve the overall health of individuals. Now it is a generic term for healthcare payment systems that attempt to control costs through utilization monitoring; health maintenance organizations and preferred provider organizations are examples. In the old cost-plus world, physicians as clinicians (not clinicians and businesspersons) had free unrestricted control over treatment plans and resource allocation for their patients. This system, focused on physicians and, arguably, hospitals, involved a complete arbitrariness to clinical decision making, and if science (as in evidence-based medicine) was involved, all the better. Imagine a world where the faith and trust in the physician as provider were sacrosanct. Depending on the age of the reader, probably you cannot imagine it, even in your wildest dreams. Also beyond the imagination for some, there was a time when insurance companies paid for resources used without much, if any, review processes for appropriateness of treatment.

Managed care, now considered an economic success and a social nightmare, has in fact reduced healthcare costs to society by tying clinical decisions to economic ones that previously were mutually exclusive. In these arrangements, a hospital or group of doctors agrees to provide services in exchange for third-party payment. Managed care networks make available to their members only those providers authorized by the plan. Often, this designation is geographically derived, thereby restricting individuals' choices to go to what they see as the "best" orthopedic or cancer care hospital or doctor if unavailable locally. It is worth mentioning that individuals still have free choice (lots of it)—if they are willing to get out their checkbook! This statement is a positivist (or factual) one amid the rhetoric of concerns from individual patients and physicians about how things used to be or ought to be. The way things "used to" or "ought to" be was inflationary, and there isn't an informed health consumer around who doesn't know this.

In managed care, the provider (physician, nurse in advanced practice, or hospital) provides covered services at a discounted rate in exchange for a steady revenue stream. If the novice reading this wonders why providers would "settle for less" by receiving a discounted rate, consider the alternative. Providers would have an uncertain revenue stream that challenges their abilities to cover the basic costs of doing business (reduces uncertainty), plus there are few, if any, alternative ways of conducting business, generally speaking. Stated another way, consider what is known as the first rule of finance: A dollar today is worth more than a dollar tomorrow as a result of the time value or opportunity cost of money. That is, any entity that gains revenue in a timely manner not only can retire debt (an asset) but invest; hence, the time value of money is realized. Remember that fee-for-service medicine has all but disappeared, taking with it the old model of the solo-practice physician, and patients who pay out of pocket are rare.

Under a per diem rate agreement, the managed care plan pays the hospital a fixed rate for each day of care, when in fact nurses are in a particularly strategic position to observe that costs per diem to the institution can be (very) variable for one patient stay. Consider the surgical patient who consumes relatively few resources on the morning of admission for a procedure that afternoon. Once the patient enters the operating room, costs to the institution soar steeply and remain high as the patient travels to the postanesthesia recovery room, not to mention more if intensive care is involved. For a monthly fee, the hospital must provide the specified services to the third-party payer's enrollees such as this patient. Under this arrangement, the hospital is ensured money in a relatively timely fashion (based on the average consumption of patients within that diagnosis-related group and other clinical factors) and the patient–consumer knows he or she will be covered for surgeries that are preapproved.

The overall aim of managed care is to make the patient a better healthcare customer, evaluating whether she or he is getting what she or he is paying for (assuming the individual pays health insurance premiums, which most do). Also, the burden of prevention and wellness increases in importance for the patient, and, presumably, physicians and advanced practice nurses share in this responsibility by virtue of recent changes in medical and nursing education. In this system, the patient has less control over selection of the doctor or hospital and may be responsible for higher deductibles and copayments as well as penalties for services done outside the network.

From a positive (or factual) point of view, the real cost savings to the healthcare system and society at large is through reduction and elimination of unnecessary services, tests, and procedures and time delays through the authorization process where untold numbers of individuals drop off, or attrition out of, the care-seeking process. It needs to be said that to the extent that costs are held down by reduction in necessary services, tests, procedures, and premature hospital discharge, there are, in fact, real detriments to patients and to society. Many healthcare professionals and consumers are now claiming that the term *managed care* translates to "discounted care," but adhering to the intent of this chapter, the positive or factual view of healthcare business operations, the author looks disparagingly upon this rhetorical and editorial change.

PROFIT MOTIVE AND PATIENT CARE

Amid the rhetoric and hysteria regarding hospitals and profit, not enough is said about why a hospital exists. A hospital exists to satisfy the needs of its various stakeholders. Among these are physicians, nurses, and other employees; patients and their families; consumers; researchers; schools of medicine and nursing; and the community at large, to name a few. Although many agree that today's hospital exists for the provision of sick care, this is not to say there are no other compelling reasons for it to subsist. It is a business entity, and, as such, it responds to many demands from the players, or stakeholders. Among these demands are the volume and morbidity of patients, requests from physicians and nurses in advanced practice for necessary equipment and efficient flow of patients, concerns from patients and families about inefficient or substandard care, training opportunities for students of medicine and nursing, and an outright appeal for more nurses from basically anyone! The profit motive drives all of these.

In an influential book in its time, *The Profit Motive and Patient Care* (Gray, 1991), the author made the previously unexplored claim that two unique accountability factors exist in health care that do not exist in other organizations: the vulnerability of the consumer (patient) being served, and the absence of payers at the point of service. He goes on to state:

> In many different ways the profit motive—on the part of organizational providers of health care, suppliers of their capital, physicians, employers who provide benefits for their employees, and organizations that administer health benefits plans and monitor the performance of health care providers—has come to shape the behavior of all parties. An ethos that emphasizes trust, community service, professional autonomy, and devotion to interests of individual patients is being replaced with undisguised self-interest, commercialization, competition, and the management of care by third parties. . . . These shifts will shape how providers and purchasers of service respond to the two great accountability problems. (p. xi)

A cursory reading through these remarks prompts one to believe there is a lament here—perhaps about "the way things ought to be." Yet on closer examination, it appears that Gray, instead, is making logical positivist (factual) remarks. His explanation of whom the important players (stakeholders) are and how they are motivated to perform has far-reaching implications for the overall philosophical and business approaches that healthcare providers, such as nurses, might take. His was among the first credible writings to shake the foundations of why a hospital exists as well as to articulate the important forces shaping the behavior of the stakeholders.

In this section, it is necessary to debunk some myths still prevailing in certain sections of our society, sometimes even among healthcare providers (some of whom should know better!):

Myth 1: We are a nonprofit entity; we don't have profit.

Myth 2: We are here to provide the highest possible quality of care.

These are among the most important misconceptions forwarded by many stakeholders, among them nurses. Replacing what might be our wishes (myths) with factual statements helps us understand the pervasive economic forces shaping our work and provides resolve for nursing research aims and hypotheses.

Getting the Word *Profit* Back

The first myth—that of no profit—has hung around for decades. First, it is important to clarify our terminology. As to profit status, hospitals are now classified as either investor owned (IO), formerly known as "for-profit," or not-for-profit (NFP), formerly known as "nonprofit." All hospitals have profit, and each of them chases profit as fast and furiously as the next, period. They may differ on many other factors, chiefly how they approach profit optimization as well as descriptive characteristics such as public versus private ownership, urban versus rural, small-margin versus large-margin, safety-net versus non-safety-net, high-mortality versus low-mortality, and teaching versus non-teaching, to name some. A number of these factors may, in fact, covary with profit status. For example, major teaching hospitals tend to be NFP hospitals, and nearly all IO hospitals are private, but it is thought that the variable of profit status, and possibly outcomes, is the prime mover of organizational behavior.

Profit, loosely defined as the excess of revenues over expenses, is as necessary to hospitals, irrespective of profit status, as oxygen is to the living system. Almost no hospital could survive without it because the hospital could not remain liquid or solvent. Without it, a hospital eventually goes out of business just like any other entity, leaving services unprovided and employees out of jobs. Profitability, as a construct, is measured by these variables: total margin ratio, operating profit margin, non-operating gain ratio, and return on equity. As you continue reading the next section on the cost inputs for varying levels of quality, keep in mind that costs to the hospital (what is expensed on the hospital's income statement) relative to revenue (money given to the hospital in lieu of care provided) are nearly synonymous with profitability, at least in the short run.

Finally, an accounting note about the differences in IO versus NFP hospitals. In lay terms, the key differences between these two sets of hospitals on the matter of profit goes like this: All that matters is where you put it, what you call it, and what you do about it! Restating this old joke another way, the dollar line item of profit is found on the income statement of general funds for NFPs versus the profit and loss statement for the corporation; profit is called "profit" in the IO world versus a "positive fund balance" in the NFP one; and the IO distributes profit (after taxes) at year's end to the shareholders, whereas the NFPs cycle profits back into facility maintenance or expansion after paying no taxes. This partly whimsical look at what the terms mean (and do not mean) causes this author to conclude "I want the word *profit* back!" given that, although there is a cost–quality trade-off (see next section), there is not necessarily a cost–profit trade-off.

Quality of Care: At What Level? At What Cost?

In this chapter's discussion of competition, it was stated that a hospital is not in the business of providing the best care money can buy but that a hospital is in the business of providing quality of care at a certain acceptable level where reimbursement is received. It is time to examine why.

Measurement of the costs of providing care quality, long a perplexing problem, is a function of the cost of providing quality and the costs of failing to do so.

Lowering quality also has costs to the organization. Besides reimbursement losses, this lowers the quality of care for patients. This can bring about more detrimental effects for patients to deal with, including death, and the organizational reimbursement and reputation suffer; and remember, reputation is an asset. So, as lowering quality occurs, this erodes the

hospital's competitive position and thus longer-term viability.

This cost–quality trade-off explains the behavior of firms in every competitive industry, including the hospital firm in health care. Although seemingly abstract constructs, hospital decision makers use this paradigm as freely as a living system uses carbohydrate for fuel in the cell.

In conclusion, what can be said about the profit motive and patient care? Profit, as an incentive, is here to stay. Profit is not a dirty word. Further, cost–quality trade-offs drive operational (day-to-day) decisions in all organizations in a competitive industry. Also, cost shifts (costs to the hospital, or expenses) might be borne by the individual, or perhaps the employer, if the individual is discharged prematurely and too sick to resume employment. Revenues would shift from one governmental organization such as CMS to another if they could. And dramatically changing one variable, such as RN staffing, necessitates significant changes in another, such as expenses for other personnel—a topic that will prove essential to our national debate about hospital staffing.

QUALITY PATIENT CARE

The discussion of profit motive demonstrated how a hospital comes to provide not the best care money can buy but instead an acceptable level of quality. The acceptable level of quality is driven by its cost. Next, to compete on a quality of care basis, the hospital must report measurable aspects of quality of care—patient outcomes (presumably at an acceptable level)—to various governmental (state health departments and federal agencies) and nongovernmental organizations, such as The Joint Commission. Through processes such as these, the information about the quality of care in one facility is said to be perfect information, a cornerstone of a competitive industry. The information can also be characterized as symmetric in that both the buyer (the insurer) and the seller (the providers) have access to it.

The old quality assurance model, now nearly extinct, was limited in at least two ways: Quality cannot be ensured, and the information, or knowledge, was asymmetric, known to the seller (a provider hospital), but not necessarily to the buyer. Therefore, under this old model, it was practically impossible for hospitals to modify their care provision processes in a competitive way because they had no information about the performance of their rival hospitals.

Given the preponderance of information-reporting requirements, it is assumed that hospitals have numerous opportunities for improvement—assuming that these many reporting requirements translate to internal care-improvement processes. Next, through the movement now known as transparency (symmetric knowledge), hospitals can bid competitively to purchasers, boasting superior quality outcomes. A third quintessentially important thing this information preponderance gives us is the incentive for public programs (e.g., Medicare) and private insurers to reward and reimburse quality of care and efficiency.

This incentive program has the overall goal of making hospitals miss reimbursement when they err with never events. It is essential to note that the quality and availability of the information to both buyers and sellers make hospital nonprice competition possible.

Information on Quality and the Risk-Adjustment Process

A time-honored claim that hospitals and other providers have made regarding quality measures in general is that their patient populations contain more risk factors than others, hence the appearance of "not looking good" to the state or inspection agency. Granted, patient populations from hospital to hospital (or even from doctor to doctor) likely always differ on factors other than the care provided, but, arguably, meaningful points of comparison have been devised by clinical and biostatistical experts within many agencies.

One such agency is California's Office of Statewide Health Planning and Development (OSHPD). California was among the first states to develop a database of risk-adjusted quality measures, and the California Hospital Outcome Project reported to the public for the first time in 1995 and has continuously updated and improved its risk-adjustment processes ever since. The project worked first with a common and costly condition, acute myocardial infarction, by reporting risk-adjusted mortality; discharge abstracts served as the basis for data collection for more than 400 hospitals representative of more than 68,000 patients.

Biostatisticians know that databases this large do, indeed, allow for meaningful points of comparison across hospitals for reasons to be explained in advanced texts of statistics and econometrics. Generally speaking, risk-adjusted measures of quality of care, such as acute myocardial infarction mortality, are in fact useful tools for the comparison of hospitals on the quality of care provided, but imperfectly so. In the California hospital project, the mortality measure was defined as the observed number of deaths from acute myocardial infarction divided by the number of qualifying persons admitted with this primary diagnosis multiplied by the statewide rate. The risk-adjustment process is described in detail in workbooks provided to all by the state (again, the information is symmetric; Office of Statewide Health Planning and Development [OSHPD], 1996a, 1996b). By making the process known to all, agencies such as this assert they have satisfactorily responded to providers' claim about disparate findings based on (unmeasured) risk factors. In fact, on a yearly basis as the press releases come out about new editions of the data, the project offers the opportunity for hospital providers to respond in writing about why their facility "looked worse than expected" in the measures. This way, the project measures are refined yearly in part on the basis of the responses of participating hospitals. Since inception of this project, the agency has made available other outcome measures, all risk adjusted, that are reflective of common and costly conditions. These include complication rates of cervical and thoracic discectomy, maternal admissions, hip fractures, and community-acquired pneumonia.

Earlier, this chapter expressed the thought that for our profession to be seated at the table of quality initiatives in the context of the hospital business entity, we need expert knowledge of the economic and quality measures being discussed. Further, societal decision makers and gatekeepers, such as the OSHPD and CMS, would benefit from nursing representation to make the hospital measures, now used for reimbursement, meaningful. Fortunately, through the years, as nursing acquired a critical mass of administratively prepared nurses, it has become common for nurse executives from hospitals and representatives of our professional societies to be invited to such tables where the decisions are made. Because this was not always the case, it could be considered progress of the profession through acquisition of the same knowledge and the same financial language spoken by lay administrators that made this possible.

HEALTHCARE POLICY: THE STAFFING RATIOS DEBATE

The relationship between nurse staffing and patient safety is reasonably well established, especially when patient outcomes such as medical-surgical mortality rates (Aiken, Smith, & Lake, 1994), acute myocardial infarction mortality rates (Schultz, van Servellen, Litwin, McLaughlin, & Uman, 1997), community-acquired pneumonia mortality rates (Schultz, 2008), failure to rescue (Needleman, Buerhaus, Mattke, Stewart, & Zelevinsky, 2002), and shorter lengths of stay (Lang, Hodge, Olson, Romano, & Kravitz, 2004), to name a few, are considered. How patients fare has long been thought to be to the result of the number of professional nurse staff available as well as their preparation, visibility, and experience. Additional organizational variables known

to be important are leadership style of the nurse manager, the overall quality of leadership in the institution, whether staffing and other operational decisions are decentralized, physician satisfaction with nursing care, and the nature of the information system used for patient care. Research on hospital characteristics and their relationships to patient outcomes has broadened to include additional variables important in the complex relationships of people and technology relative to quality. For instance, positive cultures are less expensive and achieve better outcomes. It is the opinion of the author that as these associations are identified and contextualized clearer policy implications can be investigated.

Mandated minimum nurse-to-patient staffing ratios were legislated in California in 1999 and implemented January 1, 2004. Also being considered is the importance of having patient classification system data to support the appropriate RN staff requirements. Some of the impetus for the movement toward mandating nurse staffing ratios through governmental and scientific imperatives comes from the challenging conclusions offered by the Institute of Medicine's (2002) report *To Err Is Human*. This report shook both the scientific and lay communities with its most memorable finding: Between 44,000 and 98,000 deaths occur each year as a result of medical errors. There is hardly a scientific journal that focuses on these types of organizational studies that does not report the influence of nurse staffing, often in the form of RN hours per patient day or RN to all staff hours.

The beginner in politics and policy might ask, "Isn't this a no-brainer? More nurses equals better patient care, right?" Only a fool would disagree, and certainly, more nurses sound as good as motherhood and apple pie! But so, too, do more police in a neighborhood and fewer pupils per teacher in schools. The following subsections provide the novice nurse–politician some food for thought on the potential implications, or consequences, of such legislation in the context of the (1) operation of a hospital within a community or (2) market for hospitals as a whole. The implications can be summarized in four parts: hospital operations, including closure; feasibility and the nursing shortage; political opportunity costs; and costs to society. The implications, economic consequences of legislation addressing what staffing should be (normative economics), are couched in positive economics, or what is, factually.

Hospital Operations and Closure

As mentioned previously, the healthcare workforce accounts for at least 50% of a hospital's costs (Kazahaya, 2005). Most of this is nursing personnel costs. Starting with the assumption that some hospitals staff significantly better than the minimum staffing ratios suggest while some staff significantly lower as a baseline, there is a variance around the regulated minimum ratio (also known as "the floor" ratio). Hospitals staffing well below this floor ratio will experience a rapid rise in operating expenses and lost reimbursement and a subsequent drop in operating profit margin. This endangers the hospital's liquidity (ability to meet short-term obligations) and solvency (ability to meet maturing obligations as they become due). Hospitals staffing well above the floor ratio have an incentive to drop nurse staffing levels depending on the cutoff point of where reimbursement is negatively affected as well as the ultimate response of their rivals, that is, whether neighboring hospitals can afford to remain in business after enactment of this law. Finally, hospitals staffing at about the mandated level may experience no significant change in their financial and, subsequently, business activities, so their staffing may continue as is.

Consider other hospital operations that are disrupted as a consequence of what many nurses thought was a great idea. As reported in *Medical News Report* (2004):

■ Elective procedures have been postponed, canceled, or moved to a nearby facility.

■ Community hospitals have a more difficult time transferring patients to tertiary care facilities because beds cannot always be staffed.

■ Emergency room (ER) wait times have increased.

■ ERs have increasingly switched (or requested to switch) to diversion status.

■ Night shifts are nearly impossible to staff.

■ There is a huge shift to contract (agency or registry) nursing staff, causing a significant rise in expenses, often tens of millions of (unforeseen) dollars in a year.

■ The regulations make the hospital increasingly vulnerable to lawsuits, especially on the occasion when staffing is less than required.

■ When the regulations allow for "licensed" nurses in the equation, RN unions block the effort to fill a void with licensed practical nurse hours, thereby inflating union-to-union conflict.

Evidence supporting the view that this mandate was too costly for hospitals to continue operating is seen in the number of hospitals that closed in the years during implementation phase-in of the California law. Twenty hospitals closed (9 in 2003, 8 in 2004, 3 in 2006; OSHPD, 2006), citing factors on the revenue side of the profitability equation (drop in inpatient revenue and utilization issues). The costs to hospitals of the mandate cannot be underestimated. It is important to note that many forces, both internal and external, cause a business to close and that many of these factors, when they occur simultaneously, push the firm close to the "edge," or, more specifically, to the margin. Usually, a hospital firm that closes had both failing business (patient care processes) and economic activities (on both revenue and expenditure sides) in the preceding years that ultimately caused its demise. To date, no one empirical effort has isolated the impact of such a law on a hospital's propensity to close because of the complexity of the issues.

Recall from the discussion of profit that when expenses rise in one category, pressure is exerted in the hospital system (or any business) to (1) reduce expenses in another category, (2) make up the expensed activity with an increase in revenue, or (3) both. To formulate a guiding principle on hospital profit-maximizing behavior, Needleman (2008) suggests these questions to consider:

- How much would it cost to increase nurse staffing?
- Would these costs be offset by cost savings from better reimbursement, reduced LOS, and fewer complications?
- Would the hospital realize these cost savings, or, because of how the hospital is paid, would these savings be captured by payers?
- Can the hospital attract additional profitable patients on the basis of its nurse staffing?
- Are there cost savings other than those achieved via better patient care that might also be realized if nurse staffing is increased?

So, it should be clear that changing a regulation on the most significant personnel expenditure a hospital budget contains, RN hours, has far-reaching consequences for both hospital business and economic activities. This subsection looks at the core organizational dynamics of a single hospital, which is a very limited aspect of the staffing ratios laws. Even looking at these activities in all hospitals in a state or the nation offers only a partial view of the consequences of mandated ratios as described here. Read on to see how a hospital's behavior cannot be viewed in such a microcosm because of its essential bond to the other subcategories, such as the sporadic nursing shortage.

Feasibility and the Sporadic Nursing Shortage

In the past, hospitals, lawmakers, providers, consumers, and society as a whole were increasingly concerned about the international nursing shortage and its subsequent impact on the quality of care. After implementation of California's safe-staffing law, RN hours per patient day on medical-surgical units rose significantly, perhaps by as much as 21% (Donaldson et al., 2005). Yet the nursing shortage, predicted to be a deficit of 400,000 RNs by 2020 (Buerhaus, Needleman, Mattke, & Stewart, 2002), continued to raise the question of where the nursing hours came from. Over decades, it was a long-standing principle of hospital staffing to "borrow" nurse hours from unit to unit to (1) satisfy short-term patient care demands, for example, a number of new admissions arriving at the same time as intensive care unit transfers, and (2) satisfy regulatory and reporting requirements. Patient care demands may have been met, whereas regulatory and reporting requirements almost certainly were.

Many obstacles hinder compliance with mandated staffing requirements. Consider these real-world examples from *Medical News Report* (2004):

> Hospitals may start a shift in compliance but may not end that shift in compliance.
>
> Hospitals may start and end a shift in compliance, but the middle of the shift is in question.
>
> Nurse recruitment efforts have been accelerated but often are not associated with the desired result of satisfactory staffing.
>
> California's law requires nurses to be on standby to cover breaks for bedside nurses, which is a requirement that is practically impossible to meet.
>
> Penalties exist for noncompliance.
>
> Nurses increasingly report not taking their breaks, given the lack of coverage while they are to be gone.
>
> Hospitals could be held criminally liable for adverse outcomes in the context of staffing that is less than required by mandate, even in view of evidence of the intent to comply.

These remarks point to regional shortages within one hospital carrying yet another set of concerns for patient safety. Chiefly, these concerns are costs associated with noncompliance, nurse recruitment (especially as nurses from outside the country are involved), and legal defense. Also, there were no accompanying changes in the revenue side of the hospitals' profit equation. The examples offered in this subsection highlight merely a few of the difficulties hospitals are having with the mandate. Additional issues include workplace safety, nurse injuries, nurse dissatisfaction, turnover, and propensity to stay in current positions. This subsection—not a comprehensive review for all issues related to a hospital's nurse pipeline—emphasizes some of the more immediate feasibility issues posed by such regulations. And this does not take into account how this will affect reimbursement.

Political Opportunity Costs for Nursing

Highly publicized political wars have taken place, most notably in California and New York, over the staffing ratios debate. Both states had nurse unions that were successful in getting legislation sponsored that evolved into statewide acute care hospital staffing mandates, but at what political cost? California's 12-year battle (California Nurses Association, n.d.) spanned the reign of two governors, and New York's campaign (Gerardi, 2006) was similarly protracted, both being punctuated by statewide town hall meetings, numerous "call to action" alerts to other professional societies, consumption of resources of nursing associations of all types, and bad press labeling nurses as unyielding and self-serving. In California, such ill will attracted national attention when Governor Arnold Schwarzenegger summarily dismissed both the nurse union's leadership and membership as well as nurses in general by calling nurses "a special interest group" that is just angry because "I kick their butt" (Marinucci, 2004).

These campaigns occurred just as the state of the research was judged not to categorically support the thesis of better care provision through more RNs in each case. In fact, the research results are mixed (Burnes Bolton et al., 2007), reporting that although a clear and consistent rise in nurse staffing did exist postregulation in California, it was not accompanied by a commensurate rise in quality as measured by significantly fewer falls or pressure ulcers. In a study reported by Mark and Harless (2007), a superior distribution of outcomes (mortality and length of stay [LOS]) with a lower level of RN staffing was found. In sum, the evidence points to the prevailing conclusion that there is a strong, but not yet totally conclusive, case for an impact of nurse staffing on mortality (Needleman & Buerhaus, 2003) and other adverse outcomes. This is not unlike the teachers union advocating for better teacher-to-student ratios, having to defend the national outcry (and some empiricism) that we are a nation of people who lack necessary reading, writing, and critical thinking skills.

If you believe, as some do, that science drives policy and legislation—and that's a leap—you have now identified a gap between just what we recommend on the matter of staffing mandates (the normative economic view) and a recommendation accompanied by a cogent economic rationale (the positive economic position) and plan. Stated another way, consider the words of Keepnews (2007):

> Ongoing research on the impact of nurse staffing regulation can yield important information that can guide continued staffing policy efforts. Understanding the impact of such efforts should include evaluating the outcomes of recent legislation in Oregon and Illinois as well as continued examination of staffing ratios in California. Successful efforts will need to transcend traditional boundaries between researchers, policy analysts, advocates, and organizations. (p. 236)

Costs to Society

Social policy is the domain that aims to improve human welfare and to meet human needs for education, health, housing, and social security. It is that part of public policy that has to do with social issues; among them is health. There was a time when health was considered the absence of disease. Couple this limited definition of health with the Hippocratic admonition "to do no harm" to identify what the public expects from a hospital: to emerge from the experience with an improved state of health or, at a minimum, to avoid increased morbidity as a result of seeking hospital care. Although it is touted as a modern concept, we would do well to remember that the Hippocratic admonition regarding harm emerged centuries ago (Hippocrates, n.d./2004). Previously, it was noted that, at a minimum, quality care is identified as the absence of adversity or the absence of adverse events.

The costs to society of this adversity are understudied or underreported in modern health services research. The costs to society include, but are not limited to, the alternative use of hospital resources in a community (e.g., feeding the poor, housing the homeless), consumption of a tax basis (in the case of NFP hospitals) for same, the costs of ill health for individuals and employers such as the opportunity cost of lost time and productivity at work, unreimbursed expenses related to caring for the underinsured or the uninsured, as well as the alternative use of people and technology resources in other employment.

This subsection briefly lists some questions for further study in the context of the costs to society of mandated staffing ratios with respect to the latter two factors—the function and purpose of safety-net hospitals and the opportunity realized in the operation of a hospital in a community context.

Safety-Net Hospitals

Defined as hospitals disproportionately serving vulnerable, including financially vulnerable,

populations, safety-net hospitals also experienced a sustained significant rise in nurse hours after enactment of safe staffing ratios. To assume that a higher nurse-to-patient ratio affects the financial structure of hospitals the same way across the board is folly. Safety-net hospitals are at-risk institutions, by definition. They have consistently been financially vulnerable organizations when viewed from the revenue side of the profit equation. With large numbers of underinsured or uninsured patients, they have no position from which to compete on price and may not have the resources to compete on the basis of quality. It would stand to reason that although they budget for bad debt expense, this line item varies considerably because it is volume dependent and sensitive to changes in the macroeconomic condition. In short, when the region of its location "has a bad year," this institution, among all institutions there, has an even worse one! It is close to impossible for such a hospital to court more attractive (paying) patients not only because of geography but because of poor internal economic conditions, including liquidity crises.

A study done by Conway and associates (2008) reported that nurse staffing ratios in California hospitals were relatively unchanged from 1993 to 1999, and then showed a sharp significant increase in 2004, the year of the ratios implementation. The study reported that hospitals more likely to be below the minimum had high Medicaid/uninsured patient populations and were government owned, nonteaching, urban, and located in more competitive markets. Most of these hospitals were considered part of the safety net that "catches" uninsured and underinsured patient populations, which, presumably, have poorer health outcomes as a baseline. Also, these hospitals are thought to be extraordinarily sensitive to governmental mandates on staffing, with safety-net hospitals reporting significantly fewer professional staff relative to patients in the years after the Balanced Budget Act of 1997

(Lindrooth, Bazzoli, Needleman, & Hasnain-Wynia, 2006).

Having just stated that the competitive position of these hospitals is weak to begin with (they are less able to compete on the basis of price or quality), it stands to reason that they run a high risk of closure, particularly in view of the fact that the mandate obliges them to spend more on nurse staffing. With this loss of flexibility to vary nursing skill mix come inefficient allocation of scarce resources and an inability to make trade-offs in other hospital services. The subsequent drop in operating profit margin (and perhaps other measures of profitability) could easily cause negative consequences for patients such as premature discharge, recidivism, and higher complication rates. With the Medicare pay-for-performance structure, it is easy to see the handwriting on the wall for such environments, with closure looming in the future.

Nowhere more apparently is the strain felt than in the ER of a safety-net hospital. Long a point of entry for the financially strapped patient, the ER at hospitals such as the Los Angeles Memorial Hospital (Inglewood, California) found it necessary to divert patients to a neighboring hospital, Centinela Freeman, of the same Centinela Freeman Health Care System. Memorial's ER was the 10th to close in Los Angeles County in the 2001–2006 period. Memorial Hospital had lost $30 million in that time frame, and the hospital's executive said the closure was necessary to help the system save money (Quinones, 2006). Meanwhile, Centinela Freeman's ER saw a majority of nonurgent cases, approximately 60% of the total clientele, which raises the following societal questions: Where should those patients have gone for more cost-effective care to begin with? Where will they go now and in the future? Why did the hospital's leadership not redirect its activities given the staggering loss of $30 million over 5 years?

As providers, especially safety-net hospital providers, struggle with these enmeshed issues of geographic limitations, a tangible floor in revenue, and dropping profit margins in light of rising bad debt expenses, it is no wonder that the hospital executive has an eye on cash flow relative to debt (cash-flow-to-debt ratio) because it is the prime predictor of hospital closure. Once again, without a margin there is no mission, despite outcries from community leaders in Inglewood and elsewhere that health care is a right. Is it? If yes, who pays for it?

A Hospital Firm Within a Community Context

Recall that in the subsections on hospital operations and the nursing shortage, a number of questions were raised relevant to reducing or delaying services (diversion to neighboring ERs), the potential for a hospital to realize other cost savings as RN hours rise (better reimbursement, some economies of scale, perhaps, with nursing duties in common with nonlicensed personnel), and the costs to the hospital of recruiting and retaining nurses—all of which are accentuated in a regulatory climate in which RN ratios are mandated. Here are some questions posed by the author when considering the impact of such a government intervention on small-margin hospitals. Bear in mind that small-margin hospitals include those considered safety-net hospitals or those classified as rural.

- Will there be a drop in the employees' total compensation package, say, a reduction in health benefits or a rise in premium prices, in an effort to offset the rise in operating expenditures?

- As the line item for RN hours increases, what happens to the expenditures for nonprofessional nurses and ancillary nursing personnel?

- As these nonprofessional nurse budgets get trimmed, will it be necessary to start outsourcing programs in preparation for layoffs?

- As resources become more constrained, what is the subsequent impact on measurable levels of quality? On reimbursement?

- What is the effect of the change in levels of quality on managed care contract negotiations? In short, will the insurer continue to send covered lives to a facility thought or known to be substandard?

- As measurable levels of quality are affected, what is the impact of this on the hospital's creditworthiness?

- As the hospital's creditworthiness is adversely affected, how compromised is the hospital in borrowing, even in the short term, to meet economic obligations such as employee wages and other compensatory line items? How will a hospital's payment to its suppliers be affected?

- If the hospital does, in fact, close, what is the impact of this event on the unemployment rate in the surrounding community, especially if the hospital is the largest employer around?

- If the hospital closes, what are the costs to society of airlifting or otherwise transporting the most critical of cases to the appropriate environment of care?

As decision makers in small-margin hospitals, including the nurse executive, wrestle with these tough questions, it remains in the mind's eye of the observer whether the charge "well, it's a hospital that should have closed anyway" is defensible. This discussion does not provide an answer to such normative queries. Instead, the measures (or variables) necessary to construct an individual answer are offered from the logical positivist (factual) economic view.

In concluding this discussion of one of the most challenging healthcare policy questions of modern times, mandated nurse staffing ratios, I remind you to remember some guiding principles from positive economics, that is, costs shift, revenues shift, and this will always be the case. Costs and revenues shift both within and outside the hospital firm. As in the case of borrowing nurse hours from unit to unit to "look good" or claim compliance with such

mandates, what is the subsequent impact on patient care on the unit from which the borrowing occurred? As each hospital chases profit as fast and furiously as the next or neighboring competitor, how long will it continue to play the shell game of shifting ER patients from one safety-net hospital to another or allowing premature discharge? This last causes recidivism that results in no reimbursement if patients are readmitted within a month for the same problem. Finally, as far as costs to society are concerned, how is the health of a region or the nation affected by the loss of hospitals that fail seemingly from the economic or quality point of view?

THE BUSINESS CASE: ELECTRONIC MEDICAL RECORD SYSTEMS IN HOSPITALS

Although information systems, including the electronic medical record (EMR), are considered essential to the quality and efficiency of our healthcare system as a whole, the high cost of these systems is prohibitive in successful widespread implementation, especially in hospitals. Vital to daily operations, these systems bring many benefits such as safety, accessibility, retrievability, and convenience. They are a major organizational investment, especially with respect to start-up costs (the initial one-time expenses). This section discusses some costs, some benefits, the relationship of these costs and benefits, and the elements of a successful business case for a hospital's EMR system. As done previously, this section offers readers some measures (variables) to consider when idealizing that healthcare systems, especially hospitals, ought to have a computerized record-keeping and decision-support system.

Clinical information systems that computerize documentation of physicians, nurses, and other care providers, now nearly 20 years old, hold the promise of numerous benefits—for the healthcare system or hospital, for the patient, and for the health of the nation. Among them are patient safety, accessibility, legibility, process-adherence evidence, data-mining capabilities (Manjoney, 2004), retrievability, convenience, and a reduction in indirect care time. The downside is that privacy issues, costs (including upgrades), data transfer inaccuracies, implementation problems, and so forth occur. Like the previous section on legislative mandates for professional nurse staffing, the desirability of successful EMR implementation (accompanied by ongoing maintenance and subsequent upgrades) ensure that the integrity of the system is intact. This could be considered a no-brainer in that more time could be devoted to bedside care and patient outcomes, such as fewer medication errors and increased patient satisfaction, would occur. However, this is more complex because of ongoing maintenance and subsequent upgrades (including staff time and additional expense) that ensure the integrity of the system.

Costs for the Hospital

The major costs in acquiring an EMR system include the costs of hardware, software, networking, maintenance, installation, and training as well as opportunity costs (Agrawal, 2002). Direct costs such as training are expensed on the hospital's income statement, and big-ticket items such as the hardware and contracted software are listed as assets on the balance sheet and depreciated over their useful life. This is a way of spreading out the tremendous cost outlay over time. This is also a way to pair these economic activities with the business or strategic plans the organization might have to determine an asset's future benefits. For example, an EMR system is known to be associated with increasing patient satisfaction and reductions in risk-adjusted mortality or complication rates. It is possible that these improved patient outcomes could be leveraged in a hospital's managed care contract negotiations with insurers. This matching of economic and business activities begins the process of identifying the benefits of the technology relative to its costs.

Other direct costs are for hardware, software, training time, and salary and support fees. Indirect costs, those expenses associated with ongoing operational costs, include software maintenance and support fees, salaries for support staff, fees related to space and utilities (Nahm, Vaydia, Ho, Scharf, & Seagull, 2007), and the expenses of safety/security measures. Note that all costs mentioned thus far are borne by the healthcare-providing institution, in this case, the hospital. The next section, however, discusses that the benefits are shared by more than just this one entity.

Benefits for the Hospital and Patients

Implementation of a system has both tangible and intangible benefits, further complicating a discussion of the dynamics of benefits and costs. Some tangible benefits are concrete measurable gains derived directly from the EMR system, further expanded in the next paragraph. The intangible, or hard-to-quantify, benefits are such things as patient and user satisfaction and safety, increased compliance with federal or state regulations, decreased staff turnover, future leverage derived from the same, and hospital reputation.

Other difficult-to-calculate benefits include reduced resource use (partially from reduced LOS), improved quality through convenient access to information at the point of care, enhanced data capture, enhanced business management, and improved legal compliance with subsequent reduction in claims. In an econometric model making the business case for EMR implementation, Kaiser Permanente justified the costs for an inpatient EMR system through such benefits as increased RN and medical records efficiency; decreased RN overtime; reduced lab expenses, chart review time, and physical therapy wait time along with reduced inappropriate admissions, avoidable days, ER diverts, forms expenses, and medical records supplies; fewer adverse drug events; and redeployment of space (Garrido, Raymond,

Jamieson, Liang, & Wiesenthal, 2004). On the revenue side, improved coding accuracy for Medicare risk was mentioned.

Here is where we see a shared-benefit situation. In the case of adverse drug events, the hospital realizes as much as a 2.2-day reduced LOS for those events associated with injury. The patient is spared the inconvenience of the same amount of time plus the reduced opportunity cost of further morbidity from hospital-acquired conditions and, presumably, a shortened recuperation time with subsequent earlier return to work or productivity. At this point, the patient, the family, and the employer begin to share the benefits that resulted from costs incurred by only the hospital in the business case model. Yet if this is in keeping with a hospital or healthcare organization's mission (as is certainly the case for Kaiser Permanente), the business model is said to be a successful one.

Many different ways of calculating the hospital's return on investment (ROI), the benefits in relation to costs, exist. (See **Figure 10-2**.) Among these are net present value (NPV), payback analysis, and break-even analysis. In each of these, many other influences must be assessed simultaneously, making the ROI analysis, by definition, very complicated. Among these are inflation, deflation, changes in business and strategic goals, shifts in healthcare management methods, and changes in Medicare reimbursement rates. Well beyond the scope of this chapter, econometric models identifying the multiple simultaneous influences on a successful analysis of this sort yield a partial solution for justifying the enormous outlay of costs for such information technology projects as EMR. Executive administration would do well to cost-out both sides of the analysis in the short, intermediate, and long terms.

Conventional wisdom leaves little doubt about the ability of information technology to improve clinical outcomes, but equally compelling evidence of the positive financial return of the same has yet to be established. Because the trend in reimbursement mechanisms continues to move toward outcomes achieved, technology may prove to be beneficial. However, equally compelling is pay for performance limiting reimbursements, the downturn in the U.S. economy, and security issues and other unexpected negative side effects of technology. Large purchases may continue not to be good business decisions. This means that there are currently inadequate incentives for hospitals to act on this important aspect of the hospital infrastructure, especially when many of the benefits are difficult to quantify and forecast, not to mention government intervention. This also means that as incentive programs to reward

---

FIGURE 10-2   Definitions.

Cost-to-benefit analysis compares the cost of program goals that are being considered to the cost of implementing the proposed venture's benefits. If the benefits are greater than the cost, you have a positive cost benefit. A cost-benefit example can be found in Trepanier and colleagues (2012).

Return on investment (ROI) simply calculates the bottom line from your investments in the assets used for the investment, for example, positive ROI of 6% on the investment. Examples of ROI can be found in Pine and Tart (2007).

Break-even analysis identifies the cost and number of units that must be sold at a minimum to recover the fixed costs.

early adoption of technology or other innovations and quality of care are realized, they will act as a catalyst for the implementation of large-scale EMR projects in hospitals everywhere.

Kaiser's Business Case

In the account of a successful business case for a large-scale multihospital adoption of electronic medical records, Garrido and associates (2004) describe how Kaiser Permanente is investing $3 billion over 10 years to enhance the quality of care for its members. This is a marketing effort so that providers will continue to use Kaiser as the HMO of choice for employees. Kaiser Permanente HealthConnect is an EMR system for both inpatient and outpatient information management. The authors identified 36 categories of quantifiable benefits that contribute to a positive cash flow within 8.5 years. However, this business case is contingent upon other simultaneous factors, some of which are assumptions: leadership commitment, timely implementation, partnership with labor, coding compliance, and workflow redesign.

To be phased in over 3 years, theirs is a system that integrates the clinical record with appointments, registration, and billing. It is a system that includes workflow procedures, charting tools, and decision-support rules that will be shared by all Kaiser Permanente regions in 37 hospitals and 533 medical offices. To calculate NPV (net present value), two time lags were accounted for. The first was the implementation lag, the time between installation, training, and actual use. The second was the benefit realization lag, accounting for benefits such as malpractice liability reductions that may not manifest until years after full use is realized.

Net cash flow, the difference between the quantifiable benefits of the system and its costs of implementation and support, was projected for part way through the eighth year of phase-in. More than $2 billion realized cash flow is anticipated from the $1 billion investment over the investment horizon. Projected payback of the system within its 10-year life confirms the potential for it to generate long-term return on investment. Process improvements enabled by the project affect LOS, a key driver of savings where approximately 35% of net benefits are identified. Other significant areas of savings include lower transcription costs, timely manner of changes in care delivery (e.g., processing of physician orders), 30–50% reduction in medical record supplies and non-payroll expenses, and reduction in off-site medical record storage.

The difficult-to-quantify benefits include the adoption of care management protocols and best practices known to improve health outcomes. Again, entities other than the one outlaying the expenses—the hospital—are the patients and their families who benefit from streamlined care delivery and more efficient and informed admission and discharge processes. Although the strategic benefits from these enhancements are significant, the value attributed to them is difficult to measure. These, along with quality improvement, patient safety, continuity of care, and patient centeredness, are all part of Kaiser Permanente's strategic plan, so the business case can account for goals within those plans being met. Kaiser anticipates this system will be associated with higher nurse satisfaction, reduced burnout, and subsequent decreased turnover—so much so that intermediate and longer-term nurse recruitment expenses could be reduced. Another yet-to-be-quantified benefit will likely be a related reduction in registry nurse expenses as well as reductions in new nurse orientation, education time, and expense. Finally, a societal benefit is the rich flow of information for clinical, epidemiologic, and health services research. The data could be used for benchmarking, identification of best practices, and clinical outcome studies. There may be unidentified surprises as they continue along this path.

In conclusion, healthcare information systems play a central role in both the quality of care and daily operations (Nahm et al., 2007).

They are extraordinarily expensive, even when the potential benefits are considered. Recall some of the lessons learned in this chapter's discussion of profit seeking: Costs shift, revenues shift, and this will always be the case. Costs and revenues shift both within and outside the hospital firm, as do costs and benefits, as shown. This is the factual view for any big-ticket item that a hospital might consider (such as substantially increasing professional nurse staffing or EMR implementation). This chapter does not provide an answer to normative queries on whether an EMR system should be implemented. Instead, the measures (or variables) necessary to construct an individual answer are offered from the logical positivist (factual) economic view.

As each healthcare organization addresses the issue of widespread implementation of an EMR, it will be increasingly important for decision makers to evaluate the nuances of their own business cases. Given that many factors obscure the construction of a clear business case for EMR, hospitals are forced to consider the avoidance of an expense (e.g., future litigation costs, less reimbursement if pay-for-performance mandates are not met) as parallel with actual expense reduction (including less reimbursement, if that has already occurred), especially in the short term. Similarly, they are forced to identify benefits that are realized by the hospital as well as those gained by the individual patient, his or her employer, or society as a whole. The propensity of a hospital to invest this way will likely be enhanced by the changing CMS rules on nonreimbursement for selected hospital complications. Forcing a hospital to pay for its own mistakes, such as certain hospital-acquired infections, raises the question of what type of electronic system it will take to capture the processes associated with these adverse outcomes for purposes of both quality improvement and revenue sustainability.

SUMMARY

Hospitals, wrote Lewis Thomas (1983) in *The Youngest Science*, are "held together, glued together, enabled to function . . . by the nurses" (pp. 66–67). This chapter offers background information on the nature of competition and why it is important in the market for hospital care. In the discussion of profit motive and patient care, the reader was asked to join in debunking some myths about why a hospital exists to fulfill its purpose—to satisfy the needs of various stakeholders such as employees and the community at large, as well as patients and providers such as physicians and nurses. The regulatory arena was addressed last in the context of the hospital system as a dynamic microcosm of activity affected, sometimes dramatically, by legislative and societal mandates such as safe staffing laws. All of this reflects the complexity of the system.

Some of this monetary analysis is, in fact, a brand new way of thinking for those who have not studied formally in the fields of economics, accounting, or finance. It is hoped that, through this examination of what it takes for a hospital firm to survive competitive circumstances, future cohorts of nurses can preserve the only sustained hospital foundation—the practice of professional nursing. As stated by Buerhaus and associates (2002), "Nursing matters greatly in the hospitals' ability to provide quality of care and prevent avoidable adverse outcomes" (p. 130). The prevention of avoidable adversity is going to contribute most significantly to the survival of hospital firms through the coming years.

Most of the statements on hospital conditions and the business activities therein are from the domain of positive economics ("what is" or "what exists"), leaving the reader to draw his or her conclusions in the normative economic ("what should be") field of endeavor. Nursing's history, of course, has been to embrace the mission of caring, often with less investment in the impact of the ideals such as safe staffing on the hospital's margin.

DISCUSSION QUESTIONS ───────

1. Support or refute the statement "Well, supply and demand . . . it just doesn't work in health care!"

2. Discuss how margin and mission are related in the hospital environment, or aren't they?

3. Frame arguments for or against the policy of mandated minimum staffing ratios in the positive versus normative economic dichotomy.

4. Are hospitals competing on the basis of price, quality, or both? Explain.

5. Is hospital care overly regulated? Why or why not?

6. What is healthcare regulation and what are some of its costs?

7. Why is the provision of sick-care (hospital) services said to be a derived demand?

8. Should there be minimum safe staffing ratios—from the standpoint of the patient? Why or why not?

9. Should there be minimum safe staffing ratios—from the standpoint of the hospital? Why or why not?

10. Should there be minimum safe staffing ratios—from the standpoint of the profession? Why or why not?

11. From an economic perspective describe the cost of regulation in the healthcare environment.

12. What is your definition of profit?

REFERENCES ───────

Agrawal, A. (2002). Return of investment analysis for a computer-based patient record in the outpatient clinical setting. *Journal of the Association for Academic Minority Physicians, 13*(3), 61–65.

Aiken, L., Smith, H., & Lake, E. (1994). Lower Medicare mortality among a set of hospitals known for good nursing care. *Medical Care, 32,* 771–787.

American Organization of Nurse Executives. (2005). *The AONE Nurse Executive Competencies.* Retrieved from http://www.aone.org/resources/leadership%20tools/PDFs/AONE_NEC.pdf

Berlin, L., & Sechrist, K. (2002). The shortage of doctorally-prepared nurse faculty: A dire situation. *Nursing Outlook, 50,* 50–56.

Buerhaus, P., Needleman, J., Mattke, S., & Stewart, M. (2002). Strengthening hospital nursing. *Health Affairs, 21,* 123–132.

Burnes Bolton, L., Aydin, C., Donaldson, N., Brown, D., Sandhu, M., Fridman, M., & Aronow, H. U. (2007). Mandated nurse staffing ratios in California: A comparison of staffing and nursing-sensitive outcomes pre- and postregulation. *Policy, Politics & Nursing Practice, 8,* 238–250.

California Nurses Association. (n.d.). CNA's 12-year campaign for safe RN staffing ratios. Retrieved from http://www.nationalnursesunited.org/page/-/files/pdf/ratios/12yr-fight-0104.pdf

Conover, C. (2004, October 4). Health care regulation: A $169 billion hidden tax. *Policy Analysis, 527.* Retrieved from http://www.cato.org/pubs/pas/pa527.pdf

Conway, P., Tamara Konetzka, R., Zhu, J., Volpp, K., & Sochalski, J. (2008). Nurse staffing ratios: Trends and policy implications for hospitalists and the safety net. *Journal of Hospital Medicine* (Online), *3,* 193–199.

Donaldson, N., Bolton, L., Aydin, C., Brown, D., Elashoff, J., & Sandhu, M. (2005). Impact of California's licensed nurse-patient ratios on unit-level nurse staffing and patient outcomes. *Policy, Politics & Nursing Practice, 6,* 198–210.

Dunham-Taylor, J., & Pinczuk, J. (2015). *Financial management for nurse managers: Merging the heart with the dollar* (3rd ed.). Burlington, MA: Jones & Bartlett.

Enthoven, A. (1986). Managed competition in health care and the unfinished agenda. *Health Care Financing Review, 8*(Suppl.), 105–119.

Garrido, T., Raymond, B., Jamieson, L., Liang, L., & Wiesenthal, A. (2004). Making the business case for hospital information systems—a Kaiser Permanente investment decision. *Journal of Healthcare Finance, 31*(2), 16–25.

Gerardi, T. (2006). Staffing ratios in New York: A decade of debate. *Policy, Politics & Nursing Practice, 7,* 8–10.

Gray, B. (1991). *The profit motive and patient care: The changing accountability of doctors and hospitals.* Cambridge, MA: Harvard University Press.

Harris, K., Huber, D., Jones, R., Manojlovich, M., & Reineck, C. (2006). Future nursing administration graduate curricula, Part 1. *Journal of Nursing Administration, 36,* 435–440.

Herrin, D., Jones, K., Krepper, R., Sherman, R., & Reineck, C. (2006). Future nursing administration graduate curricula, Part 2: Foundation and strategies. *Journal of Nursing Administration, 36,* 498–505.

Hippocrates. (n.d./2004). Book 1, Section 2. (F. Adams, Trans.). In *Of the epidemics* (p. 5). Whitefish, MT: Kessinger Publishing.

Institute of Medicine. (2002). *To err is human: Building a safer health system.* Washington, DC: National Academy Press.

Kazahaya, G. (2005). Harnessing technology to redesign labor cost management reports. *Healthcare Financial Management, 59*(4), 94–100.

Keepnews, D. (2007). Evaluating nurse staffing regulation. *Policy, Politics & Nursing Practice, 8,* 236–237.

Lang, N. (2003). Reflections on quality health care. *Nursing Administration Quarterly, 27,* 266–272.

Lang, T., Hodge, M., Olson, V., Romano, P., & Kravitz, R. (2004). Nurse–patient ratios: A systematic review on the effects of nurse staffing on patient, nurse, employee, and hospital outcomes. *Journal of Nursing Administration, 34,* 326–337.

Langley, M. (1998, January 7). Nuns' zeal for profits shapes hospital chain, wins Wall Street fans. *Wall Street Journal,* pp. A1, A11.

Lemire, J. (2000). Redesigning financial management education for the nursing administration graduate student. *Journal of Nursing Administration, 30,* 199–205.

Lindrooth, R., Bazzoli, G., Needleman, J., & Hasnain-Wynia, R. (2006). The effect of changes in hospital reimbursement on nurse staffing decisions at safety net and nonsafety net hospitals. *Health Services Research, 41,* 701–720.

Manjoney, R. (2004). Clinical information systems market—an insider's view. *Journal of Critical Care, 19,* 215–220.

Marinucci, C. (2004, December 8). At tribute for women, Schwarzenegger angers nurses. *San Francisco Chronicle,* p. A1.

Mark, B., & Harless, D. (2007). Nurse staffing, mortality, and length of stay in for-profit and not-for-profit hospitals. *Inquiry, 44,* 167–186.

Medical News Report. (2004, February). Nurse staffing plans and ratios. Retrieved from http://www.nursingworld.org/MainMenuCategories/Policy-Advocacy/State/Legislative-Agenda-Reports/State-StaffingPlansRatios

Nahm, E., Vaydia, V., Ho, D., Scharf, B., & Seagull, J. (2007). Outcomes assessment of clinical information system implementation: A practical guide. *Nursing Outlook, 55,* 282–288.

Needleman, J. (2008). Is what's good for the patient good for the hospital? Aligning incentives and the business case for nursing. *Policy, Politics & Nursing Practice, 9,* 80–87.

Needleman, J., & Buerhaus, P. (2003). Nurse staffing and patient safety: Current knowledge and implications for action. *International Journal for Quality in Health Care, 15,* 275–277.

Needleman, J., Buerhaus, P., Mattke, S., Stewart, M., & Zelevinsky, K. (2002). Nurse-staffing levels and the quality of care in hospitals. *New England Journal of Medicine, 346,* 1715–1722.

Office of Statewide Health Planning and Development. (1996a). *Study overview and results summary.* Sacramento, CA: Author.

Office of Statewide Health Planning and Development. (1996b). *Technical appendix.* Sacramento, CA: Author.

Office of Statewide Health Planning and Development. (2006). Hospital closures in California. Retrieved from http://www.calhealth.org

Pine, R., & Tart, K. (2007, January–February). Return on investment: Benefits and challenges of a baccalaureate nurse residency program. *Nursing Economic$, 25*(1), 13–19, 39.

Quinones, S. (2006, September 22). Closure of Memorial ER is protested. *Los Angeles Times,* p. B4.

Rollins, G. (2008). CNO burnout. *Hospitals & Health Networks, 82*(4), 30–34.

Rudan, V. (2002). Where have all the nursing administration students gone? Issues and solutions. *Journal of Nursing Administration, 32,* 185–188.

Schultz, M. (2008, July). *The association of hospital structural and financial characteristics to mortality from community-acquired pneumonia.* Paper presented at the Congress on Nursing Research of Sigma Theta Tau International, Singapore.

Schultz, M., van Servellen, G., Litwin, M., McLaughlin, E., & Uman, G. (1997). Can hospital structural and financial characteristics explain the variations in hospital mortality caused by acute myocardial infarction? *Applied Nursing Research, 12,* 210–214.

Thomas, L. (1983). *The youngest science: Notes of a medicine-watcher.* New York, NY: Penguin.

Trepanier, S., Early, S., Ulrich, B., & Cherry, B. (2012, July–August). New graduate nurse residency program: A cost-benefit analysis based on turnover and contract labor usage. *Nursing Economic$, 30*(4), 207–214.

CHAPTER 11

Government Regulation: Parallel and Powerful

Jacqueline M. Loversidge

CHAPTER OBJECTIVES

1. Review the history of the role of advanced practice nursing in health-care regulation.

2. Determine the role of the state board of nursing on the regulation of advanced practice nursing.

3. Understand the methods of professional credentialing for advanced practice nurses.

4. Explore the role of professional self-regulation for the advanced practice nurse and its influence on patient safety.

5. Realize how federal regulation influences payment mechanisms for advanced practice nurses.

6. Discuss strategies that the advanced practice nurses can employ to influence regulatory changes for effective patient care delivery.

INTRODUCTION

Regulation of the U.S. healthcare delivery system and practicing healthcare providers is extraordinarily complex. The vastness of the industry, the manner of healthcare financing, and the proliferation of laws and regulations that govern practice and reimbursement in the interest of public welfare contribute to that complexity.

This chapter focuses on major concepts associated with the regulation of healthcare professionals, with emphasis on advanced practice registered nurses (APRNs). An understanding of licensure and credentialing processes, and their impact on advanced practice nursing, is fundamental. Understanding how the healthcare system and individual providers are regulated empowers the APRN to advocate on behalf of the profession and consumers. Note that all healthcare professionals in every state are licensed within a defined scope of practice. Practice-specific boards or commissions (e.g., the Ohio Board of Nursing) or multiprofessional boards (e.g., Michigan's Department of Licensing and Regulatory Affairs) are government agencies that regulate each profession with the goal of protecting the public. Although the processes are similar, each professional is legally bound by the regulations in his or her own state.

REGULATION VERSUS LEGISLATION

The legislative and regulatory processes are parallel; both are public processes and are equally powerful. Together, legislation and regulations shape the way public policy is implemented. It is important for the APRN to understand both processes and how they are influenced. Major differences between the two processes are described here.

The legislative process is the first step in the production of laws and rules. Lawmakers in Congress, or in the state legislatures, introduce bills and conduct them through the lawmaking process. If they are passed by both houses, bills are signed into law by the president or governor. Once signed into law, implementation generally occurs in administrative agencies that are part of the executive branch of government.

Legislation (laws) and regulations (rules) are constructed differently. Note the terms *legislation* and *law* are synonymous, as are the terms *regulation* and *rule*; these synonyms are used interchangeably. Law is written using broad language to provide for flexibility and adaptability in application over time. The administrative agencies are charged, by the laws that govern them, with the responsibility to amplify those laws by writing regulations that describe,

in detail, how the administrative agency will put the law into practice.

> EXAMPLE: One provision in the nurse practice act (NPA) provides that a duty of the board of nursing is to develop criteria applicants must meet to be eligible to sit for licensure examinations, and for issuing and renewing licenses. The regulations amplifying that provision of law specify the criteria for eligibility, application procedures, the approved examination, renewal procedures, and fees.

Several details are worthy of note. First, the administrative agency's authority to write rules is specified by the law. Regulation must always tie directly to a section of law; an administrative agency is not permitted to promulgate rules that exceed its statutory authority. Second, both law and regulation have the same force and effect of law. From here forward the term *law* will be used instead of legislation, but *regulation* and *rule* will be used interchangeably. There are uses for which the word *rule* is preferable (e.g., rule-making authority).

The first step in establishing a new law or revising an existing law is the introduction of a bill by a legislator or group of legislators (sponsors) during a legislative session. The sponsor(s) may introduce legislation to address an issue or concern presented by constituents, or an administrative agency may seek a legislative sponsor to modify its practice act for a variety of reasons. If an administrative agency finds its regulations are inadequate to serve the needs of the public, it may seek statutory modification to add a section that allows additional rule-making authority in the law. Any bill introduced during a legislative session must pass in the session in which it is introduced, or else it "dies" and must be reintroduced in a subsequent session.

The regulatory process differs from the legislative process in a number of ways. Regulations can be promulgated at any time during the year by an administrative agency because rulemaking is not dependent on legislative session schedules. Some states require periodic review of regulations by the agency responsible for administering those regulations, in an effort to assure that regulations remain current and reflect changes in the environment. Some states revise regulations on a predictable schedule. Regulation promulgation, like lawmaking, is also a public process and requires disclosure of draft language, a period of time for public comment, and often a public hearing. Draft regulations may be amended by the issuing agency based on public input prior to publication of the final regulation. The administrative agency working on the regulation has discretion in determining what amendments, if any, are made. However, public comment may be very influential in determining the final outcome.

State governmental structures also have systems in place to assure checks and balances during the rule-making process. For example a body separate from the state agency, such as a Legislative Services Commission (LSC) may be charged with reviewing all administrative regulations to assure that: (1) the administrative agency does not exceed its statutory authority, and (2) proposed regulations do not encroach on other laws or regulations. The time frame for implementation of new or revised regulations varies according to the administrative procedures act (APA) of the state, but effective dates are generally within 30 to 90 days of publication of the final regulation.

HEALTH PROFESSIONS REGULATION AND LICENSING

Definitions and Purpose of Regulation

Regulation, as defined in *Black's Law Dictionary*, means "the act or process of controlling by regulation or restriction" (Garner, 2009, p. 1398). Health professions regulation provides for ongoing monitoring and maintenance of an acceptable standard of practice for the professions, with the goal of protecting the interests of public welfare and safety.

Regulation is needed as a mechanism to protect the public because of the complexity of the healthcare system. Diversity in educational credentialing, proliferation of types of providers, lack of public information about healthcare provider competency, and the bundling of healthcare services make it difficult for the public to understand and evaluate options. Nursing requires independent decision making based on specialized knowledge, skills, and abilities. Nurses provide care at all points of service in a complex and rapidly evolving healthcare system. Laypersons cannot ordinarily judge the competency of a health professional, or whether the care delivered to them meets acceptable and prevailing standards of care. For these reasons, because of the potential risk for harm, and also because of the intimate nature of nursing care, states protect the public by establishing laws to regulate the professions (Russell, 2012).

The laws that credential and govern a profession are called *practice acts*. Practice acts vary by state, but all include the same basic elements: (1) creation of a board that serves as the decision-making body; (2) the definitions, standards, and scopes of practice; (3) the extent and limits of the board's power and authority and its composition; (4) standards for educational programs; (5) types of titles, licensure, and certification; (6) title protection; (7) licensure requirements; and (8) grounds for disciplinary action, including due process (remedies) for the licensee charged with violation of the practice act or regulations (Russell, 2012). The basis for mandatory continuing education and/or competency requirements for licensure or relicensure also are found in practice acts. The extent of the board's rule-making authority is also specified in the practice act.

A board of nursing's rule-making authority is found in the section that describes its power and authority; it is the rules, or regulations, that amplify the practice act and specify detail. Rules specify details related to provisions such as initial licensing requirements, standards of practice and delegation, requirements for the registered nurse (RN) and licensed practical nurse or licensed vocational nurse (LPN/LVN) educational programs, advanced practice registered nurse (APRN) standards and requirements for practice and prescribing, disciplinary procedures, and standards for continuing education. Some states regulate both continuing education and competence. Because continuing competence is a difficult outcome to measure, most states require mandatory continuing education instead. Regulations also define the methods the governing authority will use to enforce an existing law.

Regulations cannot be instituted by an administrative agency without the expressed intent of law. It cannot be presumed that silence of the law on an issue implies legislative intent. When there is no prior statutory authority or legislative precedent to address an issue, the legislative process must be initiated to allow the agency authority to promulgate new, specific regulations.

> EXAMPLE: An APRN petitions the board of nursing to clarify whether prescriptive authority for Schedule II controlled substances is within the scope of practice for the APRN. The board's staff refers the APRN to a provision in the statute that allows the APRN to "prescribe drugs and therapeutic devices" as long as the APRN's practice is in collaboration with a physician as required by law and rules, and is practicing in a way consistent with the nurse's education and certification. The staff conclude that "prescribe drugs and therapeutic devices" may include Schedule II controlled substances if permitted in the approved written protocols of the nurse and physician collaborator. No specific language is found in the law that authorizes the prescribing of Schedule II controlled substances. When the medical board receives the board of nursing's opinion, an attorney general's opinion is requested. The attorney general concludes that the board of nursing may not extend the scope of practice of the APRN through either opinion or regulation. The expressed will of the legislature in regard to the scope of practice for the

APRN must be sought using the legislative process. Subsequently, a legislative sponsor is sought to introduce a bill permitting APRNs to specifically prescribe Schedule II controlled substances. Note that not all state boards of nursing are granted statutory authority to express formal opinions; some must rely on the express language in the practice act and regulations, the official opinions of attorney general's office, or court decisions.

History of Health Professions Regulation

Physicians were the first healthcare professionals to gain legislative recognition for their practice. Most states had physician licensing laws in place by the early 1900s. Nursing followed; North Carolina was the first state to establish a regulatory board for nurses in 1903, and by the 1930s state licensing had been enacted by 40 states (Hartigan, 2011). Physician scopes of practice are very broad, and may include any act (or attempt) to diagnose or treat any individual with a physical injury or deformity. Some medical practice acts establish no scope of practice limits whatsoever. Herein lies the problem faced by APRNs and other nonphysician healthcare providers—how to define a scope of practice that delineates their roles, particularly those that may overlap with medicine's. The history of nursing regulation is characterized by efforts to accommodate this medical preemption (Safriet, 1992).

The early regulation of nurses was permissive (voluntary). Systems developed allowing nurses to register with a governing board, hence the title "registered nurse." In some states, nurses were registered by the medical board prior to establishment of a separate board of nursing. Registration is a minimally restrictive form of state regulation, and does not usually require entrance qualification (e.g., examination). Between the 1930s and 1950s, states enacted mandatory licensure laws, or nurse practice acts (NPAs), requiring that anyone practicing nursing obtain licensure with the state regulatory agency. These early NPAs defined nursing as a dependent practice, primarily involving the implementation of physician orders. In 1955, the American Nurses Association model definition was published, which laid the groundwork for NPA revisions to define independent functions for nurses, although the model reaffirmed that medical diagnosis and prescribing were prohibited (Hartigan, 2011).

Boards of nursing (BONs) began to establish licensure criteria, including board-approved courses of nursing education, and board-constructed licensure examinations. Board examinations could include multiple-choice or essay questions, performance examinations, or a combination; during that time, each BON set its own examination passing standard. BONs gained statutory authority to regulate schools of nursing and established requirements for structure, faculty, and curricula. Because interstate mobility was becoming more common, states developed *reciprocity* agreements with other states; these reciprocity agreements no longer exist today. The National Council of State Boards of Nursing (NCSBN) Nurse Licensure Compact has made interstate mobility, new technologies, and telehealth more feasible, but not all states participate, and this complex process should not be confused with the obsolete two-state reciprocal arrangements (Hartigan, 2011; National Council of State Boards of Nursing [NCSBN], 2014b).

By the 1940s the need for a standardized licensure exam became apparent. The State Board Test Pool Examination (SBTPE) was established by the National League for Nursing (NLN) in 1944. The SBTPE assured examination standardization and relieved state BONs of the burdens associated with writing and administering the examination. Over the years, questions about potential for conflict of interest were raised. Although individual BONs set their own passing standards, authority for the creation and control of the examination had been absorbed by a professional association. Concurrently, BON leaders created a forum in which they could meet and discuss matters of common interest, but that forum was structured as a council of the American Nurses Association (ANA). This created conflict between BONs' prescribed governmental duty to establish licensure standards and professional associations' rights and responsibilities to remain independent of governmental influence. To address these issues, the NCSBN was formed in 1978 with the assistance of a Kellogg Foundation grant. The NCSBN governance and voting body consist of representation from BONs; it is autonomous, and represents the states' interests rather than those of organized nursing (Hartigan, 2011). The NCSBN is not a governmental agency but serves as a forum for discussion and advice to BONs.

History of Advanced Practice Registered Nurse Regulation

The 1960s set the stage for the expansion of nursing practice and regulation of APRNs. The birth of the federal entitlement programs, Medicare and Medicaid, increased the number of individuals with access to government-subsidized health care. With a shortage of primary care physicians predicted, the first formal nurse practitioner programs were opened (Safriet, 1992).

Idaho became the first state to legally recognize diagnosis and treatment as part of the scope of practice for the APRN in 1971. The regulation of APRNs was accomplished through joint agreements between the state boards of nursing and medicine, and was specific for each "permissible" act of diagnosis and treatment. The model of regulation established in Idaho set a precedent for subsequent state regulation of APRNs to include some form of joint nursing and medical board oversight. The joint regulation model was designed to compensate for the broad definition of the practice of medicine, and was based on the determination that advanced practice nursing was a "delegated medical practice," necessitating some degree of medical board oversight. The struggle to define APRN scope of practice and determine whether medical board oversight is necessary continues in many states.

Since 1971, every state has developed some form of legal recognition of the APRN. Both the ANA and the NCSBN have proposed model rules and regulations for the governing of advanced practice nursing. However, practice acts are a product of individual states' political forces, so titles, definitions, criteria for entrance into practice, scopes of practice, reimbursement policies, and models of regulation are unique to each state.

Since 1988, *The Nurse Practitioner* has published a summary of annual survey data from each state's board of nursing and nursing organizations relative to the legislative status of advanced practice nursing. Significant advances have been made by many states, particularly with regard to APRN practice independent of direct physician supervision. Currently, 18 states report that nurse practitioners (NPs) are regulated solely by a board of nursing and have both independent scope of practice and prescriptive authority; these 18 states report no requirement for physician collaboration, delegation, or supervision, with Nevada and Rhode Island appearing as the newest additions. In the remaining 32 states, APRNs are regulated either by the board of nursing alone with the addition of medical board oversight or jointly by the board of nursing and medical board. In jointly regulated states APRNs generally find their licensure "home" with the board of nursing. In either model, medical board oversight may include requirements for physician collaboration, consultation, and delegation or supervision circumscribing the nurse practitioner's authority to practice, prescribe, or both (Phillips, 2014). All states have allowed some form of prescriptive authority for more than 20 years (Pearson, 2002).

Methods of Professional Credentialing

Health professions regulation is facilitated through a variety of credentialing methods. The method is determined by the state government and is based on at least two variables: (1) the potential for harm to the public if safe and acceptable standards of practice are not met, and (2) the degree of autonomy and accountability

for decision making that is considered standard practice for a particular profession. The least restrictive form of regulation to accomplish the goal of public protection should be selected (Gross, 1984; Pew Health Professions Commission, 1994). Four credentialing methods are used in the United States; each credentials and regulates the individual provider. Credentialing methods are described in the following sections, moving from the most restrictive to the least restrictive method.

Licensure

A license is "a permission ... revocable, to commit some act that would otherwise be unlawful" (Garner, 2009, p. 1002). The licentiate is "one who has obtained a license or authoritative permission to exercise some function, esp. to practice a profession" (Garner, 2009, p. 1005). Licensure is the most restrictive method of credentialing and requires anyone who practices within the defined scope of practice to obtain the legal authority to do so from the appropriate administrative state agency.

Licensure implies competency assessment at the point of entry into the profession. Applicants for licensure must pass an initial licensing examination, and then comply with continuing education requirements or undergo competency assessment by the legal authority charged with assuring that acceptable standards of practice are met. Because competency is unique to the individual professional it is difficult to measure; most licensing agencies require mandatory continuing education in lieu of continued competency assessment for license renewal. Licensees are also held to practice act provisions and relevant regulations. Licensure offers the public the greatest level of protection by restricting use of the title and the scope of practice to the licensed professional who has met these rigorous criteria. Unlicensed persons cannot call themselves by the title identified in the law, and they cannot lawfully perform any portion of the scope of practice.

The administrative agency holds the licensee accountable for practicing according to the legal, ethical, and professional standards of care defined in law and regulations. A licensee holds a greater public responsibility than a non-licensed citizen. Disciplinary action, through an administrative disciplinary procedure, may be taken against licensees who have violated provisions of law or rule. State administrative practice acts (APAs) assure that licensees subject to disciplinary action are provided due process. However, the fact that a license is revocable means that the legal authority (BON) may divest the licensee of the license if it is deemed that the license holder has violated law or regulations, and that it is in the best interest of the public to rescind a license. Health professions are largely regulated by licensure because of the high risk of potential for harm to the public if unqualified or unsafe practitioners are permitted to practice.

Registration

Registration is the "act of recording or enrolling" (Garner, 2009, p. 1397). Registration provides for a review of credentials to determine compliance with the criteria for entry into the profession, and permits the individual to use the title "registered." Registration serves as title protection, but does not preclude individuals who are not registered from practicing within the scope of practice, so long as they do not use the title or hold themselves out to be a "registered" professional.

Registration does not necessarily imply that prior competency assessment has been conducted. Some state laws may have provisions for removing incompetent or unethical providers from the registry, or "marking" the registry when a complaint is lodged against a provider. However, removing the person from the registry may not necessarily protect the public, because the individual is permitted to practice without use of the title. A registration exemplar is the states' Nurse Aide Registry, which tracks individuals who have met criteria to be certified for employment in long-term care settings; this registry was required by the Omnibus Budget Reconciliation Act of 1987.

Certification

A certificate is "a document certifying the bearer's status or authorization to act in a specified way" (Garner, 2009, p. 255). In nursing, certification is generally thought of as the voluntary process that requires completion of requisite education, competency assessment, and practice hours. This type of certification in nursing is granted by proprietary professional or specialty nursing organizations and attests that the individual has achieved a level of competence in nursing practice beyond entry-level licensure. Certification, like registration, is a means of title protection. Certification awarded by proprietary organizations does not have the force and effect of law.

However, the term *certification* may also be used by state government agencies as a regulated credential; states may offer a "certificate of authority" or an otherwise-titled certificate to practice within a prescribed scope of practice. In this case, certification is required by law for practice in the specific role. For example, an APRN may need to hold a certificate as a nurse practitioner (NP) from a proprietary organization to qualify for a certificate of authority from a state board of nursing to practice as an NP in that state. Most states have enacted regulations requiring nationally recognized specialty nursing certification for an APRN to be eligible to practice in the advanced role.

In addition, states may offer certification to otherwise unlicensed assistive personnel, such as dialysis technicians or medication technicians. Astute consumers may ask whether a provider is certified, as a means of assessing competency to practice. Employers also use certification as a means of determining eligibility for certain positions or as a requirement for internal promotion.

Recognition

Recognition is "confirmation that an act done by another person was authorized ... the formal admission that a person, entity, or thing has a particular status" (Garner, 2009, p. 1385). Official recognition is used by several boards of nursing as a method of regulating APRNs, and implies the board has validated and accepted the APRN's credentials for the specialty area of practice. Criteria for recognition are defined in the practice act and may include requirements for certification.

Professional Self-Regulation

Self-regulation occurs within a profession when its members establish standards, values, ethical frameworks, and safe practice guidelines exceeding the minimum standards defined by law. This voluntary process plays a significant role in the regulation of the profession, equal to legal regulation in many ways. Professional standards of practice and codes of ethics exemplify professional self-regulation. National professional organizations set standards of practice for specialty practice. By means of the certification process, these organizations determine who may use the specialty titles within their purview. Continuing education requirements and documentation of practice competency or re-examination are usually required for periodic recertification. Standards are periodically reviewed and revised by committees of the membership to assure current practice is reflected.

Although professional organizations develop standards of practice, they have no legal authority to require compliance by certificate holders; only legal regulation provides a mechanism for translating standards of practice into enforceable regulatory language, for monitoring the actions of licensees, and for taking action against licensees if regulations are violated. Administrative agencies regulating professions generally recognize prevailing professional standards of practice when making decisions about what constitutes safe and competent care. Legal regulation and professional self-regulation are two sides of the same coin, working together to fulfill the profession's contract with society.

Regulation of Advanced Practice Registered Nurses

The evolution of APRN practice across the United States has been inconsistent because the U.S. Constitution gives states the right to establish laws governing professions and occupations. As a result, titles, scopes of practice, and regulatory standards are unique to each state. To bring some uniformity to the regulation of advanced nursing practice, the NCSBN, at the behest of its board of nursing membership, convened the Advanced Practice Task Force in 2000. The NCSBN joined with the American Association of Colleges of Nursing (AACN) to facilitate a consensus-building process to develop the *Consensus Model for Regulation: Licensure, Accreditation, Certification, and Education (LACE)*. This report is the outcome of the work of the APRN Consensus Work Group and the NCSBN APRN Advisory Committee. It defines APRN practice, titling, and education requirements; describes an APRN regulatory model and new APRN roles/population foci; and offers strategies for implementation (APRN Joint Dialogue Group, 2008). At the time of its publication, 40 nursing organizations endorsed the Consensus Model; only one was a state board of nursing. Although state boards of nursing are interested, most maintain a position of neutrality that is standard practice for government agencies in such matters and work through their legislatures to effect change.

National specialty nursing organizations and their affiliate certifying organizations play an important role in the professional regulation of APRNs. Specialty certifying organizations are nongovernmental bodies that develop practice standards and examinations to measure the competency of nurses in an area of clinical expertise. Most boards of nursing require the

APRN to hold a graduate degree in nursing and national certification in the specialty area relevant to their educational preparation. Boards of nursing promulgate regulations allowing acceptance of national certification examinations for purposes of state advanced practice certification, if predetermined criteria are met. A document published by the NCSBN (2002) serves as a guide for state boards of nursing in determining those criteria. It is imperative that criteria for evaluating the eligibility of national certification examinations as a part of the APRN application to practice be established in regulation, because boards of nursing may not abdicate regulatory authority by passively accepting examinations from independent bodies without having conducted a thorough evaluation of the examination's regulatory sufficiency and legal defensibility (NCSBN, 1993). The basis for regulatory sufficiency and legal defensibility of any licensure or certification examination includes: (1) the ability to measure entry-level practice, based on a practice analysis that defines job-related knowledge, skills, and abilities; and (2) development using psychometrically sound test construction principles.

The NCSBN developed *The Requirements for Accrediting Agencies and Criteria for APRN Certification Programs* in 1995. This document has since been updated, and serves as a guide for state boards of nursing in their review of advanced practice certification examinations' suitability for meeting regulatory standards. It also serves as a means to advance greater standardization in establishing certification criteria at the state level (NCSBN, 2009).

The criteria can be located on the NCSBN website at http://www.ncsbn.org.

National organizations that prepare certification examinations for APRNs include the following:

- American Academy of Nurse Practitioners
- American Association of Nurse Anesthetists Council on Certification
- American College of Nurse–Midwives Certification Council
- American Nurses Credentialing Center
- National Certification Board of Pediatric Nurse Practitioners
- National Certification Corporation for the Obstetric, Gynecologic, and Neonatal Nursing Specialties

THE STATE REGULATORY PROCESS

The 10th Amendment of the U.S. Constitution specifies that all powers not specifically vested in the federal government are reserved for the states. One of these powers is the duty to protect its citizens (police powers). The power to regulate the professions is one way states exercise responsibility to protect the health, safety, and welfare of its citizens. State laws, specifically practice acts, create administrative agencies that implement practice acts and assume responsibility for regulation of the professions. These agencies are given referent authority by their governments to promulgate regulations and enforce both the law and regulations for which they are responsible. Administrative agencies have been called the "fourth branch" of government because of their significant power to execute and enforce the law.

Boards of Nursing

Each state legislature designates a board or similar authority to administer the practice act for the profession. Nurse practice acts vary by state, but all NPAs include the major provisions, or elements, discussed earlier in this chapter. Provisions included in NPAs focus on a central mission—protection of the public safety and welfare.

There are 60 boards of nursing (BONs) in the United States, including in the 50 states, U.S. territories, and the District of Columbia; each of these is known as a *jurisdiction*. Each BON is a member of the NCSBN. Some states have separate boards for licensing RNs and licensed practical nurses/licensed vocational nurses (LPNs/LVNs). As members of the NCSBN, BONs represent the interest of public safety with regard to the construction and administration of the National Council Licensure Examinations (NCLEX), are allowed the privilege of using the examinations, and meet to discuss and act on matters of common interest (NCSBN, 2008).

Some states do not have a single board for RNs and/or LPNs/LVNs. Multiprofessional boards are found in several states. These types of boards have jurisdiction over a variety of licensed professionals such as physicians, nurses, dentists, and the like.

Composition of the Board of Nursing

Boards of nursing are generally composed of licensed nurses and consumer members. In most states the governor appoints members, although in at least one state, North Carolina, elections are held to fill board vacancies. Nurses who are interested in serving as board members may be helped to gain appointment to those positions by securing endorsements from their professional associations and support from their district legislators.

Some state laws designate board member representation from specific practice areas, from advanced practice nursing, and in the case of joint boards, representation from LPN/LVNs in addition to RNs/APRNs. In other states, criteria for appointment only require licensure in the profession and state residency. Information on vacancies can be obtained directly from the BON or from the governor's office. Knowing the composition of the board and its vacancy status allows professional organizations to politically influence representation on the board. Information related to serving on boards and commissions is found later in this chapter.

Board Meetings

All state government agencies must comply with open meeting or "sunshine" laws that permit the public to observe and/or participate in board meetings. Board meetings may vary in degree of formality. Public participation is usually permitted, but an open dialogue between board members and the public is not generally invited. The opportunity to address the board may be scheduled on the meeting agenda (e.g., during an open forum time). Board policies may require advance notification from individuals who wish to address the board during a meeting, so their name, topic, and the organization they represent (if applicable) can be identified on the agenda. Boards generally go into closed executive session for reasons specified in the state's APA (e.g., to obtain legal advice, conduct contract negotiations, and discuss disciplinary or personnel matters). Boards must comply with APA regulations regarding subject matter that may be discussed in executive session and report out of executive session when public session resumes. All voting is a matter of public record, and board action occurs only in open public session.

Most state APAs require the board to post public notice of meetings and make the agenda available, usually 30 days prior to the meeting. Sometimes the notice of meeting is published in major state newspapers or it may be posted on the board's website. Agendas are often updated immediately prior to the meeting date.

Board meeting participants include board members, board staff, and legal counsel for the board. Legal counsel advises the board on matters of law and jurisdiction. Some boards may have "staff" counsel, but many state boards receive advice only from an assigned representative of the state attorney general's office, known as an assistant attorney general (AAG). Staff and invited guests may present reports during the meeting, and individuals or organization representatives may provide testimony to the board on matters of interest.

Board members must take several factors into consideration when they vote. These include implications for the public welfare and safety, the legal defensibility of the outcome of the vote, and the potential statewide impact of the decision. First and foremost, the board must act only within its legal jurisdiction. Because all board actions are a matter of public record, BONs must make major actions taken during meetings available to the public. BONs may publish newsletters, which include action summaries, and may also include articles written by board members and staff that explain sections of law and rule. BON newsletters typically include disciplinary action taken against licensees, including nurses' names, license numbers, offense, and the specific disciplinary action (e.g., permanent revocation, suspension, practice restrictions). Some states mail newsletters to all licensees, or they may be available only on request. Many BONs make newsletters available to the public on their website.

Monitoring the Competency of Nurses: Discipline and Mandatory Reporting

The licensed nurse is accountable for knowing the laws and regulations governing nursing in the state of licensure and for adhering to legal, ethical, and professional standards of care. Some state regulations include standards of practice; other states may refer to professional or ethical standards established by professional associations. Employing agencies also define standards of practice through policies and procedures, but these are separate from, in addition to, and superseded by the state's NPA and regulations. When a nurse violates provisions of the NPA or regulations, the BON has authority to conduct an investigation and take possible action on the license. In the case of an APRN, the BON's authority includes the license or certificate to practice as an APRN and prescriptive authority.

Because the BON's most critical role is to assure the public safety, most NPAs include provisions for mandatory reporting that require employers to report violations of the NPA or regulations to the BON. Licensed nurses also have a moral and ethical duty to report unsafe and incompetent practice to the BON. The NPA defines acts of misconduct and provides a system for investigating complaints against licensees that assures due process for the license holder. Procedures for filing complaints, conducting investigations, and issuing sanctions for violations are enumerated in regulations. A nurse who holds a multistate license (i.e., a license that permits a nurse to practice in more than one state in accordance with a multistate compact agreement) is held accountable for knowing and abiding by the laws of the state of original licensure as well as the compact state in which the nurse practices. Multistate regulation is discussed in more detail later in this chapter. Nurses with multistate licenses should be aware that ignorance of the law in any state of licensure and/or practice does not excuse misconduct.

Most state NPAs and regulations are now available online, either directly from the BON website or linked from the board's website to a state law register website. The NCSBN also provides links to state boards of nursing (see http://www.ncsbn.org).

Instituting State Regulations

A state agency has the authority and duty to promulgate regulations amplifying its law, so long as rule-making authority has been granted in that law. Because law is created through an act of the legislature and is general in nature, rule-making authority allows state agencies to add the process details required for implementation of the law. The APA of each state specifies the process for promulgating and ratifying regulations, including requirements for public notification of proposed regulations and for providing an opportunity for public comment. State processes differ; some states designate government commissions or committees as the authorities for review and approval of regulations, whereas other states submit regulations to the general assembly or to committees of the legislature. Certain elements are common to the promulgation of regulations. These include: (1) public notice that a new regulation or modification of an existing regulation has been proposed, (2) opportunity to submit written comment or testimony, (3) opportunity to present oral testimony at a rules hearing, and (4) publication of the final regulation in a state register or bulletin. It is important that the APRN becomes familiar with all phases of rule promulgation, particularly the process for providing comment.

In some states, a fiscal impact statement is required. This statement provides an estimate of the costs that will be incurred as a result of the rule, both to the agency and to the public. In states where the rule promulgation process is overseen by a commission of legislators, the commission's role is to ensure that the regulatory agency filing the rule: (1) has the statutory authority to do so, (2) does not exceed the scope of its rule-making authority, and (3) does not draft rules that would conflict with its own law or that of any related discipline. For example, in the case of nursing, legislative commissions would cross-check other health professions' laws and regulations.

Monitoring State Regulations

Administrative agencies promulgate hundreds of regulations each year. Regulations that affect advanced nursing practice may be implemented by a variety of agencies. Knowing which agencies regulate health care, healthcare delivery systems, and professional practice, and monitoring legislation and regulations proposed by those agencies is important for safeguarding APRN practice.

Chief among the agencies APRNs should consider tracking are the health professions licensing boards, including medicine, pharmacy, and counselors and therapists. In addition, state regulations determining reimbursement for government programs should be monitored (e.g., Medicare and Medicaid). In this rapidly changing healthcare environment, conflicts related to scopes of practice, definitions of practice, right to reimbursement, and requirements for supervision and collaboration may occur.

Exhibit 11-1 provides some key questions to consider when analyzing a regulation for its impact on nursing practice.

It is critical for APRNs to be aware of regulations that mandate benefits or reimbursement

---

EXHIBIT 11-1   QUESTIONS TO ASK WHEN ANALYZING REGULATIONS

- Which agency promulgated the regulation?

- What is the source of authority (the statute that provides authority for the regulation to be promulgated)?

- What is the intent or rationale of the regulation? Is it clearly stated by the promulgating agency?

- Is the language in the regulation clear or ambiguous? Can the regulation be interpreted in different ways by different

  individuals? Discuss advantages of language that is clear versus ambiguous.

- Are there definitions to clarify terms?

- Are there important points that are not addressed? That is, are there omissions?

- How does the regulation affect the practice of nursing? Does it constrain or limit the practice of nursing in any way?

- Is there sufficient lead time to comply with the regulation?

- What is the fiscal impact of the regulation?

CASE STUDY 11- 1   Board of Pharmacy

Assume the board of pharmacy has drafted the following definition of the practice of pharmacy: The practice of pharmacy includes, but is not limited to, the interpretation, evaluation, and implementation of medical orders; the dispensing of prescription drug orders; initiating or modifying drug therapy in accordance with written guidelines or protocols previously established and approved by a practitioner authorized to independently prescribe drugs; and the provision of patient counseling as a primary healthcare provider of pharmacy care.

DISCUSSION POINTS

1. Use the questions in Exhibit 11-1 to analyze the proposed regulation. Based on your analysis, do you consider this a "good" or "bad" regulation? What could you do to improve the regulation?

2. This definition requires that anyone responsible for "initiating or modifying drug therapy in accordance with written guidelines or protocols" must be licensed as a pharmacist by the board of pharmacy. If this definition were to be included in the pharmacy practice act, how would this affect the practice of nursing, especially APRN practice?

3. The definition in this case study is an example of a scope of practice definition that could have significant overlap with the advanced practice of nursing and result in practice restrictions for APRNs. It may be that the authors of the definition had not considered the infringement on APRN practice. Develop talking points to initiate a conversation between the representatives of the nurse organization, pharmacy representatives, and the regulation's authors to negotiate a solution; the addition of an exemption for APRNs in the pharmacy practice act would suffice.

policies and to lobby for inclusion of APRNs. Several states have instituted open-panel legislation, known as "any willing provider" and "freedom of choice" laws. These bills mandate that any provider who is authorized to provide the services covered in an insurance plan must be recognized and reimbursed by the plan. Insurance company and business lobbyists oppose this type of legislation. As managed care contracts are negotiated, APRNs must ensure that APRN services are given fair and equitable consideration. Other important areas include workers' compensation participation and reimbursement provisions, and liability insurance laws.

In summary, health professions licensing boards and state agencies that govern licensing and certification of healthcare facilities, administer public health services (e.g., public health, mental health, and alcohol and drug agencies), or govern reimbursement are agencies that may potentially promulgate regulations that could have implications for APRN practice.

Serving on Boards and Commissions

One way to actively participate in the regulatory process is to seek an appointment to the state BON or other health-related board or commission. Participation in the political process, especially during times of rapid change and reform, will ensure that APRNs have a voice in setting the public policy agenda.

Appointments to boards and commissions should be sought strategically. It is important to select an agency with a mission and purpose consistent with your interest and expertise. Because most board appointments are gubernatorial or political appointments, it is important for the APRN to obtain endorsements from legislators, influential community leaders, and his or her professional associations. Individuals seeking appointment are more likely to acquire endorsements if they have an established history of service to the professional community.

Letters of support should document the APRN's primary area of practice and contributions to professional and community service. Delineate involvement in local, state, and national organizations. A letter from the employer is recommended, as both an indication of the employer's willingness to support time away from work to fulfill the responsibilities of the position during the term of office and as an endorsement of professional merit; the letter should speak to both. A personal letter from the APRN seeking appointment should include the rationale for volunteering to serve on the particular board or commission, evidence of a good match between one's expertise and the role of that board or commission, and expression of a clear interest in serving the public. A résumé or curriculum vitae should be attached. Letters should emphasize desire to serve over self-interest; ideally, appointment decisions are based on a determination of the individual's potential contributions to the work of the board or commission. This kind of public service requires a substantial time commitment, so it is wise to speak to other members of the board or call the executive director/agency administrator to determine the extent of that commitment.

THE FEDERAL REGULATORY PROCESS

The federal government has become a central factor in health professions regulation. A number of forces have influenced this trend; however, one of the most significant was the advent of the Medicare and Medicaid programs. Federal initiatives that have grown from these programs include cost containment initiatives (prospective payment), consumer protection (combating fraud and abuse) (Jost, 1997; Roberts & Clyde, 1993), and the initiatives and programs written into the Affordable Care Act and Health Care and Education Reconciliation Act of 2010 (U.S. Department of Health and Human Services [DHHS], 2014).

A significant change occurred in July 2001 when the Centers for Medicare & Medicaid Services (CMS) was created to replace the former Health Care Financing Administration (HCFA). The reformed agency provides an increased emphasis on responsiveness to beneficiaries, providers, and quality improvement. Three business centers were established as part of the reform: Center for Beneficiary Choices, Center for Medicare Management, and Center for Medicaid and State Operations (Centers for Medicare & Medicaid Services, 2014). In 2003, President George W. Bush signed the Medicare Prescription Drug, Improvement, and Modernization Act (MMA) into law. The act created a prescription drug benefit for Medicare beneficiaries and established the Medicare Advantage program (O'Sullivan, Chaikind, Tilson, Boulanger, & Morgan, 2004), effectively providing seniors with prescription drug benefits and more choice in accessing health care.

The practice of APRNs has been influenced by the changes in Medicare reimbursement policy as it has continued to evolve. In 1998, Medicare reimbursement reform was enacted, allowing APRNs to be directly reimbursed for provision of Medicare Part B services that, until that time, had been provided only by physicians. In addition, the reform lifted the geographic location restrictions that had limited patient access to APRNs. More recent revisions to the required qualifications, coverage criteria, billing, and payment for Medicare services provided by APRNs are specific, depending on whether the APRN is a certified registered nurse anesthetist (CRNA), nurse practitioner (NP), certified nurse–midwife (CNM), or clinical nurse specialist (CNS). Reimbursement for APRNs has generally improved; for example, nurse practitioner services are now paid at 85% of the amount a physician is paid (DHHS & CMS, 2011). Because of their education, experience, and practice, APRNs in many states are working toward reimbursement at 100% of the amount paid to physicians.

Relationships between the state and federal regulatory systems are continuously evolving. Responsibilities once assumed by the federal government have been shifted down to the state level, including administration and management of the Medicaid and welfare programs. The perspective that states are better equipped to make decisions about how best to assist their citizens, coupled with a public sentiment that generally seeks to diminish federal bureaucracy and its accompanying tax burden, have been instrumental in shifting the placement of authority to the states. However, although states have primary authority over regulation of the health professions, federal policies continue to have a significant effect on healthcare workforce regulation. Policies related to reimbursement and quality control over the Medicare and Medicaid programs are promulgated by the U.S. Department of Health and Human Services (DHHS) and administered through its financing agency, CMS. APRNs should familiarize themselves with other federal laws that have a regulatory impact on healthcare providers:

- Clinical Laboratory Improvement Amendments of 1988 (CLIA 88)
- Occupational Safety and Health Act of 1970 (OSHA)
- Mammography Quality Standards Act of 1987 and 1992 (MQSA 87 and 92)
- Omnibus Budget Reconciliation Act of 1987 and 1990 (OBRA 87 and 90)
- Americans with Disabilities Act of 1990 (ADA)

- North American Free Trade Agreement of 1993 (NAFTA, effective date January 1, 1994)
- Telecommunications Act of 1996
- Health Insurance Portability and Accountability Act of 1996 (HIPAA)
- Patient Protection and Affordable Care Act (ACA, effective date March 23, 2010)

The Veterans Health Administration, the Indian Health Service, and the uniformed armed services are regulated by the federal government. Large numbers of health professionals, many of whom are nurses/APRNs, are employed by these federal agencies and departments. Health professionals who are federally employed must be licensed in at least one state/jurisdiction. These individuals are subject to the laws of the state in which they are licensed, as well as the policies established by the federal system in which they are employed. However, the state of licensure need not correspond with the state in which the federal agency or department resides, because practice that occurs on federal property is not subject to state oversight.

The Supremacy Clause of the U.S. Constitution, Article VI, Paragraph 2, establishes that federal laws generally take precedence over state laws (Legal Information Institute, n.d.). State laws in conflict with federal laws cannot be enforced. At times, the courts may be asked to determine the constitutionality of a law or regulation to resolve jurisdictional disputes.

The Commerce Clause of the U.S. Constitution limits the ability of states to erect barriers to interstate trade (Gobis, 1997). Courts have determined that the provision of health care constitutes interstate trade under antitrust laws, and this sets the stage for the federal government to preempt state licensing laws regarding the practice of professions across state boundaries if future circumstances make this a desirable outcome for the nation.

The impact of technology on the delivery of health care, for example telehealth, allows providers to care for patients in remote environments and across the geopolitical boundaries defined by traditional state-by-state licensure. This raises the question as to whether the federal government would have an interest in interceding in the standardization of state licensing requirements to facilitate interstate commerce. If this occurred, the federal government would be in the position of usurping what is presently the state's authority. Licensing boards have an interest in avoiding federal intervention, and are beginning to identify ways to facilitate the practice of telehealth, while simultaneously preserving the power and right of the state to protect its citizens by regulating health professions at the state level. One approach to nursing regulation that addresses this conundrum is multistate regulation, which is discussed later in this chapter.

The most recent federal initiative is the Patient Protection and Affordable Care Act (ACA). The enactment of this law in 2010 represented progress toward comprehensive and far-reaching national healthcare system reform. The ACA represents the broadest revamping of health care since the Medicare and Medicaid programs were created in 1965. The provisions of this law, which is being implemented over a 5-year period (through 2015), include requirements for consumer protection, improvement of healthcare quality, lowering of healthcare costs, increased access to affordable care, and greater insurance company accountability (Commonwealth Fund, 2014; HealthCare.gov, 2010). Note that changes in the ACA have been evolving since its inception. That is the nature of the process of legislation and regulation; few laws are written perfectly, and many are altered during implementation.

The ACA also includes a number of provisions related to nursing, many of which are applicable or specific to the APRN. Among these are increased funding for a primary care workforce, grants for funding nurse-managed health centers through DHHS, and clarification of the funding of advanced practice nursing education to include accredited nurse–midwifery education. In addition, the Nurse Corps Loan Repayment Program, the Nurse Scholarship Program, and Faculty Loan Repayment Program have been expanded. Even more specifically applicable to APRNs are provisions related to the inclusion of nurse practitioners and clinical nurse specialists as accountable care organization (ACO) professionals. ACOs are legally formed structures composed of a group of providers and suppliers who are responsible for managing and coordinating care for Medicare fee-for-service beneficiaries. The law also authorizes DHHS to establish a grant program for states or designated entities to establish community-based interprofessional teams to support primary care practices, increases Medicare payments for primary care practitioners, and increases reimbursement rates for certified nurse-midwives. There are numerous other provisions in this law; a complete list of key provisions related to nursing may be found on the American Nurses Association website (http://www.nursingworld.org).

Promulgating Federal Regulations

The federal regulatory process is established by the federal Administrative Procedures Act. A notice of proposed rulemaking (NPRM) is published in the proposed regulation section of the *Federal Register*, which includes information for the public about the substance of the intended regulation. The notice also provides information about public participation in the regulatory process, including procedures for attending meetings or hearings, or providing comment. Once public comment has been received it is given careful consideration by the agency, and amendments to the draft regulations are made, if warranted. The agency issues final regulations by means of publication in the rules and regulations section of the *Federal Register*. The rules become effective 30 days after publication (see **Figure 11-1**).

Emergency Regulations

Provisions for promulgating emergency regulations are defined at both the state and federal

FIGURE 11-1 The federal rule-making process.

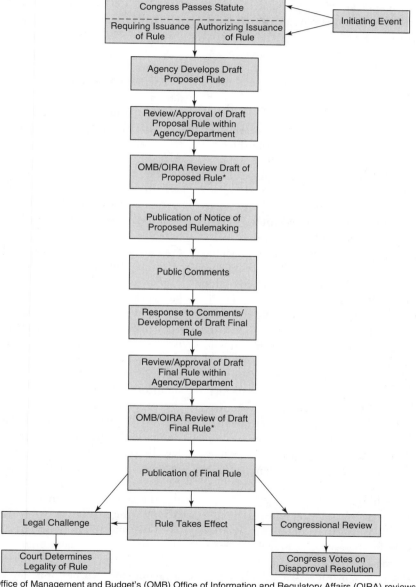

* The Office of Management and Budget's (OMB) Office of Information and Regulatory Affairs (OIRA) reviews only significant rules, and does not review any rules submitted by independent regulatory agencies

Source: Reproduced from Carey, M. P. (2013, June 17). The federal rulemaking process: An overview. Congressional Research Service Report RL32240. Retrieved from http://www.fas.org/sgp/crs/misc/RL32240.pdf

levels. Emergency regulations are enacted if an agency determines that the public welfare is in jeopardy and the regulation will serve as an immediately enforceable remedy. Emergency regulations often take effect upon date of publication, are generally temporary, and are effective for a limited time period (usually 90 days), with an option to renew. Emergency regulations must be followed with permanent regulations that are promulgated in accordance with APA procedures.

Locating Information

The *Federal Register* is the federal government's bulletin board, or newspaper. It is published on the U.S. Government Printing Office website and updated daily, Monday through Friday, except for federal holidays. It contains executive orders and presidential proclamations, rules and regulations, proposed rules, notices from federal agencies and organizations, sunshine act meetings, and corrections to previous copies of the *Federal Register*. Daily issues of the *Federal Register* also include a table of contents alphabetized by federal department. Daily issues may be downloaded in their entirety, or documents particular to a federal department of interest may be searched. Department-specific information begins with a heading including the name of the department, relevant information (e.g., the Code of Federal Regulations title), and a content synopsis. Deadlines for comments or effective dates are provided, as is contact information and other supplementary information. The *Federal Register* may be accessed online via the Government Printing Office (GPO) website at http://www.gpoaccess.gov/fr/index.html.

The Code of Federal Regulations (CFR) is the official compilation of all final regulations issued by the executive branch agencies of the federal government. The CFR consists of 50 titles representing broad subject areas. The CFR is updated annually on a staggered basis, and is available for download from the CFR website. The Electronic Code of Federal Regulations (e-CFR) is an unofficial, editorial compilation of the CFR material and *Federal Register* amendments that is produced by the National Archives and Records Administration Office of the Federal Register (OFR) and the GPO. The OFR updates the e-CFR daily. Titles may be browsed using a drop-down list. The Code of Federal Regulations is found online at the GPO website at http://www.gpoaccess.gov; the e-CFR is found at http://www.ecfr.gov.

Each state government publishes similar documents that identify proposed regulations, notices, final regulations, and emergency regulations. The publication is usually called the State Register or the State Bulletin, and the publication cycle can be obtained by accessing the state legislative printing office/website or the state legislative information system office/website. Hard copies of these documents may be available at local libraries; however, most states make these documents available on the state's government website.

State and federal agencies promulgate numerous regulations. It is in the APRN's best interest to belong to at least one professional nurse organization because most large organizations employ professional lobbyists who track legislation and report to their membership. Specialty organization newsletters and journals, legislative subscription and monitoring services, and bulletins summarizing proposed regulations are also resources that are helpful for monitoring legislation and regulations. Subscription services that track legislation and proposed agency regulation revisions provide summaries of the bill or regulation's substance and progress reports showing the status of the measure in its journey through the legislative or regulatory process. Both free and subscription legislative information services are available online.

In addition, numerous private services are available and can be found by searching the Internet. Several nursing and healthcare associations also feature relevant updates and information on current legislative and public policy issues (see **Exhibit 11–2**).

EXHIBIT 11-2 Selected Websites of Interest

http://www.statenet.com Legislative and regulatory reporting services from all 50 states and Congress. A subscription service that provides comprehensive and timely information on legislation.

http://thomas.loc.gov Thomas Legislative Information System, sponsored by the U.S. Library of Congress. Summarizes bills and provides the full text of bills and the *Congressional Record*, information on the legislative process, and U.S. government Internet resources.

http://www.ahrq.gov Agency for Healthcare Research and Quality. Provides information on healthcare research, evidence reports, clinical practice guidelines, and consumer health information; part of the U.S. Department of Health and Human Services.

http://www.ctel.org Center for Telehealth and e-Health Law. Information on the latest findings in the regulation of telehealth and e-health, and state-by-state updates on telehealth legislation.

http://www.nursingworld.org American Nurses Association. Access to all ANA services and the *Online Journal of Issues in Nursing*, which is jointly prepared with Kent State University.

http://www.ncsbn.org National Council of State Boards of Nursing (NCSBN). Information on all NCSBN services and committee activities, access to state nurse practice acts, and information on the progress of multistate regulation.

http://www.hhs.gov U.S. Department of Health & Human Services. Access to all agencies within the department, including the Centers for Disease Control and Prevention (CDC), CMS, Health Resources and Services Administration (HRSA), and National Institutes of Health (NIH). Includes consumer and policy information.

http://www.hschange.com Center for Studying Health Systems Change. A Washington, D.C.–based research organization dedicated to studying the nation's healthcare systems and the impact on the public.

http://www.nurse.org State-by-state display of advanced practice nursing organizations, links to related sites that contain legislative and regulatory information, and NP Central (a comprehensive site for APRN continuing education offerings, salary information, and job opportunities).

http://www.nursingethicsnetwork.org Nursing Ethics Network. A nonprofit organization committed to the advancement of nursing ethics. Site contains ethics research findings and online inquiry.

http://www.aanp.org American Association of Nurse Practitioners. Comprehensive site for this NP membership organization featuring information on the latest trends and issues affecting APRN practice and regulation, advocacy, continuing education, and professional development.

http://www.cms.gov Centers for Medicare & Medicaid Services. Provides the latest legislative and regulatory information on reimbursement and HIPAA implementation.

http://www.hhs.gov/ocr/hipaa Office for Civil Rights. Fact sheets, sample forms, and frequently asked questions (FAQs) on HIPAA implementation, along with related links and educational materials.

http://www.iom.edu Institute of Medicine. Provides objective, evidence-based information helpful for advancing science and health policy. A leading and respected authority on health issues. Access to published reports.

Providing Public Comment

There is a small window of opportunity for public input into the development of regulations. Most comment periods last 30 days from the date of publication of the proposed regulation, although sometimes an NPRM will provide for a longer comment period if the agency anticipates the issue has strong public interest or involves controversy. It is important that APRNs remain vigilant with regards to tracking comment period deadlines.

Public hearings are held by the agency proposing the regulation. Public agencies must comply with APA regulations regarding public hearings. Federal agencies are generally required to hold hearings when a numeric threshold is reached (i.e., a certain number of individuals or agency/organization representatives make requests to offer testimony). Written comments received by the agency are made a part of the permanent record and must be considered by the agency's board or commission members prior to publication of the final regulation. A final regulation can be challenged in the courts if the judge determines the agency did not comply with the APA or ignored public comments.

The *Federal Register* provides agency contact information on its website, making it reasonably easy for the public to provide comment on proposed regulations. Only written comments are included in the public record, although it is permissible to call the agency and provide comments orally if time is of the essence. Instructions for submitting electronic comments or written submissions by mail, hand delivery, or courier are generally included on the filing agency's *Federal Register* webpage. It is imperative to meet the deadline posted in the *Federal Register*; comments received after the comment period is closed can be legitimately disregarded by the agency.

When providing comment in writing, or written/oral testimony at a hearing, it is important for the APRN to:

- Be transparent about identity, background, and representation status; that is, the APRN should be clear about whether comments/testimony are representative of an organization's position or are representative of the individual APRN's position.

- Be specific regarding whether the position you are representing is in support of or opposition to the regulation. Give examples using brief scenarios or experiences when possible.

- Have credible evidence to back the position. Explain major points using common language; avoid nursing/medical jargon.

- Know the opposition's position and respond to these concerns.

- Convey a willingness to negotiate or compromise toward mutually acceptable resolutions.

- Demonstrate concern for the public good, rather than self-interest.

- Be brief and succinct. Limit remarks to one or two pages, or 5 minutes for oral testimony.

Regulatory agencies charged with public protection are more likely to address concerns that are focused on how the public may be harmed or benefited rather than concerns that give the impression of turf protection and professional jealousy. Demonstrate support for your position by asking colleagues who represent a variety of organizations, professions, and interests to submit comments; interprofessional solidarity projects a powerful message. In addition, if a significant number and variety of professionals and organizations form a coalition around a single issue, this demonstrates the degree of concern and a high level of commitment toward finding a solution. In this way, the volume and breadth of interest expressed in a proposed regulation can serve as the deciding factor in assisting an agency to assess support or nonsupport for the proposed regulation.

Strengths and Weaknesses of the Regulatory Process

The regulatory process is much more ordered than the legislative process, in that the state or federal APAs direct the respective processes. APA process guarantees opportunity for comment and public input. The regulatory process also includes built-in delays and time constraints that slow the process. On the other hand, administrative agencies are able to exert a great deal of control over the rule-drafting process. Agency staff generally draft proposed regulations; staff have an interest in assuring the final regulation has sufficient detail that it can be reasonably enforced. However, it is possible that agency staff, although skilled regulators, may not be knowledgeable about a regulation's impact from the practitioner point of view. If the agency did not invite stakeholders to assist with the original drafting of the regulation, then public input during the comment period is especially important.

In addition to enforcement, administrative agencies may have legislative authority to interpret regulations. Be aware that regulations may be misinterpreted by the agency staff or board members, resulting in the imposition of a new meaning that is not aligned with the original intent of the regulation.

New interpretations of existing laws and regulations may occur over time. These interpretations may be published as opinions, interpretive statements, and/or declaratory rulings of the board, attorney general opinions, or opinions of the court. Official opinions carry the force and effect of law even though they are not promulgated according to the APA. There is a fine line between the duty to interpret existing laws and regulations and establishing new regulations without complying with the APA or new laws without going through the formal legislative process. In some states, official interpretations of law or regulation are only permitted by the attorney general's office or the courts. BONs may be able to offer interpretive statements to facilitate licensee/consumer understanding of a section of a law or regulation, but nothing stronger or enforceable. The courts have been known to revoke board rulings that were made without statutory authority, or unofficial BON "opinions" that were not "properly filed" as rules. If this occurs, the BON unofficial opinion may be rescinded by court order and appropriate means to obtain enforcement authority must be sought. This may require legislation if a change in the practice act is required, or rule-making if legislative intent for a new rule or rule amplification already exists in the practice act.

CURRENT ISSUES IN REGULATION AND LICENSURE

Regulation in a Transforming Healthcare Delivery System

Healthcare professionals are regulated based on a longstanding system of regulating the individual licensee. As new healthcare occupations and professions have developed, there has been increasing professional debate about scopes of practice. Overlapping scopes of practice have naturally emerged in nursing, medicine, pharmacy, social work, physical therapy, respiratory therapy, and other licensed health professions. The overlap may be appropriate when areas of educational preparation and competency are substantially equivalent in more than one profession, but restrictive practice acts have made overlap a source of debate. Questions have been raised as to whether a system regulating individual licensees by means of separate practice acts serves the interests of public protection, or whether the system has become a means to protect the professions and create monopolies for services (Gross, 1984; Pew Health Professions Commission, 1994).

In 1995, the Pew Health Professions Commission published a sweeping report that began to change thinking about existing regulatory systems. The report suggested that the current system, based on a century-old model, was out of sync with the nation's healthcare delivery systems and financing structures. The Pew Health Professions Commission suggested that major reform was needed, and asked states to review regulatory processes with the following questions in mind (Dower & Finocchio, 1995, p. 1):

- Does regulation promote effective health outcomes and protect the public from harm?
- Are regulatory bodies truly accountable to the public?
- Does regulation respect consumers' rights to choose their own healthcare providers from a range of safe options?
- Does regulation encourage a flexible, rational, and cost-effective healthcare system?
- Does regulation allow effective working relationships among healthcare providers?
- Does regulation promote equity among providers of equal skill?
- Does regulation facilitate professional and geographic mobility of competent providers?

Workforce regulation has a significant impact on healthcare cost and accessibility. Restrictive scopes of practice limit the ability of comparably prepared health professionals to provide care. Boundary disputes within and across the health professions create tension and are counterproductive to efforts to improve interprofessional collaboration. A workforce response to regulatory restrictions has been to increase the use of unlicensed assistive personnel (UAP), who are unregulated and less expensive, in both acute and primary care settings. In many employment settings, UAPs are used appropriately. However, when employers misunderstand the roles of these unlicensed individuals or expand their job descriptions in an effort to provide more and less costly care, there is a risk that UAPs may be asked to function in a way that approaches nursing practice without the education or license to do so. Potential dangers include unsafe patient care, when UAPs are asked to function beyond their capacity; liability for nurses who, because of their employment situations, feel forced to delegate more nursing tasks to UAPs than safe standards of delegation would dictate; and

infringement on professional nursing practice by unlicensed workers.

The Pew Task Force on Health Care Workforce Regulation challenged state and federal governments to respond to the complex health professions education and regulation issues identified in the report. The task force made 10 recommendations to improve state regulatory systems' responsiveness to changes in the nation's healthcare system. Recommendations addressed the use of standardized and understandable language, standardization of entry-to-practice requirements, assurance of initial and continuing competence of healthcare practitioners, and the redesign of professional boards, including the creation of super-boards with a majority of consumer representatives. The report also called for better methods of assessing the achievement of objectives and improved disciplinary processes (Pew Health Professions Commission, 1995). Since the 1995 task force report, the Institute of Medicine (IOM) has issued a number of reports related to safety in healthcare systems, known as the Quality Chasm Series. In its first report, *To Err Is Human*, the IOM called for licensing and certification bodies to pay greater attention to safety-related performance standards and expectations for health professionals (Kohn, Corrigan, & Donaldson, 2000).

A consensus report, focused singularly on nursing, was jointly issued by the Robert Wood Johnson Foundation (RWJF) and the IOM in October 2010. This report, *The Future of Nursing: Leading Change, Advancing Health*, provides four key messages to guide changes and remove barriers that prevent nurses from being able to function effectively in a rapidly evolving healthcare system (IOM, 2010). These are that nurses should be enabled to practice to the full extent of their education and training, should be able to access higher levels of education and training in an improved education system that allows for academic progression, should be full partners in the interprofessional redesign of the

U.S. healthcare system, and finally that effective workforce planning and policymaking need better data collection and information infrastructures. Eight recommendations for fundamental change are found in the report, along with related actions for Congress, state legislatures, CMS, the Office of Personnel Management, and the Federal Trade Commission and Antitrust Division of the Department of Justice. These are: (1) remove scope-of-practice barriers, (2) expand opportunities for nurses to lead and diffuse collaborative improvement efforts, (3) implement nurse residency programs, (4) increase the proportion of nurses with a baccalaureate degree to 80 percent by 2020, (5) double the number of nurses with a doctorate by 2020, (6) ensure that nurses engage in lifelong learning, (7) prepare and enable nurses to lead change to advance health, and (8) build an infrastructure for the collection and analysis of interprofessional healthcare workforce data (Institute of Medicine, 2010).

The Josiah Macy Jr. Foundation, an organization dedicated to improving the health of the public through the advancement of health professions education, has been instrumental in providing direction for regulatory reform. In 2013, the foundation held a consensus conference with health professions education leaders to discuss a vision for a joint future of healthcare practice and education. Conference participants made recommendations for immediate action in five areas; one of these was to "revise professional regulatory standards and practices to permit and promote innovation in interprofessional education and collaborative practice" (Josiah Macy Jr. Foundation, 2013, p. 2).

The sum total of these reports and recommendations provides a body of evidence substantive enough to leverage for reform of health professions regulation that can serve the needs of the 21st century. APRNs have a window of opportunity and must be open to the notion that collaboration with other health professions is essential if new regulatory models are to emerge. Regulation determines who has access to the patient, who serves as gatekeeper in a managed care environment, who is reimbursed, and who has autonomy to practice. APRNs must be visible participants in the political process to shape a dynamic, evolving system that is responsive to the healthcare environment, authorizes APRNs to practice to the full extent of their education in a collaborative environment as equal team members, and ensures consumer choice and protection.

Multistate Regulation

State BONs have made progress facilitating interstate mobility for nurses. Cumbersome licensure processes across geopolitical boundaries make seamless transition difficult or impossible, particularly for APRNs. The Nurse Licensure Compact (NLC) model was adopted by the NCSBN delegate assembly in 1997 during the same timeframe the Consensus Model (LACE) was in development. The NLC is nursing's mutual recognition model of multistate licensure. States adopting the model voluntarily enter into an interstate compact to legally recognize the licensure policies and processes of a licensee's home state and permit practice in a remote state without obtaining an additional license (NCSBN, 1998). The NLC requires the licensee to comply with the NPA in each state. Nurses are subject to those NPA provisions and regulations, and therefore are accountable and subject to discipline in the state of practice, whether it is the original state of licensure or the remote compact state. To implement the mutual recognition model, the cooperating states' legislatures must enact the interstate compact provisions into law. APRNs have not been included in the compact agreements to date, so although the compact may apply to a nurse's RN license, it does not extend to cover advanced practice. Therefore, the APRN must apply for licensure in each state of practice.

A number of states moved quickly to enter the compact when it was instituted, but many states remain independent. As of July 2014, 24 states are participating as compact states and 3 states have NLC legislation pending (NCSBN, 2014a). To promote APRN participation in multistate regulation and APRN competitive advantages in a global market, state NPAs would need to be revised to include the Uniform APRN Requirements. Alternatively, the NLC would need to be expanded to include APRNs.

THE FUTURE OF ADVANCED PRACTICE NURSE REGULATION

Much of the discussion in this chapter has focused on ways regulatory systems affect APRNs. However, not all challenges associated with practice limitations and patient access are external to the profession; some dilemmas have been created from within. The lack of common APRN role definitions, growing numbers of advanced practice specializations, deliberations about credentials and scopes of practice, and inconsistency in educational standards and state regulations have contributed to public confusion and limited patient access to APRNs as care providers (NCSBN, 2010).

A number of forces within the profession are working independently to address these issues. These forces could coalesce to potentially remedy some of the challenges faced by APRNs. They are: (1) the development of an APRN Consensus Model that has been widely endorsed by nursing organizations; (2) individual states' progress toward Consensus Model implementation through legislation; (3) consolidation of APRN nursing organizations, in particular the two national nurse practitioner organizations; (4) advancing the future of postgraduate APRN education to a level equivalent with other healthcare providers, specifically the practice doctorate; and (5) directions in research on credentialing in nursing.

The NCSBN 2006 draft vision paper, *The Future Regulation of Advanced Practice Nursing*, was the subject of considerable debate among advanced practice nursing organizations and

the American Association of Colleges of Nursing (AACN) (Nelson, 2006; NCSBN, 2006). The final report of the Consensus Work Group and the NCSBN Advisory Committee, the *Consensus Model for APRN Regulation: Licensure, Accreditation, Certification, and Education* (Consensus Model), referred to as LACE, was a major step in reaching a level of agreement between stakeholders in organized nursing (APRN Joint Dialogue Group, 2008). Note that the Consensus Model and LACE are not one and the same. The APRN Consensus Model is a stand-alone product of the NCSBN APRN Advisory Committee and the APRN Consensus Work Group, whereas LACE is a mechanism to engage interested stakeholders who are necessarily communicating about and implementing the Consensus Model. The Consensus Model provides detailed definitions for four APRN roles, the certified registered nurse anesthetist, certified nurse–midwife, clinical nurse specialist, and certified nurse practitioner. Realization of the Consensus Model is dependent on how quickly its recommendations, including the merged adult-gerontology foci for NP and CNS curricula, are embedded in educational programs to assure continued graduate eligibility to sit for national certification, and how quickly states are able to enact legislation actualizing recommendations in the NPA. The Consensus Model target date for full implementation is 2015; however, not all APRN groups are on the same timeline, so some variation in timing will occur. The NCSBN document *APRN Consensus Model Frequently-Asked Questions* clarifies questions APRNs may have about implications for their roles, titles, practice, grandfathering, specialization, population foci, and timelines (NCSBN, 2010). In 2008, the NCSBN revised the *Model Nursing Practice Act* and *Model Nursing Administrative Rules* to reflect the Consensus Model (NCSBN, 2011).

The status of implementation of the Consensus Model by each state is unique. The NCSBN has developed a grid to track states' status in adopting elements of the model. Elements tracked include titles, roles, license, education, certification, and whether practice and prescribing is independent for each of the four APRN titles. The grid assigns points to each element enacted; a color-coded map of the United States is periodically updated on the NCSBN website as APRN laws change. As of May 2014, the states that have achieved 100 percent implementation are Idaho, Montana, Nevada, New Mexico, North Dakota, Utah, Minnesota, and Vermont (NCSBN, 2014a).

The voice of APRNs is stronger when it is unified and consistent. The American Academy of Nurse Practitioners and American College of Nurse Practitioners (2012) have consolidated to better position a single organization, the American Association of Nurse Practitioners, to capitalize on growth in NP demand; direct NP legislative and policy agendas; achieve the goals and objectives of NPs; provide enhanced resources for education, research, and grant writing; increase public awareness; and work toward globalization.

Directions in the education of advanced practice nurses parallel changes in regulation. The national standard in health professions education is moving toward the clinical doctorate; pharmacy, physical therapy, and other health professions have advanced the level of graduate education required for entry accordingly. In 2004, the AACN Board of Directors endorsed a *Position Statement on the Practice Doctorate* in nursing, which calls for a change from masters-level educational preparation to the clinical doctorate for APRNs by 2015 (American Association of Colleges of Nursing, 2004). The AACN cites the need for change in graduate nursing education as a response to the increasing complexity of the nation's healthcare environment, and points to national calls to action from the IOM, The Joint Commission (an independent company that accredits healthcare organizations and programs), and the 2005 National Institutes of Health (NIH) report calling for the development of

nonresearch (clinical) doctorates in nursing. As of May 2014, 235 DNP programs in the United States enrolled students and more than 100 others were under development (AACN, 2014a).

Finally, credentialing bodies play a crucial role in advancing the profession. Quality in credentialing speaks to the value of creating a system that aims to improve the performance and healthcare outcomes of its credential holders. In 2012, the American Nurses Credentialing Center (ANCC) announced the formation of an Institute of Medicine Standing Committee on Credentialing Research in Nursing. Among other activities, the committee discusses short- and long-term strategic planning, maintains surveillance of the credentialing field, and serves as a public venue of communication for relevant stakeholders. It is within the committee's purview to address the following topics: priorities for nursing credentialing research; relevant research methodologies, measures, and outcomes assessment related to the impact of credentialing in nursing on healthcare quality improvements; and strategic planning for advancing research in nursing credentialing. The ANCC is the primary sponsor of this activity (American Nurses Credentialing Center, 2012; Institute of Medicine, 2014).

Reimbursement

Significant breakthroughs are being made in reimbursement policy for APRNs, largely as a result of the formation of grassroots lobbying efforts and coalitions of APRN specialty nursing organizations. With the passage of federal legislation in 1997 allowing APRNs to bill Medicare directly for services, consumers' access to care provided by APRNs has improved. Managed care markets value efficiency and provider effectiveness. Understanding the concept of market value has motivated APRNs to become more skilled in costing out services and winning contracts in a competitive market.

Discrepancies in Medicare APRN reimbursement still exist, and the reimbursement structure for comparable services is arbitrary. Calls to achieve pay parity have suggested the CMS lead demonstrations of market-based, population-based, and performance-based initiatives to facilitate recognition of NPs as eligible providers (Naylor & Kurtzman, 2010).

Impact of the Nurse Shortage on Regulation and Licensure

Supply and demand projections substantiate that the shortage of nurses will continue well into the next decade. Factors driving the shortage include: (1) the fact that nurse education capacity is not growing rapidly enough to meet the projected demands, in part because of nurse faculty shortages; (2) the aging of the nurse workforce, resulting in a large cohort of retiring nurses; (3) a growth in the aging population, resulting in an increased number of individuals who will require complex care; and (4) insufficient staffing levels and stressful job environments, which are motivating nurses to leave the profession (AACN, 2014b). In December 2013, the U.S. Department of Health and Human Services announced $55.5 million in funding in FY 2014 to strengthen health professions education and increase the size of the healthcare workforce. The majority of funding, $45.4 million, was earmarked to support nursing workforce development. Areas targeted included: (1) increasing the number of nurse faculty, (2) improving diversity in nursing, (3) increasing traineeships in nurse anesthesia and supporting advanced practice nurse education, and (4) supporting the development of interprofessional collaborative practice models (DHHS, 2013). It is expected that nursing workforce issues will continue to fuel policy on work environment issues across the nation.

Although projections in job growth are expected, the nurse workforce able to fill vacant or new positions continues to decline. Several issues bear monitoring during this period. They include the following:

- *Comprehensive U.S. healthcare reform:* Provisions in the ACA will increase access for the nation's under- and uninsured, estimated at more than 50 million. It is also estimated that in more than 6,400 shortage areas in the United States, 66 million Americans are limited in access to primary care (American Nurses Association [ANA], 2011). The need for APRNs in a variety of settings, but particularly in primary care, will be enormous, but their usefulness is dependent on the lifting of practice restrictions in their state of licensure.

- *Delegation and supervision of unlicensed assistive personnel (UAP):* Utilization of UAPs will continue to be debated and expanded as the shortage of licensed nurses makes it difficult to meet the public's demands for care. Providing safe and effective care while delegating care tasks appropriately to a potentially growing cadre of UAPs will place additional responsibilities on the licensed nurse.

- *Mandatory overtime legislation:* The IOM report, *Keeping Patients Safe: Transforming the Work Environment of Nurses* (2003) presented a body of evidence associating the nurses' work environment and patient safety. Nurses commonly work extended hours; this work environment factor was found to be associated with diminished work performance, increased risk of errors, and potential patient harm. Employers have coerced nurses to remain on duty against their will by threatening termination, using the concept of patient abandonment as "cause." Employers follow coercion with threats of reporting the alleged patient abandonment to the licensing board. Disciplinary sections in NPAs typically read in such a way that the employers' threats are empty; most state boards do not consider refusal to work additional consecutive shifts as an incident that constitutes patient abandonment. Fourteen states have protected nurses from this kind of employer threat by enacting restrictions on the use of mandatory overtime in law, and two states have included provisions in regulation (ANA, 2014).

- *Staffing ratios:* In some states, nurses have organized to pass legislation implementing staffing ratios based on patient acuity. Staffing ratios have both positive and negative implications. Although staffing ratio regulations may require a facility to employ a certain minimum number of nurses, or staff units with a minimum number of nurses, employers may interpret the regulated minimum ratios as the maximum number of nurses that *must* be employed, and subsequently place a cap on hiring.

- *Foreign nurse recruitment:* Employers may seek to recruit foreign-educated nurses during acute nurse shortages. Deregulation of licensure and examination standards has historically been enacted during these periods. Few countries outside the United States have nurse education systems equivalent in academic breadth or rigor, or in clinical requirements. The nurse community must be vigilant to these attempts to lower the standards for licensure, which could lead to increased risk for patients and a change in public perception of the profession.

- *Proliferation of new nursing education programs:* Colleges, universities, and other legitimate, accredited public and private educational institutions are finding the business of nurse education is becoming more attractive. The number of qualified applicants for nursing programs far exceeds the number of available seats. However, proprietary organizations are also seeing nursing education as an opportunity for profit, and may not consider the infrastructure and support systems necessary to carry out a quality program. State BONs are challenged to strike a balance between the concept of an open marketplace and a desire to protect the stretched interests of existing programs that are struggling to maintain a cadre of qualified faculty and ensure clinical placements for their students.

Other trends and issues will surface over the next several years that may affect the regulation of nurses and APRNs. It will be increasingly important to stay abreast of legislative and regulatory initiatives, and to affiliate with professional organizations to preserve and protect professional standards.

CONCLUSION

The capacity to adapt is crucial in an era of rapid change. Healthcare reform is transforming healthcare delivery systems, but it is also providing momentum for fundamental changes in APRN practice and regulation. A window of opportunity has presented itself for politically astute APRNs to shape public policy by working with coalitions of nurses, other health professionals, and consumers to advocate for regulations that will allow the public greater access to affordable, quality health care. It is essential for APRNs to develop skills to capitalize on the chaos present in the healthcare and political environments and create opportunities to advance the profession.

Familiarity with the regulatory process will give APRNs the tools needed to navigate with confidence. Knowing how to access the status of critical issues involving scopes of practice, licensure issues, and reimbursement will allow the APRN to influence outcomes. Participation in specialty professional nurse organizations is especially advantageous. Participation builds a membership base, providing the foundation for strong coalition building and a power base from which to effect change in the political and regulatory arenas. Participation also presents members with access to a colleague network, legislative affairs information, and professional and educational opportunities. Although supporting the profession through participation is central, it is equally important to remember that each APRN has the ability to make a difference.

DISCUSSION QUESTIONS _____

1. Compare and contrast the legislative and regulatory processes.

2. Describe the major methods of credentialing. List the benefits and weaknesses of each method from the standpoint of public protection, and protection of the professional scope of practice.

3. Discuss the role of state BONs in regulating professional practice.

4. Compare the role of state BONs with the role of professional organizations in regulating professional practice.

5. Obtain a copy of a proposed or recently promulgated regulation. Using Exhibit 11–1, analyze the regulation for its impact on nursing practice.

6. Assume the BON has promulgated a regulation requiring all APRNs to have 20 contact hours of continuing education credit in pharmacotherapeutics each year to maintain prescriptive authority. Write a brief (no more than two pages) testimony supporting or opposing this proposed regulation.

7. Describe the federal government's role in the regulation of health professions. Do you believe the role will increase or decrease over time? Explain your rationale.

8. Discuss the pros and cons of multistate regulation. Based on your analysis, defend a position either for or against multistate regulation.

9. Prepare written testimony for a public hearing defending or opposing the need for a second license for APRNs.

10. Contrast the BON and the national or state nurses association vis-à-vis mission, membership, authority, functions, and source of funding.

11. Identify a proposed regulation. Discuss the current phase of the process, identify methods for offering comments, and submit written comments to the administrative agency.

12. Download at least one resource from one of the websites listed in Exhibit 11–2 and evaluate the credibility of the author (the "author" may be the organization), the most recent update, and the appropriateness of the data. Share the resources with colleagues.

13. Evaluate the APRN section of the nurse practice act in your state using the *NCSBN Model Nursing Practice Act* (2011).

14. Identify the states that have implemented nurse-staffing ratios. List some of the obstacles one of the states has encountered in the implementation phase.

REFERENCES _____

American Academy of Nurse Practitioners & American College of Nurse Practitioners. (2012, July 3). *Two national nurse practitioner organizations announce plans to consolidate*. Retrieved from http://www.aanp.org/28-press-room/2012-pressreleases/996-plans-to-consolidate

American Association of Colleges of Nursing (AACN). (2004). *AACN position statement on the practice doctorate in nursing*. Retrieved from http://www.aacn.nche.edu/DNP/DNPPositionStatement.htm

American Association of Colleges of Nursing (AACN). (2014a). *DNP program schools*. Retrieved from http://www.aacn.nche.edu/dnp/program-schools

American Association of Colleges of Nursing (AACN). (2014b). *Nursing shortage fact sheet*. Retrieved from http://www.aacn.nche.edu/media-relations/NrsgShortageFS.pdf

American Nurses Association. (2011). *Advanced practice nursing: A new age in health care*. American Nurses Association Backgrounder. Retrieved from http://www.nursingworld.org/functionalmenucategories/mediaresources/mediabackgrounders/aprn-a-new-age-in-health-care.pdf

American Nurses Association. (2014). *Mandatory overtime*. Retrieved from http://www.nursingworld.org/MainMenuCategories/ThePracticeofProfessionalNursing/NurseStaffing/OvertimeIssues/Overtime.pdf

American Nurses Credentialing Center. (2012, September). *American Nurses Credentialing Center announces members of the IOM committee on credentialing research in nursing*. Retrieved from http://www

.nursingworld.org/FunctionalMenuCategories /MediaResources/PressReleases/2012-PR/IOM -Committee-on-Credentialing-Research-in -Nursing.pdf

APRN Joint Dialogue Group. (2008). *Consensus model for APRN regulation: Licensure, accreditation, certification & education.* Retrieved from www.aacn.nche .edu/education-resources/APRNReport.pdf

Centers for Medicare & Medicaid Services. (2014). *History.* Retrieved from http://www.cms.gov /About-CMS/Agency-Information/History.Index .html

Commonwealth Fund. (2014). Affordable care act reforms. Retrieved from: http://www .commonwealthfund.org/topics/affordable-care -act-reforms

Dower, C., & Finocchio, L. (1995). Health care workforce regulation: Making the necessary changes for a transforming health care system. *State Health Workforce Reforms, 4,* 1–2.

Garner, B. A. (2009). *Black's law dictionary* (9th ed.). St Paul, MN: Thompson West.

Gobis, L. J. (1997). Licensing & liability: Crossing the borders with telemedicine. *Caring, 16*(7), 18–24.

Gross, S. (1984). *Of foxes and hen houses: Licensing and the health professions.* Westport, CT: Quorum.

Hartigan, C. (2011). APRN regulation: The licensure-certification interface. *AACN Advanced Critical Care, 22*(1), 50–65.

HealthCare.gov. (2010). *About the law: Patient protection and Affordable Healthcare Act.* Retrieved from http://www.healthcare.gov/law/about/Index.htm

Institute of Medicine (2003). *Keeping patients safe: Transforming the work environment of nurses.* Washington, DC: National Academies Press.

Institute of Medicine. (2010). *The future of nursing: Leading change, advancing health.* Retrieved from http://www.iom.edu/~/media/Files/Report%20 Files/2010/The-Future-of-Nursing/Future%20 of%20Nursing%202010%20Recommendations.pdf

Institute of Medicine. (2014). *Standing committee on credentialing research in nursing.* Retrieved from http://www.iom.edu/Activities/Workforce /NursingCredentialing

Josiah Macy Jr. Foundation. (2013). *Transforming patient care: Aligning interprofessional education with clinical practice redesign.* Conference recommendations. Retrieved from http://macyfoundation.org/publications /publication/aligning-interprofessional-education

Jost, T. S. (1997). *Regulation of the health professions.* Chicago: Health Administration Press.

Kohn, L. T., Corrigan, J. M., & Donaldson, M. S. (Eds.). (2000). *To err is human: Building a safer health care system.* Institute of Medicine of the National Academies. Washington, DC: National Academies Press.

Legal Information Institute. (n.d.). *Supremacy clause.* Retrieved from http://www.law.cornell.edu/wex /supremacy_clause

National Council of State Boards of Nursing. (1993). *Regulation of advanced nursing practice position paper.* Retrieved from https://www.ncsbn .org/1993_Position_Paper_on_the_Regulation_ of_Advanced_Nursing_Practice.pdf

National Council of State Boards of Nursing. (1998, April). *Multi state regulation task force communiqué.* Chicago: Author.

National Council of State Boards of Nursing. (2002). *Uniform advanced practice registered nurse licensure /authority to practice requirements.* Retrieved from https://www.ncsbn.org/APRN_Uniform_require-ments_revised_8_02.pdf

National Council of State Boards of Nursing. (2006). *Draft—Vision paper: The future regulation of advanced practice nursing.* Retrieved from https://www .ncsbn.org/Draft__Vision_Paper.pdf

National Council of State Boards of Nursing (NCSBN). (2008). *Contact a board of nursing.* Retrieved from https://www.ncsbn.org/515.htm

National Council of State Boards of Nursing. (2009). *Requirements for accrediting agencies and criteria for APRN certification programs.* Retrieved from https: //www.ncsbn.org/428.htm

National Council of State Boards of Nursing. (2010). *APRN consensus model: Frequently-asked questions.* Retrieved from https://www.ncsbn.org/aprn.htm

National Council of State Boards of Nursing. (2011). *NCSBN model nursing practice act and model nursing administrative rules: Introduction to revised models.* Retrieved from https://www.ncsbn.org/nlc.htm

National Council of State Boards of Nursing. (2014a). *Map of NLC states.* Retrieved from http: //www.ncsbn.org/nlc

National Council of State Boards of Nursing. (2014b). *Nurse practice act, rules & regulations.* Retrieved from https://www.ncsbn.org/1455.htm

Naylor, M. D., & Kurtzman, E. T. (2010). The role of nurse practitioners in reinventing primary care. *Health Affairs, 29*(5), 893–899. doi: 10.1377 /hlthaff.2010.0440

Nelson, R. (2006). NCSBN 'vision paper' ignites controversy. *American Journal of Nursing, 106*(7), 25–26.

O'Sullivan, J., Chaikind, H., Tilson, S., Boulanger, J., & Morgan, P. (2004). *Overview of the Medicare Prescription Drug, Improvement and Modernization Act of 2003.* Congressional Research Service. Order Code RL31966. Washington, DC: Library of Congress.

Pearson, L. J. (2002). Fourteenth annual legislative update. *Nurse Practitioner, 27*(1), 10–15.

Pew Health Professions Commission. (1994). *State strategies for health care workforce reform.* San Francisco: UCSF Center for the Health Professions.

Pew Health Professions Commission. (1995). *Report of task force on health care workforce regulation* (executive summary). San Francisco: UCSF Center for the Health Professions.

Phillips, S. J. (2014). 26th annual legislative update. *Nurse Practitioner, 39*(1), 29–52.

Roberts, M. J., & Clyde, A. T. (1993). *Your money or your life: The health care crisis explained.* New York: Doubleday.

Russell, K. A. (2012). Nurse practice acts guide and govern nursing practice. *Journal of Nursing Regulation, 3*(3), 36–42.

Safriet, B. J. (1992). Health care dollars and regulatory sense: The role of advanced practice nursing. *Yale Journal of Regulation, 9*(2), 419–488.

U.S. Department of Health and Human Services. (2013). *HHS awards $55.5 million to bolster America's health care workforce.* Retrieved from http://www .hhs.gov/news/press/2013pres/12/20131205a .html

U.S. Department of Health and Human Services. (2014). *The Affordable Care Act, section by section.* Retrieved from http://www.hhs.gov/healthcare /rights/law/

U.S. Department of Health and Human Services & Centers for Medicare & Medicaid Services. (2011). *Information for advanced practice registered nurses, anesthesiologist assistants, and physician assistants.* Medical Learning Network. ICN901623. Retrieved from http://www.cms.gov/Outreach -and-Education/Medicare-Learning-Network -MLN/MLNProducts/APNPA.html

PART 3

Quality, Safety, and Information Systems for Advanced Practice Nurses

With specialized knowledge and practical application of that knowledge to influence patient outcomes, nurses in advanced practice have the fiduciary responsibility not only to provide and manage quality care but also to take leadership roles within the practice setting to promote a culture of quality and safety. As described in Part 2, quality is one of the major components of the healthcare triad, along with cost and access. In Part 3, we consider quality issues and the intersection of quality, patient safety, and information technology.

There are many definitions of quality and many perspectives on what healthcare quality means. Consumers, providers, payers, and regulators may all have different viewpoints about what healthcare quality is and how it should be measured and reported. However, with the national, healthcare industry, and societal interest in the costs of health care and the outcomes of that care, the Institute of Medicine's definition (IOM, 2001) of quality is a well-accepted one and the one used for this book. This agency defines healthcare quality as "The degree to which health services for individuals and populations increase the likelihood of desired health outcomes and are consistent with current professional knowledge."

Further, in its report titled *Crossing the Quality Chasm*, the IOM (2001) described six quality aims for health care. Specifically, health care should be

1. Safe
2. Effective
3. Patient centered
4. Timely
5. Efficient
6. Equitable

These characteristics of quality should be foremost in mind as readers study Part 3.

Patient safety is one of the top—if not the top—current quality issues politically and professionally. Nevertheless, it is essential to think broadly about healthcare quality, going beyond just safety, and to keep foremost in one's thinking all of the aforementioned characteristics of quality. For instance, a patient may experience a safe healthcare episode, but if the providers do not consider the patient's preferences and beliefs, it would not be defined as a quality encounter.

With the recent emphasis on patient safety as a result of the IOM (1999) report *To Err Is Human,* a concerted, ongoing effort focused on assessing and improving patient safety has been a major driver in health care. In this report, the IOM documented the serious and pervasive nature of the United States' overall patient safety problem, concluding that more than 98,000 deaths per year occurred due to medical error and stating that the U.S. healthcare system had a severe problem.

In 2008, the Robert Wood Johnson Foundation (RWJF) and the IOM realized the need to assess and transform the nursing profession. The 2-year initiative resulted in the 2010 IOM consensus report entitled *The Future of Nursing: Leading Change and Advancing Health.* Through extensive dialogue, the committee developed four goals linked to policy, safety, and education:

1. Nurses should practice to the full extent of their education and training.

2. Nurses should achieve higher levels of education and training through an improved education system that promotes seamless academic progression.

3. Nurses should be full partners, with physicians and other healthcare professionals, in redesigning health care in the United States.

4. Effective workforce planning and policy-making require better data collection and information infrastructure.

With the passage of the 2010 Affordable Care Act and the national recognition that nurses work on the front lines of patient care,

collaborative efforts will be made to ensure that the U.S. healthcare system provides seamless, affordable, quality care that is accessible to all and leads to improved health outcomes. In this part, we examine how the advanced practice nurse can meet this challenge.

Chapter 12 sets the foundation and introduces the reader to the concept of continuous quality improvement that can be applied not only to direct patient care in primary care or hospital settings but also to disease prevention and population initiatives in public health. These applications are characterized by continuous, ongoing learning and sharing among disciplines about ways to use CQI philosophies, processes, and tools. In this chapter, the authors discuss factors and processes that facilitate or impede the implementation of CQI as a dynamic programmatic innovation within a healthcare setting.

Despite a strong political, consumer, and industry response to the *To Err Is Human Report* (IOM, 1999) and a national will to decrease medical errors, the results have been poor. A recent study suggests that between 210,000 and 440,000 medical errors occur annually, making medical errors the third highest cause of death (James, 2013). The next two chapters acknowledge this concern and provide recommendations to mitigate adverse events and medical errors.

In Chapter 13, the authors review the foundation of patient safety by exploring the historical events that have shaped patient safety as it is known today. By examining the issues health care faces and the history of patient safety in America, they argue that a more cohesive and united effort is needed to have a meaningful effect on both quality of care and patient safety. In Chapter 14, the authors suggest three approaches to accelerate the patient safety movement: (1) establish a mandatory standard of patient safety performance; (2) initiate specific interventions to improve the healthcare workplace and the safety of workers and patients; and (3) upgrade the knowledge and skills of healthcare leaders and workers to build organizational cultures of safety.

The last two chapters in Part 3 are dedicated to the use of information technology and electronic health records—factors that are transforming the U.S. healthcare environment into a more technologically sophisticated field and possibly creating positive impact on quality and safety. Improving patient safety and the quality of health care are tied to technology in three ways: (1) Without databases at the local, state, and national levels we could not get the information to determine whether there is a problem and the scope of the problem. (2) Technology can assist the delivery of care in a myriad of ways such as with bar-coded medication administration, the electronic health record, and medical devices, to name few. (3) Without technology it would be difficult to measure outcomes and the effectiveness of practice changes. In Chapter 15, Kroth provides an overview of health information technology (HIT), including its history, present state, and future challenges. This chapter provides the reader a foundation to build on for the application of information technology to improving quality and safety. Chapter 16 discusses the implications of adoption of the electronic health record (EHR).

This trend is being driven by legislation—specifically, the passage of the American Recovery and Reinvestment Act of 2009 (ARRA), including the HITECH Act, which offers incentives to health organizations and providers to become "meaningful users" of EHRs. The eight components of an EHR are reviewed: (1) health information and data; (2) results management; (3) order entry management; (4) decision support; (5) electronic communication and connectivity; (6) patient support; (7) administrative processes; and (8) reporting and population health management (IOM, 2003).

REFERENCES

Institute of Medicine. (1999). *To err is human: Building a safer health system.* Washington, DC: Author.

Institute of Medicine. (2001). *Crossing the quality chasm: A new health system for the 21st century.* Washington, DC: Author.

Institute of Medicine. (2003). *Key capabilities of an electronic health record system.* Washington, DC: Author.

Institute of Medicine. (2010). *The future of nursing: Leading change and advancing health.* Washington, DC: Author.

James, J. T. (2013). A new, evidence-based estimate of patient harm associated with hospital care. *Journal of Patient Safety, 9*(3), 122–128.

CHAPTER 12

Factors Influencing the Application and Diffusion of CQI in Health Care

William A. Sollecito and Julie K. Johnson

© A-R-T/Shutterstock

CHAPTER OBJECTIVES

1. Define continuous quality improvement (CQI) and list its characteristics.

2. Gain an appreciation of the complexity of healthcare organizations and the difficulty in diffusing innovation in the industry.

3. Describe the current state of quality in health care.

4. Identify problems regarding implementation of CQI in the local practice setting.

5. Describe the factors that have influenced the rate of diffusion and spread of CQI in health care in general and in the advanced nurse practitioner's setting specifically.

INTRODUCTION

Continuous quality improvement (CQI) has gained acceptance within all sectors of health care and across geographic and economic boundaries. It has evolved as a global strategy for improving health care in a variety of settings, spanning a broad number of issues and improving services to a variety of customers, ranging from individual patients to communities. The spectrum of applications covers not only direct patient care in primary care or hospital settings but also disease prevention and population initiatives—such as HIV, childhood obesity, and influenza vaccination programs—under the domain of public health agencies at the local, national, and international levels. These applications are characterized by continuous, ongoing learning and sharing among disciplines about ways to use

CQI philosophies, processes, and tools in a variety of settings. New applications continue to emerge, but at the same time, there are new challenges to the broad application of CQI. In this chapter, we examine the factors and processes that facilitate or impede the implementation of CQI as a dynamic programmatic innovation within a healthcare setting.

DEFINITION OF CONTINUOUS QUALITY IMPROVEMENT

What was originally called *total quality management* (TQM) in the manufacturing industry evolved into *continuous quality improvement* as it was applied to healthcare administrative and clinical processes. Over time the term continued to evolve, and now the same concepts and activities are referred to as *quality improvement* or *quality management*, or even sometimes simply as *improvement*. To focus on the unique challenges within health care, the term *CQI* is used primarily throughout this chapter.

In health care, CQI is defined as a structured organizational process for involving personnel in planning and executing a continuous flow of improvements to provide quality health care that meets or exceeds expectations. CQI usually involves a common set of characteristics, which include the following:

- A link to key elements of the organization's strategic plan
- A quality council made up of the institution's top leadership
- Training programs for personnel
- Mechanisms for selecting improvement opportunities
- Formation of process improvement teams
- Staff support for process analysis and redesign
- Personnel policies that motivate and support staff participation in process improvement
- Application of the most current and rigorous techniques of the scientific method and statistical process control

The Dynamic Character of CQI: The Case of the Safe Surgery Checklist

As a natural consequence of the scientific method, CQI methodology and applications continue to evolve and also continue to be challenged and debated before they are fully accepted as evidence-based practice. A recent example is a reemphasis on the use of a simple tool—the checklist—to improve patient safety. Checklists are a good example of the use of CQI philosophies and processes. They demonstrate leadership and interdisciplinary teamwork, using a form of the Plan, Do, Study, Act (PDSA) improvement cycle to test, learn, and improve by enlisting a broad range of expertise to improve safety on a global scale. The World Health Organization (WHO) initiative to promote use of the Surgical Safety Checklist is an excellent example of both the evolutionary process of spreading CQI in health care and, at the same time, the challenges to full diffusion and institutionalization of CQI (Gawande, 2009).

The process for developing and proving the value of the surgical checklist was long and arduous. Checklists first contributed to improvements in safety and quality in other fields, most notably aviation, where they have made a dramatic impact on the testing and development of new aircraft as well as the safety of the thousands of people who travel by air on a daily basis (Gawande, 2009). The successful use of checklists in the aviation industry led to the initial efforts by Pronovost et al. (2006) to test the use of checklists to reduce central line infections and other adverse events in intensive care units (ICUs). This effort, which started in 2001, was successful and led to experimentation within medical care to extend the use of checklists to attack other inpatient medical safety issues, again following the same evolutionary model that has led to the expansion of CQI in other healthcare areas.

Following on the successful applications of Pronovost et al. to reduce central line infections, a global initiative was launched under the auspices of the WHO to develop and apply checklists to improve surgical safety. Enlisting safety and surgery experts from multiple countries and applying techniques learned from various medical applications, a quasi-experimental study was undertaken that encompassed a large number of medical facilities practicing surgery under a wide range of conditions. As a result, Haynes, Weiser, and Berry (2009) demonstrated a statistically significant ($p < .001$) overall reduction in complication rates from 11.0% at baseline to 7.0% and a statistically significant ($p < .003$) reduction in death rates from 1.5% to 0.8% with the introduction of the surgical safety checklist in eight hospitals in eight cities, worldwide.

Similar results were demonstrated in a study of six hospitals in the Netherlands (the SURPASS Collaborative Group) that included almost 4,000 surgical patients observed before and after implementation of a surgical checklist, extending the checklist process to activities both within and outside the operating room. Findings included a statistically significant ($p < 0.001$) decrease in the proportion of patients with one or more complications, from 15.4% to 10.6% (de Vries et al., 2010). The findings from both of these studies replicate earlier findings demonstrating reduction in catheter-related bloodstream infections associated with the use of checklists in ICUs (Pronovost et al., 2006).

Despite the successful adaptation of checklists from industry to health care, significant questions about the application of checklists and the adaptation and diffusion of quality improvement methods remain:

- Why aren't more healthcare providers using CQI tools and processes?
- Why is the gap between knowledge and practice so large?
- Why don't clinical systems incorporate the findings of clinical science or copy the "best known" practices reliably, quickly, and even gratefully into their daily work simply as a matter of course?

The answers to these questions, which have been raised by CQI leaders such as Dr. Brent James (Leonhardt, 2009) and Dr. Donald Berwick (2003), are multifaceted. For example, critics of checklists assert that the overemphasis on simple tools like the checklist is not without risks and instead advocate pursuing more complex system solutions for ensuring patient safety and the highest quality of care (Bosk, Dixon-Woods, Goeschel, & Pronovost, 2009).

The checklist example is only one very limited application but a good current illustration of some of the key issues surrounding the diffusion of CQI in health care. It is the tip of the iceberg for a set of much broader issues. These broader issues include, but are not limited to, process versus outcome, and cost versus benefit versus value. Also important in this debate are scientific issues regarding the minimum standards to define evidence for change, such as the use of double-blind randomized trials versus quasi-experimentation. These issues are the direct result of the traditions of the scientific process guiding all we do in health care; this rich tradition requires rigor but also imposes buffers to quick decisions, including complex assumptions, different interpretations of causality, and, more simply, differences of opinion about findings. Also related is the question of how to influence practitioners to adopt new ideas and the broader topic of diffusion of innovation in health care.

The remainder of this chapter addresses several questions:

1. What is the current state of quality in health care, and what are the problems regarding implementation of CQI in health care?

2. Given the widespread application of CQI in recent years, what are the factors that contribute to the implementation of CQI across industries and settings?

3. Specifically for our application in health care, what are the factors that have influenced the rate of diffusion and spread of CQI in health care?

To answer these questions, we will consider the current state of health care, and we will consider the parallels between CQI and more general factors associated with the diffusion of innovation in health care, including factors associated with the business case for the use of CQI in health care.

THE CURRENT STATE OF CQI IN HEALTH CARE

Despite progress since the publication of the Institute of Medicine's landmark reports *To Err Is Human* (2000) and *Crossing the Quality Chasm* (2001), and the interprofessional as well as global dispersion of CQI techniques in various segments of health care, major gaps still exist in the quality of care and the functioning of the health care system. For example, qualitative assessments have characterized, or "graded," the progress of the patient safety movement to close the gap as a B– in 2009, compared to the C+ awarded 5 years earlier (Wachter, 2010). This qualitative assessment has been supported by numerous studies that present quantitative data confirming this lack of progress. For example, a 2010 study documented that little change occurred in "patient harms" during a 6-year review (from 2002 to 2007) of more than 2,300 admissions in 10 hospitals in North Carolina, a state chosen for study because it had shown a high level of engagement in patient safety efforts (Landrigan et al., 2010).

In a recent, and now frequently cited, study by James (2013), the author argues that the initial report by the Institute of Medicine (2000) on hospital deaths due to medical error, which estimated 98,000 deaths per year, was most likely underestimated. In the new study the investigator reports that preventable deaths from avoidable adverse events is between 210,000 and 400,000, being the third largest cause of death in the United States.

Although there is evidence that these are global trends, a group of learned and experienced experts assess the situation in the United States as follows:

> U.S. health care is broken. Although other industries have transformed themselves using tools such as standardization of value-generating processes, performance measurement, and transparent reporting of quality, the application of these tools to health care is controversial, evoking fears of "cookbook medicine," loss of professional autonomy, a misinformed focus on the wrong care, or a loss of individual attention and the personal touch in care delivery. . . . Our current health care system is essentially a cottage industry of nonintegrated, dedicated artisans who eschew standardization. . . . Growing evidence highlights the dangers of continuing to operate in a cottage-industry mode. Fragmentation of care has led to suboptimal performance. (Swensen et al., 2010, p. e12[1])

These statements were made at a time when the United States was launching the most major health reform in its history, amid great opposition. The challenge of the coming years is how to fix this broken system.

Rather than assume that we have any easy answers—which we do not—some time will be devoted in this chapter to further describe the scope of the problem, with a particular focus on CQI philosophies and processes and why they have not been more widely adopted. Hopefully, this will give us some direction toward a set of ideas to expand the implementation of CQI across a broader range of providers.

Dr. Brent James is executive director of the Institute for Health Care Delivery Research and vice president of Medical Research and Continuing Medical Education at Intermountain Health Care. He has demonstrated leadership in improving health care in many ways, not the least of which is his leadership by example at Intermountain Health Care. In an interview with *The New York Times*, Dr. James gives several examples of how Intermountain Health Care has led the way to value-based care through the use of CQI processes. He identifies the lack of widespread change as being directly related to the complexity of the healthcare system; a clear symptom of the depth of problems that persist is that the American healthcare system is vastly more expensive, but not vastly better, than the health systems of other countries (Leonhardt, 2009).

Dr. Donald Berwick founded the Institute for Healthcare Improvement (IHI) more than 20 years ago and in 2010 was appointed by President Obama as administrator of the Centers for Medicare and Medicaid Services (CMS). In 2003, he noted that "Americans spend almost 40% more per capita for health care than any other country, yet rank 27th in infant mortality, 27th in life expectancy, and are less satisfied with their care than the English, Canadians, or Germans" (Berwick, 2003, p. 1969). He is one of many to point out the gravity of this situation due to the fact that little change has occurred between 2003 and 2010. Two of the important issues at the heart of this problem, complexity and cost, were also key factors in the debate about health reform in the United States in 2009; as will be shown later in this chapter, they are also contributors to the explanation of why CQI has not been more widely adopted.

The complexity of the healthcare system is both a challenge and a source of ideas for how to make improvements (Plsek & Greenhalgh, 2001). Health care is a complex adaptive system, a concept that has implications for how to improve the system. For example, the importance of leadership is critical, as are incentives for improvement. As a complex adaptive system, health care can only be designed to a certain extent and cannot be designed around minimizing costs; rather, the focus must be on maximizing value (Rouse, 2008).

CQI AND THE SCIENCE OF INNOVATION

Although health care is unique in many ways, one commonality that it has with other complex endeavors is the difficulty surrounding diffusion of innovation, starting with simple resistance to change but including many other complex factors. Understanding these issues helps to provide pathways toward greater diffusion of CQI in health care.

The research and principles that are specific to diffusion of innovation of health services are summarized in a systematic review of the literature presented by Greenhalgh, Robert, Macfarlane, Bate, and Kyriakidou (2005). From this review, it is noted that there is a wide range of literature using a variety of concepts and approaches that describe how to move along the spectrum from the initiation of a concept for change to the spread, diffusion, and institutionalization of innovation.

Diffusion theory is useful in understanding the factors that thwart or support the adoption of CQI in health care. Because of the complexity of health care and the added complexity of CQI, as alluded to earlier in this chapter, there are no simple answers about how to move CQI innovations into the mainstream of health care more quickly and efficiently. Complexity must be considered in understanding innovation. Although there are competing theories about how and why, innovation clearly does happen in "complex zones." There is some evidence that while innovation may not be susceptible to being managed, it is possible to design and control organizational conditions that "enhance the possibility of innovation occurring and spreading" (Greenhalgh et al., 2005, p. 80). Addressing this complexity requires, first and foremost, leadership, but also the creation of a receptive and even enthusiastic culture; one excellent example of how this has been accomplished in CQI in health care is the formation of quality improvement collaboratives, such as the SURPASS Collaborative Group, mentioned earlier in regard to the successful application of surgical checklists to improve patient safety (de Vries et al., 2010). These ideas and examples are discussed further in this context later in this section.

The speed and overall adoption of any change, including CQI, can be influenced by the characteristics of the change and how it is perceived by those responsible for implementation. These characteristics include relative advantage, compatibility, simplicity, trialability, and observability (Rogers, 1995). All of these characteristics relate to changes and improvements in health care, and two in particular are directly relevant to the checklist example: compatibility, which relates to how closely the change ideas align with the existing culture and environment, and trialability, which addresses how the changes can be adapted and tested in the new environments in which they are being spread.

A further extension of these change concepts yields the following seven rules for dissemination of innovation in health care (Berwick, 2003):

1. Find sound innovations.
2. Find and support innovators.
3. Invest in early adopters.
4. Make early adopter activity observable.
5. Trust and enable reinvention.
6. Create slack for change.
7. Lead by example.

All of these rules are applicable to innovations around CQI; leadership, trust, and reinvention are fundamental. Reinvention has to do with the cross-disciplinary learning concept that has permeated CQI and is responsible for its evolution across industries and around the globe. CQI cannot be a top-down mandate. It must be part of the vision of an organization and accepted by all who must implement CQI, thus requiring trust at all levels, which comes from leadership, teamwork, and Deming's concept of "constancy of purpose." Top leadership must be involved, supporting and communicating the vision for innovation and change; however, participation, buy-in, and support from opinion leaders at all levels within an organization are critical for successful implementation and the process to reinvention.

One size will not fit all. As described by Berwick (2003), "To work, changes must be not only adopted locally, but also locally adapted" (p. 1974). Berwick asserts that for this to happen, there must be reinvention. In his words, "Reinvention is a form of learning, and, in its own way, it is an act of both creativity and courage. Leaders who want to foster innovation . . . should showcase and celebrate individuals who take ideas from elsewhere and adapt them to make them their own" (p. 1974).

Once again, the checklist example cited at the beginning of this chapter is a clear illustration of this process of reinvention and leadership. It was adapted from the airline and other industries, first to intensive care and later to surgery, with trusted leaders in their fields using scientific media and disseminating their ideas and successes. The fact that these evidence-based tools are not fully accepted and used returns us to the point that health care is complex and requires diligence to spread the improvement process. The systematic review of diffusion of innovation in health services identifies complexity as one of the key elements that is inversely associated with successful diffusion. Quite often, because of the complex nature of healthcare systems, equally complex quality improvement strategies are required, thus lessening their quick and easy adoption. This helps to explain why simpler quality improvement processes, such as the use of PDSA cycles, have enjoyed broad success. However, resistance to the use of simple checklists defies this explanation.

A prospective study of the attributes of 42 clinical practice recommendations in gynecology (Foy et al., 2002) may help to explain this resistance to some degree. After review of almost 5,000 patient records, findings indicate two outcomes of relevance to the checklist example. First, recommendations that were compatible with clinician values and did not require changes to fixed routines (to some, the surgical checklist may be contrary to both of these notions) were associated with greater compliance. Second, initial noncompliance could be reversed after audit and feedback stages were carried out (indicating that perhaps more time will yield greater compliance). Although these findings may bode well for the long-term acceptance of the surgical checklist and the ICU checklist developed in 2006 by Pronovost et al., there is insufficient evidence at the time of this writing to make firm conclusions.

THE BUSINESS CASE FOR CQI

Healthcare delivery systems are large, decentralized, and complex, yet at their core they involve a fundamental personal relationship between providers and patients. Moreover, if this were not a sufficient challenge, rapid and uncertain changes in the structure and processes of providing and paying for care make measuring the effect of any single management intervention over time very difficult, if not impossible. Although evidence has been accumulated from both controlled trials (Goldberg, Wagner, & Finh, 1998; Mehta et al., 2000; Solberg, 1993) and survey data (Shortell, Bennett, & Byck, 1998) on the implementation process and perceived impact, much of the evidence remains anecdotal (Arndt & Bigelow, 1995). Leatherman et al. (2003), for example, argue that the "business case" for quality improvement is yet to be proven, even while evidence mounts for the overall societal and economic benefits:

> A *business case* for a health care improvement intervention exists if the entity that invests in the intervention realizes a financial return on its investment in a reasonable time frame, using a reasonable rate of discounting. This may be realized as "bankable dollars" (profit), a reduction in losses for a given program or population, or avoided costs. In addition, a *business case* may exist if the investing entity believes that a positive indirect impact on organization function and sustainability will accrue within a reasonable time frame. (p. 18)

These arguments continue; the economic case includes the returns to all the actors, not just the individual investing business unit. The social case, as they define it, is one of measuring benefits, but not requiring positive returns on the investment. That has been overriding the consideration in the battle to control medical variation and medical errors (McGlynn, Asch, & Adams, 2003). The business case for quality improvement suffers from the same negative factors as the business case for other preventive healthcare measures—namely, all or part of the benefits accruing to other business units or patients, and delayed impacts that get discounted heavily in the reckoning (Leatherman et al., 2003). The regulatory arguments for quality improvement efforts have generally been justified on the basis of social and economic benefits such as lives saved and overall cost reductions, but these arguments are not necessarily profitable to the investor. These authors also present a whole array of public policy measures that would overcome the barriers to a positive business case and encourage wider and more assertive implementation of quality improvement methods. Clearly, economics alone does not provide an argument strongly for or against the use of CQI, but it does add to the complexity that pervades the wider and more rapid implementation of CQI in health care.

In summary, this brief overview indicates that a strong business case for CQI in health care cannot be made. Looking back over the past 40 years, Robert Brook (2010), UCLA professor of Medicine and Health Services and director of the Health Sciences Program for the RAND Corporation, observes, "Although there are some examples in the literature to support the concept that better quality of care is less expensive, few studies have produced information that could be generalized across time and institutional settings" (p. 1831). Building on the traditional business concepts that have been discussed and in consideration of the limited evidence to support the business case for CQI, a transformation that may support greater diffusion of CQI and the continuing need to bridge the quality chasm is to consider a more value-based approach to CQI in health care. This approach argues for simultaneous goals of higher quality and lower cost, which will only be achieved when there is a reorientation among CQI proponents that includes a thorough understanding of how to achieve a positive return on investment (Brook, 2010).

FACTORS ASSOCIATED WITH SUCCESSFUL CQI APPLICATIONS

Despite the need for greater diffusion of CQI in health care, much progress has been made, suggesting a broad array of factors that can be associated with successful CQI implementation. The key to greater diffusion is understanding and emphasizing those factors that do work while exploring new concepts, such as the value focus described previously. This analysis starts with motivational factors but also includes regulatory (e.g., accreditation) factors and finally organizational factors such as leadership, organizational culture, and teamwork.

Motivational Factors

A number of motivational factors contribute to the sustained interest and enthusiasm for CQI in health care. These factors have an impact on the motivation of the management of the organization and its employees. The first argument for CQI is its direct impact on quality, usually a net gain to the customer and to the employees of the organization, the external and internal customers. The second argument relates to the set of benefits associated with a plan that empowers employees in health care through participation in decision making. These factors represent benefits for employees and management that can be classified as follows.

Intrinsic motivation: The vast majority of healthcare workers support the concept of quality care and would like to see improvements and participate in a meaningful quality improvement process. Allowing personnel to work on their own processes, permitting them to "do the right thing," and then rewarding them for that behavior is almost sure to increase

intrinsic motivation in employees, if done properly. It is a classic case of job enrichment for healthcare workers.

Capturing the intellectual capital of the workforce: Industrial managers are increasingly recognizing that frontline workers know their work processes better than the management does. Therefore, management encourages workers to apply that knowledge and insight to the firm's processes. This is especially true in health care, where the professionals employed by or practicing in the institution control the technological core of the organization. Management that does not capitalize on this available pool of professional and specialized knowledge within the organization is naive at best.

Reducing managerial overhead: Some companies have been able to remove layers of management as work groups have taken responsibility for their own processes. Healthcare organizations are actually already limited in the number of staff positions, mostly because the professionals rather than the corporate staff have clinical process knowledge. Indeed, one might view the new investments in CQI as a catching-up process for the lack of process-oriented staff that are involved in process enhancement in most other industries. This is but another example of how the incentives in health care are misaligned. Because physicians are not employees in most community hospitals, they are not at risk when processes are suboptimal, unless the situation is so bad that it prompts a lawsuit.

Lateral linkages: Healthcare organizations are characterized by their many medical specialties, each organized into its own professional fiefdom. Specialization is just one response to an information overload in the organization (Galbraith, 1973). By specializing, each unit tends to learn more and more about less and less. One way to offset the effects of this specialization is to provide lateral linkages—coordinators, integrating mechanisms—to get the information moving across the organization as well as up and down the chain of command (Galbraith, 1973; Lawrence & Lorsch, 1967). So far, that has proved very difficult in healthcare institutions. CQI, however, through its use of interdisciplinary teams and its focus on a broader definition of process and system as it affects customers rather than professional groups, presents one way to establish linkages. The technology of CQI focuses as much on coordination of the change process as on its motivation. In modern medicine, as practiced in the twenty-first century, this coordination and motivation of CQI is bolstered by the need for greater coordination in medical care in general and is therefore quite natural. There is a greater emphasis on interdisciplinary care, which leads to fostering interdependence and, in turn, better teamwork, including greater employee engagement and improvements in the patient experience and the financial performance of practices (Swensen et al., 2010).

Regulatory Agencies and Accreditation

Regulatory mechanisms such as accreditation are key factors that have led to greater diffusion of CQI and will continue to do so in the future as a direct result of mandated measurement and improvement of the quality of care.

In the United States, the efforts of The Joint Commission (TJC) and CMS have led to the implementation of a series of initiatives that require hospitals to report on quality measures; after a period of strong resistance, routine reporting of key metrics is now commonplace and required for accreditation by TJC. Likewise, CMS generates extensive CQI activities and associated reporting of findings via the efforts of Quality Improvement Organizations (QIOs). QIOs represent a clear example of diffusion of CQI in health care and continue to play an important role in ensuring the highest quality of care to the 46 million beneficiaries covered by Medicare in the United States. QIOs are a clear example of diffusion, as they grew from what were in 1972 termed Professional Standards Review Organizations (PSROs). In fact, QIOs may also provide a good model for how to ensure quality in a national health plan such as that being initiated in the United States. Also, accreditation initiatives at the national and state levels have served as an impetus for CQI in public health agencies in the United States.

The processes for each of these regulatory mechanisms provide evidence for factors to be considered, as well as lessons learned, in regard to further diffusion of CQI in health care. For example, the impact of the measurement requirements has been notable. In a review published by members of TJC, this impact was described as being due to the use of robust, evidence-based measures, which link process performance and patient outcomes (Chassin, Loeb, Schmaltz, & Wachter, 2010). Despite extensive documentation of successes in the article, these authors also note the need and define a direction for further improvement, centered around process measurement. They point out that the focus of this measurement process is entirely on hospital care, leaving much to be done in regard to ambulatory care. They also note that the measures in place are process measures, not outcome measures. In the spirit of continuous improvement, they offer guidance in improving the measures that are currently in place.

Once again, this program, while not without problems, is a good model for further diffusion of CQI; early resistance to measurement no longer exists, and now the issue is more about finding the most effective measures, with little resistance from hospitals and physicians expected. In the language of diffusion of innovation, TJC has passed the early adoption stage and is now well into the institutionalization stage, at least in the hospital sector, and relative to a subset of process measures.

However, despite their optimism about the progress that has been made and the value of their proposed measurement framework, Chassin et al. (2010) close their discussion of these new accountability measures by realistically pointing out that perpetual vigilance is required to review and improve the measurement process via feedback from internal and external customers. So, a partial answer to our question of how to "fix the broken system" is provided by accreditation, and much has been accomplished, with some guidance from TJC on what to do next.

However, these comments are specific to measurement of processes in hospitals, and a more general answer is still needed to truly address the broader healthcare system and its subcomponents.

Transformational Leadership, Teamwork, and a Culture of Excellence

Throughout the history of the application of CQI, one of the most important factors associated with successful applications of CQI has been the interaction of leadership, organizational culture, and teamwork. Transformational leadership, distinguished by its reliance on vision, is a starting point and a consistent factor in motivating change and improvement. To ensure CQI, the most important role of a leader is transformation (Deming, 1993), which starts with a motivating vision that must be developed, communicated, and embraced by all in the organization, which in turn leads to high levels of commitment to the vision of change and improvement (Melum & Sinioris, 1993; Tichy & Devanna, 1986). Leaders ensure commitment to the vision by shaping a culture that not only accepts but embraces change (Balestracci, 2009; Schein, 1991). **Figure 12-1** describes the way in which this is accomplished in an organization that is dedicated to CQI and thereby defines a set of factors that are critical to the greater diffusion of CQI in health care.

The development of a vision and the commitment to that vision lead to what Deming called constancy of purpose for all in the organization, referring to a clear sense of where the organization is going or what a system is

FIGURE 12-1   Factors influencing successful CQI implementation.

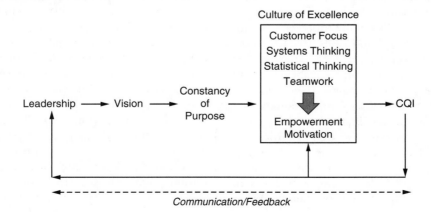

intended to accomplish (Deming, 1986). The type of culture that is needed to succeed in an organization whose goal is to continuously improve can be called a "culture of excellence." This concept is similar to a "safety culture," defined as a culture in which "a commitment to safety permeates all levels of the organization from frontline personnel to executive management" (AHRQ Patient Safety Network, 2011). Similarly, a culture of excellence is one that ensures excellence and high quality at every customer interface and in which a commitment to the highest quality—and CQI, in particular—is shared by all in the organization. Underlying the creation of a culture of excellence is a need for a systems view. A systems view of health care emphasizes the importance of adding value and the importance of leadership rather than management, influence rather than power, and the alignment of incentives focused on quality rather than quantity of services (Rouse, 2008). A culture of excellence embraces this view, is performance oriented, and at a minimum adopts a CQI philosophy. It exemplifies the following elements outlined in Figure 12-1:

Customer focus: Emphasizing the importance of both internal and external customers

Systems thinking: Maintaining a goal of optimizing the system as a whole and thereby creating synergy (Deming, 1986; Kelly, 2007)

Statistical thinking: Understanding causes of variation and the importance of learning from measurement; having the ability to use data to make decisions (Balestracci, 2009)

Teamwork: Teams of peers working together to ensure empowerment, thereby creating the highest levels of motivation to ensure alignment of the organization, the team, and the individual around the CQI vision (Grove, 1995)

Communication and feedback: Maintaining open channels of communication and feedback to make adjustments as needed, including modifying the vision to achieve higher levels of quality in a manner consistent with a learning organization (Senge, 1990), including feedback that is fact based and given with true concern for individuals' organizational success (Balestracci, 2009)

Leadership and Diffusion

In discussing factors that support the implementation of CQI, the theory of diffusion of innovation clearly supports the important role of leadership in CQI. Innovativeness, as described in the literature of organizational psychology, is seen as critically dependent on good leadership; one of the key factors to the implementation and routinization of innovation once adopted is the consultation and active involvement of leaders. Furthermore, organizational leadership is critical to the development of a culture that fosters innovation (Greenhalgh et al., 2005). CQI is a form of change and innovation that also requires cultural change driven by leadership. As Greenhalgh et al. (2005) explain, "Leaders within organizations are critical firstly in creating a cultural context that fosters innovation and secondly, establishing organizational strategy, structure, and systems that facilitate innovation" (p. 69). This perspective ties directly back to Deming's point about leadership; leaders must know and understand the processes they are responsible for and lead by example, acting as part of the improvement effort and on the "corrections" required (Deming, 1986). This point was emphasized by Gawande (2009) in describing how the initial adoption of surgical checklists was accomplished:

> Using the checklist involved a major cultural change, as well—a shift in authority, responsibility, and expectations about care—and the hospitals needed to recognize that. We gambled that their staff would be far more likely to adopt the checklist if they saw their leadership accepting it from the outset. (p. 146)

LEADERS AT ALL LEVELS

Various types of leaders can contribute to (or detract from) the innovation process. Traditional organizational and team leaders are most often associated with CQI initiatives; however, in regard to innovations, the terminology of "leader" can be expanded to include opinion leaders, champions, and boundary spanners.

Opinion leaders represent a broad range of leaders "within the ranks" as well as those at the top level. In clinical settings, opinion leaders have influence on the beliefs and actions of their colleagues, either positive or negative in regard to embracing innovation. Opinion leaders may be experts who are respected for their formal academic authority in regard to a particular innovation; their support represents a form of evidence-based knowledge. Opinion leaders may also be peers who are respected for their know-how and understanding of the realities of clinical practice (Greenhalgh et al., 2005). Unlike opinion leaders, who may support or oppose an innovation, champions persistently support new ideas. They may come from the top management of an organization, including technical or business experts. Champions include team and project leaders and others who have perseverance to fight both resistance and indifference to promote the acceptance of a new idea or to achieve project goals (Greenhalgh et al., 2005).

Boundary spanners represent a combination of these various types of leaders and are distinguished by the fact that they have influence across organizational and other boundaries (Greenhalgh et al., 2005; Kaluzny, Veney, & Gentry, 1974). Boundary spanners play an important role in multiorganizational innovations and quality improvement initiatives, such as quality improvement collaboratives. Each of these types of leaders is found in the adoption of quality improvement initiatives in health care, and often these various types of leaders are found in combination.

Teamwork

CQI in health care is a team game. These teams are composed of peers who are highly trained technical experts supporting each other and empowered to take a leadership role as required to meet the needs of customers. Teamwork is one of the most important components of all successful CQI initiatives; team building centers on the ability to create teams of empowered and motivated people who are leaders themselves and who will take the lead as needed to foster change, innovation, and improvement (Byham & Cox, 1998; Grove, 1995; Kotter, 1996). The glue that holds a culture of excellence together and that ensures there will be quality at every interface is the link between leadership and teamwork—with leadership exhibited as called for at all levels within a team. As Deming (1986) states, "There is no substitute for teamwork and good leaders of teams to bring consistency of effort along with knowledge" (p. 19).

Inherent in teamwork is a high level of empowerment of team members, which in turn leads to high levels of motivation. Empowerment implies that levels of authority match levels of responsibility and training. For example, suggestions and interventions can be made to allow improvements and prevent problems or errors; this initiative goes beyond simply allowing team members to speak up, but means providing comfort in speaking up when something seems wrong (Byham & Cox, 1998; Deming, 1986; Grove, 1995). This is illustrated in the surgical checklist example, which emphasizes that all members of the surgical team are responsible for the outcome, not just the surgeon, and all members have a role in preventing errors, which implies the empowerment to question traditional authority and take actions (Gawande, 2009).

Improved motivation is the direct result of empowerment, and both interact to lead to higher quality; but to work, these elements require another aspect of cultural change and associated leadership responsibility—building a culture of trust. Deming (1986) explains, "No one can put in his best performance unless he feels secure. . . . Secure means without fear, not afraid to express ideas, not afraid to ask questions" (p. 59). This ties directly back to the surgical checklist example as well as the airline safety tradition, where use of a checklist implies responsibility to communicate and question each other as part of the checklist process, regardless of the team member's rank. A leader's goal must be to create a culture where people are empowered to do their jobs to the best of their abilities, with trust and a clear understanding of the vision that creates the constancy of purpose needed to achieve the highest quality.

Training is critical to the success of leaders and the ability to achieve constancy of purpose, not only training of employees in the skills required to do their jobs but also training the future leaders of the organization. Training of future leaders is one of the most important responsibilities of a leader (Tichy, 1997). For example, the emphasis on quality improvement in the curriculum for the education of nurses is a critical goal to ensure that nurses, because of their close interaction with patients, can take a greater leadership role in ensuring the quality of care provided to patients and take more direct responsibility for identifying and leading, not merely participating in, quality improvement initiatives. Gawande (2009) addresses this issue in describing the process for testing and implementing the surgical safety checklist. Despite the obvious key role of the surgeon, it was decided that the "circulating nurse" on the surgery team would be the one to start the checklist process at the beginning of a surgery. This was done for several reasons, but one of the most important was "to spread responsibility and the power to question" (p. 137).

Examples of Leadership and Teamwork in CQI

The linkage between leadership and teamwork to ensure success in quality improvement in health care has been demonstrated in many instances, including the very successful implementation of quality improvement collaboratives (QICs). QICs represent a form of virtual organizations (Byrne, 1993) whose effectiveness has been demonstrated in industry for many years. Part of the success of QICs can be tied to this effective team structure. For example, in describing the successful application of a QIC using the IHI Breakthrough series (Kilo, 1998) in 40 U.S. hospitals to reduce adverse drug events, Leape et al. (2000) identify strong leadership and teamwork among their most important success factors: "Success in making significant changes was associated with strong leadership, effective processes, and appropriate choice of intervention. Successful teams were able to define, clearly state, and relentlessly pursue their aims, and then chose practical interventions and moved early into changing a process" (Greenhalgh et al., 2005, p. 165).

In summary, leadership, effective teamwork, and the empowerment of teams have been critical factors in the evolution of CQI in health care and are directly related to the pace and broad adoption of CQI in health care in recent years.

USING THE CHANGE MODEL IN CQI

A model (see Table 5-1) for making organizational changes was presented earlier in this text and can be used in the CQI process. The discussion of leadership, organizational culture, and teamwork presented previously described "what is" the type of culture that is needed to implement successful CQI initiatives. The change model describes "how to" implement major change and also provides guidance on traditional errors to avoid. These two approaches are closely related. There is clear overlap between the change model and the factors defined in Figure 12-1, which describe the culture of excellence. These common elements include empowerment, communication, feedback loops to produce more change, and, most important, the central role of vision and anchoring change in the culture.

One key point of the change model that is worthy of more discussion here is the first step. This effort relates to an earlier point about how long it takes, or should take, to implement CQI concepts. The emphasis is not that decisions should be rushed, but that complacency is to be avoided. Complacency may be due to many reasons that can be associated with the need for CQI in health care. These include, according to Kotter (1996), "too much past success, lack of visible crises, low performance standards, [and] insufficient feedback from external constituencies.... Without a sense of urgency, people won't give that extra effort that is essential. They won't make needed sacrifices. Instead they cling to the status quo and resist initiatives from above" (p. 5). This point directly relates to CQI in health care; the importance of ensuring safety and quality in health care requires a sense of urgency.

CONCLUSIONS

The factors associated with successful CQI applications have been clearly identified, from its earliest applications in industry and throughout its evolution into health care. Most notable among these factors are leadership and teamwork and their synergistic role in developing a vision that leads to a culture of excellence, embracing CQI. This has led to widespread use of CQI in health care and the emergence of a new set of leaders who lead by example, teach others, and continue to develop and expand both the philosophy and processes of CQI.

Despite the widespread use of CQI methods and a good understanding of the leadership and teamwork processes that make it work, its effectiveness and its further adoption in health care remain subjects of ongoing research and continue to meet challenges; most notably, there has been lack of documentation of substantial progress in improving quality of health care and, most importantly, reducing harm to patients (Landrigan et al., 2010; Wachter, 2010).

The literature on diffusion of innovation suggests some guidelines to understand factors that influence the adoption of CQI. Most notable is the fact that complexity inhibits further adoption, just as it does for other forms of innovation. Understanding the factors that enable or influence adoption of CQI, as well as the factors that present barriers, is particularly important as more countries around the world, including resource-poor countries, are utilizing CQI to solve health challenges and as national health plans are being modified or introduced around the world, including in the United States.

Overall, despite the need for wider diffusion of CQI in health care, current trends indicate a continuation of cross-disciplinary learning and significant interprofessional spread of CQI. So, while it is important to understand the factors that inhibit the broader use of CQI and the problems affecting the improvement in health care overall, it is more important to review what works so that others may learn. These factors and approaches illustrate how the new sectors within health care that are enthusiastically adopting the CQI philosophy and processes may improve their performance within the healthcare system.

DISCUSSION QUESTIONS _____

1. Attempt to make a business case for a continuous improvement project you would envision for your practice setting. Why was this difficult to do?

2. As a leader without formal managerial authority, you can influence change as an opinion leader, champion, or boundary spanner. Consider how you may apply each to your role in your setting.

3. Discuss the following statement: There is some evidence that although innovation may not be susceptible to being managed, it is possible to design and control organizational conditions that "enhance the possibility of innovation occurring and spreading" (Greenhalgh et al., 2005, p. 80).

REFERENCES

AHRQ Patient Safety Network. (2011). Glossary: Safety culture. Retrieved from http://psnet.ahrq .gov/popup_glossary.aspx?name=safetyculture

Arndt, M., & Bigelow, B. (1995). The implementation of total quality management in hospitals. *Health Care Management Review, 20,* 3–14.

Balestracci, D. (2009). *Data sanity: A quantum leap to unprecedented results.* Englewood, CO: Medical Group Management Association.

Berwick, D. M. (2003). Disseminating innovations in health care. *Journal of the American Medical Association, 289,* 1969–1975.

Bigelow, B., & Arndt, M. (1995). Total quality management: Field of dreams? *Health Care Management Review, 20,* 15–25.

Bosk, C. L., Dixon-Woods, M., Goeschel, C. A., & Pronovost, P. J. (2009). Reality check for checklists. *Lancet, 374,* 444–445.

Brook, R. H. (2010). The end of the quality improvement movement: Long live improving value. *Journal of the American medical Association, 304*(16), 1831–1832.

Byham, J. C., & Cox, J. (1998). *Zapp! The lightning of empowerment—how to improve quality, productivity and employee satisfaction.* New York, NY: Fawcett Ballantine.

Byrne, J. (1993). The virtual corporation. *Business Week, 3304,* 98–102.

Chassin, M. R., Loeb, J. M., Schmaltz, S. P., & Wachter, R. M. (2010). Accountability measures: Using measurement to promote quality improvement. *New England Journal of Medicine, 363,* 683–688.

Deming, W. E. (1986). *Out of the crisis.* Cambridge: Massachusetts Institute of Technology Center for Advanced Engineering Study.

Deming, W. E. (1993). *The New Economics for Industry, Government, Education.* Cambridge: Massachusetts Institute of Technology Center for Advanced Engineering Study.

de Vries, E. N., Prins, H. A., Crolla, R. M., den Outer, A. J., van Andel, G., van Helden, S. H., . . . Boermeester, M. A. (2010). Effect of a comprehensive surgical safety system on patient outcomes. *New England Journal of Medicine, 363,* 1928–1937.

Foy, R., MacLennan, G., Grimshaw, J., Penney, G., Campbell, M., & Grol, R. (2002). Attributes of clinical recommendations that influence change in practice following audit and feedback. *Journal of Clinical Epidemiology, 55,* 717–722.

Galbraith, J. (1973). *Designing complex organizations.* Reading, MA: Addison-Wesley.

Gawande, A. (2009). *The checklist manifesto.* New York, NY: Metropolitan Books.

Goldberg, H. I., Wagner, E. H., & Finh, S. D. (1998). A randomized controlled trial of CQI teams and academic detailing: Can they alter compliance with guidelines? *Joint Commission Journal of Quality Improvement, 24,* 130–142.

Greenhalgh, T. E., Robert, G., Macfarlane, F., Bate, P., & Kyriakidou, O. (2005). *Diffusion of innovations in health services organizations: A systematic review of the literature.* Oxford, England: Blackwell.

Grove, A. S. (1995). *High output management.* New York, NY: Vintage Books.

Haynes, A. B., Weiser, T. G., & Berry, W. R. (2009). A surgery safety checklist to reduce morbidity and mortality in a global population. *New England Journal of Medicine, 360,* 491–499.

Institute of Medicine. (2000). *To err is human: Building a safer health system.* Washington, DC: National Academies Press.

Institute of Medicine. (2001). *Crossing the quality chasm: A new health paradigm for the 21st century.* Washington, DC: National Academies Press.

Kaluzny, A., Veney, J. A., & Gentry, J. T. (1974). Innovation of health services: A comparative study of hospitals and health departments. *Milbank Quarterly, 52,* 51–82.

Kelly, D. L. (2007). *Applying quality management in healthcare: A systems approach* (2nd ed.). Chicago, IL: Health Administration Press.

Kilo, C. M. (1998). A framework for collaborative improvement: Lessons from the Institute for Healthcare Improvement's Breakthrough series. *Quality Management in Health Care, 6,* 1–13.

Kotter, J. P. (1996). *Leading change.* Boston, MA: Harvard Business School Press.

James, J. (2013). A new evidenced-based estimate of patient harms associated with hospital care. *Journal of Patient Safety, 9*(3), 122–128.

Landrigan, C. P., Parry, G. J., Bones, C. B., Hackbarth, A. D., Goldmann, D. A., & Sharek, P. J. (2010). Temporal trends in rates of patient harm resulting from medical care. *New England Journal of Medicine, 363*(22), 2124–2134.

Lawrence, P. R., & Lorsch, J. W. (1967). *Organization and environment.* Boston, MA: Harvard University Press.

Leape, L. L., Kabcenell, A. I., Gandhi, T. K., Carver, P., Nolan, T. W., & Berwick, D. M. (2000). Reducing adverse drug events: Lessons from a breakthrough series collaborative. *Joint Commission Journal on Quality Improvement, 26,* 321–331.

Leatherman, S., Berwick, D., Iles, D., Lewin, L. S., Davidoff, F., Nolan, T., & Bisognano, M. (2003). The business case for quality: Case studies and an analysis. *Health Affairs, 22*(2), 17–30.

Leonhardt, D. (2009, November 24). Making health care better. *New York Times,* pp. 1–14.

McGlynn, E. A., Asch, S. M., & Adams, J. (2003). The quality of health care delivered to adults in the United States. *New England Journal of Medicine, 348,* 2635–2645.

Mehta, R. H., Das, S., Tsai, T. T., Nolan, E., Kearly, G., & Eagle, K. A. (2000). Quality improvement initiative and its impact on the management of patients with acute myocardial infarction. *Archives of Internal Medicine, 160,* 3057–3062.

Melum, M. M., & Sinioris, M. K. (1993). *Total quality management—the health care pioneers.* Chicago, IL: American Hospital Publishing.

Plsek, P., & Greenhalgh, T. (2001). The challenge of complexity in health care. *British Medical Journal, 323*(7313), 625–628.

Pronovost, P., Needham, D., Berenholtz, S., Sinopoli, D., Chu, H., Cosgrove, S., . . . Goeschel, C. (2006). An intervention to reduce catheter-related bloodstream infections in the ICU. *New England Journal of Medicine, 355,* 2725–2732.

Rogers, E. (1995). *Diffusion of innovations.* New York, NY: Free Press.

Rouse, W. B. (2008). Health care as a complex adaptive system. *Bridge, 38,* 17–25.

Schein, E. H. (1991). *Organizational culture and leadership.* San Francisco, CA: Jossey-Bass.

Senge, P. (1990). *The fifth discipline: The art and practice of a learning organization.* New York, NY: Doubleday.

Shortell, S. M., Bennett, C. L., & Byck, G. R. (1998). Assessing the impact of continuous quality improvement on clinical practice: What will it take to accelerate programs. *Milbank Quarterly, 76,* 593–624.

Solberg, L. (1993). *Improving disease prevention in primary care.* AHCPR Working Paper. Washington, DC: Agency for Health Care Policy and Research.

Swensen, S. J., Meyer, G. S., Nelson, E. C., Hunt, G. C., Jr., Pryor, D. B., Weissberg, J. I., . . . Berwick, D. M. (2010). Cottage industry to postindustrial care: The revolution in health care delivery. *New England Journal of Medicine, 362,* e12(1)–e12(4).

Tichy, N. M. (1997). *The leadership engine.* New York, NY: Harper Business.

Tichy, N. M., & Devanna, M. A. (1986). *The transformational leader.* New York, NY: Wiley.

Wachter, R. M. (2010). Patient safety at ten: Unmistakable progress, troubling gaps. *Health Affairs, 29,* 165–173.

CHAPTER 13

© A-R-T/Shutterstock

Patient Safety Movement: The Progress and the Work That Remains

Manisha Shaw and Karla M. Miller

CHAPTER OBJECTIVES

1. Appreciate the historical foundation of the patient safety movement and how it has shaped current policy and practice.

2. Define a culture of safety and list the elements that support it.

3. Assess the advanced practice nurse's setting against Agency for Healthcare Research and Quality criteria for a culture of safety.

INTRODUCTION

One need only turn on the news to see that health care is still at the forefront of national consciousness.

Fifteen years after the release of the landmark Institute of Medicine (IOM) report, *To Err Is Human: Building a Safer Health System*,[1] preventable errors continue to occur, systemic frailties in every aspect of the healthcare delivery system exist, and seemingly simple solutions gain limited traction.[2] It is difficult to determine whether media coverage has caused or increased consumer concern or whether the public's desire for information prompts the media to scrutinize events more closely. What is certain is that keeping patients safe is now an expectation in health care.

Accountability to ensure safety of all patients is expected at all levels of leadership, from individual clinicians to national legislators who oversee healthcare regulations. Recent events have ensured that patient safety is never far from the minds of caregivers, patients, payers, and regulators.[2] Although advances in patient safety have been made, countless numbers of patients continue to suffer preventable medical errors. More and more attention is being paid to system issues. Wachter graded the progress from a C+ in 2004 to a B– in 2010, noting advancement in many areas such as error reporting and involvement by leaders. However, he also noted a lack of progress in areas such as health information technology and malpractice system reform.[3]

Efforts to improve patient safety are not limited to hospitals and healthcare institutions. Healthcare institutions are not the only ones coming under scrutiny; the public is growing wary of medical device manufacturers and the pharmaceutical industry. The existence of several device recall registries, the fact that often the labeling practices of drugs have been shown to be one of the root causes of many medical errors, and the fact that product recalls make the news on a regular basis attest to the fact that device malfunctions and drug safety are not isolated incidents.[4]

Much progress has been made in patient safety over the past decade. Yet, as an industry, health care has only scratched the surface. This chapter reviews the foundation of patient safety by exploring the historical events that have shaped patient safety as it is known today. We discuss critical issues that continue to gain attention. By examining the issues health care faces and the history of patient safety in the United States, we will show that a more cohesive and united effort is needed to have a meaningful effect on both quality of care and patient safety.

A HISTORY OF PATIENT SAFETY

The frequency and magnitude of avoidable adverse patient events was not well known until the 1990s, when multiple countries reported staggering numbers of patients harmed or killed by medical errors. Recognizing that healthcare errors affect 1 in every 10 patients around the world, the World Health Organization called patient safety an endemic concern.[5]

The first big step toward improving patient safety was the formation of the Institute of Medicine (IOM). Established in 1970, the IOM is the health arm of the National Academy of Sciences, chartered under President Abraham Lincoln in 1863.[6] The IOM asks and answers the nation's most pressing questions about health and health care. The Institute's goal is to provide unbiased, reliable information about health care, especially as it pertains to public health and policy. Information is furnished primarily by committees in the form of formal reports. The IOM arranges forums for sharing information and conducts its own research.[5] Information and research provided by the IOM have been invaluable for advancing the cause of patient safety. As a nonprofit, nonpartisan organization, policy makers highly regard and give considerable weight to findings from the IOM. *To Err Is Human* is one of the recognized contributions from the IOM. Additionally, because the IOM has completed numerous studies and reports on issues pertaining to patient safety, it is an excellent source of information for those advocating for safer care both at the patient and the provider levels. Many of the studies that the IOM undertakes begin as specific mandates from Congress, whereas others are requested by federal agencies and independent organizations.

The IOM tackles questions about general patient safety and quality, whereas the newer FDA MedWatch (developed in 1993) focuses more on medical products, such as medications and devices.[7] MedWatch provides medical product safety alerts, recalls, withdrawals, and important labeling changes that may affect the health of all Americans via its website and the MedWatch E-list. MedWatch allows healthcare professionals and consumers to report serious problems that they suspect are associated with the drugs and medical devices they prescribe, dispense, or use. It also has played a pivotal role in incorporating consumers into improving patient safety.

The catalyst for addressing patient safety concerns was initiated by three major publications put out by IOM: *To Err Is Human* (1999),[1] *Crossing the Quality Chasm* (2001),[8] and *Preventing*

Medication Errors (2006).[9] The first report sent shock waves through the industry and the nation by awakening everyone to the level of preventable medical errors occurring in the United States. *To Err Is Human* was the inspiration for the Institute for Healthcare Improvement's 100,000 Lives Campaign,[10] which in 2006 claimed to have prevented an estimated 124,000 deaths in a period of 18 months through patient safety initiatives in more than 3,000 hospitals. *Crossing the Quality Chasm*[8] urgently called for changes to healthcare system processes to improve patient care. It analyzed this dilemma and explored potential ways in which change could be implemented in the healthcare delivery system at all levels. These two documents were instrumental in raising patient safety awareness in health care and among policy makers. Most recent, the report *Preventing Medication Errors*[9] put forth a national agenda for reducing medication errors predicated on estimates of the incidence and cost of such errors and presented evidence on the efficacy of various prevention strategies. This report proved to be more of a call to action than were the other two, providing specific strategies for medication safety improvement rather than more general information detailing the errors in health care and specific patient safety concerns.

Efforts to improve patient safety have been made in the past, and the report built on this earlier work. In the early part of the twentieth century, two important pieces of legislation were passed: the Biologics Control Act and the Food, Drug and Cosmetics Act.[6] The former, passed in 1902, was spurred by the deaths of 13 children who had received a diphtheria vaccine. It regulated the production of biological products to ensure the safety of consumers.[8] The latter, passed in 1938, required that drugs be proven safe before being advertised to the public, set quality standards for packaged products, and authorized inspections of production facilities.[6] The importance of this legislation

cannot be overstated. Medications and vaccines are indispensable for consumer health but can do more harm than good if not properly regulated. The legislation of 1902 and 1938 set precedents for product regulation and demonstrated the willingness of the government to step in on behalf of consumers.

The next landmark event in patient safety occurred in 1951 with the founding of The Joint Commission (TJC, formerly the Joint Commission on Accreditation of Healthcare Organizations, or JCAHO).[11] At its inception, TJC provided accreditation to hospitals based on adherence to its published standards. In 1965, adherence to TJC standards became mandatory for hospitals that wished to participate in Medicare or Medicaid, ensuring compliance by even more institutions. Over time, standards became more complex, and councils were formed to oversee accreditation for mental health facilities, facilities for persons with disabilities, hospice facilities, and long-term care facilities, among others.[10] Although accreditation is an important part of its mission, TJC also conducts research on patient safety and healthcare quality, provides tools to help hospitals measure performance, and periodically issues reports on the state of patient safety.[12]

Two decades after the founding of the IOM, another critical piece of legislation was passed. The Safe Medical Devices Act was passed in 1996 and gave the FDA power to regulate the medical device industry. The law stipulates that hospitals and other healthcare providers must report and track undesirable events related to medical devices. Additionally, manufacturers must create tracking methods for each device they produce, such as a unique serial number or bar code.[13] This legislation greatly expanded the regulatory capabilities of the FDA and officially brought medical devices into the realm of patient safety concerns.

In 1994, *Error in Medicine* was published, drawing attention to the need for human factors research in the prevention of medical errors.[14]

In 1997, the National Patient Safety Foundation[15] was created with a singular mission of ensuring safe care of patients.[14] Several other organizations, such as the Agency for Healthcare Research and Quality,[16] the Institute for Healthcare Improvement (IHI),[17] and the Leapfrog Group,[18] have as central to their missions the improvement of quality and patient safety.

Although much was accomplished before *To Err Is Human* was published, the report spurred a wave of interest and action in the realm of patient safety and established it firmly as a movement rather than a collection of isolated efforts. In 2002, TJC created the National Patient Safety Goals program to help organizations target areas most in need of improvement.[19] The following year, in 2003, the National Quality Forum (NQF) published a set of guidelines called Safe Practices for Better Healthcare, an evidence-based list of 30 practices to be employed by all healthcare facilities to increase safety and quality.[20] The guidelines address topics such as safety culture, transfer of information, and medication safety and suggest ways to improve them.

Two years later, another important piece of legislation was passed, the Patient Safety and Quality Improvement Act (PSQIA) of 2005.[21] This law led to the creation of the patient safety organizations with the goal of learning from collated event data to improve patient safety. This law laid a framework in which providers and organizations could collect patient safety data without fear of legal retribution. Malpractice suits are a serious concern for healthcare organizations and providers; for them to be forthcoming about errors, a certain level of protection needed to be ensured. The PSQIA also emphasized the need for a comprehensive database of adverse safety events.[15] It is hoped that ultimately this reporting initiative will collect information in a standardized way and will be useful to compare geographic regions and track national trends.[15]

The latest development in patient safety is the creation of the Partnership for Patients program.[22] Launched in 2011, the Partnership has two main goals: to reduce patient harm in healthcare environments and to improve transitions from hospitals to less-acute care settings to lessen the rate of readmission. To accomplish these goals, the Partnership for Patients has identified nine specific areas of concentration: adverse drug events, catheter-associated urinary tract infections, central line–associated bloodstream infections, inpatient falls, adverse obstetrical events, pressure ulcers, surgical-site infection, venous thromboembolism, ventilator-associated pneumonia, plus other unspecified hospital-acquired conditions.[23] If the goals of this program are met, the federal government estimates that $35 billion and 60,000 lives could be saved over the next 3 years.[16]

The preceding organizations and legislation are testimony to the leadership and movement in patient safety. Despite the consistent efforts of many in health care, this industry continues to be faced with critical issues that have a profound effect on patient outcomes. We discuss some of these critical issues and their prevalence later in this chapter in more detail. Creating a culture of safety is considered to be the foundation for all patient safety activities and perhaps, given the tradition and hierarchy in our healthcare delivery system, has proven to be one of the most challenging issues.

CREATING A CULTURE OF SAFETY

According to the Institute of Medicine,[1] changing patient safety culture is the biggest impediment to improving outcomes. Workplace culture makes a difference in clinical outcomes. All healthcare organizations must recognize that patient safety is a top priority and make decisions based on that priority. Several omnipresent elements that support a culture of safety include a blame-free work environment, transparency, and a process designed to prevent errors. A just and fair culture of transparency is essential to empowering employees to create safe processes and improve the safety of the care they deliver. In organizations committed to patient safety, leadership must recognize patient safety as its top priority and describe the factors that must be present in an organization to support a culture of safety. Among these factors are a pervasive commitment to patient safety, which is evident in all decisions made by leadership; open communication, where everyone in the organization feels free to report potential safety concerns; a blame-free environment, where such reporting is rewarded rather than ignored; and the use of tools, techniques, and processes that have been proven to prevent future errors.

Safety culture can be defined as the set of values, beliefs, and norms about what is important, and how to behave and what attitudes are appropriate when it comes to patient safety in a work group.[24] Many organizations measure patient safety culture through the use of the Safety Attitude Questionnaire, developed by the Agency for Healthcare Research and Quality (AHRQ).

The dimensions measured by the AHRQ patient safety culture tool are as follows:

- Supervisor/manager expectations and actions promoting patient safety
- Organizational learning—continuous improvement
- Openness of communication
- Feedback and communication about errors
- Hospital management support for patient safety
- Nonpunitive response to error (blame-free environment or a *just* culture)
- Staffing
- Teamwork within units
- Teamwork across hospital units
- Hospital handoffs and transitions

The University of Texas Patient Safety Attitudes Questionnaire is also frequently used to assess safety culture. Healthcare organizations can use the survey to measure caregiver attitudes about six patient safety-related domains to compare themselves to other organizations, to prompt interventions to improve safety attitudes, and to measure the effectiveness of these interventions.[25]

Assessing the culture of patient safety allows organizations to delineate the areas where improvement is needed. At present, these are the most standardized tools available for assessing culture. It must be noted that questionnaires are somewhat subjective because they collect data on the perceptions of respondents, not on their actual activities or habits.

Currently, there are few proven interventions that have been successful in completely changing the culture of a healthcare organization. However, a nonpunitive, blame-free culture is essential as a foundation for a culture of safety.

MOST COMMON PATIENT SAFETY CONCERNS

Over the past 12 years, research specific to patient safety has accelerated, and though clearly we have yet to fully operationalize the solutions, we have a much clearer understanding of the problems. Analysis of specific event types is bringing us closer to the development of specific strategies for reducing or eliminating these patient safety risks.

Medication Errors

One of the most common preventable medical errors relates to the ordering, dispensing, preparing, and administering of medication. Medication errors injure 1.5 million people per year and amass $3.5 billion in additional healthcare costs.[8] According to the National Coordination Council for Medication Error Reporting, a medication error is any preventable event that may cause or lead to inappropriate medication use or patient harm while the medication is in the control of the healthcare professional, patient, or consumer. Such events may be related to professional practice, healthcare products, procedures, and systems, including prescribing; order communication; product labeling, packaging, and nomenclature; compounding; dispensing; distribution; administration; education; monitoring; and use.[26] An adverse medication event denotes some type of harm, from unexpected side effects to serious injury and death. Some medication errors result from patients taking their medications incorrectly, but others result from errors by healthcare providers. Examples of these errors include errors in transcription, errors in dispensing, errors in prescribing, and errors in administering drugs. Together, errors by clinicians and patients send more than 282,500 people to the emergency department each year. Of those, 98,000 are children, 177,000 are elderly, and 7,500 are middle aged.[27] Clearly, the elderly are at the most risk, but this may also be because they take the most medications and fill the most prescriptions of any age group.

Research has identified many of the reasons for medication errors, which include hard-to-read paper prescriptions, confusing labeling or packaging, unclear directions, low health literacy, and an unwillingness of patients to ask questions about their medications. Means of prevention include bar-coded medications, electronic medical records, rewriting medication directions so they are easier to understand, higher health literacy in general, and closer monitoring of at-risk groups, such as infants and the elderly. Establishing standards by which to identify and assess gaps in the medication management process is a first step to prevention of medication errors.

Hospital-Acquired Infections

Hospital-acquired infection (HAI), also referred to as a nosocomial infection, is an infection acquired during the course of treatment at a healthcare facility that was not present prior to the visit. The infection often occurs within 48 hours of admission, but infections that occur after discharge are also considered HAIs if the pathogen was acquired during the patient's stay.[28]

The World Health Organization estimates that approximately 8.7% of hospital patients worldwide have an HAI at any given time.[29] In the United States, 1 out of 20 hospitalized patients contracts an HAI and 100,000 die each year,[30] but as of 2010 only 27 states had laws requiring hospitals to report their rates of infection.[31] For patients, the cost of an HAI is high: the length of the hospital stay increases by seven to nine days and they pay $40,000 more on average. For the healthcare system as a whole, HAIs add between $4.5 billion and $5.7 billion each year to medical costs.[32] There are many types of HAIs, but the most common are central line–associated bloodstream infections, catheter-associated urinary tract infections, and ventilator-associated pneumonia. Although surgical-site infections and MRSAs (methicillin-resistant *Staphylococcus aureus*) are also grave concerns, the aforementioned infections account for more than two-thirds of all HAIs.[33]

Fortunately, HAIs are preventable. The World Health Organization (WHO)[27] and the Centers for Disease Control and Prevention (CDC)[34] recommend several steps to reduce infection: hand washing of the proper length and frequency, proper cleaning and sterilization of the patient's environment, proper staff attire, and reduction of unnecessary injections and surgical procedures.[35] It has been demonstrated through clinical research that strict adherence to these recommendations has the potential to prevent infections or reduce infection rates to extremely low levels. Ensuring that the recommendations are followed correctly and uniformly, however, has proved difficult.

Surgical-Site Errors

Surgical-site errors result in procedures being performed on the wrong site, correct procedures performed on the wrong person, incorrect procedures being performed at a site, and procedures that are more invasive than intended or necessary. Causes vary, but some are cited by TJC as risk factors because of their prevalence in cases where wrong-site surgeries have occurred. These include time constraints (caused by emergency surgery or a full schedule), room or staffing changes, multiple procedures being performed, and patient characteristics, such as obesity or physical deformities, that prompted a change in operating room setup.[36]

Wrong-site surgeries, though uncommon, are preventable. Between 1995 and 2010, 956 wrong-site incidents were reported to The Joint Commission.[37] However, these numbers are believed to represent only 10% of actual occurrences because reporting to TJC is voluntary.[34] One study surveyed surgical procedures from 28 hospitals and found the incidence of wrong-site surgeries to be approximately 1 in 112,994 procedures. For the average hospital, this means one error every 5 to 10 years. This study also surveyed the costs of these incidents to the hospitals. The median payment to the patient was $12,000, and the cost of defense was $1,500, for a total of $13,500 per case on average.[38]

To address the problem of surgical-site errors, The Joint Commission chaired a summit that produced the "Universal Protocol for Preventing Wrong Site, Wrong Procedure, and Wrong Person Surgery." The Protocol makes three central recommendations to prevent errors: a preprocedure verification, marking the procedure site clearly, and taking a time-out before the surgery to conduct a final check.[34]

Device Malfunctions

According to the Food and Drug Administration (FDA), a medical device is any object used for the diagnosis, prevention, or treatment of disease in humans or animals.[39] The device can be internal or external but excludes substances metabolized by the body, commonly known as drugs or pharmaceuticals.[40] A device malfunction is any function of a device that causes harm or is unintended even if the patient is not injured. Adverse events of this type are required

to be reported to the FDA because its Center for Devices and Radiological Health oversees the regulation of medical devices. Unfortunately, not all adverse events are reported, and of those reported, the FDA releases information only about products that could cause patients to be seriously injured or to die. In the year 2011, 27 such press releases were issued by the FDA in addition to those done by the manufacturers themselves.[41] In almost all cases, recalls are initiated by the company and completed voluntarily; the difficulty lies in getting information about recalled items out to the affected consumers.

Error in Diagnosis

Misdiagnosis is of serious concern to both patients and their doctors. Besides the cost in patient lives, misdiagnosis—defined as an incorrect diagnosis, an incomplete diagnosis, errors in testing, and mishandling of lab or diagnostic test data—places heavy financial costs on the healthcare system. In 2004 alone, $4.2 billion was paid out for malpractice lawsuits, and of these, the vast majority were brought for misdiagnosis or failure to diagnose.[42] The threat of misdiagnosis and its aftermath keeps malpractice insurance premiums and healthcare costs high. The possibility of such a suit is particularly high for primary care physicians because they are often the first healthcare providers patients present to deal with a problem. The primary care physician is often responsible for the patient's course of care.

The effects on patients are even more sobering because early detection and a proper course of treatment are crucial for fighting chronic conditions such as cancer, diabetes, asthma, and other autoimmune disorders. Meta-analyses have shown the diagnostic error rate to be between 4.1% and 49.8%, with 4% of cases displaying preventable, lethal errors. Diagnostic error is difficult to study, however, because it often goes undetected or unreported.[43] Present studies rely heavily on autopsy findings and malpractice suits for data, which is problematic because such methods preferentially select for a population that has already been seriously harmed by errors. Nonetheless, the effects of diagnostic error—poor prognoses, lost productivity, increase in costs for patients and healthcare systems—are known, but the scope and prevalence are yet to be determined.

THE IMPACT OF LITERACY ON PATIENT SAFETY

It is well acknowledged that informed patients make better decisions. The ability to obtain and analyze information pertaining to health and wellness is called health literacy. Health literacy is necessary to navigate the healthcare system and to make decisions about one's health care; unfortunately, many Americans have low health literacy. This has negative consequences for patient safety for several reasons. First, patients with low health literacy are more likely to misunderstand medical instructions or ignore advice from their doctors. This can lead to adverse medication events, a worsening of medical conditions, and repeat visits to the hospital for the same problem. Second, patients with low health literacy are less likely to speak up or ask a question when something is amiss, which removes a source of protection against clinician errors.

Finally, patients with low health literacy incur more costs than do those with high literacy. This places an additional strain on already strapped health systems and diverts money from improvement initiatives.[44]

Health literacy is recognized as an important facet of patient safety, and improvements are already under way. Centers for health literacy have been created as a part of existing organizations and as free-standing groups. With these centers has come the position of consumer health librarian, an individual who creates community partnerships and teaches people to access and understand health information. Another point of focus is on making healthcare materials—prescription information, device recalls, and websites—simpler and easier to understand. Most sources of healthcare information are written at a college level, and many Americans' reading comprehension is below this. Advocates hope that by conducting outreach and making materials more accessible, the public can make better healthcare decisions.[42]

MAKING CARE SAFER THROUGH RESEARCH

It is impossible to overstate the importance of research to patient safety. One can speculate about the causes and consequences of medical errors, but scientific research provides a more concrete basis for large-scale changes in law and policy. Research also helps solve problems because it can answer questions about the nature, scope, and prevalence of an issue, as well as determine whether a certain process or policy is effective at preventing error. From preliminary investigations to meta-analyses, research is helping to improve patient safety. There is still much to be done, however. The importance of research for patient safety is well recognized, but the resources are limited. A large amount of research has been done, but there are still questions left to be answered and future projects that will require analysis.

EMERGING TRENDS

As an industry, health care is testing new tools to help improve patient safety. Risk management has historically focused on ameliorating damage once it occurs and minimizing legal retributions. Safety officers and risk management experts are focusing more on prevention as a result of the new emphasis on patient safety, being proactive and learning from close calls and near misses. Sharing these outcomes is imperative to improving the safe care of patients.

Many industries have identified teamwork as a critical factor in developing a culture of safety. Rather than praising clinicians exclusively for their individual skills and encouraging them to solve problems on their own, healthcare systems are emphasizing teamwork skills as important for clinical outcomes and preventing medical errors. Utilizing skills from other industries, healthcare facilities have made team building an important tool. Working in teams puts an emphasis on an interdisciplinary approach to providing care to patients. Instead of working in silos, the emphasis is on collaborative care among physicians, patients, and the entire healthcare team.

Before the patient safety movement, responsibility for medical errors was considered to be solely the clinician's. Slowly, this mindset is changing and there is a realization that breakdowns in the system are to be blamed for most medical errors.

TECHNOLOGY

From electronic health records to palm-scanning devices, many believe that new technology can help prevent medical errors. The Obama administration passed the Health Information Technology for Economic and Clinical Health (HITECH) Act as part of the stimulus bill, demonstrating its support of health information technology (HIT) as a means of addressing quality and cost issues.[45] The government has allocated $19.2 billion to motivate increased use of electronic health records, which in turn shall improve the processes of healthcare delivery documentation and record keeping for safer care. However, there is skepticism too that the lack of a completely integrated health information technology system is a risk to patient safety. The infrastructure does not allow for the plethora of systems to seamlessly integrate data, hence creating a gap in the patient record. An infrastructure to enable multiple care settings and systems to integrate data is the key to safer care.

CONCLUSIONS: WHERE WE STAND TODAY

Improving patient safety is a daunting task, not least of all because the well-being of millions is at stake. Most can agree on the importance of keeping patients safe, but the agreement often ends there. There is a plethora of proposed solutions, and we continue to search for solutions that will be accepted by all stakeholders. Compounding the problem is the fact that the body of knowledge gleaned from research is not always consistent. It varies tremendously in source, scope, and reliability. This is in part due to the nature of what we are trying to study—behavior is intensely subjective both for the performer and the observer—and in part because different research groups are seeking different results. It is commonly understood that being observed changes the nature of an action and that the way in which a question is phrased determines the nature of the answer received. Therefore, the different interests of stakeholder groups create different understandings of patient safety and different ideas about what action is necessary. The problem of patient safety can be stated thus: the pursuit of an understanding of the full scope of the problem and exact solutions remains a work in progress.

Despite these hurdles, the patient safety movement has made great strides. The central issues have been identified, which means that the healthcare industry now has a direction in which to focus in terms of research and policy developments. The system-level weaknesses are evident; now the industry must agree on concrete solutions for conditions to change considerably. Additionally, there is a growing realization across different sectors that everyone has a stake in and responsibility for patient safety. There is an increasing emphasis on patient safety in areas such as patient engagement, health literacy, medication management, safer devices, and prevention of healthcare-acquired infections and hospital-acquired conditions. This development shows that different sectors of the healthcare industry are beginning to consider their roles in improving safety and understand how critical it is at each system juncture.

Creating change is always difficult. For all striving to create a sustainable culture of safety, the following provides a solid foundation. The inaugural meeting of the Lucian Leape Institute (LLI) at the National Patient Safety Foundation (NPSF) cast the vision for the transformation of the healthcare delivery system by proposing five key areas: transparency, care integration, consumer engagement, restoration of joy and meaning in work, and medical education reform.[46] Stakeholders must be honest with themselves about shortcomings and must be willing to compromise with one another to make the necessary changes. It won't be easy, but with acceptance of the problem, transparency, cultural evolution, and a blame-free environment, patient safety will improve drastically.

DISCUSSION QUESTIONS

1. Using the dimension used on the AHRQ survey of patient safety culture, discuss how your practice setting is performing on each, its strengths, and where improvement is needed.

2. Of the most common patient safety concerns discussed in this chapter, which are most pertinent to your practice setting?

3. What preventative, proactive measures might you take to ensure patient safety in your setting?

REFERENCES

1. Kohn LT, Corrigan JM, Donaldson MS, eds. *To Err Is Human: Building a Safer Health System*. Committee on Quality of Health Care in America, Institute of Medicine. Washington, DC: National Academy Press; 2000.

2. Partnerships for Patients. Available at: http://partnershipforpatients.cms.gov. Accessed September 30, 2014.

3. Wachter RM. Patient safety at ten: unmistakable progress, troubling gaps. *Health Aff (Millwood)*. 2010;29(1):165–173.

4. US Food and Drug Administration. List of device recalls. Available at: http://www.fda.gov/MedicalDevices/Safety/RecallsCorrections Removals/ListofRecalls/default.htm. Accessed September 30, 2014.

5. World Alliance for Patient Safety. Available at: http://www.who.int/patientsafety/worldalliance/en.

6. National Institutes of Health. A short history of the National Institutes of Health: biologics. Available at: http://history.nih.gov/exhibits/history/docs/page_03.html. Accessed September 30, 2014.

7. US Food and Drug Administration. Significant dates in U.S. food and drug law history. Available at: http://www.fda.gov/AboutFDA/WhatWeDo/History/Milestones/ucm128305.htm. Accessed September 30, 2014.

8. Institute of Medicine, Committee on Quality of Health Care in America. *Crossing the Quality Chasm: A New Health System for the 21st Century*. Washington, DC: National Academy Press; 2001.

9. Institute of Medicine. *Preventing Medication Errors*. Quality Chasm Series; July 2006. Available at: http://www.iom.edu/~/media/Files/Report%20Files/2006/Preventing-Medication-Errors-Quality-Chasm-Series/medicationerrorsnew.pdf.

10. Institute for Healthcare Improvement. About us. Available at: http://www.ihi.org/about/Pages/InnovationsContributions.aspx.

11. The Joint Commission. *The Joint Commission History*. Available at: http://www.jointcommission.org/assets/1/6/Joint_Commission_History.pdf. Accessed September 30, 2014.

12. The Joint Commission. Facts about The Joint Commission. Available at: http://www.jointcommission.org/facts_about_the_joint_commission/. Accessed September 30, 2014.

13. Alder HC. Safe Medical Devices Act: management guidance for hospital compliance with the new FDA requirements. *Hosp Technol Ser*. 1993;12(11):1.

14. Leape LL. Error in medicine. *JAMA*. 1994;272(23):1851–1857.

15. National Patient Safety Foundation. Mission and vision. Available at: http://www.npsf.org/about-us/mission-and-vision. Accessed September 30, 2014.

16. Agency for Healthcare research and Quality. Mission and budget. Available at: http://www.ahrq.gov/cpi/about/mission/index.html. Accessed September 30, 2014.

17. Institute for Healthcare Improvement. About us. Available at: http://www.ihi.org/about/pages/default.aspx. Accessed September 30, 2014.

18. The Leapfrog Group. About Leapfrog. Available at: http://www.leapfroggroup.org/about_leapfrog. Accessed September 30, 2014.

19. The Joint Commission. *2011 Hospital National Patient Safety Goals.* Available at: http://www.jointcommission.org/assets/1/6/HAP_NPSG_6-10-11.pdf. Accessed September 30, 2014.

20. Agency for Healthcare Research and Quality. *Safe Practices for Better Health Care Fact Sheet.* AHRQ Publication No. 05-P007. Rockville, MD: Agency for Healthcare Research and Quality; March 2005.

21. The Patient Safety and Quality Improvement Act of 2005. Available at: http://www.ahrq.gov/qual/psoact.htm. Accessed September 30, 2014.

22. The Health Foundation. *Making Care Safer.* London, England: Health Foundation; 2011. Available at: http://www.health.org.uk/public/cms/75/76/313/2568/Making%20care%20safer.pdf?realName=SWOwwl.pdf. Accessed September 30, 2014.

23. Partnerships for Patients. Available at: http://partnershipforpatients.cms.gov. Accessed September 30, 2014.

24. Nieva VF, Sorra J. Safety culture assessment: A tool for improving patient safety in healthcare organizations. *Qual Saf Health Care.* 2003;12:ii17–ii23.

25. Sexton JB, Helmreich RL, Neilands TB, et al. The Safety Attitudes Questionnaire: psychometric properties, benchmarking data, and emerging research. *BMC Health Services Res.* 2006;6:44. doi:10.1186/1472-6963-6-44.

26. National Coordinating Council for Medication Error Reporting and Prevention. What is a medication error? Available at: http://www.nccmerp.org/aboutMedErrors.html. Accessed September 30, 2014.

27. Hafner JW, Belknap SM, Squillante MD, Buchelit KA. Adverse drug events in emergency department patients. *Ann Emerg Med.* 2002;39(3):258–267.

28. Custodio HT. Hospital-acquired infections. Medscape; 2014. Available at: http://emedicine.medscape.com/article/967022-overview. Accessed September 30, 2014.

29. World Health Organization. About WHO. Available at: http://www.who.int/about/en. Accessed September 30, 2014.

30. Healthcare-associated infections: the burden. Available at: http://www.who.int/gpsc/country_work/burden_hcai/en. Accessed September 30, 2014.

31. National Conference of State Legislatures. Methicillin-resistant *Staphylococcus aureus* (MRSA) and other healthcare-associated infections. Available at: http://www.ncsl.org/default.aspx?tabid=14084. Accessed September 30, 2014.

32. de Lissovoy G, Fraeman K, Hutchins V, Murphy D, Song D, Vaughn B. Surgical site infection: incidence and impact on hospital utilization and treatment costs. *Am J Infect Control.* 2009;37:5:387–397.

33. Centers for Disease Control and Prevention. Healthcare-associated infections: types of healthcare-associated infections. Available at: http://www.cdc.gov/HAI/infectionTypes.html. Accessed September 30, 2014.

34. Centers for Disease Control and Prevention. Healthcare Infection Control Practices Advisory Committee (HICPAC). Available at: http://www.cdc.gov/hicpac/pubs.html. Accessed September 30, 2014.

35. Ducel G, Fabry J, Nicolle L, eds. *Prevention of Hospital-Acquired Infections: A Practical Guide.* 2nd ed. Geneva, Switzerland: World Health Organization; 2002.

36. Mulloy DF, Hughes RG. Wrong-site surgery: a preventable medical error. In: Hughes RG, ed. *Patient Safety and Quality: An Evidence-Based Handbook for Nurses.* Rockville, MD: Agency for Healthcare Research and Quality Publishing; 2008:chap. 36.

37. The Joint Commission. Total number of sentinel events. Available at: http://www.jointcommission.org/assets/1/18/Stats_with_all_fields_hidden30September2010_(2).pdf. Accessed September 30, 2014.

38. Kwaan MR, Studdert D, Zinner M, Gawande A. Incidents, patterns and prevention of wrong-site surgery. *Arch Surg.* 2006;141:353–358.

39. US Food and Drug Administration. Is the product a medical device? Available at: http://www.fda.gov/MedicalDevices/DeviceRegulationandGuidance/Overview/ClassifyYourDevice/ucm051512.htm?utm_campaign=Google2&utm_source. Accessed September 30, 2014.

40. US Food and Drug Administration. Is the product a medical device? Available at: http://www.fda.gov/MedicalDevices/DeviceRegulationandGuidance/Overview/ClassifyYourDevice/ucm051512.htm?utm_campaign=Google2&utm_source. Accessed September 30, 2014.

41. US Food and Drug Administration. List of device recalls. Available at: http://www.fda.gov/Medi calDevices/Safety/RecallsCorrectionsRemovals /ListofRecalls/default.htm. Accessed September 30, 2014.

42. McDonald C, Hernandez MB, Gofman Y, Schreier W. The five most common misdiagnoses: a meta-analysis of autopsy and malpractice data. *Internet J Fam Prac.* 7(2). Available at: http://ispub .com/IJFP/7/2/5537. Accessed September 30, 2014.

43. Pennsylvania Patient Safety Authority. Diagnostic error in acute care. *Pa Patient Saf Advis.* 2010;7(3):76–86. Available at: http://www .patientsafetyauthority.org/ADvISORIES /AdvisoryLibrary/2010/Sep7(3)/Pages/76.aspx. Accessed September 30, 2014.

44. National Network of Libraries of Medicine. Health literacy. Available at: http://nnlm.gov /outreach/consumer/hlthlit. Accessed September 30, 2014.

45. Health Information Technology for Economic and Clinical Health (HITECH) Act, 42 USC §300jj (2009).

46. Leape L, Berwick D, Clancy C, et al. Lucian Leape Institute at the National Patient Safety Foundation. Transforming healthcare: a safety imperative. *Qual Saf Health Care.* 2009;18(6):424–428.

CHAPTER 14

Accelerating Patient Safety Improvement

Thomas R. Krause and John Hidley

CHAPTER OBJECTIVES

1. Discuss the benefits and challenges of implementing a mandatory standard of patient safety performance.
2. Consider specific interventions to improve the healthcare workplace and the safety of workers and patients.
3. Discuss the need for organizational cultures of safety in healthcare organizations.

INTRODUCTION

In this chapter, we argue that despite much activity, patient safety improvement has been surprisingly sluggish, and we describe an integrated strategic policy designed to accelerate improvement. The approach has three concurrent components: (1) establish a mandatory standard of patient safety performance that is valid, reliable, and universal in its application; (2) initiate specific interventions to improve the healthcare workplace and the safety of workers and patients; and (3) upgrade the knowledge and skills of healthcare leaders and workers to build organizational cultures of safety.

To pick up the pace of patient safety progress, execution of all three components is essential. To execute just one or two leaves gaps in reporting, gaps in safe and productive work environments, or gaps in cultural imperatives.

SLOW PROGRESS

At a recent conference for healthcare board members and CEOs, one of the conference organizers—a physician and CEO of one of the largest healthcare organizations in the United States—said the following: "My father is having surgery in the next month. I will be at the hospital and in his room because I fear that he will not receive the optimal care he deserves. I do not fear for his medical condition or the ability of his doctors to treat it, but I do fear for his safety in the hospital."

This is not an exceptional point of view among healthcare workers. The year 2009 marked the 10-year anniversary of the groundbreaking *To Err Is Human* report, published by the U.S. Academy of Sciences' Institute of Medicine (IOM).[1] The milestone report triggered assessments of how the healthcare industry has responded to the 1999 report's call for a national effort to reduce medical errors. Frustration, disappointment, and concern are the major findings:

- Lucian Leape et al.[2] laments that "the slow progress is not for want of trying."
- The Consumers Union[3] summarizes the situation this way: "Ten years later, we don't know if we've made any real progress, and efforts to reduce the harm caused by our medical care system are few and fragmented."
- Stevens[4] says that health care is running out of excuses and notes that "the prescription from . . . patient safety leaders . . . seems to collide with inertia that defies explanation."

The picture is not entirely bleak. Perhaps Wachter's[5] is the most positive of the progress reports. He writes that patient safety at the 10-year mark has made "unmistakable progress," and he gives "safety efforts a grade of B–, a modest improvement since 2004 (the five-year anniversary)." He specifically praises The Joint Commission for developing its National Patient Safety Goals, the National Quality Forum for developing its *never events* list as the scaffolding for more robust and insightful reporting systems, and the 27 states that now require hospitals to report never events.

Wachter mentions other significant milestones as well:

- In 2004 the World Health Organization formed the World Alliance for Patient Safety (later renamed WHO Patient Safety).

- The Institute for Healthcare Improvement launched two massive nationwide campaigns to promote the use of patient safety interventions.
- The U.S. Congress authorized the creation of patient safety organizations to promote voluntary error reporting.
- The *New England Journal of Medicine* published the Michigan ICU study, which demonstrated significant reductions in catheter-related bloodstream infections through the use of an observation checklist and other interventions.
- In 2008 Medicare initiated its *no pay for errors* policy, the first use of the payment system to promote patient safety.

But note that most of these accomplishments are at the governmental level and have yet to drive universal patient safety improvement at the level of the individual healthcare institution, be it the system, hospital, or private practice.

Perhaps the intervention that has produced the most widespread benefit at the level of individual hospital practice is The Joint Commission's ongoing endeavor to institute and improve performance measures. In The Joint Commission's 2010 annual report on quality and safety,[6] substantial improvement is apparent among The Joint Commission accredited hospitals in their performance of their 24 accountability measures. Although these process measures represent only a narrow slice of patient safety exposure—they cover only five issues—the improvement they demonstrate is real. Nevertheless, the report also indicates that improvement is uneven and concludes that more improvement is needed.

One issue may be that hospital CEOs are not always comfortable in their role as patient safety leaders. A 2008 survey of hospital CEOs found few "feel strongly confident about practices in place to prevent or manage" patient safety incidents.[7] Seventy percent of the CEOs agreed that consumer concerns about safety in hospitals are justified and that very few patient safety interventions have focused on educating CEOs.

To summarize, although effort is being expended to improve patient safety, progress is slow. Too many healthcare institutions are deficient in the cultural values needed for patient safety improvement: mutual respect, teamwork, and transparency.[2] Healthcare leaders are far too timid about organizational cultural transparency. Workforce and training issues have been "surprisingly inert in recent years," and progress in nursing safety has been "surprisingly sparse."[8] These problems have resulted in calls to accelerate what Leape et al. describe as "sputtering progress."[2]

GETTING IN GEAR

Leaders understand the need for patient safety improvement. What is hard to understand is why change is so slow in coming. One way to understand this sluggish response is that broad societal norms implicitly condone the status quo, norms such as those manifested in comments like these:[9]

- The so-called patient safety crisis is exaggerated; we don't have a problem here.
- Health care is not like other industries; what works there won't necessarily work here.
- Medicine is an art; you can't just impose cookbook solutions.
- There may be a problem, but fixing it is not my job.
- The problem is complex and needs more study.
- We are already doing everything we can.
- Some adverse events are unavoidable.

To get beyond the status quo requires both healthcare and policy leadership committed to improvement. Leaders in other industries know that leaders create culture and what gets measured gets done. These truisms lead to three practical recommendations for shifting patient safety improvement into high gear:

(1) establish a mandatory standard of patient safety performance that is valid, reliable, and universal in its application; (2) initiate specific interventions to improve the safety of workers and patients and the healthcare workplace; and (3) upgrade the knowledge and skills of healthcare leaders and workers to build organizational cultures of safety.

All three components of this approach are essential and should be implemented concurrently. As previously noted, utilizing only one or two would leave gaps in reporting, safe and productive work environments, or cultural imperatives. Nevertheless, urgency is such that no one component should wait on the others.

The rationale for this strategy rests on three principles:

1. A mandatory, universal, and publicly accessible patient safety performance reporting metric, parallel in concept to the U.S. Bureau of Labor Statistics' annual report on workplace injuries and illnesses, will set the bar for driving improvement in both patient safety and worker safety.

2. Emphasizing the well-being of healthcare workers and their work conditions will engage workers in the effort and create needed consistency in safety climate and culture, at the same time improving quality of care and patient safety.[10]

3. Although the first two prongs of this strategy underwrite the development of a culture that fosters patient safety, building culture requires skills, knowledge, and abilities that local leaders may not have.

The use and ultimate success of this approach depends on the willingness of healthcare and policy leaders to confront and correct these issues:

- The lack of a nationally mandated, universal metric for patient safety performance[3] forfeits the meaningful context within which to drive patient safety performance.

- Health care is plagued by high rates of work injuries and illnesses, particularly back injuries and falls. These produce absences from work or restricted duty and affect operations, organizational culture, quality of care, and patient safety.[11]

- Barriers exist to institutional and physician commitment to patient safety, such as the absence of strong market incentives, lack of a budget line item for patient safety, lack of reimbursement to physicians for time spent on patient safety, vague guidelines about what constitutes a patient safety activity, insufficient physician and/or administrator buy-in regarding the magnitude of the problem, and malpractice liability concerns and the litigious culture of blame that has a chilling effect on error reporting.[12]

A UNIVERSAL METRIC FOR PATIENT SAFETY

The 1999 Institute of Medicine's (IOM) report, *To Err Is Human*, propelled medical errors into the spotlight of public and policy-maker awareness. Among the report's strong recommendations was the proposal to create a mandatory reporting system for medical adverse events.[1] Today, variability remains rampant in the quality and utility of the healthcare safety measures used across geographic locations and delivery institutions.[13,14] There is no mandatory reporting system. We believe the lack of adequate metrics is a major impediment to patient safety progress and will remain so, absent a mandatory, standardized performance statistic.

Contrast this circumstance to the same need for standardization and benchmarking in almost any manufacturing, agricultural, maritime, construction, or service industry. Companies are required under the 1970 Occupational Safety and Health Act[15] to maintain a standard log and are periodically surveyed for their employee illness and injury statistics. These data encompass work-related deaths, injuries, and illnesses.

When the Department of Labor's Bureau of Labor Statistics (BLS) was delegated responsibility for developing this employee safety measurement system, it was not obvious how different types of injuries should be categorized and summarized. How should the severity of different types of injuries be handled? How should the variance in exposure between and within industries be dealt with? Many factors can influence counts and rates of injuries and illnesses in a given year.[15] Variability includes not only the year's injury and illness experience but also employer understanding of record-keeping guidelines. The number of injuries and illnesses reported in a given year can also be affected by changes in the level of economic activity, working conditions and practices, and worker demographics, experience, and training.

Despite such obstacles—which are notably similar to those faced today in patient safety—a system was developed and successfully implemented. Neither the inherent difficulty of this task nor difficulties due to variability of the data have impeded private industry's acceptance and use of the data. Today, information collected under this system is valued by industry, policy makers, the safety community, and employees.

The effect of the employee health and safety record-keeping and reporting mandate can be viewed in historical terms. From 1940 to 1970, work-related injury rates improved 45%, but after the creation of the Occupational Safety and Health Administration and its record-keeping requirements, rates improved by 75% from 1970 to 2000.[16] The earlier period saw a 42% improvement in work-related fatalities, but the subsequent OSHA-led period bested that with 78% improvement.[17]

Incidence rates permit comparison and fair competition in safety performance. Rates express various injury and illness events in terms of a constant: hours of exposure to the work environment (for example, 200,000 employee hours or the equivalent of 100 full-time employees working for one year). This creates a common statistical base across industries regardless of size or level of activity.[15] Rates are also useful for trending safety performance over time and comparing geographic variations in an industry's safety record.

National and state policy makers use the survey as an indicator of the magnitude of occupational safety and health problems. OSHA uses the statistics to help determine which industries clearly need to improve safety programs. The agency annually sends approximately 15,000 letters to workplaces with the highest rates of severe injuries and illnesses, namely, those resulting in days away from work, restricted work activities, or job transfers. This metric is known as the DART rate. Employers receiving the letters are provided copies of their injury and illness data, along with a list of the most frequently cited OSHA standards for their specific industry. The letter offers assistance in reducing workplace injuries and illnesses by suggesting, among other things, the use of OSHA's free safety and health consultation services for small businesses provided through the states.[18]

OSHA also uses the data for targeted industry- or hazard-specific inspection programs, called national emphasis programs (NEP) and regional/local emphasis programs (REPs/LEPs). In July 2009, OSHA was operating seven NEPs focusing on amputations, lead, crystalline silica, shipbreaking, trenching/excavations, petroleum refinery process safety management, and combustible dust. OSHA also conducted approximately 140 REPs/LEPs.[19]

Within organizations, both labor and management use the estimates in evaluating safety programs. The log serves as an important source of information for employees regarding the safety and healthfulness of their workplace. OSHA requires that employees have direct access to the log and that companies post the summary of injuries and illnesses by February 1 of each year.[20] Other users include insurance carriers involved in workers' compensation, industrial hygienists, manufacturers of safety equipment, researchers, and others concerned with job safety and health.[15]

Within the industrial safety world these measures are viewed as essential. They provide support for or directly enable the following:[21,22]

- Distinguishing safety approaches that work from those that do not
- Tracking progress over time
- Pinpointing the effect on safety performance of organizational and process changes
- Analyzing cost–benefit performance
- Making judicious use of scarce resources
- Gaining and maintaining employee, management, and leadership support
- Pinpointing incidents that require further investigation and prioritizing issues that require attention
- Benchmarking with others with similar exposures and issues
- Supporting safety accountability processes

Health care likewise needs a mandatory metric to drive patient safety improvement and enable benchmarking.[1] We believe a widely shared patient safety metric will facilitate fair patient safety accountability and vigorous comparison and competition across organizations, just as the BLS data have generated for employee safety and health. We need the metric so we can set patient safety targets and create plans and budgets to achieve them, just like we do in occupational safety and health. We need it to measure progress, both within healthcare institutions and between them. And the metric needs to be mandatory. The IOM recognized that practitioners might be reluctant to voluntarily report medical mistakes. At the time of the IOM report, underutilization was a recognized, serious problem for error-reporting programs,[23] and in many institutions underreporting remains a serious problem today.

In the face of the missing mandatory metric, delivery organizations that are serious about improving patient safety improvise, but improvisation generates a hodgepodge of indicators that defy performance comparison across and within organizations, and fails to provide the many benefits of a standard metric described previously. These measures range from simple incident counts to complex dashboards that allow for the aggregation and trending of data over time.

The mandatory metric for patient safety should be a simple set of standard outcome measures. An outcome metric is one that quantifies performance against the desired end result. Profit is an example of a financial outcome measure. One could not successfully operate a business without a measure of profit. Patient outcome measures are what the public needs to judge performance and what institutions need to drive performance and to develop and maintain a clear picture of their standing among peer organizations.[24] The rate of sentinel events is an example of a patient safety outcome metric. The sentinel event rate and several other measures like it should be standardized and mandated. Doing this properly requires refining a taxonomy for adverse events with operational definitions and classification decision rules. Considerable work in this direction has already been accomplished. For example, excellent work has been done to develop chart-auditing protocols (trigger tools) that result in reliable incident counts for specific types of adverse events. Although time consuming and resource intensive when performed manually, this method can be automated in systems that use electronic health records, and it provides the raw incident data from which standard event rates can be computed.[25]

HEALTHCARE WORKER SAFETY

Employee safety metrics already exist and are well tested in industry to quantify how well the organization performs on dimensions of worker safety outcomes. Health care, like all industries, tracks these measures. But, unlike other industries, health care does not use them effectively to drive organizational improvement.[10]

Access to health care is a recognized problem in the industry. There is increasing recognition that patient safety performance and access to health care are linked through healthcare worker well-being. Both the access problem and patient safety difficulties are compounded by staff shortages due to morale problems and time lost to injuries, illness, and long-term disability, as well as by the increased demands on staff of quarantines for hospital-acquired infections.[10]

Joseline Sikorski, president and CEO of the Ontario Safety Association for Community and Healthcare (OSACH), states:[26]

> The health care sector must make a fundamental shift to equate worker safety with patient safety. It must also make this shift a strategic priority if it is to deliver exemplary patient care and ensure the health and safety of workers, patients and the public. Failure to do so puts the sector at risk and makes it vulnerable to crises.

In the United States, more than three-quarters of respondents in a 2001 survey conducted by the American Nurses Association indicated that unsafe conditions interfere with nurses' ability to deliver high-quality care.[27] Bureau of Labor Statistics data on healthcare worker safety underline the extent of the problem and highlight the need to focus time and resources on employee health and safety. In 2008, hospitals had a total recordable incidence rate of 7.6 cases per 100 equivalent full-time workers. That is double the national average for all of private industry (which is only 3.9 cases).[19] The total recordable case rate for nursing and residential care facilities is even higher: 8.4 cases per 100 full-time workers.

Moreover, injuries and illnesses in health care are more serious than in other industries. The DART rate (injuries requiring days away from work or job restriction or transfer) for hospital employees is 3.0 per 100 workers compared to only 2.0 for workers in other industries. For nursing and residential care facilities, the

DART rate is 5.0. Nursing aides, orderlies, and attendants suffered more DART cases (44,610) in 2008 than construction workers (31,310) and required a median of five days to recuperate. This clearly represents a substantial unnecessary drain on staffing.

Of particular concern in health care are injuries involving musculoskeletal disorders (MSD). Healthcare support occupations were one of seven occupational categories with an MSD-related DART case rate three times greater than the all-worker rate. Among healthcare workers, MSD cases relating to the back caused on average 5 lost workdays; the shoulder, 8; the arm, 8; the wrist, 6; and the knee, 11. Lifts and transfers of patients using awkward postures, adverse psychosocial aspects of work such as high job demands with low decision authority and job control, and low social support and low job satisfaction at work are all deemed to contribute.[10]

For many years, other industry sectors have recognized a connection between a safe, engaged workforce and excellent customer care.[22] These sectors have pursued systems and processes to ensure employee safety and well-being, often implementing the *hierarchy of controls*. This model, which is enforced by OSHA, calls for first engineering out the hazard. If that is not feasible, administrative controls such as rotating employees in and out of jobs with hazardous exposures should be used. If administrative controls are not feasible, the last line of defense is the use of personal protective equipment.

These methods are often not standard practice in health care. Reasons for this include the following:[26]

■ Workplace health and safety is infrequently understood or addressed as a strategic priority by healthcare boards of directors, leadership, and management.

■ Often there is limited sustained leadership commitment and allocation of adequate health and safety resources.

■ Health and safety resources often are not aligned with corporate planning and the budgeting cycle.

■ Health care has a well-entrenched, hierarchical, and tradition-bound professional and organizational culture that does not view safety as an important value.

■ There is often fragmented accountability and inadequate communication of health and safety matters in healthcare settings.

■ Often there is an absence of comprehensive corporate analysis to identify, monitor, mitigate, and manage health and safety risks.

■ The healthcare workplace has complex, trained groups of professionals who have experienced different training and who are used to working independently and in silos.

■ There is limited cross-enterprise communication on solution management.

More research on the linkages between employee and patient safety are needed, and some studies are indeed under way. Projects include investigating the effect of working conditions in ICUs on elderly patient outcomes and the safety and health of healthcare workers, and assessing how staffing levels and other organizational parameters act as risk factors for injury for both patients and workers in acute- and long-term care facilities.[28]

In terms of intervention, performance improvement requires systematic feedback, whether the performance area is patient or employee safety.[9,24] Methods from industrial engineering can be adapted to health care to improve both quality of care and employee safety.[29] By viewing patient and employee safety as different manifestations of the same issue, health care would benefit from increased employee engagement in patient safety, higher employee morale, intervention synergies, a more cohesive culture, more coherent vision of safety, and greater bang for the intervention buck.

A HEALTHCARE CULTURE OF SAFETY

Measurement, as we have stressed, plays a central role in driving performance. But it is not the sole driver.[2] Culture is pivotal to both a high level of performance and its sustainability. Creating a culture of safety is a difficult leadership challenge,[8] and part of the challenge consists of leadership understanding culture and how leadership practices shape organizational culture.[9] The first step in culture change is not to give another survey on the climate for safety but to understand what unspoken assumptions are being made that create the culture leaders want to change.

What unspoken assumptions underlie the lack of attention to patient and worker safety? Such assumptions involve what healthcare institutions expect from their people and from leadership. "Medical practitioners have their own view of the world," writes Dr. Robert Wachter and Dr. Kaveh G. Shojania in *Internal Bleeding*. "We speak of the art of medicine . . . teamwork, checklists, standard operating procedures, systems thinking—none of that comes naturally to us."[30] Many physicians are dead set against giving up their autonomy and authority for what some call *cookbook medicine*, although this is emphatically not what patient and employee safety actually requires of them.

Interestingly, the first author found a similar cultural dynamic at NASA after the *Columbia* tragedy. At NASA we found brilliant scientists who were genuinely motivated to accomplish nearly impossible tasks, who took on challenges with enthusiasm, and who inadvertently compromised safety in the process.[22] Wachter calls these same traits in medical personnel "hubris, elitism, and wishful thinking."[30] In health care, as at NASA, these sentiments are understandable, and they have served a purpose in fostering individual rigor and dedication among healthcare providers. They explain why many healthcare providers take personal responsibility for medical errors, why they are personally demanding, prone to blame, and

inclined to fire employees who make mistakes. These traits produce individual excellence but are maladaptive for optimal health care as a system, and they set up a culture that supports heroes but impedes safety.[9,30,31] The good news in all this is that worker safety and patient safety are inextricably linked and can be used to motivate culture change.

The leading attributes of organizational culture that influence operational performance—the credibility of management, procedural justice, and receptiveness to upward communication—also drive outcomes in both patient and worker safety.[32-34] Improvement tools needed to address patient safety are the same tools and strategies needed to address worker safety, and both can be used by leaders with cultural know-how to foster and sustain an organizational culture that supports safety: root cause analysis, behavioral observation and feedback, assessment of safety leadership capability, cultural diagnostics, and powerful intervention design.

CONCLUSION

The opportunity exists to shift patient safety into drive with the three-pronged strategic policy described here. A universal and mandatory patient safety outcome metric is required, and health institutions should transparently post worker and patient incident frequencies. Reinvigorated initiatives to improve worker safety and combine or coordinate them with patient safety will engage patient well-being and improve quality of care and employee well-being. The third and crucial element of the strategy is supporting leadership's systematic analysis of the organization's culture and upgrading the culture-shaping skills of leaders.

DISCUSSION QUESTIONS ————

1. Applying the concept of microsystems to patient safety initiatives, consider why the national efforts have not been successful in reducing medical errors.

2. Do you agree that having a national mandatory reporting system will result in fewer medical errors? Why or why not?

3. Why is there a link between worker safety and patient safety?

4. The authors argue that organizations must have a culture of safety. How does this apply to your role? How can you influence such a culture in your workplace?

REFERENCES

1. Kohn L. T., Corrigan, J. M., Donaldson, M. S. (Eds.), for Committee on Quality of Health Care in America and Institute of Medicine. (1999). *To err is human*. Washington, DC: National Academies Press.

2. Leape, L., Berwick, D., Clancy, C., Conway, J., Gluck, P., Guest, J., . . . Isaac, T. (2009). Transforming healthcare: A safety imperative. *Quality & Safety in Health Care, 10*, 424–428.

3. Consumers Union Safe Patient Project. *To err is human—To delay is deadly: Ten years later, a million lives lost, billions of dollars wasted*. Retrieved from http://cu.convio.net/site/PageNavigator /spp_To_Delay_Is_Deadly_Executive_Summary

4. Stevens, D. P. (2010). Safe healthcare: We're running out of excuses. *Postgraduate Medicine Journal, 86*, 129–130.

5. Wachter, R. M. (2010). Patient safety at ten: Unmistakable progress, troubling gaps. *Health Affairs, 29*(1), 1–9.

6. The Joint Commission. (2010). *Improving America's hospitals—The Joint Commission's annual report on quality and safety*. Retrieved from http://www .jointcommission.org/annualreport.aspx

7. VHA Foundation. (2008, May 6). *New survey finds that hospital CEOs recognize patients' safety concerns, but lack confidence about best ways to create safer environment*. Retrieved from http://www.psqh.com /enews/0508d.shtml

8. Wachter, R. M. (2008). *Understanding patient safety*. New York, NY: McGraw-Hill.

9. Krause, T. R., & Hidley, J. H. (2009). *Taking the lead in patient safety: How healthcare leaders influence behavior and create culture*. Hoboken, NJ: Wiley.

10. Yassi, A., & Hancock, T. (2005). Patient safety-worker safety: Building a culture of safety to improve healthcare worker and patient well-being. *Healthcare Quarterly, 8*, 32–38.

11. U.S. Department of Labor, Bureau of Labor Statistics. (2009). Workplace injury and illness summary. Retrieved from http://www.bls.gov/news .release/osh.nr0.htm

12. Devers, K. J., Pham, H. H., & Liu, G. (2004). What is driving hospitals' patient-safety efforts? *Health Affairs, 23*(2), 103–115.

13. U.S. Department of Health and Human Services, Agency for Healthcare Research and Quality. (2008). *2007 national healthcare quality report*. Retrieved from http://archive.ahrq.gov/qual /nhqr07/nhqr07.pdf

14. U.S. Department of Health and Human Services, Agency for Healthcare Research and Quality. (2008). *2007 national healthcare disparities report*. Retrieved from http://archive.ahrq.gov/qual /nhdr07/nhdr07.pdf

15. U.S. Department of Labor, Bureau of Labor Statistics. (1997). Chapter 9: Occupational safety and health statistics. In *BLS Handbook of Methods*. Retrieved from http://www.bls.gov/opub/hom /homch9.htm

16. National Safety Council. *Injury facts: 2008 edition*. Itasca, IL: National Safety Council. Retrieved from https://www.usw12775.org/uploads/Inju ryFacts08Ed.pdf

17. National Safety Council. *Accident facts: 1997*, p. 49. Itasca, IL: National Safety Council.

18. U.S. Department of Labor, Occupational Safety and Health Administration. (2010, March 9). US Labor Department's OSHA notifies 15,000 workplaces nationwide of high injury and illness rates. Retrieved from https://www.osha .gov/pls/oshaweb/owadisp.show_document?p_ table=NEWS_RELEASES&p_id=17238

19. U.S. Department of Labor, Occupational Safety and Health Administration. (2009). *Site-specific targeting 2009* (SST-09). Retrieved from https://www.osha.gov/OshDoc/Directive_pdf /CPL_02_09-05.pdf

20. Seligman, P. J., Sieber, W. K., Pedersen, D. H., Sundin, D. S., & Frazier, T. M. (1988). Compliance with OSHA record-keeping requirements. *American Journal of Public Health, 78*(9), 1219.

21. Petersen, D. (2006). The problem with macro measures. *Industrial Safety & Hygiene News, 40*(10), 110.

22. Krause, T. R. (2005). *Leading with safety*. Hoboken, NJ: Wiley.

23. Yale Journal of Health Policy, Law, and Ethics Editorial Staff. (2008). A national survey of medical error reporting laws. *Yale Journal of Health Policy, Law, and Ethics, IX*(1), 202–286.

24. Pronovost, P., Nolan, T., Zeger, S., Miller, M., & Rubin, H. (2004). How can clinicians measure safety and quality in acute care? *Lancet, 363,* 1064.

25. For example, see Eckstrand, J. A., Habib, A. S., Williamson, A., Horvath, M. M., Gattis, K. G., Cozart, H., & Ferranti, J. (2009). Computerized surveillance of opioid-related adverse drug events in perioperative care: A cross-sectional study. *Patient Safety in Surgery, 3,*18.

26. Sikorski, J. (2009). Connecting worker safety to patient safety: A new imperative for healthcare leaders. *Ivey Business Journal.* Retrieved from http://iveybusinessjournal.com/topics /leadership/connecting-worker-safety-to-patient -safety-a-new-imperative-for-health-care-leaders# .VCsCDmddWSo

27. American Nurses Association. (2002). *Analysis of American Nurses Association staffing survey.* Warwick, RI: Cornerstone Communications Group.

28. U.S. Department of Health and Human Services, Agency for Healthcare Research and Quality. (2002). Impact of working conditions on patient safety. Retrieved from http://www.ahrq.gov /news/workfact.htm

29. Brennan, T. A., & Berwick, D. M. (1996). *New rules: Regulation markets and the quality of American health care.* San Francisco, CA: Jossey-Bass.

30. Wachter, R. M., & Shojania, K. G. (2004). *Internal bleeding: The truth behind America's terrifying epidemic of medical mistakes.* New York, NY: Rugged Land.

31. Bohmer, R. M. J. (2009). *Designing care: Aligning the nature and management of health care.* Cambridge, MA: Harvard Business Press.

32. Coyle-Shapiro, J., Kessler, I., & Purcell, J. (1985). Reciprocity or "it's my job": Exploring organizationally directed citizenship behavior in a national health service setting. *Journal of Applied Psychology, 70,* 777–781.

33. Mark, B., & Hoffman, D. A. (2006). An investigation of the relationship between safety climate and medication errors as well as other nurse and patient outcomes. *Personnel Psychology, 9,* 847–869.

34. Katz-Navon, T., Naveh, E., & Stern, Z. (2005). Safety climate in healthcare organizations: A multidimensional approach. *Academy of Management Journal, 48,* 1075–1089.

CHAPTER 15

Health Information Technology

Philip J. Kroth

CHAPTER OBJECTIVES

1. Review the major historical developments in the evolution of health information technology.

2. Discuss government initiatives to support the implementation of health information technologies.

3. State both benefits and challenges of using this new technology and progress in implementation to date.

4. Consider the benefits and challenges of health care technology to the role of the advanced practice nurse.

HISTORICAL OVERVIEW

Applying modern information technology (IT) to the health care system to improve its quality and reduce its costs is not new. On April 27, 2004, President Bush created the Office of the National Coordinator for Health Information Technology (ONCHIT or "the ONC") by Executive Order as the first step to create the Nationwide Health Network.[1] On February 17, 2009, President Obama signed the American Recovery and Reinvestment Act (ARRA) that designated $20.8 billion through the Medicare and Medicaid reimbursement systems to incentivize providers and health care organizations to adopt and achieve "Meaningful Use" of electronic health records (EHRs).[2]

These programs are the latest in a long history of government health information technology (HIT) initiatives. One of the earliest government inquiries into the potential benefits of HIT occurred in the Kennedy administration in the early 1960s. A report from the President's Science

Advisory Committee, "Some New Technologies and Their Promise for the Life Sciences," was optimistic about the benefits HIT would bring to biomedical research and the health care system. Ironically, the report written a half century ago is still relevant to current HIT issues:

> The application of computer technology to the recording, storage, and analysis of data collected in the course of observing and treating large numbers of ill people promises to advance our understanding of the cause, course, and control of disease. The need for a general purpose health information technology stems in large part from increasingly rapid changes in the pattern of illness in the United States and from equally significant changes in the way medicine is practiced. The acute infectious diseases from which the patient either recovered or died have largely given place to chronic disorders which run an extremely variable course dependent on many factors both in the environment and within the patient himself. Within any sizable community there are numerous administrative organizations charged with providing health services. It is not uncommon for a single patient to be cared for by a large number of agencies in a single city, and workers in any one agency usually cannot find out about the activities of others; sometimes they even fail to learn that other agencies are active at all. . . . Modern data processing techniques make it possible to assemble all the necessary information about all the patients in a given geographical or administrative area in one place with rapid access for all authorized health and welfare agencies. Such a system would produce an immediate and highly significant improvement in medical care with a simultaneous reduction in direct dollar costs of manual record processing and an even greater economy in professional time now wasted in duplicating tests and procedures.[3]

To date, despite a half century of government programs and technological advancement, the best and most current scientific evidence indicates that the benefits of HIT on the quality and cost of health care are, at best, mixed.[4] This chapter will explore the history of how HIT has evolved and the imprint HIT has made on the current health care system and will speculate about how HIT will likely influence the future of health care and the health care system as a whole.

Using computers to improve health care in many ways parallels the development of modern IT. The late 1960s and early 1970s saw several pioneering efforts at a small number of universities to apply IT to various aspects of the health care delivery process. Early systems were not the Web-based, interactive systems of today but were usually a hybrid of computer and paper integrated into a clinical work process. One early example was a system at Indiana University where a small army of data entry clerks manually entered data into a computer on key parts of all patients' medical records.

The night before a patient's clinic appointment, a one-page, paper encounter form was printed for the appointment listing the patient's name, record number, medical problem list (i.e., the known diagnoses and medical problems), medication list, medication allergies, and suggestions based on the data in the computer system. A suggestion was printed on the list when the computer software detected any of 290 agreed upon patient care protocols or conditions defined by rules applied to the computer's database. When a physician saw the patient in the clinic, he or she would handwrite encounter notes on the appropriate section of the paper encounter form and manually annotate the computer-printed problem list, medication list, and other items. The next day, a team of data entry clerks would review all encounter forms and update the computer data to reflect the physician's orders and updates to the patient's condition. The paper form would then be filed to the patient's chart. The Indiana group conducted a study demonstrating a 29% improvement in adherence to agreed upon treatment protocols in the group of physicians who received the computer "suggestions" for recommended treatment protocols on the encounter forms versus those who did not.[5]

With the introduction of the IBM PC in the late 1970s and early 1980s, paper forms were mostly eliminated and physicians began interacting with the patient's EHR in real time on the video screen. Similar experimental systems were designed and built during the same time period at a number of other U.S. universities, including the University of Pittsburgh,[6] the University of Utah,[7,8] Vanderbilt University,[9,10] Duke University,[11] and Harvard University/Massachusetts General Hospital.[12] These early systems were custom designed, built, and maintained by in-house dedicated teams of computer programmers and systems engineers. Because of the custom designs, the unique work process that existed at each institution, and the advanced nature of these early systems, they were not portable and could not be transplanted to other institutions without extensive software design rework. More importantly, because each of these early systems had a unique design, they were incapable of electronically transferring any of the patients' records to any other system. Despite these limitations, the pioneering works done with these early systems laid the foundation for modern EHR design.

It was not until the 1990s that commercially produced comprehensive EHR systems were marketed and sold to health care institutions in high volume. These commercially produced systems allowed hospitals to implement EHRs without the prohibitive expenses of building custom systems. Instead, hospitals could buy an "off-the-shelf" system that, although not completely customized to institutional work flows, could be configured to meet most of their perceived HIT institutional needs. However, as with the pioneering EHR systems at academic institutions, the off-the-shelf, commercially produced EHRs of today still require extensive configuration to accommodate the unique and varying work processes at each institution. The configuration differences between institutions are often so significant that even institutions with the same commercial EHR systems cannot electronically exchange patients' records without customized software. The ONC Website reports that there are a total of 2,648 certified ambulatory EHR products and a total of 878 inpatient products currently on the Certified HIT Product List.[13] While many of these are merely different versions of the same software, there are at least 200 unique systems. None of these systems is designed to interface with another system for patient data sharing across different software platforms. Due to this lack of standardization, regional health information organizations (RHIOs) have been created to facilitate the exchange of patient data among different health care institutions to support improved patient care. RHIOs and health information exchanges (HIEs) are discussed in more detail later in this chapter.

The 2009 HITECH Act created several programs to incentivize individual physicians and health care organizations to buy, install, and adopt EHR systems in the hope that this will yield significant benefits by reducing the cost and improving the quality of care.[2] "The provisions of the HITECH Act are specifically designed to work together to provide the necessary assistance and technical support to providers, enable coordination and alignment within and among states, establish connectivity to the public health community in case of emergencies, and assure the workforce is properly trained and equipped to be meaningful users of EHRs."[14] The following brief descriptions of programs created and supported by the HITECH Act provide an overview of its comprehensive approach to HIT implementation:[14]

- Beacon Community Program to assist communities in building their HIT infrastructures and exchange capabilities
- Consumer eHealth Program to help empower Americans to access their personal health information and to use this as a tool to gain more control over their health

- State Health Information Exchange Cooperative Agreement Program to support states in establishing HIE capabilities among health care providers and hospitals in their jurisdictions
- HIT Exchange Program to establish regional extension centers for education and training of health providers in use of EHRs
- Strategic Health IT Advanced Research Projects to fund research advances to overcome major barriers to EHR adoption

While the HITECH Act and its funding provide a new thrust toward EHR adoption, the state of EHR technology does not allow most systems to interface with each other. Despite this large government investment and more than half a century of technological development, U.S. health care system HIT still consists of a large number of disparate "siloed" systems that cannot electronically exchange patient records in an efficient and secure manner.

HISTORICAL CHALLENGES IN IMPLEMENTING HIT

Figure 15-1 illustrates the three essential components required for successful HIT implementation.

The first essential component is the technology. Organizations often focus on this first component with the mistaken belief that merely selecting the "right" technology or the "right EHR" is the most important aspect of HIT implementation. The essential technologies needed to implement an EHR system are a relational database, a computer network, and computer workstation. All three technologies have existed for more than 40 years, raising the question of why adoption of HIT in the clinical environment has been so slow compared to the adoption of IT in other industries such as the airline industry's reservation system. The second component of successful implementation, work policies and procedures, makes implementing HIT systems in the clinical environment extremely challenging because of wide variations in work policies and procedures among different organizations and institutions.

An organization's policies and procedures describe and define the processes through which work is carried out. The process component is complex, because it requires HIT system implementers to fully understand all existing work processes. Many such processes are not written or formalized, having evolved over the years to accommodate the unique characteristics of a particular organization. Often existing work processes are significantly different from those officially documented or assumed to be in place, while many critical work processes

---

FIGURE 15-1 The three essential components of a successful HIT implementation.

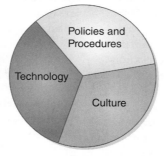

are not documented at all. When a HIT system is implemented, it is common for many of the undocumented processes to become apparent for the first time.[15] Undocumented or unknown work processes have been the root cause for many HIT implementation failures.[16]

In addition, it is well known that the most significant component of HIT implementation is the institutional and organizational culture—what people are willing to do.[17] This is the most critical, least studied, and least understood of the HIT implementation components.[18] Ash and Bates summarized the importance of organizational culture with regard to EHR adoption:[19]

> The organizational culture must be ready to support adoption by the individuals within it. There has been a period when clinicians have not experienced a sense of collaboration and trust between them and hospital administration. Consequently, if clinicians believe the administration wants to force them to use computerized physician order entry (CPOE), for example, they may dig in their heels. They may be more resistant to arguments based on safety and patient care benefit if the level of trust is not there. On the other hand, if the impetus comes from the clinical staff, other clinicians may be more apt to adopt sooner, and readiness will be at a higher level. One gauge of readiness is the extent to which certain categories of people hold positions within the organization. In particular, administrators at the highest level must offer both moral and financial support and demonstrate that they really believe in the patient care benefits of the systems. There must be clinical leaders, including a chief medical information officer if at all possible, who understand the fine points of implementation strategies, and opinion leaders among the clinical staff members. In addition, there need to be sufficiently skilled implementation, training, and support coordinators who understand both clinical and technical issues.*

* Reproduced from the *Journal of the American Medical Informatics Association*, "Factors and forces affecting EHR system adoption: report of a 2004 ACMI discussion," by JS Ash and DW Bates, Issue 12.1, pages 8–12, © 2005, with permission from BMJ Publishing Group Ltd.

There is a significant publication bias in the biomedical literature against publishing on HIT implementation failures. Because of the human tendency to avoid publicizing individuals' mistakes, the body of literature is strongly skewed toward successful implementations and studies. Unfortunately, this has made it difficult to study and understand causes of HIT implementation failures. A significant advance for the HIT industry as a whole would be a shift in its culture toward not only reporting HIT failures but viewing them as valuable learning opportunities rather than events to be downplayed and forgotten.

One major example of a HIT implementation failure occurred at the prestigious Cedars Sinai Hospital in Los Angeles, California, in 2002. After implementing a new $34 million HIT system, several hundred physicians refused to use the new system 3 months after it was turned on. Cedars Sinai attempted to implement a new electronic medical record that changed the way physicians ordered patient treatments and tests in the hospital. Prior to implementing the new system, physicians wrote their orders on paper forms in the patients' paper charts. After new patient orders were written, physicians gave the chart to nurses or ward clerks to read and implement the orders. The new system required physicians to type orders directly into a computer workstation, where the software provided the physicians with immediate feedback if they attempted to enter an order that the computer either did not understand or interpreted as a mistake. An article in the *Washington Post* reported:[20]

> A veteran physician at the prestigious Cedars Sinai Medical Center here had been mixing up a certain drug dosage for decades. Every time he wrote the prescription for 10 times the proper amount, a nurse simply corrected it, recalled Paul Hackmeyer. The computers arrived—and when the doctor typed in his medication order, the machine barked at him and he barked back. . . . "What we discovered was that for 20 years he was writing the wrong dose."

This failure illustrates the three principal HIT implementation components described earlier. Technology: With physicians required to enter orders directly to the computer system, time required to enter orders became dependent on the computer's ordering input format and system response time. Process: Many undocumented processes in the old system were not carried to the new system. In this example, the nurse's automatic correction of an obvious dosage error was a critical, undocumented, process step—a check on the orders' accuracy. Although the new system caught the error, the physician user in this case could no longer rely on the nurse's checking and correcting his orders. Culture: The new system required physicians to interact with a computer, which took more time than did writing orders on paper forms. The new system required physicians to change the way they practiced medicine in the hospital, and, as is common, people dislike change. This was a significant change in physicians' work culture in which nurses had routinely checked and corrected physician orders without communicating the corrections. Physicians also had to deal with a barrage of system alerts when they were imprecise or inaccurate in entering their orders. While possibly enhancing patient safety, responding to the system alerts increased the time required for physicians to place orders.

Another historical barrier to broad implementation of HIT is the chasm between those who bear the costs of the technology and those who receive its benefits. The purchase and operation of an EHR system represent a major investment for large health care organizations and especially for small private physicians groups. Not only must physicians groups bear the costs of the hardware and software but also they must support ongoing IT maintenance, staff training, and software upgrade costs. Because small practice groups often have no experience or expertise with IT issues, they also experience anxiety about making decisions necessary to convert from paper to electronic

charting. While economies of scale make the marginal costs of adopting EHR technology somewhat lower for large health care organizations, these organizations often do not realize cost savings from their investment. For example, a health care system participating in a HIE may reduce the number of duplicate laboratory and imaging tests, saving the patient and the payer significant expense, but the health care system may actually lose money by not receiving revenue for the duplicate tests. As with large health care systems, small practices that invest in EHR technology may not directly benefit from the technology. Patients may receive better age-appropriate screening[21,22] and preventative care[23] as well as reduced duplicate testing because of physician access to HIEs and patient records from outside of the practice group or health system.[24] However, from a practice financial perspective, these factors actually may produce a significant disincentive for adopting EHRs.

THE FEDERAL GOVERNMENT'S RESPONSE TO HIT IMPLEMENTATION CHALLENGES

The federal government's financial incentive programs for large health care organizations and private practices that adopt and demonstrate "meaningful use" of EHRs are an effort to bridge the chasm between costs and benefits. On April 27, 2004, President Bush created the ONCHIT or "the ONC" by Executive Order.[1] In 2009, the ONC was also tasked in the Health Information Technology for Economic and Clinical Health Act (HITECH Act)[25] to be "the principal Federal entity charged with coordination of nationwide efforts to implement and use the most advanced HIT and the electronic exchange of health information."[26] The ONC's mission is to promote the development of a nationwide HIT infrastructure, provide leadership in the development of standards, provide the certification of HIT products, coordinate

FIGURE 15-2   ONC organizational structure.

ONC Organization

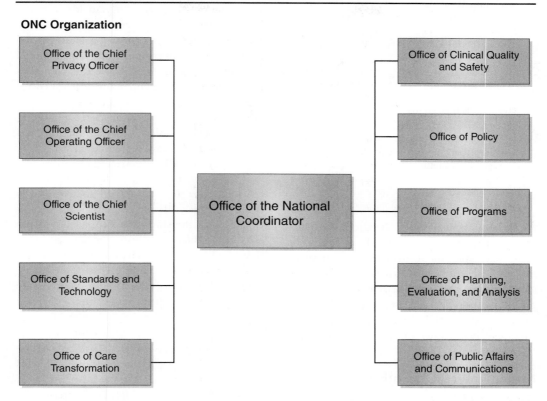

Source: Reproduced from Office of the National Coordinator for Health Information Technology Newsroom, http://www.healthit.gov/newsroom/about-onc.

HIT policy, perform strategic planning for HIT adoption and HIE, and establish the governance for the Nationwide Health Information Network. **Figure 15-2** depicts the ONC's organizational structure.[27]

The ONC employs 191 full-time staff and operated with an annual budget of $66 million in fiscal year 2013, excluding the $20.8 billion in HITECH funding in incentive payments for providers and health care organizations administered through the Centers for Medicare and Medicaid Services for achieving meaningful use of EHRs. In addition to these resources, the HITECH Act created a HIT Policy Committee and a HIT Standards Committee under the auspices of the Federal Advisory Committee Act. Both committees have multiple workgroups with representatives from payers, academia, and the health care industry. They address a variety of HIT-related issues including certification/adoption, governance, HIE, meaningful use, privacy and security, quality measures, implementation, and a HIT vocabulary standards committee.[28]

The Health IT Policy Committee will make recommendations to the National Coordinator for Health IT on a policy framework for the development and adoption of a nationwide health information infrastructure, including standards for the exchange of patient medical information. The American Recovery and Reinvestment Act of 2009 (ARRA) provides that the Health IT Policy Committee shall at least make recommendations on the areas in which standards, implementation specifications, and certifications criteria are needed in eight specific areas.

The Health IT Standards Committee is charged with making recommendations to the National Coordinator for Health IT on standards, implementation specifications, and certification criteria for the electronic exchange and use of health information.

As noted previously, the ONC also has funded several programs to facilitate the adoption of EHRs. Examples include training programs to increase the number of professionals with IT skills required in the health care domain. Other programs fund the development of HIE standards across multiple EHR vendor platforms. The ONC also funds annual surveys to track HIT adoption.

Meaningful Use Incentives

The $20.8 billion included in the HITECH Act created the Medicare and Medicaid EHR incentive programs for eligible professionals (individual providers in solo or multiprovider practice groups) and hospitals as they adopt, implement, upgrade, or demonstrate meaningful use of certified EHR technology to improve patient care.[20]

Eligible professionals may receive up to $44,000 through the Medicare EHR Incentive Program and up to $63,750 through the Medicaid EHR Incentive Program. Eligible professionals may participate in either the Medicare or Medicaid EHR Incentive Programs, but not both. Eligible hospitals can participate in both the Medicare and Medicaid incentive programs.[29] Each hospital incentive includes a base payment of $2 million plus an additional amount determined by a formula based on the number of discharges per year.[30,31] The Medicare Program is a 5-year program administered through the federal government, while the Medicaid program is a 6-year program funded by the federal government but administered through individual states. **Table 15-1** compares Medicare and Medicaid adoption incentive programs for eligible professionals and hospitals.[29-37] CMS also publishes a flow chart to help eligible professionals determine qualifications to meet program requirements.[32]

To receive EHR incentive payments, providers and hospitals must demonstrate that they are "meaningfully using" their EHRs by meeting thresholds for several specific objectives. In a partnership with the ONC, CMS has established the objectives for "meaningful use" that eligible professionals and eligible hospitals must meet in order to receive incentive payments.[38] The CMS meaningful use criteria are developed by the experts who compose the various workgroups in the ONC's Health IT Policy Committee. The level of evidence for the majority of meaningful use objectives is only at the expert opinion level. The science of HIT awaits rigorous research studies to validate the choices and designs of the meaningful use criteria.

To receive incentive payments, eligible professionals and health care organizations must meet specific meaningful use criteria in three stages. Stages 1 and 2 have been defined, but stage 3 is yet to be developed. Stage 1 includes objectives for capturing patient data and sharing data in a standardized format with patients and other health care professionals. Stage 2 includes objectives for advanced clinical processes. Stage 3 will reportedly be related to measuring and reporting clinically relevant patient outcomes.

To receive the full Medicare incentive, providers and hospitals were required to apply for Stage 1 certification by 2012 or the maximum amount of the Medicare incentive payments

TABLE 15-1	Comparison of Medicare and Medicaid Adoption Incentive Programs for Eligible Professionals (Individual Providers in Solo and Group Practices) and Hospitals (Including Critical Access Hospitals)[29-37]	

	Medicare Program	Medicaid Program
Eligible Professionals	■ Administered by CMS ■ $44,000 Maximum per physician (over 5-year period) ■ 90% or more of practice must be outpatient based ■ Cannot participate in Medicaid Program if ■ enrolled in Medicare Program ■ Must apply for Stage 1 Meaningful Use by 2012 ■ to obtain the maximum incentive ■ Medicare imposes payment penalty on those ■ failing to demonstrate Meaningful Use by 2015	■ Administered by State Medicaid Agency ■ $63,750 Maximum per physician participate (over 5 years) ■ Must have ≤30% Medicaid patient volume or ≤20% Medicaid patient volume and be a pediatrician or practice predominantly in a Federally Qualified Health Center or Rural Health Clinic and have ≤30% patient volume attributable to needy individuals ■ ≤90% of practice must be outpatient based ■ Cannot participate in Medicare Program if enrolled in Medicaid Program ■ Can begin to certify for Meaningful Use by 2016 and still receive full incentive ■ Non-participants exempt from Medicaid payment reductions
Hospitals (including Critical Access Hospitals)	■ Administered by CMS ■ Can begin receiving incentive FY 2011 to FY 2015, but payments will decrease for hospitals that start receiving payments in FY 2014 and later ■ Medicare and Medicaid Program eligible ■ Must apply for Stage 1 Meaningful Use by FY 2013 to receive maximum incentive ■ Hospitals that do not successfully demonstrate Meaningful Use will be subject to Medicare payment penalties beginning in FY 2015	■ Administered by State Medicaid Agency ■ Acute care hospitals (including critical access and cancer hospitals) with at least 10% Medicaid patient volume are eligible ■ Children's hospitals are eligible regardless of their Medicaid volume ■ Can apply for both Medicare and Medicaid Programs ■ Incentive payments are based on a number of factors, beginning with a $2 million base payment

(continues)

TABLE 15-1	Comparison of Medicare and Medicaid Adoption Incentive Programs for Eligible Professionals (Individual Providers in Solo and Group Practices) and Hospitals (Including Critical Access Hospitals)[29-37] *(continued)*

- Incentive payments are based on several factors, beginning with a $2 million base payment

Sources: Data from Centers for Medicare and Medicaid Services. Eligible hospital information. 2012; http://www.cms.gov/Regulations-and-Guidance/Legislation/EHRIncentivePrograms/Eligible_Hospital_Information.html. Accessed September 30, 2014; Centers for Medicare and Medicaid Services. *EHR Incentive Program for Medicare Hospitals: Calculating Payments.* 2012; http://www.cms.gov/Outreach-and-Education/Medicare-Learning-Network-MLN/MLNProducts/downloads/EHR_TipSheet_Medicare_Hosp.pdf. Accessed September 30, 2014; Centers for Medicare and Medicaid Services. *Flow Chart to Help Eligible Professionals (EP) Determine Eligibility for the Medicare and Medicaid Electronic Health Record (EHR) Incentive Programs.* 2012; https://www.cms.gov/Regulations-and-Guidance/Legislation/EHRIncentivePrograms/downloads/eligibility_flow_chart.pdf. Accessed September 30, 2014; Centers for Medicare and Medicaid Services. EHR incentive programs. 2012; http://www.cms.gov/Regulations-and-Guidance/Legislation/EHRIncentivePrograms/index.html?redirect=/ehrincentiveprograms/. Accessed September 30, 2014; Centers for Medicare and Medicaid Services. Medicare Electronic Health Record Incentive Program for Eligible Professionals. 2012; http://www.cms.gov/Outreach-and-Education/Medicare-Learning-Network-MLN/MLNProducts/Downloads/CMS_eHR_Tip_Sheet.pdf. Accessed September 30, 2014; Centers for Medicare and Medicaid Services. *An Introduction to the Medicaid EHR Incentive Program for Eligible Professionals.* 2012; http://www.cms.gov/Regulations-and-Guidance/Legislation/EHRIncentivePrograms/downloads/Beginners_Guide.pdf. Accessed September 30, 2014; Centers for Medicare and Medicaid Services. *An Introduction to the Medicare EHR Incentive Program for Eligible Professionals.* 2012; http://www.cms.gov/Regulations-and-Guidance/Legislation/EHRIncentivePrograms/Downloads/Beginners_Guide.pdf. Accessed September 30, 2014; Centers for Medicare and Medicaid Services. Medicaid Electronic Health Record Incentive Payments for Eligible Professionals. 2012; http://www.cms.gov/Outreach-and-Education/Medicare-Learning-Network-MLN/MLNProducts/Downloads/EHRIP_Eligible_Professionals_Tip_Sheet.pdf. Accessed September 30, 2014.

decreases each year until 2015 when the Medicare incentive stops.[39] The Medicaid incentive payments for eligible professionals are higher under the Medicaid EHR Incentive Program. Unlike the Medicare EHR Incentive Program, the Medicaid EHR Incentive Program does not penalize those who begin to certify meaningful use after 2012. In fact, an eligible professional can begin to certify meaningful use in the Medicaid Program as late as 2016 and still receive the same total incentive payment as those who began to certify in 2011. Those eligible professionals who begin to certify under the Medicaid Program after 2016 will receive no incentive. Regardless of which of the two programs certifies an eligible professional, beginning in 2015, Medicare will impose payment penalties upon providers who fail to demonstrate meaningful use. **Table 15-2** summarizes the timetable for meaningful use criteria implementation.[40]

Detailed information on the meaningful use requirements for Stage 1 is available for eligible professionals[41] and eligible hospitals.[42] Some examples of meaningful use requirements for Stage 1 for eligible professionals include the following:

CPOE

Drug–Drug Interaction and Drug–Allergy Checking

Up-to-Date Problem List of Current and Active Diagnoses

Electronic or "e-prescribing" (of at least 40% of prescriptions)

TABLE 15-2	Meaningful Use Implementation Timeline

	Stage 2: 2014	Stage 3: 2016
Meaningful use criteria focus on:	Meaningful use criteria focus on:	Meaningful use criteria focus on:
■ Electronically capturing health information in a standardized format ■ Using that information to track key clinical conditions ■ Communicating that information for care coordination processes ■ Initiating the reporting of clinical quality measures and public health information ■ Using information to engage patients and their families in their care	■ More rigorous health information exchange (HIE) ■ Increased requirements for e-prescribing and incorporating lab results ■ Electronic transmission of patient care summaries across multiple settings ■ More patient-controlled data	■ Improving quality, safety, and efficiency, leading to improved health outcomes ■ Decision support for national high-priority conditions ■ Patient access to self-management tools ■ Access to comprehensive patient data through patient-centered HIE ■ Improving population health

Source: HealthIT.gov. Meaningful use regulations. http://www.healthit.gov/policy-researchers-implementers /meaningful-use. Accessed September 30, 2014.

Maintaining an Active Medication List

Record and Chart Changes in Vital Signs

Recording Smoking Status for Patients 13 Years and Older

Reporting Ambulatory Clinical Quality Measures to CMS and States

Implementing Clinical Decision Support

Providing Patients with an Electronic Copy of Their Health Information upon Request

Providing Clinical Summaries to Patients for Each Office Visit

Stage 1 also includes a "menu" of requirements from which providers must achieve a total of 5. Examples of requirements include the capability to generate lists of patients by specific conditions, proactively sending reminders to patients for preventive/follow-up care, providing patients with electronic access to health information, reconciling patient medication lists, and producing summaries of records for transitions of care. Stage 2 requirements build on those of Stage 1 and contain 17 required objectives and a menu of 6 items from which 3 can be chosen. The complete list of meaningful use objectives and metrics for individual providers and health care organizations is available.[43,44] The list of meaningful use objectives to attain Stage 3 compliance is not yet published but is scheduled for release in time for the first Stage 3 certifications in 2016.

HIT OPPORTUNITIES: IMPROVING HEALTH CARE DELIVERY QUALITY, EFFECTIVENESS, AND EFFICIENCY

With mediocre evidence to date for HIT goals to improve health care quality and reduce costs, the question looms: What is the driving

FIGURE 15-3 Why EHRs have potential to improve quality and reduce costs.

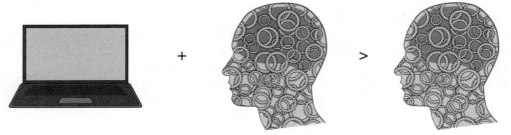

Source: Modified from Friedman CP. A "Fundamental Theorem" of Biomedical Informatics. *J Am Med Inform Assoc.* 2009;16:169-170.

force behind the U.S. quest to implement HIT? The answer resides in understanding the limitations of the human brain and attention span. A healthy human's performance begins to measurably decrease in about 40 minutes while monitoring a continuous process.[45] These limitations explain regulations for work-time breaks for air traffic controllers and anesthesiologists and work-hour limitations for airplane pilots and commercial truck drivers, and more recently work-hour limitations for medical students and residents.[46] These regulations recognize that human performance is limited by innate biology and physiology and that fatigue degrades performance; no amount of training or willpower can overcome these biological and physiological limitations. These acknowledgments apply to health care delivery where a provider in a busy outpatient clinic or inpatient ward is much like an air traffic controller monitoring a continuous process. Patients are tightly scheduled with additional patients often "doubled booked" at the last minute because of acute illness. Every patient must be seen and volumes of data accessed, processed, and synthesized to formulate a diagnosis and a plan of care. At the same time, the provider must document the encounter in detail, complete all required forms and

insurance paperwork, respond to electronic pages and phone calls, speak with consultants, manage correspondence, and in many cases supervise midlevel providers, nursing, and office staff. Stead and Hammond have shown that the amount of data accessed and used by clinicians per medical decision is increasing exponentially despite the fact that providers' ability to cope with the higher information load remains constant.[47] The driving concept behind EHRs' potential to improve the quality and reduce the cost of health care is represented by **Figure 15-3**.[48]

The ultimate goal is to combine the intuitive strengths of humans and data retention strengths of computers to create a hybrid system that is intuitive with a tireless data processing capability. The computer reminds providers to do what they already know how to do, and what they want to do, in a manner that makes it easy to implement. Meeting these parameters results in an efficacious computerized decision support system (CDSS). For CDSS to work, the computer system must provide the right information at the right place and at the right time. If any of these three requirements is missing, the system will tend to fail. With EHRs, the right place and time are often when the provider is entering patient orders at a computer workstation, a process termed CPOE. At this place and time, the provider's mind is focused on the patient just seen or the patient the provider is currently thinking about. It is also this place and time when it is easiest for the provider to take action, such as writing new orders that result in timely follow-through for a patient's care.

For example, when a provider has completed a patient interview and examination and is using an EHR to enter prescriptions that will be sent securely over the Internet to the patient's pharmacy, the computer can present the provider with a popup "reminder" that the patient is allergic to the medication being prescribed. It can also indicate that the prescribed requires at least annual kidney function monitoring and that the last record of kidney function laboratory work is more than a year old. In this event, the system can present the provider with an option to order the appropriate laboratory work or to ignore the warning with one keystroke or mouse click. Most decision support is designed with these "soft stops" or interventions that allow the provider to heed or ignore the warning as he or she believes to be most appropriate. CDSS "hard stops" do not allow provider options to ignore a warning. An example of a "hard stop" could be the use of a very expensive, broad spectrum antibiotic that by hospital policy can be ordered only by an infectious disease specialist. In this case, the CDSS would not allow the provider to order the medication but would inform the provider that an infectious disease consult is required and would make ordering that consult a mouse click away. A nonmedical example of a "hard stop" is the automobile design preventing the shift of an automatic transmission out of Park and into Drive unless the brake petal is depressed. This was implemented after reports of multiple accidental injuries and deaths attributed to unanticipated automobile movements. In this, like the medical example, the decision support

system prevents the operator from making an error with high probability of significant adverse consequences.

Like the first example that used a computer–paper hybrid system in the 1970s, CDSS reminds the provider to do what they already know how to do—at the right place and time and in the most convenient manner possible. Because the computer never fatigues, the reminders compensate for providers' biological limitations, and the human–computer hybrid system outperforms what either could accomplish alone.

Hundreds of studies and randomized controlled trials published in the peer-reviewed, biomedical literature have demonstrated how CDSS can have a dramatic impact on improving provider performance in myriad health care venues. CDSS similarly designed to produce popup warnings and recommendations to providers have been shown to improve the ordering of age-appropriate screening tests,[21,22] appropriate antibiotic prescribing for inpatients,[49] appropriate advance directive discussions with patients,[50] the use of preventative care for hospitalized patients,[21] appropriate weaning of patients from mechanical ventilators,[51] appropriate reductions of inpatient resource utilization,[52] the prevalence of methicillin-resistant *Staphylococcus aureus* (MRSA) in a community,[53] the isolation rates of patients admitted to the hospital with drug-resistant infections,[54] the screening for sexually transmitted diseases in the emergency department,[55] the accurate capture and recording of patient temperatures by nurses in the inpatient setting,[56] and many others. Despite these very promising studies, until recently, most of these studies were performed at major university health care centers that had custom-designed and maintained EHR software systems, maintained by local IT departments with relatively large IT support budgets compared with smaller community hospitals' budgets.[18] In 2006, Chaudhry et al. published a systematic review of 257 CDSS studies published up to 2005 that concluded 25% of the studies were from four major academic institutions that all had custom-designed systems and "only 9 studies evaluated multifunctional, commercially developed systems."[18] Therefore, while there are hundreds of studies demonstrating the potential for CDSS to improve the quality of care, reduce its costs, or both, the appropriateness of this research to typical health care settings in other than large academic institutions is mostly unknown.

The Agency for Healthcare Research and Quality commissioned the most systematic, rigorous, and comprehensive CDSS review of prior studies to date and published the results in 2012.[57] The systematic review analyzed 311 studies in the biomedical literature and found moderately strong evidence confirming three previously reported factors associated with successful CDSS implementation:

1. Automatic provision of decision support as part of clinician workflow
2. Provision of decision support at time and location of decision making
3. Provision of a recommendation, not just an assessment

The study also identified six additional factors that were correlated with the successful implementation of CDSS:

1. Integration with charting or order entry system to support workflow integration
2. No need for additional clinician data entry
3. Promotion of action rather than inaction
4. Justification of decision support via provision of research evidence
5. Local user involvement in development process
6. Provision of decision support results to patients as well as providers

The study found a high strength of evidence for CDSS to improve the ordering and completing of preventative care and ordering and prescribing recommended treatments "across academic, VA, and community inpatient and ambulatory settings that had both locally and commercially developed CDSS systems."[57]

There was a moderate strength of evidence that CDSS improves appropriate ordering of clinical studies, reduces patient morbidity and cost of care, and increases health care provider satisfaction.

Studies demonstrated a low strength of evidence for CDSS impact on efficiency of the user, length of hospital stay, mortality, health-related quality of life, and "adverse events" or medical errors.

The study also pointed out some significant voids in the current biomedical literature. None of the studies addressed the impact of CDSS on health care delivery organization changes, on the number of patients seen per unit of time, on user knowledge, on system cost effectiveness, or on provider workload.

In summary, the current cumulative evidence for the benefits of EHRs with CPOE and CDSS is mixed. Even in areas where there is a high strength of evidence such as improvement in the ordering and completing of preventative care, the effective magnitude of the improvement is small, even though statistically significant.[57]

HEALTH INFORMATION EXCHANGES

Virtually none of the commercially available EHR systems available in today's market or the custom-designed systems at large academic institutions can easily exchange patients' health information with care providers outside of their institutions. Despite 50 years of efforts, patients' health information remains siloed, and "it is not uncommon for a single patient to be cared for by a large number of agencies in a single city, and workers in any one agency usually cannot find out about the activities of others; sometimes they even fail to learn that other agencies are active at all."[3] Barriers to sharing patient information across multiple providers often become immediately apparent when a patient with a significant illness sees a number of different specialty providers and attempts to coordinate the flow of information among them. Unlike other industries such as the airlines that have cooperated to create a standardized ticketing system, the health care system has been marginally successful in designing a common platform or standard to allow a patient's records to be compatible with multiple vendor systems. In addition, health domain data are orders of magnitude larger and more complex than data for ticketing in the airline industry. In addition, the Health Insurance Portability and Accountability Act (HIPAA) regulations have had a chilling effect on health care institutions' willingness to share data with other institutions because they are responsible for patient privacy and the security of patient data.

These and other factors led to development of HIEs with their corresponding administering organizations, Regional Health Information Organizations (RHIOs). RHIOs attempt to create systems, agreements, processes, and technology to manage these factors in order to facilitate the appropriate exchange of health care information between institutions and across different vendor platforms. While most all states and regions of the United States have RHIOs, the actual state of implementation and real data exchange varies widely. For example, some states have active RHIOs that are in the planning stages of establishing relationships with all key stakeholders, creating administration agreements, creating governance structures, securing funding, attempting to develop business models for sustained funding of the organization, and so forth. Other RHIOs have functioning HIEs where medical data are actually being exchanged between institutions and across disparate software EHR platforms. The ONC has funded many RHIOs to develop and test the national standards for HIE with the ultimate goal of creating the "Nationwide Health Information Network" that would be a network of regional networks. Despite the testing and demonstration projects to date, actively functioning HIEs exist only at regional levels.[58]

Each vendor's building toward one common standard would significantly reduce the technical complexity of data exchange. Unfortunately, vendors' products are still not being built toward one national standard to facilitate electronic HIE. Despite these limitations, there have been significant accomplishments in implementing the data and IT standards necessary to facilitate the exchange of health information among multiple EHR platforms. Today, most institutions participating in HIEs must build or configure "interface engines" that convert the institution's data format to the form used by the HIE. This is a major challenge as there is no single standard that provides sufficient specification of data formats and communication protocols. Rather, there are a number of standards that address various domains of data management. In addition, the voluminous scope of modern health care and continuous advancements in knowledge and technology make managing data in the health care domain extremely dynamic and complex.

As an example of this complexity, the Logical Observations Indexes Names and Codes (LOINC) standard was developed in the 1990s to solve a problem with an older health information communication protocol that specified how clinical data should be identified for transmission between computer systems. LOINC uniquely defines codes for information such as blood chemistry laboratory tests and clinical observations, such as patient blood pressure that can be recorded in many different formats. There are currently more than 70,000 LOINC-defined codes for uniquely reporting laboratory tests and clinical observations.[59] For example, there are 419 different codes for reporting blood pressure. With its unique codes for laboratory tests and clinical observations, LOINC enables computer systems receiving the data to generate exact interpretations. This is called semantic interoperability. Semantic interoperability is essential for patient record transmission from one EHR system to another so that the meaning of the critical data contained within the records is not at risk of erroneous interpretation.

Because new laboratory tests are constantly being developed and existing assays are being improved, LOINC creates and disseminates new codes so that semantic interoperability can be maintained. Old codes are not deleted from the system, ensuring that researchers using prior clinical databases can retrieve prior results comparable with new codes. LOINC is supported by the National Library of Medicine (NLM), a division of the National Institutes of Health. The LOINC Committee publishes quarterly updates and holds biannual, national meetings to discuss proposed new clinical observations and laboratory tests for the assignment of new LOINC codes.

For a HIE to transfer information accurately, each EHR system must map its own internal code for each datum to a standard code to ensure that information passed from one EHR to another in the exchange is interpreted exactly the same by the receiver as it is in the sender's system. LOINC is one of the many HIT-related standards. The Systematic Nomenclature of Medicine (SNOMED) was originally developed by the College of American Pathologists (CAP) to exactly specify tissue pathologic diagnoses. The same group also developed a standard for clinical observations called SNOMED Clinical Terms (SNOMEDCT). LOINC and SNOMEDCT domain standards overlap, but their design characteristics are valuable in different situations; for example, exchanging laboratory results versus coding patient problem lists within EHRs. Similar to LOINC, CAP also provides periodic updates to SNOMEDCT codes.

To keep track of the many coding standards and the terms within, the NLM built and maintains the Unified Medical Language System (UMLS), which houses a massive "metathesaurus" and a variety of tools for mapping between and discovery of more than 200 biomedically related terminology standards.[60] Because LOINC, SNOMEDCT, and the 200 or so other standards are periodically updated, the UMLS is also regularly updated to keep the interstandard terminology mapping current and accurate.

Using HIEs, designated member groups of health care institutions exchange data in a standardized format using a combination of the previously described standards. This cooperation enables the access to a comprehensive clinical data set on individual patients across multiple institutions and multiple EHR vendor platforms.

There are two kinds of HIE architectures: "monolithic" and "federated." The monolithic architecture is a design where all member institutions periodically send copies of their clinical data to one central repository where all the data reside together in one format. The advantage of this approach is that a patient's comprehensive data can be maintained in one place and in one format. However, this approach has several disadvantages. First, the frequency with which members contribute and update copies of institutional data can vary, making the comprehensive HIE medical record potentially out of date. Second, aggregating data from multiple institutions creates administrative complexity with regard to HIPAA regulations. HIPAA requires each health care institution to maintain security of patient data. If an institution's data are "mixed" in the HIE database with data from other institutions, the responsibility of who ensures patient privacy and data security reverts to all HIE member institutions. HIPAA requirements make fulfilling health care organization obligations to insure patient privacy more difficult and complex. Third, when data are aggregated by a third party or HIE, the ability of the source institution to assert control over data contributed to the collective HIE is limited. If, for example, an institution desires

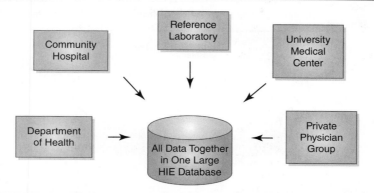

FIGURE 15-4 HIE monolithic model. Institutions periodically send copies of their clinical data to one central repository. Individual transinstitutional patient records are maintained in the central database where they can be accessed by authorized users.

to stop participating in an HIE because of concern for patient privacy and data security, it may be technically difficult and time consuming to selectively delete all data from one institution from the HIE database. The monolithic model is depicted in **Figure 15-4**.

The federated model is the most widely used design, allowing contributing institutions to maintain control over data for which they are responsible under HIPAA. In this model, institutional data resides only within each institution's system. The HIE database is small, containing only a master patient index (MPI) housing the identifiers for each patient in the form of each institution's unique patient record numbers along with only sufficient patient demographic data to facilitate accurate identification of individual patients with the same or similar names. This information is mapped to all of the institutional-specific patient identifiers in the exchange. **Figure 15-5** depicts the federated model.

For example, a patient who has medical records at more than one institution in the HIE would have all the medical record

numbers from the various institutions where clinical data are stored, linked together in the common MPI along with basic demographics such as address, date of birth, and social security number. This allows for fast and accurate identification of patients named "John Smith" because the MPI maintains only sufficient identifying information to ensure selection of the correct patient among all institutions in the exchange. "John Smith" would be identified from others with the same name by parameters such as date of birth and social security number. No clinical data are stored in the MPI. Clinical data are usually maintained in the proprietary format of the particular EHR system used by each institution. A copy of the same data is also maintained but is formatted in the standard used by all members of the HIE. For example, all HIE members could agree to code all laboratory test results using the LOINC standard described earlier. Each institution would create and maintain a database of all patients' laboratory results coded with LOINC. When a user requests a comprehensive record from the HIE, the system would query all of its

FIGURE 15-5 HIE federated model. Institutions maintain copies of their own data at their site in the format used by the health information exchange. Individual transinstitutional patient records are assembled in real time by searching all institutions' databases only when needed/requested by authorized users. Individual institutions can opt out of the HIE at any time by disabling access to their database.

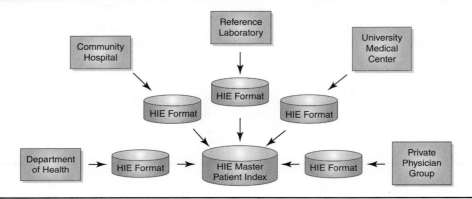

institutional members in real time to send all the data available on a particular patient as identified using the MPI. In this way, when an HIE receives a records request on a particular patient, each institution sends data on the requested patient from the database where all clinical data are in the HIE format. This process ensures that the data are collected securely, assembled into a comprehensive record, and made available to authorized users in real time. This comprehensive record is accessible only on a patient-by-patient basis for immediate patient care purposes; it is not copied to any institution's system. When the user logs out of the HIE, the comprehensive record assembled for that episode of patient care is deleted.

The federated model has several advantages over the monolithic model. With the federated model, each institution maintains complete control over its data, simplifying compliance with HIPAA regulations. If, for example, a data breach occurs in the database of an HIE

that uses the monolithic model, responsibility for the data breach is not always clear. Data breaches in a federated system are always clearly attributable to a particular institution and not the HIE (unless there is a data breach of the MPI). Another benefit of the federated system is that transinstitutional data are up-to-the-minute accurate because each time a user requests access, the clinical data from all institutions are assembled in real time. Institutional HIT administrators typically favor the federated model. With this model, HIT administrators have the option of withdrawing from the HIE at any time in order to maintain control of their responsibilities for patient information and data security under HIPAA guidelines.

While communities with HIEs generally appreciate the benefits, the current reality is that most of the operating HIEs are heavily subsidized with federal research grant funding. The RHIOs that administer the HIEs and seek funding have not developed a business model that can be used in all communities in order to sustain their HIEs independent of federal funding. Some HIEs have developed services for payers, charging them for access to the comprehensive records available in the HIE. These services allow payers to increase their claims processing efficiency. Other HIEs have developed services to generate comprehensive quality reports to sell to payers desiring to track provider and health plan outcomes or to help them meet the meaningful use requirements for CMS financial eligibility incentives. Some communities are resistant to allowing payer access to a data resource they believe should be solely dedicated to improving patient care and quality.[61] An excellent example of this is the state of Vermont's 2006 law that prevented data miners from selling providers' prescribing data to pharmaceutical companies that wanted the information to inform their marketing practices. In 2011, the law was struck down by the Supreme Court on a First Amendment basis.[62] Providers may feel uncomfortable participating in an exchange they know government, payers, or pharmaceutical companies may use for monitoring of individual practice outcomes and patterns. While the benefits of HIEs are documented and desirable, solving the cultural and business model issues will be essential to obtaining the national goal of a network of regional exchanges that will constitute the Nationwide Health Information Network.

THE VETERANS ADMINISTRATION HEALTH INFORMATION SYSTEM

No discussion of HIT, EHRs, and HIEs would be complete without noting the HIT system used by the Veterans Administration (VA). The VA is a model representing a single-payer health care system in the United States. For example, the VA HIT system supports only one payer, one pharmaceutical formulary, one provider group, and one supplier of laboratory testing. All VA providers are employees of the same organization, so new policies and practices can

be communicated, implemented, and monitored much more easily and efficiently than in a U.S. multipayer, multiformulary, siloed system. Also, key is that the VA has one, universal EHR system with CPOE and CDSS. The VA EHR is able to code all data in one format that allows veterans who move from state to state to have their entire VA medical record seamlessly follow them. All these factors have allowed the VA to offer high-quality care at a relatively reasonable cost. Until the United States creates a single payer system and uses the same EHR universally, the larger system will suffer from the enormous complexity and costs of developing and maintaining multiple data standards to support the exchange of health information among institutions and across vendor platforms.

EHR ADOPTION PROGRESS IN THE UNITED STATES

One of the legislated functions of the ONC is to perform periodic surveys of EHR adoption. The ONC performs two national surveys. One surveys physician provider offices and the other surveys hospitals. The ONC defines two levels of adoption defined as "Basic" and "Full."[63] This distinction is important because many other surveys report EHR adoption rates but do not define in any detail what "EHR adoption" means. The ONC survey uses an exacting definition of Basic and Advanced EHR adoption that produces results that are much more valid than surveys where "adoption" is not well defined. **Figure 15-6** from the January 2012 ONC report to Congress, "Update on the Adoption of Health Information Technology and Related Efforts to Facilitate the Electronic Use and Exchange of Health Information," illustrates the rate of EHR Basic adoption among non-hospital-based physicians. These results demonstrate a steady increase in the adoption of Basic EHRs:[64]

> As of 2011, 34 percent of nonhospital based physicians had adopted a "basic" EHR. This is double the adoption rate among nonhospital

FIGURE 15-6 Adoption of "basic" electronic health records among non-hospital-based physicians.

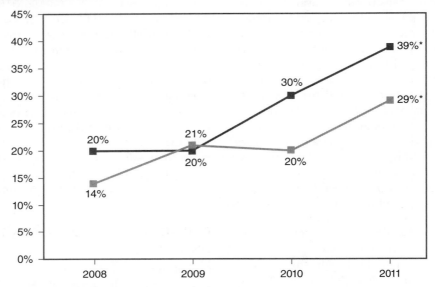

Source: Reproduced from ONC report to Congress. Update on the Adoption of Health Information Technology and Related Efforts to Facilitate the Electronic Use and Exchange of Health Information: A Report to Congress. January 2012.

based physicians in 2008. Adoption among primary care physicians, a key focus area of the HITECH Act, grew to approximately 40 percent; adoption among this same group has nearly doubled since 2008. These results are initial indications of the effects that the HITECH Act and CMS and ONC programs have had to date in accelerating the adoption of health IT and EHRs.[63]

Figure 15-7 from the ONC report noted previously illustrates the adoption rate of Basic EHRs among nonfederal acute care hospitals.[64] The report states, "Nearly 19 percent of nonfederal acute care hospitals adopted a 'basic' EHR by 2010. This represents over a 50 percent increase in adoption among hospitals since 2008."[64]

The adoption rate of electronic prescribing or "eprescribing" has been much more successful than the overall adoption of basic

EHRs. The ONC report of 2012 further noted:

> Data from Surescripts, the nation's largest electronic prescribing network, shows that the percent of nonhospital based physicians active on the Surescripts network using an electronic health record has increased more than threefold since 2008, to 44 percent. Pharmacies have reached near universal adoption of electronic prescribing at 93 percent.[64]

The report also attributes much of the increase to the CMS financial incentive program for eprescribing. **Figures 15-8** and **15-9** from the January 2012 ONC report provide the adoption rates for eprescribing by non-hospital-based physicians and retail community pharmacies.[64]

FIGURE 15-7

Adoption of "basic" electronic health records among nonfederal acute care hospitals.

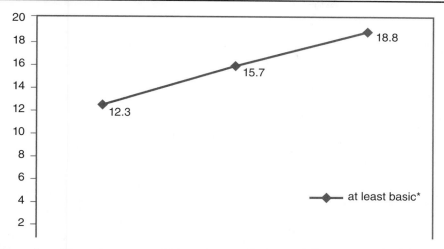

Source: Reproduced from ONC report to Congress. Update on the Adoption of Health Information Technology and Related Efforts to Facilitate the Electronic Use and Exchange of Health Information: A Report to Congress. January 2012.

FIGURE 15-8

Adoption of electronic prescribing through and electronic health record among non-hospital-based physicians.

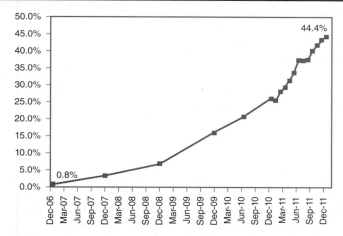

Source: Reproduced from ONC report to Congress. Update on the Adoption of Health Information Technology and Related Efforts to Facilitate the Electronic Use and Exchange of Health Information: A Report to Congress. January 2012.

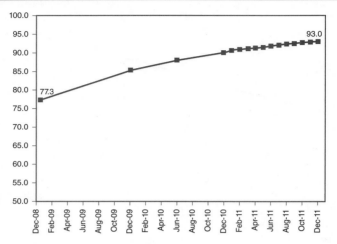

FIGURE 15-9 Adoption of electronic prescribing among retail community pharmacies.

Source: Reproduced from ONC report to Congress. Update on the Adoption of Health Information Technology and Related Efforts to Facilitate the Electronic Use and Exchange of Health Information: A Report to Congress. January 2012.

FUTURE CHALLENGES

Although there is mounting evidence supporting the value of EHRs with CPOE and CDSS in several well-defined areas such as improving preventative care delivery, the extensive meta-analyses only report the combined average results. There have been several inconclusive and negative studies, and some that have actually shown patient harm associated with the installation of CPOE. In one of the most extensively reported, the mortality rate in a neonatal intensive care unit more than doubled after a CPOE system was installed at the University of Pittsburgh.[65] Much has been written about the reasons for this negative result, and despite the finger pointing, there is virtually universal agreement that HIT can be very disruptive to work processes and work cultures, resulting in significant harm to patients.[66] Some have called for more HIT standards and regulation to prevent these negative consequences in the same way as the U.S. Food and Drug Administration regulates medical devices.[67,68]

Due to the administrative and technical difficulties of achieving the Nationwide Health Information Network, proprietary entities have offered alternate approaches to develop "personal health records" (PHRs) through which patients create their own records in a standardized format. In these approaches, patients may physically carry records or make them available to caregivers via the Internet. Microsoft, Google, and many others have built such systems but with little marketing success. Google Health announced its shutdown on June 24, 2011, after only 3 years of operation. Google joins other lesser known firms that have decided to close down PHR services.[69] Design of existing PHRs requires patients to have a high level of health literacy and computer savvy. A major reason analysts believed Google Health failed was the newness of the concept for most people and the fact that PHRs are difficult to use and that many people find the amount of data entry work necessary to complete their record to be too laborious.[70] One survey of patients found that only 7% had tried using a PHR and only about 3% continued to use them in 2011.[70] Other barriers to patient adoption include lack of personal health management tools (PHMT), the difficulty in achieving semantic interoperability such that PHMTs could be useful, problems vetting the identity of PHR users, patient privacy concerns, and, perhaps most importantly, the lack of a business model to support the long-term operation of PHRs.[69]

In addition to providers and patients affected by development and implementation of HIT, there are many other health care professionals and venues with significant complexities and characteristics that make HIT implementation challenging. Many of the same issues previously discussed in this chapter apply to these venues, such as standardized data formats to facilitate data portability, work culture barriers, system expense, training issues, and other matters. For example, some emergency medical service (EMS) providers have begun to use a variety of portable EHRs to collect data at the scenes of patient incidents with systems designed to transmit data to receiving hospitals. The same issues that complicate the ease of universal HIE between health care institutions apply to the data exchange between EMS and hospital systems and will not be easily resolved.

To achieve the HIT goals of improving health care quality and reducing costs, extensive and rigorous work remains in the research and implementation arenas. After 50 years of efforts and most notably in the past 5 years, government, industry, and academia are only now recognizing the critically important and interdependent roles that standardization, administrative processes, and work cultures play in the HIT desired outcomes.

REFERENCES

1. Bush GW. Executive Order: Incentives for the Use of Health Information Technology and Establishing the Position of the National Health Information Technology Coordinator. 2004; http://georgewbush-whitehouse.archives.gov/news/releases/2004/04/20040427-4.html. Accessed September 25, 2012.
2. One Hundred Eleventh Congress of the United States of America. *The American Recovery and Reinvestment Act*. Washington, DC: U.S. Government Printing Office; 2009.
3. The Life Sciences Panel of the President's Science Advisory Committee. *Some New Technologies and Their Promise for the Life Sciences*. Washington, DC: The White House; January 23, 1963.
4. Duke Evidence-based Practice Center. *Enabling Health Care Decisionmaking through Clinical Decision Support and Knowledge Management*. Rockville, MD: Agency for Healthcare Research and Quality, U.S. Department of Health and Human Services; 2012.
5. McDonald CJ. Protocol-based computer reminders, the quality of care and the non-perfectability of man. *N Engl J Med*. 1976;295(24):1351–1355.
6. Yount RJ, Vries JK, Councill CD. The Medical Archival System: an information retrieval system based on distributed parallel processing. *Info Proces Management*. 1991;27(4):1–11.
7. Gardner RM, Pryor TA, Warner HR. The HELP hospital information system: update 1998. *Int J Med Inform*. 1999;54(3):169–182.
8. Pryor TA, Gardner RM, Clayton PD, Warner HR. The HELP system. *J Med Syst*. 1983;7(2):87–102.
9. Higgins SB, Jiang K, Swindell BB, Bernard GR. A graphical ICU workstation. *Proc Annu Symp Comput Appl Med Care*. 1991:783–787.
10. Giuse DA, Mickish A. Increasing the availability of the computerized patient record. *Proc AMIA Annu Fall Symp*. 1996:633–637.
11. Stead WW, Hammond WE. Computer-based medical records: the centerpiece of TMR. *MD Comput*. 1988;5(5):48–62.
12. Greenes RA, Pappalardo AN, Marble CW, Barnett GO. Design and implementation of a clinical data management system. *Comput Biomed Res*. 1969;2(5):469–485.
13. United States Department of Health and Human Services. Certified health IT product list. 2012; http://oncchpl.force.com/ehrcert?q=CHPL. Accessed September 30, 2014.

14. HITECH Programs and Advisory Committees. Health IT adoption programs. http://www.healthit.gov/policy-researchers-implementers/health-it-adoption-programs. Accessed September 30, 2014.

15. Campbell EM, Guappone KP, Sittig DF, Dykstra RH, Ash JS. Computerized provider order entry adoption: implications for clinical workflow. *J Gen Intern Med.* 2009;*24*(1):21–26.

16. Bloomrosen M, Starren J, Lorenzi NM, Ash JS, Patel VL, Shortliffe EH. Anticipating and addressing the unintended consequences of health IT and policy: a report from the AMIA 2009 Health Policy Meeting. *J Am Med Inform Assoc.* 2011;*18*(1):82–90.

17. Ash JS, Stavri PZ, Dykstra R, Fournier L. Implementing computerized physician order entry: the importance of special people. *Int J Med Inform.* 2003;*69*(2–3):235–250.

18. Chaudhry B, Wang J, Wu S, et al. Systematic review: impact of health -information technology on quality, efficiency, and costs of medical care. *Ann Intern Med.* 2006;*144*(10):742–752.

19. Ash JS, Bates DW. Factors and forces affecting EHR system adoption: report of a 2004 ACMI discussion. *J Am Med Inform Assoc.* 2005;*12*(1):8–12.

20. Connolly C. Cedars-Sinai doctors cling to pen and paper. *Washington Post.* March 21, 2005:A01. http://gunston.gmu.edu/healthscience/740/Presentations/cedars-sinai%20cpoe%20washpost%203-21-05.pdf. Accessed September 30, 2014.

21. Dexter PR, Perkins S, Overhage JM, Maharry K, Kohler RB, McDonald CJ. A computerized reminder system to increase the use of preventive care for hospitalized patients. *N Engl J Med.* 2001;*345*(13):965–970.

22. Weiner M, Callahan CM, Tierney WM, et al. Using information technology to improve the health care of older adults. *Ann Intern Med.* 2003;*139*(5 Pt 2):430–436.

23. Dexter PR, Perkins SM, Maharry KS, Jones K, McDonald CJ. Inpatient computer-based standing orders vs physician provider reminders to increase influenza and pneumococcal vaccination rates: a randomized trial. *JAMA.* 2004;*292*(19):2366–2371.

24. Overhage JM, Dexter PR, Perkins SM, et al. A randomized, controlled trial of clinical information shared from another institution. *Ann Emerg Med.* 2002;*39*(1):14–23.

25. One Hundred Eleventh Congress of the United States of America. Health Information Technology for Economic and Clinical Health Act. 2009; http://www.hhs.gov/ocr/privacy/hipaa/understanding/coveredentities/hitechact.pdf. Accessed September 25, 2012.

26. The Office of the National Coordinator for Health Information Technology (ONC). About ONC. 2012; http://healthit.hhs.gov/portal/server.pt/community/healthit_hhs_gov_onc/1200. Accessed September 30, 2014.

27. The Office of the National Coordinator for Health Information Technology (ONC). ONC organizational structure. 2012; http://healthit.hhs.gov/portal/server.pt/community/healthit_hhs_gov__organization/1512. Accessed September 30, 2014.

28. United States Department of Health and Human Services. HITECH Programs and Advisory Committees. http://www.healthit.gov/facas/federal-advisory-committees-facas. Accessed September 30, 2014.

29. Centers for Medicare and Medicaid Services. Eligible hospital information. 2012; http://www.cms.gov/Regulations-and-Guidance/Legislation/EHRIncentivePrograms/Eligible_Hospital_Information.html. Accessed September 30, 2014.

30. Centers for Medicare and Medicaid Services. *EHR Incentive Program for Medicare Hospitals: Calculating Payments.* 2012; http://www.cms.gov/Outreach-and-Education/Medicare-Learning-Network-MLN/MLNProducts/downloads/EHR_TipSheet_Medicare_Hosp.pdf. Accessed September 30, 2014.

31. Centers for Medicare and Medicaid Services. *Medicaid Hospital Incentive Payments Calculations.* 2012; http://healthinsight.org/Internal/docs/2012-07-18/medicaid_hosp_incentive_payments_tip_sheets.pdf. Accessed September 30, 2014.

32. Centers for Medicare and Medicaid Services. *Flow Chart to Help Eligible Professionals (EP) Determine Eligibility for the Medicare and Medicaid Electronic Health Record (EHR) Incentive Programs.* 2012; https://www.cms.gov/Regulations-and-Guidance/Legislation/EHRIncentivePrograms/downloads/eligibility_flow_chart.pdf. Accessed September 30, 2014.

33. Centers for Medicare and Medicaid Services. EHR incentive programs. 2012; http://www.cms.gov/Regulations-and-Guidance/Legislation/EHRIncentivePrograms/index.html?redirect=/ehrincentiveprograms/. Accessed September 30, 2014.

34. Centers for Medicare and Medicaid Services. Medicare Electronic Health Record Incentive

Program for Eligible Professionals. 2012; http://www.cms.gov/Outreach-and-Education/Medicare-Learning-Network-MLN/MLNProducts/Downloads/CMS_eHR_Tip_Sheet.pdf. Accessed September 30, 2014.

35. Centers for Medicare and Medicaid Services. *An Introduction to the Medicaid EHR Incentive Program for Eligible Professionals.* 2012; http://www.cms.gov/Regulations-and-Guidance/Legislation/EHRIncentivePrograms/downloads/Beginners_Guide.pdf. Accessed September 30, 2014.

36. Centers for Medicare and Medicaid Services. *An Introduction to the Medicare EHR Incentive Program for Eligible Professionals.* 2012; http://www.cms.gov/Regulations-and-Guidance/Legislation/EHRIncentivePrograms/Downloads/Beginners_Guide.pdf. Accessed September 30, 2014.

37. Centers for Medicare and Medicaid Services. Medicaid Electronic Health Record Incentive Payments for Eligible Professionals. 2012; http://www.cms.gov/Outreach-and-Education/Medicare-Learning-Network-MLN/MLNProducts/Downloads/EHRIP_Eligible_Professionals_Tip_Sheet.pdf. Accessed September 30, 2014.

38. Centers for Medicare and Medicaid Services. 2014 Stage 1 definition of meaningful use. 2012; http://www.cms.gov/Regulations-and-Guidance/Legislation/EHRIncentivePrograms/Meaningful_Use.html. Accessed September 30, 2014.

39. Centers for Medicare and Medicaid Services. Medicare and Medicaid EHR Incentive Program Basics. 2012; http://www.cms.gov/Regulations-and-Guidance/Legislation/EHRIncentivePrograms/Basics.html. Accessed September 30, 2014.

40. United States Department of Health and Human Services. Meaningful use regulations. 2012; http://www.healthit.gov/policy-researchers-implementers/meaningful-use. Accessed September 30, 2014.

41. Centers for Medicare and Medicaid Services. *Eligible Professional Meaningful Use Table of Contents Core and Menu Set Objectives.* 2014; https://www.cms.gov/Regulations-and-Guidance/Legislation/EHRIncentivePrograms/downloads/EP-MU-TOC.pdf. Accessed September 30, 2014.

42. Centers for Medicare and Medicaid Services. *Eligible Hospital and CAH Meaningful Use Table of Contents Core and Menu Set Objectives.* 2014; http://www.cms.gov/Regulations-and-Guidance/Legislation/EHRIncentivePrograms/downloads/Hosp_CAH_MU-TOC.pdf. Accessed September 30, 2014.

43. United States Department of Health and Human Services. *Stage 1 vs. Stage 2 Comparison Table for Eligible Professionals.* 2012; http://www.cms.gov/Regulations-and-Guidance/Legislation/EHRIncentivePrograms/Downloads/Stage1vsStage2CompTablesforEP.pdf. Accessed September 30, 2014.

44. United States Department of Health and Human Services. *Stage 1 vs. Stage 2 Comparison Table for Eligible Hospitals and CAHs.* 2012; http://www.cms.gov/Regulations-and-Guidance/Legislation/EHRIncentivePrograms/Downloads/Stage1vsStage2CompTablesforHospitals.pdf. Accessed September 30, 2014.

45. Dukette D, Cornish D. *The Essential 20: Twenty Components of an Excellent Health Care Team.* Pittsburgh, PA: RoseDog Books; 2009:72–74.

46. Parthasarathy S. Sleep and the medical profession. *Curr Opin Pulm Med.* 2005;*11*(6):507–512.

47. Institute of Medicine. *Free Executive Summary: Beyond Expert-Based Practice. IOM Annual Meeting Summary: Evidence-Based Medicine and the Changing Nature of Healthcare.* Washington, DC: National Academies Press; 2008:18–19.

48. Friedman CP. What informatics is and isn't. *J Am Med Inform Assoc.* 2012;*0*:1–3.

49. Evans RS, Pestotnik SL, Classen DC, et al. A computer-assisted management program for antibiotics and other antiinfective agents. *N Engl J Med.* 1998;*338*(4):232–238.

50. Tierney WM, Dexter PR, Gramelspacher GP, Perkins AJ, Zhou XH, Wolinsky FD. The effect of discussions about advance directives on patients' satisfaction with primary care. *J Gen Intern Med.* 2001;*16*(1):32–40.

51. Gardner RM. Computerized clinical decision-support in respiratory care. *Respir Care.* 2004;*49*(4):378–386; discussion 386–378.

52. Tierney WM, Miller ME, Overhage JM, McDonald CJ. Physician-provider inpatient order writing on microcomputer workstations. Effects on resource utilization. *JAMA.* 1993;*269*(3):379–383.

53. Kho AN, Dexter P, Lemmon L, et al. Connecting the dots: creation of an electronic regional infection control network. *Stud Health Technol Inform.* 2007;*129*(Pt 1):213–217.

54. Kho A, Dexter P, Warvel J, Commiskey M, Wilson S, McDonald CJ. Computerized reminders to improve isolation rates of patients with drug-resistant infections: design and preliminary results. *AMIA Annu Symp Proc.* 2005:390–394.

55. Rosenman M, Wang J, Dexter P, Overhage JM. Computerized reminders for syphilis screening in an urban emergency department. *AMIA Annu Symp Proc.* 2003:987.

56. Kroth PJ, Dexter PR, Overhage JM, et al. A computerized decision support system improves the accuracy of temperature capture from nursing personnel at the bedside. *AMIA Annu Symp Proc.* 2006:444–448.

57. Agency for Healthcare Research and Quality. Enabling health care decisionmaking through clinical decision support and knowledge. Evidence Report/Technology Assessment Number 203. 2012; http://www.ahrq.gov/clinic/tp/knowmgttp.htm. Accessed September 30, 2014.

58. Markle Foundation. The Common Framework: Technical Issues and Requirements for Implementation. 2006; http://www.markle.org/sites/default/files/T1_TechIssues.pdf. Accessed September 30, 2014.

59. Lin MC, Vreeman DJ, McDonald CJ, Huff SM. Auditing consistency and usefulness of LOINC use among three large institutions—using version spaces for grouping LOINC codes. *J Biomed Inform.* 2012;45(4):658–666.

60. National Library of Medicine. UMLS Quick Start Guide. 2012; http://www.nlm.nih.gov/research/umls/quickstart.html. Accessed September 30, 2014.

61. Sorrell WH. Supreme Court Strikes Down Vermont Prescription Privacy Law. 2011; http://www.atg.state.vt.us/news/supreme-court-strikes-down-vermont-prescription-privacy-law.php. Accessed September 30, 2014.

62. The Supreme Court of the United States. Sorrell, Attorney General of Vermont, et al. vs. IMS Health Inc. et al. 2011; http://www.supremecourt.gov/opinions/10pdf/10-779.pdf. Accessed September 30, 2014.

63. Hsiao CJ, Hing E, Socey TC, Cai B. Electronic health record systems and intent to apply for meaningful use incentives among office-based physician practices: United States, 2001–2011. *NCHS Data Brief.* 2011;79:1–8. http://www.cdc.gov/nchs/data/databriefs/db79.htm. Accessed September 30, 2014.

64. The Office of the National Coordinator for Health Information Technology (ONC). Update on the Adoption of Health Information Technology and Related Efforts to Facilitate the Electronic Use and Exchange of Health Information: A Report to Congress. January 2012; http://www.healthit.gov/sites/default/files/rtc_adoption_of_healthit_and_relatedefforts.pdf. Accessed September 30, 2014.

65. Han YY, Carcillo JA, Venkataraman ST, et al. Unexpected increased mortality after implementation of a commercially sold computerized physician order entry system. *Pediatrics.* 2005;116(6):1506–1512.

66. Sittig DF, Ash JS, Zhang J, Osheroff JA, Shabot MM. Lessons from "Unexpected increased mortality after implementation of a commercially sold computerized physician order entry system." *Pediatrics.* 2006;118(2):797–801.

67. Miller RA, Gardner RM. Summary recommendations for responsible monitoring and regulation of clinical software systems. American Medical Informatics Association, The Computer-based Patient Record Institute, The Medical Library Association, The Association of Academic Health Science Libraries, The American Health Information Management Association, and The American Nurses Association. *Ann Intern Med.* 1997;127(9):842–845.

68. Miller RA, Gardner RM. Recommendations for responsible monitoring and regulation of clinical software systems. American Medical Informatics Association, Computer-based Patient Record Institute, Medical Library Association, Association of Academic Health Science Libraries, American Health Information Management Association, American Nurses Association. *J Am Med Inform Assoc.* 1997;4(6):442–457.

69. Rishel W, Booz RH. Google Health Shutdown Underscores Uncertain Future of PHRs. 2011; http://www.gartner.com/resources/214600/214682/google_health_shutdown_under_214682.pdf. Accessed September 30, 2014.

70. Lohr S. Google is closing its health records service. *New York Times.* June 24, 2011.

CHAPTER 16

The Electronic Health Record and Clinical Informatics

Emily B. Barey, Kathleen Mastrian, and Dee McGonigle

CHAPTER OBJECTIVES

1. Describe the common components of an electronic health record.
2. Assess the benefits of implementing an electronic health record.
3. Explore the ownership of an electronic health record.
4. Evaluate the flexibility of the electronic health record in meeting the needs of clinicians and patients.

INTRODUCTION

The significance of electronic health records (EHRs) to nursing cannot be underestimated. Although EHRs on the surface suggest a simple automation of clinical documentation, in fact their implications are broad, ranging from the ways in which care is delivered, to the types of interactions nurses have with patients in conjunction with the use of technology, to the research surrounding EHRs that will inform nursing practice for tomorrow. A basic knowledge of EHRs and nursing informatics is now considered by many to be an entry-level nursing competency.

At the Technology Informatics Guiding Education Reform (TIGER, 2010) summit on evidence and informatics transforming nursing, participants stated that "the nation is working full-speed to realize the 10-year goal of Electronic Health Records for its citizens" (p. 1). Nurses must become active participants in this effort to capture healthcare information, generate knowledge, and enhance patient care. "This is a critical juncture for nurses, who comprise

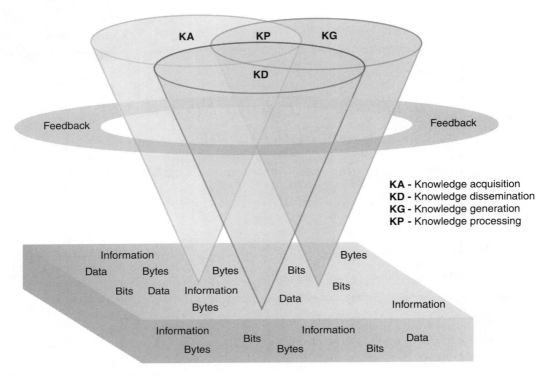

Foundation of Knowledge Model.

Designed by Alicia Mastrian.

55% of the healthcare workforce, number more than 3 million, and who must become more aware and involved at every level of the Informatics Revolution" (p. 1). Although EHR standards are evolving and barriers to adoption remain, the collective work has a positive momentum that will benefit clinicians and patients alike.

This drive to adopt EHRs has been underscored with the passage of the Health Information Technology for Economic and Clinical Health Act of 2009 (HITECH). It is essential that this competency be developed if nurses are to participate fully in the changing world of healthcare information technology.

This chapter has four goals. First, it describes the common components of an EHR. Second, it reviews the benefits of implementing an EHR. Third, it provides an overview of successful ownership of an EHR, including nursing's role in promoting the safe adoption of EHRs in day-to-day practice. Fourth, it discusses the flexibility of an EHR in meeting the needs of both clinicians and patients, including an introduction to interoperability.

SETTING THE STAGE

The U.S. healthcare system faces the enormous challenge of improving the quality of care while simultaneously controlling costs. EHRs have been proposed as one solution to achieve this goal (Institute of Medicine [IOM], 2001). In January 2004, President George W. Bush raised the profile of EHRs in his State of the Union address by outlining a plan to ensure that most Americans have an EHR by 2014. He stated that "by computerizing health records we can avoid dangerous medical mistakes, reduce costs, and improve care" (Bush, 2004). This proclamation generated an increased demand for understanding EHRs and promoting their adoption, but relatively few healthcare organizations were motivated to pursue more rapid adoption of EHRs. The Healthcare Information and Management Systems Society (HIMSS) has been tracking EHR adoption since 2005 through its "Stage 7" award and reports that most U.S. healthcare organizations (77%) are in Stage 3, reflecting only implementation of the basic components of laboratory, radiology, and pharmacy ancillaries; a clinical data repository, including a controlled medical vocabulary; and simple nursing documentation and clinical decision support (HIMSS, 2013). Higher stages of the electronic medical record adoption model include more sophisticated use of decision support tools and medication administration tools, with Stage 7—the highest level—consisting of EHRs that have data sharing and warehousing capabilities and that are completely interfaced with emergency and outpatient facilities (HIMSS Analytics, 2013).

In President Barack Obama's first term in office, Congress passed the American Recovery and Reinvestment Act of 2009 (ARRA). This legislation included the HITECH Act, which specifically sought to incentivize health organizations and providers to become meaningful users of EHRs. These incentives will come in the form of increased reimbursement rates from the Centers for Medicare and Medicaid Services (CMS); ultimately, the HITECH Act will result in payment of a penalty by any healthcare organization that has not adopted EHRs by January 2015. The final rule was published by the Department of Health and Human Services (DHHS) in July 2010 for the first phase of implementation. Stage 1 meaningful use criteria focus on data capture and sharing (DHHS, 2010). Stage 2 criteria, which were in implemented in 2014, focus on several clinical processes and promote health information exchange (HIE) and more patient control over personal data. Stage 3, which has a target implementation date of 2016, focuses on improved outcomes for individuals and populations, and introduction of patient self-management tools (Centers for Medicare and Medicaid Services, 2014).

COMPONENTS OF ELECTRONIC HEALTH RECORDS

Overview

Before enactment of the ARRA, several variants of EHRs existed, each with its own terminology and each developed with a different audience in mind. The sources of these records included, for example, the federal government (Certification Commission for Healthcare Information Technology, 2007), the IOM (2003), HIMSS (2007), and the National Institutes of Health (2006; Robert Wood Johnson Foundation [RWJF], 2006). Under ARRA, there is now an explicit requirement for providers and hospitals to use a certified EHR that meets a set of standard functional definitions to be eligible for the increased reimbursement incentive. DHHS granted two organizations the authority to accredit EHRs: the Drummond Group and the Certification Commission for Healthcare Information Technology. These bodies are authorized to test and certify EHR vendors against the standards and test procedures developed by the National Institute of Standards and Technology (NIST) and endorsed by the Office of the National Coordinator for Health Information Technology for EHRs. These bodies ceased their work in November 2014. The Office of the National

Coordinator (ONC), part of HHS, has taken over the process of certifying EHRs (HealthIT .gov, 2014).

The NIST test procedure includes 45 certification criteria, ranging from the basic ability to record patient demographics, document vital signs, and maintain an up-to-date problem list, to more complex functions, such as electronic exchange of clinical information and patient summary records (Jansen & Grance, 2011; NIST, 2010). **Box 16-1** lists the 45 certification criteria outlined by NIST.

BOX 16-1   EHR Certification Criteria

Criteria #	Certification Criteria
§170.302 (a)	Drug–drug, drug–allergy interaction checks
§170.302 (b)	Drug formulary checks
§170.302 (c)	Maintain up-to-date problem list
§170.302 (d)	Maintain active medication list
§170.302 (e)	Maintain active medication allergy list
§170.302 (f)(1)	Vital signs
§170.302 (f)(2)	Calculate body mass index
§170.302 (f)(3)	Plot and display growth charts
§170.302 (g)	Smoking status
§170.302 (h)	Incorporate laboratory test results
§170.302 (i)	Generate patient lists
§170.302 (j)	Medication reconciliation
§170.302 (k)	Submission to immunization registries
§170.302 (l)	Public health surveillance
§170.302 (m)	Patient-specific education resources
§170.302 (n)	Automated measure calculation
§170.302 (o)	Access control
§170.302 (p)	Emergency access
§170.302 (q)	Automatic log-off
§170.302 (r)	Audit log
§170.302 (s)	Integrity
§170.302 (t)	Authentication
§170.302 (u)	General encryption

BOX 16-1	EHR Certification Criteria *(continued)*

§170.302 (v)	Encryption when exchanging electronic health information
§170.302 (w)	Accounting of disclosures (optional)
§170.304 (a)	Computerized provider order entry
§170.304 (b)	Electronic prescribing
§170.304 (c)	Record demographics
§170.304 (d)	Patient reminders
§170.304 (e)	Clinical decision support
§170.304 (f)	Electronic copy of health information
§170.304 (g)	Timely access
§170.304 (h)	Clinical summaries
§170.304 (i)	Exchange clinical information and patient summary record
§170.304 (j)	Calculate and submit clinical quality measures
§170.306 (a)	Computerized provider order entry
§170.306 (b)	Record demographics
§170.306 (c)	Clinical decision support
§170.306 (d)(1)	Electronic copy of health information
§170.306 (d)(2)	Electronic copy of health information
	Note: For discharge summary
§170.306 (e)	Electronic copy of discharge instructions
§170.306 (f)	Exchange clinical information and patient summary record
§170.306 (g)	Reportable lab results
§170.306 (h)	Advance directives
§170.306 (i)	Calculate and submit clinical quality measures

Source: Data from National Institute of Standards and Technology (NIST). (2010). Meaningful use test method: Approved test procedures version 1.0. Retrieved from http://healthcare.nist.gov/use_testing /finalized_requirements.html

Despite the points articulated in the ARRA, the IOM definition also remains a valid reference point. This definition is useful because it has distilled all the possible features of an EHR into eight essential components with an emphasis on functions that promote patient safety—a universal denominator that everyone in health care can accept. The eight components are (1) health information and data, (2) results management, (3) order entry management, (4) decision support, (5) electronic communication and connectivity, (6) patient support, (7) administrative processes, and (8) reporting and population health management (IOM, 2003). Each of these components is described in more detail here. With the exception of EHR infrastructure functions, such as security and privacy management, controlled medical vocabularies, and interoperability standards, the 45 NIST standards easily map into the IOM categories (Jansen & Grance, 2011).

Health Information and Data

Health information and data comprise the patient data required to make sound clinical decisions, including demographics, medical and nursing diagnoses, medication lists, allergies, and test results (IOM, 2003).

Results Management

Results management is the ability to manage results of all types electronically, including laboratory and radiology procedure reports, both current and historical (IOM, 2003).

Order Entry Management

Order entry management is the ability of a clinician to enter medication and other care orders, including laboratory, microbiology, pathology, radiology, nursing, supply orders, ancillary services, and consultations, directly into a computer (IOM, 2003).

Decision Support

Decision support entails the use of computer reminders and alerts to improve the diagnosis and care of a patient, including screening for correct drug selection and dosing, screening for medication interactions with other medications, preventive health reminders in such areas as vaccinations, health risk screening and detection, and clinical guidelines for patient disease treatment (IOM, 2003).

Electronic Communication and Connectivity

Electronic communication and connectivity include the online communication among healthcare team members, their care partners, and patients, including e-mail, Web messaging, and an integrated health record within and across settings, institutions, and telemedicine (IOM, 2003).

Patient Support

Patient support encompasses patient education and self-monitoring tools, including interactive computer-based patient education, home telemonitoring, and telehealth systems (IOM, 2003).

Administrative Processes

Administrative processes are activities carried out by the electronic scheduling, billing, and claims management systems, including electronic scheduling for inpatient and outpatient visits and procedures, electronic insurance eligibility validation, claim authorization and prior approval, identification of possible research study participants, and drug recall support (IOM, 2003).

Reporting and Population Health Management

Reporting and population health management are the data collection tools to support public and private reporting requirements, including data represented in a standardized terminology and machine-readable format (IOM, 2003).

NIST has not provided an exhaustive list of all possible features and functions of an EHR. Consequently, different vendor EHR systems combine different components in their offerings, and often a single set of EHR components may not meet the needs of all clinicians and patient populations. For example, a pediatric setting may demand functions for immunization management, growth tracking, and more robust order entry features to include weight-based dosing (Spooner & Council on Clinical Information Technology, 2007). These types of features may not be provided by all EHR systems, and it is important to consider EHR certification to be a minimum standard.

ADVANTAGES OF ELECTRONIC HEALTH RECORDS

There are mixed reviews of the advantages offered by EHRs. Much has been written about the potential promise of reduced costs, improved quality, and better outcomes, but very little of this promise's realization has been substantiated except anecdotally (Sidorov, 2006). Possible methods to estimate EHR benefits include using vendor-supplied data that have been retrieved from customer systems, synthesizing and applying studies of overall EHR value, creating logical engineering models of EHR value, summarizing focused studies of elements of EHR value, and conducting and applying information from site visits (HealthIT.gov, 2012; Thompson, Osheroff, Classen, & Sittig, 2007). However, the time and effort involved in completing this work are further increased by the fact that historically there has been no standard by which to measure adoption or expected benefits (HealthIT.gov, 2012; RWJF, 2006; Thompson et al., 2007).

With the advent of ARRA, there are now 25 meaningful use objectives for eligible providers and 24 such objectives for eligible hospitals (CMS, 2010a). In addition, the final rule calls for providers to report on three required clinical quality measures and three additional quality measures of their choice from a list of 44 possible measures (CMS, 2010b). Eligible hospitals must report on 15 clinical quality measures. Although these objectives and measures will provide a universal benchmark moving forward for EHR benefits, for most healthcare organizations these outcomes alone will not provide sufficient return on investment to justify the capital investment made to implement an EHR, and additional benefits will continue to be sought.

The four most common benefits cited for EHRs are (1) increased delivery of guidelines-based care, (2) enhanced capacity to perform surveillance and monitoring for disease conditions, (3) reduction in medication errors, and (4) decreased use of care (Chaudhry et al., 2006; HealthIT.gov, 2012). These findings were echoed by two similar literature reviews. The first review focused on the use of informatics systems for managing patients with chronic illness. It found that the processes of care most positively impacted were guidelines adherence, visit frequency (i.e., a decrease in emergency department visits), provider documentation, patient treatment adherence, and screening and testing (Dorr et al., 2007).

The second review was a cost–benefit analysis of health information technology completed by the Agency for Healthcare Research and Quality (AHRQ) that studied the value of an EHR in the ambulatory care and pediatric settings, including its overall economic value. The AHRQ study highlighted the common findings already described but also noted that most of the data available for review came from six leading healthcare organizations in the United States, underscoring the challenge of generalizing these results to the broader healthcare industry (Shekelle, Morton, & Keeler, 2006). As noted previously by the HIMSS Stage 7 Awards, the challenge to generalize results persists in the hospital arena, with fewer than 1% of U.S. hospitals or eight leading organizations providing most of the experience with comprehensive EHRs (HIMSS, 2010a).

Finally, all three literature reviews cited here indicated that there are a limited number of hypothesis-testing studies of EHRs and even fewer that have reported cost data.

The descriptive studies do have value, however, and should not be hastily dismissed. Although not as rigorous in their design, they do describe the advantages of EHRs well and often include useful implementation recommendations learned from practical experience. As identified in these types of reviews, EHR advantages include simple benefits, such as no longer having to interpret poor handwriting and handwritten orders, reduced turnaround time for laboratory results in an emergency department, and decreased time to administration of the first dose of antibiotics in an inpatient nursing unit (HealthIT.gov, 2012; Husk & Waxman, 2004; Smith et al., 2004). In the ambulatory care setting, improved management of cardiac-related risk factors in patients with diabetes and effective patient notification of medication recalls have been demonstrated to be benefits of the EHR (Jain et al., 2005; Reed & Bernard, 2005). Two other unique advantages that have great potential are the ability to use the EHR and decision support functions to identify patients who qualify for research studies or who qualify for prescription drug benefits offered by pharmaceutical companies at safety-net clinics and hospitals (Embi et al., 2005; Poprock, 2005).

The HIMSS Davies Award may be the best resource for combined quantitative and qualitative results of successful EHR implementation. The Davies Award recognizes healthcare organizations that have achieved both excellence in implementation and value from health information technology (HIMSS, 2010b). One winner demonstrated a significant avoidance of medication errors because of bar-code scanning alerts, a $3 million decrease in medical records expenses as a result of going paperless, and a 5% reduction of duplicate laboratory orders by using computerized provider order entry alerting (HIMSS, 2010c). Another winner noted a 13% decrease in adverse drug reactions through the use of computerized physician order entry;

it also achieved a decrease in methicillin-resistant *Staphylococcus aureus* (MRSA) nosocomial infections from 9.8 per 10,000 discharges to 6.4 per 10,000 discharges in less than a year using an EHR flagging function, which made clinicians immediately aware that contact precautions were required for MRSA-positive patients (HIMSS, 2009). At both organizations, there was qualitative and quantitative evidence of high rates of end user adoption and satisfaction with use of the EHR.

A 2011 study of the effects of EHR adoption on nurse perceptions of quality of care, communication, and patient safety documented that nurses report better care outcomes and fewer concerns with care coordination and patient safety in hospitals with a basic EHR (Kutney-Lee & Kelly, 2011). In this study, nurses perceived that in hospitals with a functioning EHR, there was better communication among staff, especially during patient transfers, and fewer medication errors.

Without an EHR system, any of these benefits would be very difficult and costly to accomplish. Thus, despite limited standards and published studies, there is enough evidence to warrant pursuing widespread implementation of the EHR (Halamka, 2006; HealthIT.gov, 2012) and certainly enough evidence to warrant further study of the use and benefits of EHRs. **Box 16-2** describes some of the clinical information system (CIS) functions of an EHR.

BOX 16-2   The EHR as a Clinical Information System

Denise Tyler

A clinical information system (CIS) is a technology-based system applied at the point of care and designed to support care by providing instant access to information for clinicians. Early CISs implemented prior to the advent of

EHRs were limited in scope and provided such information as interpretation of laboratory results or a medication formulary and drug interaction information. With the implementation of EHRs, the goal of many organizations is to expand the scope of the early CISs to

BOX 16-2   The EHR as a Clinical Information System *(continued)*

become comprehensive systems that provide clinical decision support, an electronic patient record, and in some instances professional development and training tools. Benefits of such a comprehensive system include easy access to patient data at the point of care; structured and legible information that can be searched easily and that lends itself to data mining and analysis; and improved patient safety, especially the prevention of adverse drug reactions and the identification of health risk factors, such as falls.

TRACKING CLINICAL OUTCOMES

The ability to measure outcomes can be enhanced or impeded by the way an information system is designed and used. Although many practitioners can paint a very good picture of the patient by using a narrative (free text), employing this mode of expression in a clinical system without the use of a coded entry makes it difficult to analyze the care given or the patient's response. Free-text reporting also leads to inconsistencies of reporting from clinician to clinician and patient information that is fragmented or disorganized. This can limit the usefulness of patient data to other clinicians and interfere with the ability to create reports from the data for quality assurance and measurement purposes. Moreover, not all clinicians are equally skilled at the free-text form of communication, yielding inconsistent quality of documentation. Integrating standardized nursing terminologies into computerized nursing documentation systems enhances the ability to use the data for reporting and further research.

According to the IOM (2012), "Payers, healthcare delivery organizations and medical product companies should contribute data to research and analytic consortia to support expanded use of care data to generate new insights" (para. 2). McLaughlin and Halilovic (2006) described the use of clinical analytics to promote medical care outcomes research. The use of a CIS in conjunction with standardized codes for patient clinical issues helps to support the rigorous analysis of clinical data. Outcomes data produced as part of these analyses may include length of stay, mortality, readmissions, and complications. Future goals include the ability to compare data and outcomes across various institutions as a means of developing clinical guidelines or best practices guidelines. With the implementation of a comprehensive CIS, similar analyses of nursing outcomes could also be performed and shared. Likewise, such a system could aid nurse administrators in cross-unit comparisons and staffing decisions, especially when coupled with acuity systems data. In addition, clinical analytics can support required data reporting functions, especially those required by accreditation bodies.

SUPPORTING EVIDENCE-BASED PRACTICE

Evidence-based practice (EBP) can be thought of as the integration of clinical expertise and best practices based on systematic research to enhance decision making and improve patient care. References supporting EBP, such as clinical guidelines, are available for review at the click of a mouse or the press of a few keystrokes. The CIS's prompting capabilities can also reinforce the practice of looking for evidence to support nursing interventions rather than relying on how things have been

(continues)

BOX 16-2 The EHR as a Clinical Information System *(continued)*

done historically. This approach enhances processing and understanding of the information and allows the nurse to apply the information to other areas, increasing the knowledge obtained about why certain conditions or responses result in prompts for additional questions or actions.

To incorporate EBP into the practice of clinical nursing, the information needs to be embedded in the computerized documentation system so that it is part of the workflow. The most typical way of embedding this timely information is through clinical practice guidelines. The resulting interventions and clinical outcomes need to be measurable and reportable for further research. The supporting documentation for the EBP needs to be easily retrievable and meaningful. Links, reminders, and prompts can all be used as vehicles for transmission of this information. The format needs to allow for rapid scanning, with the ability to expand the amount of information when more detail is required or desired. Balancing a consistency in formatting with creativity can be difficult but is worth the effort to stimulate an atmosphere for learning.

EBP is supported by translational research, an exciting movement that has enormous potential for the sharing and use of EBP. The use of translational research to support EBP may help to close the gap between what is known (research) and what is done (practice).

THE CIS AS A STAFF DEVELOPMENT TOOL

Joy Hilty, a registered nurse from Kaweah Delta, came up with a creative way to provide staff development or education without taking staff away from the bedside to a classroom setting. She created pop-up boxes on the opening charting screens for all staff who chart on the computer. These pop-ups vary in color and content and include a short piece of clinical information, along with a question. Staff can earn vacations from these pop-ups for as long as 14 days by emailing the correct answer to the question. This medium has provided information, stimulation, and a definite benefit: the vacation from the pop-up boxes. The pop-up box education format has also encouraged staff to share their answers, thereby creating interaction, knowledge dissemination, and reinforcement of the education provided.

Embedding EBP into nursing documentation can also increase the compliance with The Joint Commission core measures, such as providing information on influenza and pneumococcal vaccinations to at-risk patients. In the author's experience at Kaweah Delta, educating staff via classes, flyers, and storyboards was not successful in improving compliance with the documentation of immunization status or offering education on these vaccinations to at-risk patients. Embedding the prompts, information, and related questions in the nursing documentation with a link to the protocol and educational material, however, improved the compliance to 96% for pneumococcal vaccinations and to 95% for influenza vaccinations (Hettinger, 2007).

As more information is stored electronically, nurse informaticists must translate the technology so that the input and retrieval of information are developed in a manner that is easy for clinicians to learn and use. A highly usable product should decrease errors and

BOX 16-2 The EHR as a Clinical Information System *(continued)*

improve information entry and retrieval. Nurse informaticists must be able to work with staff and expert users to design systems that meet the needs of the staff who will actually use the systems. The work is not done after the system is installed; the system must continue to be developed and improved, because as staff use the system, they will be able to suggest changes to improve it. This ongoing revision should result in a system that is mature and meets the needs of the users.

In an ideal world, all clinical documentation will be shared through a national database, in a standard language, to enable evaluation of nursing care, increase the body of evidence, and improve patient outcomes. With minimal effort, the information will be translated into new research that can be analyzed and linked to new evidence that will be intuitively applied to the CIS. Alerts will be meaningful and will be patient and provider specific. The steps required of the clinician to find current, reliable information will be almost transparent, and the information will be presented in a personalized manner based on user preferences stored in the CIS.

REFERENCES

Hettinger, M. (2007, March). *Core measure reporting: Performance improvement*. Visalia, CA: Kaweah Delta Health Care District.

McLaughlin, T., & Halilovic, M. (2006). Clinical analytics, rigorous coding bring objectivity to quality assertions. *Medical Staff Update Online, 30*(6). http://med.stanford.edu/shs/update/archives/JUNE2006/analytics.htm

OWNERSHIP OF ELECTRONIC HEALTH RECORDS

The implementation of an EHR has the potential to affect every member of a healthcare organization. The process of becoming a successful owner of an EHR has multiple steps and requires integrating the EHR into the organization's day-to-day operations and long-term vision, as well as into the clinician's day-to-day practice. All members of the healthcare organization—from the executive level to the clinician at the point of care—must feel a sense of ownership to make the implementation successful for themselves, their colleagues, and their patients. Successful ownership of an EHR may be defined in part by the level of clinician adoption of the tool, and this section reviews key steps and strategies for the selection, implementation and evaluation, and optimization of an EHR in pursuit of that goal.

Historically, many systems were developed locally by the information technology department of a healthcare organization. It was not unusual for software developers to be employed by the organization to create needed systems and interfaces between them. As commercial offerings were introduced and matured, it became less and less common to see homegrown or locally developed systems.

As this history suggests, the first step of ownership is typically a vendor selection process for a commercially available EHR. During this step, it is important to survey the organization's level of interest, identify possible barriers to participation, document desired functions of an EHR, and assess the willingness to fund the implementation (Holbrook, Keshavjee, Troyan, Pray, & Ford, 2003). Although clinicians should drive the project, the assessment should also include the needs and readiness of the executive leadership, information technology, and project management teams. It is essential that leadership understands that this type of project is as much about redesigning clinical work as it is about technically automating it and that they agree to assume accountability for its success (Goddard, 2000). In addition, this preacquisition phase should concentrate on understanding the current state of the health information technology industry to identify appropriate questions and the next steps in the selection process (American Organization of Nurse Executives, 2006). These first steps begin to identify any organizational risks related to successful implementation and pave the way for initiating a change management process to educate the organization about the future state of delivering health care with an EHR system.

The second step of the selection process is to select a system based on the organization's current and predicted needs. It is common during this phase to see a demonstration of several vendors' EHR products. Based on the completed needs assessment, the organization should establish key evaluation criteria to compare the different vendors and products. These criteria should include both subjective and objective items that cover such topics as common clinical workflows, decision support, reporting, usability, technical build, and maintenance of the system. Providing the vendor with these guidelines will ensure that the process meets the organization's needs; however, it is also essential to let the vendor demonstrate a proposed future state from its own perspective. This activity is critical to ensuring that the vendor's vision and the organization's vision are well aligned (Konschak & Shiple, n.d.). It also helps spark dialogue about the possible future state of clinical work at the organization and the change

required in obtaining it. Such demonstrations enable the organization to compare and contrast the features and functions of different systems, and they are a good way to engage the organization's members in being a part of this strategic decision.

Implementation planning should occur concurrently with the selection process, particularly the assessment of the scope of the work, initial sequencing of the EHR components to be implemented, and resources required. However, this step begins in earnest once a vendor and a product have been selected. In addition to further refining the implementation plan, this is the time to identify key metrics by which to measure the EHR's success. An organization may realize numerous benefits from implementing an EHR. It should choose metrics that match its overall strategy and goals in the coming years and may include expected improvements in financial, quality, and clinical outcomes. Commonly used metrics focus on reductions in the number of duplicate laboratory tests through duplicate orders alerting, reductions in the number of adverse drug events through the use of bar-code medication administration, meaningful use objectives and measures, and the EHR advantages mentioned earlier in this chapter. To ensure that the desired benefits are realized, it is important to avoid choosing so many that they become meaningless or unobtainable, to carefully and practically define those that are chosen, to measure before and after the implementation, and to assign accountability to a member of the organization to ensure the work is completed.

End-user adoption of the EHR is also essential to realizing its benefits. Clinicians must be engaged to use the EHR successfully in their practice and daily workflows so that data may be captured to drive the decision support that underlies so many of the advantages and metrics described. To promote adoption, a change management plan must be developed in conjunction with the EHR implementation plan. The most effective change management plans offer end users several exposures to the system and relevant workflows in advance of its use and continue through the go-live and postlive time periods. Successful prelive strategies include end-user involvement as subject-matter experts to validate the EHR workflow design and content build, hosting end-user usability testing sessions, shadowing end users in their current daily work in parallel with the new system, and formal training activities. The goal of these prelive activities is not only to ensure that the EHR implementation will meet end user needs but also to assess the impact of the new EHR on current workflow and process. The larger the impact, the more change management is required above and beyond system training. For example, simulation laboratory experiences may be offered to more thoroughly dress rehearse a significant workflow change, executive leadership may need to convey their support and expectations of clinicians about a new way of working, and generally more anticipatory guidance is required to communicate to those impacted by the changes.

Training may be delivered in a variety of media. Often a combination of approaches works best, including classroom time, electronic learning, independent exercises, and peer-to-peer, at-the-elbow support. Training must be workflow based and reflect real clinical processes. It must also be planned and budgeted for through the postlive period to ensure that competency with the system is assessed at the go-live point and that any necessary retraining or reinforcements are made in the 30 to 60 days postlive. This not only promotes reliability and safe use of the system as it was designed but also can have a positive impact on end users'

morale: Users will feel that they are being supported beyond the initial go-live period and have an opportunity to move from basic skills to advanced proficiency with the system.

Finally, the implementation plan should account for the long-term optimization of the EHR. This step is commonly overlooked and often results in benefits falling short of expectations because the resources are not available to realize them permanently. It also often means the difference between end users of EHRs merely surviving the change versus becoming savvy about how to adopt the EHR as another powerful clinical tool, such as the stethoscope (HealthIT.gov, 2012). Optimization activities of the EHR should be considered a routine part of the organization's operations, should be resourced accordingly, and should emphasize the continued involvement of clinician users to identify ways that the EHR can enable the organization to achieve its overall mission. Many organizations start an implementation of EHRs with the goal of transforming their care delivery and operations. An endeavor that differs from simply automating a previously manual or fragmented process, transformation often includes steps to improve the process so as to realize better patient care outcomes or added efficiency. Although some transformation is experienced with the initial use of the system, most of this work is done postimplementation and relies on widespread clinician adoption of the EHR. As such, it makes optimization a critical component to successful ownership of an EHR.

Box 16-3 reviews the barriers to and methods for successful acceptance of EHRs.

BOX 16-3	Resistance to Implementation

Julie A. Kenney and Ida Androwich

For an implementation to be successful, a few things need to happen. The informatics nurse specialist (INS) will need to understand and use change management theory to ensure that the implementation of the new EHR system will be

(continues)

BOX 16-3   Resistance to Implementation *(continued)*

successful. It is a well-known fact that nurses can make or break a system implementation. A nursing staff that is involved early in the implementation process has been found to be a major determinant in a successful implementation. Assessing nursing attitudes and concerns early in the process can aid the INS in determining the best way to proceed with staff education and implementation rollout. Nurses may believe that the implementation that should be making their job easier will actually make it more challenging (Trossman, 2005). Nurses who feel that the system has been forced onto them are very likely to be highly resistant to the change. This is why it is imperative that nurses be involved in the design, development, and implementation of the EHR. Nurses who have been involved in the implementation process will ensure that the product meets the needs of the staff, which will result in high end-user satisfaction (McLane, 2005).

Another challenge facing those wishing to implement an EHR is the issue that writing is nearly automatic for most, but using a computer is not. This potential problem can be overcome by ensuring that data entry and system navigation make for a system that is user friendly (Walsh, 2004). Voice data entry is an easy way to enter data into the system and may be a way for those who are not comfortable with computers to still use the system effectively (Walsh, 2004). Another way to encourage staff to accept the new EHR is

to ensure that they have received adequate training prior to the implementation as well as to provide continued support and education after the implementation.

The implementation of a new EHR system requires the staff to make significant changes to how they work and how they handle patient information. The INS who is familiar with change management and the NI process should have an integral role in the redesign of workflow processes to ensure a smooth transition from a paper record to an electronic record. Many excellent EHR systems fail after their installation due to poor implementation planning. It is imperative that nurses are employed in the information systems (IS) department (Trossman, 2005).

REFERENCES

McLane, S. (2005). Designing an EMR planning process based on staff attitudes toward and opinions about computers in healthcare. *CIN: Computers, Informatics, Nursing, 23*(2), 85–92.

Trossman, S. (2005). Bold new world: Technology should ease nurses' jobs, not create a greater work load. *American Journal of Nursing, 105*(5), 75–77.

Walsh, S. (2004). The clinician's perspective on electronic health records and how they can affect patient care. *BMJ: British Medical Journal, 328*(7449), 1184–1187.

FLEXIBILITY AND EXPANDABILITY

Health care is as unique as the patients themselves. It is delivered in a variety of settings, for a variety of reasons, over the course of a patient's lifetime. In addition, patients rarely receive all their care from one healthcare organization; indeed, choice is a cornerstone of the American healthcare system. An EHR must be flexible and expandable to meet the needs of patients and caregivers in all these settings, despite the challenges.

At a very basic level, there is as yet no EHR system available that can provide all functions for all specialties to such a degree that all clinicians would successfully adopt it. Consider oncology as an example. Most systems do not yet provide the advanced ordering features required for the complex treatment planning undertaken in this field. An oncologist could use a general system, but he or she would not find as many benefits without additional features for chemotherapy ordering, lifetime cumulative dose tracking, or the ability to adjust a treatment day schedule and recalculate a schedule for the remaining days of the plan.

Further, most healthcare organizations do not yet have the capacity to implement and maintain systems in all care areas. As one physician stated, "implementing an EMR is a complex and difficult multidisciplinary effort that will stretch an organization's skills and capacity for change" (Chin, 2004, p. 47).

These two conditions are improving every day at both vendor and healthcare organizations alike. Improvements in both areas were recently fueled by ARRA incentives (see **Box 16-4**).

ARRA has also set the expectation that despite the large number of settings in which a patient may receive care, a minimum set of data from those records must flow or "interoperate" between each setting and the unique EHR systems used in those settings. Today, interoperability exists through what is called a continuity of care document. This data set includes patient demographics, medication, allergy, and problem lists, among other things, and the formatting and exchange of the continuity of care document is required to be supported by EHR vendors and healthcare organizations seeking ARRA meaningful use incentives.

Despite this positive step forward, financial and patient privacy hurdles remain to be overcome to achieve an expansive EHR. Most health care is delivered by small community practices and hospitals, many of which do not have the financial or technical resources

BOX 16-4   Cloudy EHRs

A paradigm shift from healthcare facility-owned, machine-based computing to off-site, vendor-owned cloud computing, Web browser-based log-in accessible data, software, and hardware could link systems together and reduce costs. Hospitals with shrinking budgets and extreme IT needs are exploring the successes in this area achieved in other industries, such as Amazon's S3. As providers strive to implement potent EHRs, they are looking for cloud-based models that offer the necessary functionality without having to assume the burden associated with all of the hardware, software, application, and storage issues. However, in the face of the

HITECH Act and its associated penalties, how can we overcome the challenges to realize the benefits of this approach? Cloud computing has both advantages and disadvantages, and while they explore this new paradigm, healthcare providers must relinquish control as they continue to strive to maintain security. The vendors that are responsible for developing and maintaining this new environment are also facing challenges originating from both legislatures and healthcare providers. As the vendors and healthcare providers work together to improve the implementation and adoption of the cloud-based EHR, the sky is the limit!

to implement EHRs. DHHS recently loosened regulations so that physicians may now be able to receive healthcare information technology software, hardware, and implementation services from hospitals to alleviate the financial burden placed on individual providers and to foster more widespread adoption of the EHR.

Finally, patient privacy is a pivotal issue in determining how far and how easy it will be to share data across healthcare organizations. In addition to the Health Insurance Portability and Accountability Act privacy rules, many states have regulations in place related to patient confidentiality. The recent experience of the state of Minnesota foreshadows what all states will soon be facing. In 2007, Governor Tim Pawlenty announced the creation of the Minnesota Health Information Exchange (State of Minnesota, 2007). Although the intentions of the exchange were to promote patient safety and increase healthcare efficiency across the state, it raised significant concerns about security and privacy. New questions arose about the definition of when and how patient consent is required to exchange data electronically, and older paper-based processes needed to be updated to support real-time electronic exchange (Minnesota Department of Health, 2007). For health exchanges such as these to reach their full potential, members of the public must be able to trust that their privacy will be protected, or else the healthcare industry risks that patients may not share a full medical history or, worse yet, may not seek care, effectively making the exchanges useless.

THE FUTURE

Despite the challenges, the future of EHRs is an exciting one for patients and clinicians alike. Benefits may be realized by implementing stand-alone EHRs as described here, but the most significant transformation will come as interoperability is realized between systems. As the former national information technology coordinator in the DHHS David Brailer noted about the potential of interoperability:

> For the first time, clinicians everywhere can have a longitudinal medical record with full information about each patient. Consumers will have better information about their health status since personal health records and similar access strategies can be feasible in an interoperable world. Consumers can move more easily between and among clinicians without fear of their information being lost. Payers can benefit from the economic efficiencies, fewer errors, and reduced duplication that arises from interoperability. Healthcare information exchange and interoperability (HIEI) also underlies meaningful public health reporting, bioterrorism surveillance, quality monitoring, and advances in clinical trials. In short, there is little that most people want from health care for which HIEI isn't a prerequisite. (Brailer, 2005, p. W 5-20)

The future also holds tremendous potential for EHR features and functions that will include not only more sophisticated decision support and clinical reporting capacity but also improved biomedical device integration, ease of use and intuitiveness, and access through more hardware platforms.

Implementations of EHRs will become more commonplace in the near future, with ARRA putting pressure on healthcare organizations to move more quickly toward adoption of such records. More organizations adopting EHRs will facilitate broader dissemination of implementation best practices, with the hope of further shortening the time required to take advantage of advanced EHR features.

SUMMARY

It is an important time for health care and technology. EHRs have come to the forefront and will remain central to shaping the future of health care. In an ideal world, all nurses, from entry-level personnel to executives, will have a basic competency in nursing informatics that will enable them to participate fully in shaping the future use of technology in the practice at a national level and wherever care is delivered. Such initiatives as TIGER are imperative for adoption and ultimately more visibility of nursing in the later phases of the ARRA meaningful use standards, which are still being defined.

DISCUSSION QUESTIONS

1. What are the implications for nursing education as the EHR becomes the standard for caring for patients?

2. What are the ethical considerations related to interoperability and a shared EHR?

3. You are asked about a diagnosis with which you are unfamiliar. Where would you start looking for information? How would you determine the validity of the information?

REFERENCES

American Organization of Nurse Executives. (2006, September). AONE guiding principles for *defining the role of the nurse executive in technology acquisition and implementation*. Washington, DC: Author. Retrieved from http://www.google .com/url?sa=t&rct=j&q=&esrc=s&source=web& cd=1&ved=0CCAQFjAA&url=http%3A%2F%2F www.aone.org%2Fresources%2FPDFs%2FAONE_ GP_Technology_and_Acquisition_and_Imple mentation.pdf&ei=FjBIVNPiKImU8QHJzoH4Bg &usg=AFQjCNFgwksLDt-QyOt0v6c-Nnp56TqM kQ&sig2=lAL0Yb9k0OnjYgdM9yhs7Q&bvm=bv .77880786,d.b2U

Brailer, D. J. (2005, January). Interoperability: The key to the future healthcare system. *Health Affairs—Web Exclusive*, W 5-19–W 5-21. Retrieved from http://content.healthaffairs.org/cgi/reprint /hlthaff.w5.19v1

Bush, G. W. (2004). State of the Union address. Retrieved from http://www.washingtonpost.com /wp-srv/politics/transcripts/bushtext_012004.html

Centers for Medicare and Medicaid Services (CMS). (2010a). EHR incentive programs: Meaningful use. Retrieved from https://www.cms.gov/EHRIn centivePrograms/35_Meaningful_Use.asp

Centers for Medicare and Medicaid Services (CMS). (2010b). Quality measures: Electronic specifi cations. Retrieved from http://www.cms.gov /QualityMeasures/03_ElectronicSpecifications .asp#TopOfPage

Centers for Medicare and Medicaid Services (CMS). (2014). The official website for the Medicare and Medicaid electronic health records (EHR) incentive programs. Retrieved from http://www .cms.gov/Regulations-and-Guidance/Legislation /EHRIncentivePrograms/index.html

Certification Commission for Healthcare Informa tion Technology. (2007). Certification Com mission announces new work group members. Retrieved from http://www.cchit.org/about /news/releases/Certification-Commission -Announces-New-Work-Group-Members.asp

Chaudhry, B., Wang, J., Wu, S., Maglione, M., Mojica, W., Roth, E.,. . . Shekelle, P. (2006). Systematic review: Impact of health information technology on quality, efficiency, and costs of medical care. *Annals of Internal Medicine, 144*(10), E-12–E-22.

Chin, H. L. (2004). The reality of EMR implementa tion: Lessons from the field. *Permanente Journal, 8*(4), 43–48.

Department of Health and Human Services (DHHS). (2010). Medicare and Medicaid pro grams: Electronic health record incentive pro gram. *Federal Register, 75*(144), 44314–44590. Retrieved from http://www.gpo.gov/fdsys/pkg /FR-2010-07-28/pdf/2010-17207.pdf

Dorr, D., Bonner, L. M., Cohen, A. N., Shoai, R. S., Per rin, R., Chaney, E., & Young, A. (2007). Informat ics systems to promote improved care for chronic illness: A literature review. *Journal of the American Medical Informatics Association, 14*(2), 156–163.

Embi, P. J., Jain, A., Clark, J., Bizjack, S., Hornung, R., & Harris, C. M. (2005). Effect of a clinical trial alert system on physician participation in trial recruit ment. *Archives of Internal Medicine, 165*, 2272–2277.

Goddard, B. L. (2000). Termination of a contract to implement an enterprise electronic medical record system. *Journal of American Medical Infor matics Association, 7*, 564–568.

Halamka, J. D. (2006, May). Health information tech nology: Shall we wait for the evidence? [Letter to the editor]. *Annals of Internal Medicine, 144*(10), 775–776.

Healthcare Information and Management Systems Society (HIMSS). (2007). Electronic health record. Retrieved from http://www.himss.org/ASP/top ics_ehr.asp

Healthcare Information and Management Systems Society (HIMSS). (2009). HIMSS Davies Organi zational Award application: MultiCare. Retrieved from http://www.himss.org/files/HIMSSorg/davies/docs/2009_RecipientApplications/MultiCareConnectHIMSSDaviesManuscript.pdf

Healthcare Information and Management Systems Society (HIMSS). (2010a). HIMSS Davies awards. Retrieved from http://www.himss.org/davies

Healthcare Information and Management Systems Society (HIMSS). (2010b). HIMSS Davies awards. Retrieved from http://apps.himss.org/davies

Healthcare Information and Management Systems Society (HIMSS). (2010c). Stage 7 hospitals. Retrieved from http://www.himssanalytics.org/hc_providers/stage7Hospitals.asp

Healthcare Information and Management Systems Society (HIMSS). (2013). HIMSS 2013 iHIT Study: Executive summary. Retrieved from http://www.himss.org/ResourceLibrary/ResourceDetail.aspx?ItemNumber=17104

Healthcare Information and Management Systems Society (HIMSS) Analytics. (2013). Electronic medical record adoption model (EMRAM). Retrieved from http://www.himssanalytics.org/emram/emram.aspx

HealthIT.gov. (2012). Benefits of EHRs: Why adopt EHRs? Retrieved from http://www.healthit.gov/providers-professionals/why-adopt-ehrs

HealthIT.gov (2014). Certification programs and policies. Retrieved from http://www.healthit.gov/policy-researchers-implementers/certification-programs-policy

Hettinger, M. (2007, March). *Core measure reporting: Performance improvement.* Visalia, CA: Kaweah Delta Health Care District.

Holbrook, A., Keshavjee, K., Troyan, S., Pray, M., & Ford, P. T. (2003). Applying methodology to electronic medical record selection. *International Journal of Medical Informatics, 71,* 43–50.

Husk, G., & Waxman, D. A. (2004). Using data from hospital information systems to improve emergency care. *Academic Emergency Medicine, 11*(11), 1237–1244.

Institute of Medicine (IOM). (2001). *Crossing the quality chasm: A new health system for the 21st century.* Washington, DC: National Academies Press.

Institute of Medicine (IOM). (2003). *Key capabilities of an electronic health record system: Letter report.* Washington, DC: National Academies Press.

Institute of Medicine (IOM). (2012). Best care at lower cost. Retrieved from http://www.iom.edu/~/media/Files/Report%20Files/2012/Best-Care/Best%20Care%20at%20Lower%20Cost_Recs.pdf

Jain, A., Atreja, A., Harris, C. M., Lehmann, M., Burns, J., & Young, J. (2005). Responding to the rofecoxib withdrawal crisis: A new model for notifying patients at risk and their healthcare providers. *Annals of Internal Medicine, 142*(3), 182–186.

Jansen, W., & Grance, T. (2011). *Guidelines on security and privacy in public cloud computing.* Draft Special Publication 800-144. U.S. Department of Commerce, National Institute of Standards and Technology (NIST). Retrieved from https://cloudsecurityalliance.org/wp-content/uploads/2011/07/NIST-Draft-SP-800-144_cloud-computing.pdf

Konschak, C., & Shiple, D. (n.d.). System selection: Aligning vision and technology. Retrieved from http://www.divurgent.com/images/White%20Paper.Vendor%20Selection.vfinal.pdf

Kutney-Lee, A., & Kelly, D. (2011). The effect of hospital electronic health record adoption on nurse-assessed quality of care and patient safety. *Journal of Nursing Administration, 41*(11), 466–472. doi:10.1097/NNA.0b013e3182346e4b

McLane, S. (2005). Designing an EMR planning process based on staff attitudes toward and opinions about computers in healthcare. *CIN: Computers, Informatics, Nursing, 23*(2), 85–92.

McLaughlin, T., & Halilovic, M. (2006). Clinical analytics, rigorous coding bring objectivity to quality assertions. *Medical Staff Update Online, 30*(6). Retrieved from http://med.stanford.edu/shs/update/archives/JUNE2006/analytics.htm

Minnesota Department of Health. (2007, June). *Minnesota Health Records access legislative study.* Minneapolis, MN: Author. Retrieved from http://www.health.state.mn.us/e-health/hras/hras050113facts.pdf

National Institute of Standards and Technology (NIST). (2010). Meaningful use test method: Approved test procedures version 1.0. Retrieved from http://healthcare.nist.gov/use_testing/finalized_requirements.html

National Institutes of Health. (2006, April). *Electronic health records overview.* McLean, VA: Mitre Corporation.

Poprock, B. (2005, September). *Using Epic's alternative medications reminder to reduce prescription costs and encourage assistance programs for indigent patients.* Presented at the Epic Systems Corporation user group meeting, Madison, WI.

Reed, H. L., & Bernard, E. (2005). Reductions in diabetic cardiovascular risk by community primary care providers. *International Journal of Circumpolar Health, 64*(1), 26–37.

Robert Wood Johnson Foundation (RWJF). (2006). Health information technology in the United States: The information base for progress. Retrieved from http://www.rwjf.org/programareas/resources/product.jsp?id=15895&pid=1142&gsa=1

Shekelle, P. G., Morton, S. C., & Keeler, E. B. (2006). *Costs and benefits of health information technology. Evidence report/technology assessment, No. 132* [Prepared by the Southern California Evidence-based Practice Center under Contract No. 290-02-0003]. Agency for Healthcare Research and Quality Publication No. 06-E006. Rockville, MD: Agency for Healthcare Research and Quality.

Sidorov, J. (2006). It ain't necessarily so: The electronic health record and the unlikely prospect of reducing healthcare costs. *Health Affairs, 25*(4), 1079–1085.

Smith, T., Semerdjian, N., King, P., DeMartin, B., Levi, S., Reynolds, K., . . . Dowd, J. (2004). *Nicholas E. Davies Award of Excellence: Transforming healthcare with a patient-centric electronic health record system.* Evanston, IL: Evanston Northwestern Healthcare. Retrieved from http://www.himss.org/content/files/davies2004_evanston.pdf

Spooner, S. A., & Council on Clinical Information Technology. (2007). Special requirements of electronic health record systems in pediatrics. *Pediatrics, 119*, 631–637.

State of Minnesota, Office of the Governor. (2007). New public-private partnership to improve patient care, safety and efficiency. Retrieved from http://www.leg.state.mn.us/docs/2010/other/101582/www.governor.state.mn.us/mediacenter/pressreleases/2007/PROD008303.html

Technology Informatics Guiding Education Reform (TIGER). (2010). *AMIA Tiger Team Testimony by Bradley Malin, PhD.* Retrieved from http://www.amia.org/sites/amia.org/files/Malin-AMIA-Tiger-Team-Testimony.pdf

Thompson, D. I., Osheroff, J., Classen, D., & Sittig, D. F. (2007). A review of methods to estimate the benefits of electronic medical records in hospitals and the need for a national database. *Journal of Healthcare Information Management, 21*(1), 62–68.

Trossman, S. (2005). Bold new world: Technology should ease nurses' jobs, not create a greater work load. *American Journal of Nursing, 105*(5), 75–77.

Walsh, S. (2004). The clinician's perspective on electronic health records and how they can affect patient care. *BMJ: British Medical Journal, 328*(7449), 1184–1187.

CHAPTER 17

IOM Core Competency: Utilize Informatics

Anita Finkelman

CHAPTER OBJECTIVES

1. Discuss the Institute of Medicine competency: Utilize informatics.
2. Describe informatics and its relationship to nursing.
3. Explain the purpose of documentation and key issues related to informatics and documentation.
4. Identify informatics tools used in healthcare delivery.
5. Describe telehealth and its relationship to healthcare delivery and nursing.
6. Examine the impact of the use of biomedical equipment on nursing care.
7. Compare and contrast high-touch care with high-tech care.

INTRODUCTION

This chapter concludes the section that focuses on the Institute of Medicine (IOM) healthcare profession core competencies with a discussion of the fifth core competency: utilize informatics. Informatics/information technology (IT) is an important topic in all areas of life today; with the explosion of technology, there are many opportunities for communication and sharing of knowledge. The impact of informatics on nursing care is explored here. Other issues that need to be addressed are documentation, confidentiality and privacy of information, and telehealth. This chapter also includes content about biomedical equipment, an expanding area in healthcare technology that impacts nurses and nursing care. Some of this equipment also uses IT. Nurses today cannot avoid technology, whether it is used for communication, for care provision, or

FIGURE 17-1	Utilize informatics: Key elements.

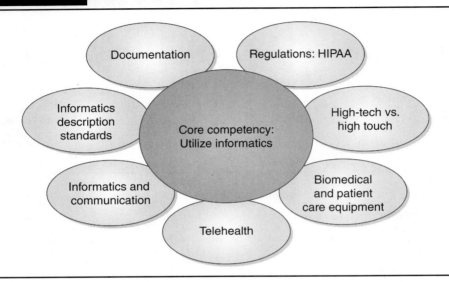

for monitoring the quality of care. The chapter concludes with a discussion about the potential conflict between high-touch care versus high-tech care and the need for nursing leadership in health informatics—important issues for nurses to consider. **Figure 17-1** identifies key elements in this chapter.

THE IOM COMPETENCY: UTILIZE INFORMATICS

The IOM's description of the fifth healthcare profession core competency is "communicate, manage knowledge, mitigate error, and support decision making using information technology" (IOM, 2003, p. 4). Informatics entails more than just understanding what health informatics technology (HIT) is; it also includes how that technology is used to prevent errors and improve care. From the initial use of computers to management of financial records to the current use of informatics, there has been a major move toward HIT application in care. Some examples are greater use of informatics to find evidence to implement evidence-based practice; use of

informatics in research; greater consumer access to information via the Internet; and more specific clinical applications, such as reminder and decision systems, telehealth, teleradiology, online prescribing, and use of e-mail for provider–provider communication and patient–provider communication. The IOM (2003, p. 63) concludes that every healthcare professional should meet the following informatics competencies:

- Employ word processing, presentation, and data analysis software.
- Search, retrieve, manage, and make decisions using electronic data from internal information databases and external online databases and the Internet.
- Communicate using e-mail, instant messaging, e-mail lists, and file transfers.
- Understand security protections such as access control, data security, and data encryption, and directly address ethical and legal issues related to the use of IT in practice.
- Enhance education and access to reliable health information for patients.

A position statement from the Healthcare Information and Management Systems Society (HIMSS, 2011) addressed the IOM report *The Future of Nursing* from the perspective of informatics. The following recommendations were made and align with the IOM report on the key points of leadership, education, and practice:

- Partner with nurse executives to lead technology changes that advance health and the delivery of health care.
- Support the development of informatics departments.
- Foster the evolution of the chief nursing informatics (NI) officer role.
- Transform nursing education to include informatics competencies and demonstrable behaviors at all levels of academic preparation.
- Promote the continuing education of all levels of nursing, particularly in the areas of electronic health records (EHRs) and HIT.
- Ensure that data, information, knowledge, and wisdom form the basis of 21st-century nursing practice by incorporating informatics competencies into practice standards in all healthcare settings.
- Facilitate the collection and analysis of interprofessional healthcare workforce data by ensuring data can be collected from existing IT systems.

The statement also indicates that nurses play a critical role in healthcare informatics and need to continue to do so.

> Nurses are key leaders in developing the infrastructure for effective and efficient health information technology that transforms the delivery of care. Nurse informaticists play a crucial role in advocating both for patients and fellow nurses who are often the key stakeholders and recipients of these evolving solutions. Nursing informatics professionals are the liaisons to successful interactions with technology in healthcare. (HIMSS, 2011)

INFORMATICS

Informatics is complex, and the fact that it is changing daily makes it even more difficult to keep current with this field. Healthcare delivery has been strongly influenced by the changes in informatics, but what is informatics?

> Technology is revolutionizing the way that healthcare is delivered with a steady infusion of new solutions into clinical environments. At the same time, outside of healthcare, both clinicians and consumers are learning to incorporate technological solutions into their daily lives with tools like high-speed data networks, smart phones, handheld devices, and various forms of patient engagement in social media exchanges. Bringing these types of technologies into the healthcare marketplace will transform the time and place for how care is provided. Having individuals who understand the unique complexities of healthcare practices along with how to best develop technological tools that positively affect safe patient care is essential. Nurses integrating informatics solutions into clinical encounters are critical for the transition to an automated healthcare environment that promotes the continuum of care across time and place, in addition to wellness and health maintenance activities. (HIMSS, 2011)

Just as mobile forms of informatics are increasing, mobile applications are used more by nurses, for example for discharge teaching and follow-up care. Nurses are also designing some of the applications for use in a variety of ways to promote patient safety and health.

Definitions and Description

Informatics has opened doors to many innovative methods of communication with patients and among providers, individuals, and healthcare organizations (HCOs) of all types. It often saves time, but can also lead to information overload. Today, physicians are using e-mail to communicate with patients (e.g., sending appointment reminders, sharing lab results, and answering questions). The Web has provided opportunities to build communities of people with common chronic diseases to help them with disease management. HCOs have developed websites to share information about their organizations with the public (a marketing tool for services). In addition, these websites provide HCOs with an effective method for internal communication; staff can access some parts of the sites with special passwords. With these changes comes greater risk of inappropriate access to information through hacking and other means. Informatics is also used to evaluate the performance of the HCO and individual healthcare providers. IT has a major impact on quality improvement; today, it is much easier to collect, store, and analyze large amounts of data that in the past were collected by hand. Insurers rely heavily on informatics to provide insurance coverage, manage data, and analyze performance, which has a direct impact on whether care is covered for reimbursement. Informatics allows governments at all levels—local, state, national, and international—to collect and use data for policy decision making and evaluation.

Informatics has its own language and is a highly specialized area. Nurses do not have to be informatics experts, but they do need to understand the basics. Some terms have become so common that the majority of people know what they are (such as *Internet* and *e-mail*). Other terms that are useful to know are highlighted here:

- Clinical data repository: A physical or logical compendium of patient data pertaining to health; an "information warehouse" that stores data longitudinally and in multiple forms, such as text, voice, and images (American Nurses Association [ANA], 2008).

- Clinical decision support systems: Computer applications designed to facilitate human decision making. Decision support systems are typically rule based. These systems use a knowledge base and a set of rules to analyze data and information and provide recommendations (ANA, 2008).

- Clinical information system: An information system that supports the acquisition, storage, manipulation, and distribution of clinical information throughout an HCO, with a focus on electronic communication. This system uses IT that is applied at the point of clinical care. Typical clinical information system components include electronic medical records (EMRs), clinical data repositories, decision support programs (such as application of clinical guidelines and drug interaction checking), handheld devices for collecting data and viewing reference material, imaging modalities, and communication tools such as electronic messaging systems.

- Coding system: A set of agreed-on symbols (frequently numeric or alphanumeric) that are attached to concept representation or terms to allow exchange of concept representations or terms with regard to their form or meaning. Examples are the Perioperative Nursing Data Set and the Clinical Care Classification System (ANA, 2008).

- Computer literacy: The knowledge and skills required to use basic computer applications and computer technology.

- Data: Discrete entities described objectively without interpretation.

- Data analysis software: Computer software that is used to analyze data.

- Data bank: A large store of information; may include several databases.

- Database: A collection of interrelated data that are organized according to a scheme to serve one or more applications. The data are stored so that several programs can use the data without concern for data structures or organization. An example is the National Database of Nursing Quality Indicators (NDNQI) (ANA, 2008).

- Data mining: Locating and identifying unknown patterns and relationships within data.

- E-mail list: A list of e-mail addresses that can be used to send an e-mail to many addresses simultaneously.

- Encryption: To change information into a code, usually for security reasons, so as to limit access to that information.

- Information: Data that have been interpreted, organized, or structured.

- Information literacy: The ability to recognize when information is needed and to locate, evaluate, and effectively use that information (ANA, 2008).

- Knowledge: Information that has been synthesized so that relationships are identified and formalized (ANA, 2008).

- Minimum data set: The minimum categories of data with uniform definitions and categories; they concern a specific aspect or dimension of the healthcare system that meets the basic needs of multiple data users. An example is the Nursing Minimum Data Set (ANA, 2008).

- Nomenclature: A system of designations (terms) that is elaborated according to preestablished rules. Examples include Systematized Nomenclature of Medicine—Clinical Terms International and International Classification for Nursing Practice (ANA, 2008).

- Security protections (access control, data security, and data encryption): Methods used to ensure that information is not read or taken by unauthorized persons.

- Software: Computer programs and applications.

- Standardized language: A collection of terms with definitions for use in informational systems databases. A standardized language enables comparisons to be made because the same term is used to denote the same condition. Standardized language is necessary for documentation in EHRs (ANA, 2008).

- Wisdom: The appropriate use of knowledge to solve human problems; understanding when and how to apply knowledge (ANA, 2008).

The role of health IT in e-measurement and quality care has become increasingly more important in recent years (Dykes & Collins, 2013). E-measurement is the secondary use of electronic data to populate standardized performance measures (National Quality Forum [NQF], 2013). The NQF is developing e-measures to make sure that data used for clinical documentation can be reused to measure patient outcomes. This endeavor, which is very complex, remains far from complete at this time. Getting the data in a consistent form into systems that can reuse the data and relate them to patient outcomes in languages that are clear and consistent will require much more work to be done.

Nursing Standards: Scope and Standards of Nursing Informatics

Nursing informatics (NI) is a specialty that integrates nursing science, computer science, and information science to manage and communicate data, information, knowledge, and wisdom in nursing practice. NI supports consumers, patients, nurses, and other providers in their decision making in all roles and settings. This support is accomplished through the use of information structures, information processes, and IT. The goal of NI is to improve the health of populations, communities, families, and individuals by optimizing information management and communication (ANA, 2008, p. 1).

This specialty area has expanded, and all nurses need to understand basic IT concepts and their application to nursing practice. Undergraduate nursing programs may include IT in the curriculum, sometimes as a course on informatics, but not all programs include this content. This omission from nursing educational programs is now a problem because of the emphasis on informatics as a healthcare professions core competency. Some schools of nursing offer master's degrees in NI.

Three major concepts related to information are important to understand (Englebardt & Nelson, 2002):

1. *Data* are discrete entities that are described objectively without interpretation.
2. *Information* is defined as data that are interpreted, organized, or structured.
3. *Knowledge* is information that is synthesized so that relationships are identified and formalized.

The flow from data to wisdom can be described as data naming, collecting, and organizing, following this pattern: (1) information—organizing and interpreting; (2) knowledge—interpreting, integrating, and understanding; and (3) wisdom—understanding, applying, and applying with compassion. **Figure 17-2** illustrates this flow.

"Wisdom is defined as the appropriate use of knowledge to manage and solve human problems. It is knowing when and how to apply knowledge to deal with complex problems or specific human needs" (Nelson & Joos, 1989, p. 6). "While knowledge focuses on what is known, wisdom focuses on the appropriate application of that knowledge. For example, a knowledge base may include several options for managing an anxious family, while wisdom would help decide which option is most appropriate for a specific family" (ANA, 2008, p. 5). Nurses first need to understand the importance of data collection and data analysis, and then need to understand how to apply data and knowledge—leading to wisdom. Data are important to the delivery of nursing care. In hospitals, data can be used to evaluate outcomes, identify problems for a specific group of patients, and assist in making plans for change to improve care. In the community, aggregated data are often collected to better understand the health issues in a population or community and to formulate a plan of action.

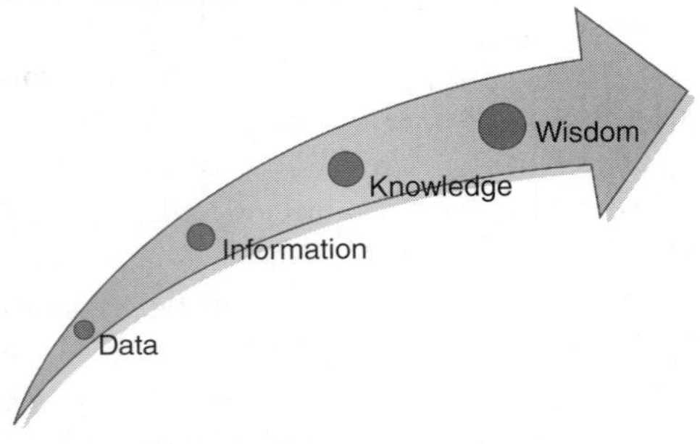

Certification in Informatics Nursing

Nurses who practice in the area of informatics can be certified if they meet the eligibility criteria and complete the certification examination satisfactorily. The following list provides examples of application eligibility criteria required for the informatics certification exam sponsored by the American Nurses Credentialing Center (ANCC, 2014). The nurse must:

- Hold a current, active registered nurse license within a state or territory of the United States or the professional, legally recognized equivalent in another country
- Have practiced the equivalent of 2 years full time as a registered nurse
- Hold a baccalaureate or higher degree in nursing or a baccalaureate degree in a relevant field
- Have completed 30 hours of continuing education in informatics within the last 3 years
- Meet one of the following practice hour requirements:

  a. The nurse must have practiced a minimum of 2000 hours in informatics nursing within the last 3 years.

  b. The nurse must have practiced a minimum of 1000 hours in informatics nursing in the last 3 years and must have completed

FIGURE 17-2 From Data to Wisdom

a minimum of 12 semester hours of academic credit in informatics courses that are a part of a graduate-level NI program.

c. The nurse must have completed a graduate program in NI containing a minimum of 200 hours of faculty-supervised practicum in informatics.

These are not simple criteria; they take time to meet, and they provide a good overview of the need for expertise in this area. All criteria must be met before a nurse can apply for the ANCC certification examination.

The informatics nurse is involved in activities that focus on the methods and technologies of information handling in nursing. Informatics nursing practice includes the development, support, and evaluation of applications, tools, processes, and structures that help nurses to manage data in direct care of patients as well as in nursing education and research. The work of an informatics nurse can involve any and all aspects of information systems, including theory formulation, design, development, marketing, selection, testing, implementation, training, maintenance, evaluation, and enhancement. "Informatics nurses are engaged in clinical practice, education, consultation, research, administration, and pure informatics" (ANCC, 2014). It is clear that a nurse who wants to function in this specialty area must have excellent computer skills, understand practice needs for information, and know how best to apply IT to nursing practice. The nurse must also be able to work collaboratively in interprofessional teams and demonstrate leadership. By speaking for the needs of the practicing nurse, the informatics nurse represents all nurses in practice—clinical, education, and research—as applies to the specific situation.

Informatics: Impact on Care

The IOM recommendations indicate that informatics can lead to safe, quality care—and it

truly can. Application of informatics, however, does not guarantee perfection.

> There is a perception that technology will lead to fewer errors than strategies that focus on staff performance; however, technology may in some circumstances lead to more errors. This is particularly true when the technology fails to take into account end users, increases in staff time, replicates an already bad process or is implemented with insufficient training. The best approach is not always clear, and most approaches have advantages and disadvantages. (Finkelman & Kenner, 2012, p. 192)

Nurses need to assume an active role in the development of HIT for patient care and not wait to be asked to participate. When an HCO is choosing a system for an EMR, nurses need to be involved to ensure that the system meets nursing care documentation requirements and that relevant data can be collected to assist nurses in providing and improving care. Nurses may serve in key IT roles to guide development and implementation, and they may have special training or education in informatics. Nurses may also serve as resources in identifying needs and testing systems to ensure that the systems are nurse user friendly. Many nurses who provide feedback about systems do not have special IT training; they review the system to determine if it is user friendly for nurses who have limited informatics knowledge and help to determine if the system meets documentation needs and standards. All nurses need be skilled in managing and communicating information, and they are primarily concerned with the content of that information.

In today's dynamic healthcare environment, coordination of care is very important. One of the barriers to seamless coordination is the lack of interoperable computerized records (Bodenheimer, 2008). In 2007, only 34.8% of physician offices used computerized records, though this was a major increase from 2005, when that proportion was only 23.9%; also in 2007, 49.8% of U.S. hospitals had adopted the

EMR, with more embracing this technology each year. Data for 2009 (U.S. Department of Health and Human Services [HHS], 2013) indicate that 41% of office-based physicians and 81% of hospitals planned on taking advantage of the federal incentive payments for adoption and meaningful use of certified EHR technology. To improve information sharing and coordination of care, ideally this percentage should be 100%, but implementing the EMR is a costly, complex process of change (National Center for Health Statistics, 2010). Nevertheless, the federal government's incentive program may make a significant difference in adoption of this critical healthcare informatics technology. From 2012 to 2013, the number of hospitals using EHRs tripled, with 4 out of every 10 hospitals now employing such records (Thompson, 2013). "HHS has met and exceeded its goal for 50 percent of doctor offices and 80 percent of eligible hospitals to have EHRs by the end of 2013" (HHS, 2013). A continuing problem is that information can rarely be shared from one system to another, which is a limitation that needs to be resolved for better coordination of care. For example, it should be possible to share current information among healthcare providers in private practice and clinics and the hospitals when it is needed.

Innovative methods to improve coordination that focus on informatics have been developed. One method is to use electronic referral (e-referral.) This approach allows a healthcare provider to send an e-mail to another provider, such as a specialist, with information about the patient and to ask for consultation. In many situations, such communication eliminates the need to see the patient. The specialist reviews information such as lab reports, surgical reports, and so on, and can share his or her opinion with the other healthcare provider. It is critical that reimbursement be provided for this type of service, or it will not be used. Health Insurance Portability and Accountability Act (HIPAA) requirements must also be considered, with all parties working together to ensure patient privacy. Timely information flow from the hospital to posthospital care should improve patient coordination. Not having this is a major drawback; even though the technology to improve it is available, it is not freely used.

Implications for Nursing Education and Nursing Research

Informatics is important not only for practice, but also for nursing education and nursing research. Today, there is greater use of IT in nursing education than was the case in the past. The increased use of online courses throughout the nursing curriculum, at both the undergraduate and graduate levels, has revolutionized nursing education. It has required that faculty consider more interactive learning methods. Informatics also impacts simulation, allowing faculty to create complex learning scenarios that use the computer and computerized equipment. Moreover, as students use more technology in their personal lives, they expect correspondingly greater use of IT in education. Such tools as iPods, tablets, and smartphones, and Internet tools and apps such as Facebook, Instagram, and Twitter provide instant information and can be very interactive. These methods can also be used to increase student–faculty communication and have the potential to provide different means of student–faculty supervision in the clinical area. This is particularly true in areas such as community health, when students visit multiple sites and faculty move from site to site to see students.

Nursing research uses informatics in data collection and analysis; it saves time and improves the quality of data collection and analysis.

> The capacity for a mega-repository of clinical and research findings will allow for a richer science derived from multiple perspectives. Nurses have the responsibility to initiate practice-based inquiry, participate in clinical

nursing research, and use nursing research to enhance patients' well-being and contribute to the body of nursing knowledge. (Appleton, 1998, as cited in Richards, 2001, p. 10)

This quote is not current, but the message is the same today, though we have yet to really reach this status.

DOCUMENTATION

Over time, nursing documentation has increased in terms of its relevance to nurses and to other healthcare professionals, thus increasing its impact on patient care and patient outcomes.

> Clear, accurate, and accessible documentation is an essential element of safe, quality, evidence-based nursing practice. Nurses practice across settings at position levels from the bedside to the administrative office; the registered nurse (RN) and the advanced practice registered nurse (APRN) are responsible and accountable for the nursing documentation that is used throughout an organization. This may include either documentation on nursing

care that is provided by nurses—whether RN, APRN, or nursing assistive personnel—that can be used by other non-nurse members of the health care team or the administrative records that are created by the nurse and used across organization settings. (ANA, 2010, p. 3)

According to the ANA (2010), nursing documentation is used for the following purposes:

- Communicate within the healthcare team
- Communicate with other professionals
- Verify credentialing—to monitor performance
- Provide legal support
- Learn about regulation and legislation—to provide data for audits and monitoring
- Receive reimbursement—determine services for reimbursement
- Support research—data for studies
- Conduct quality process and performance improvement

The ANA principles for nursing documentation are found in **Exhibit 17-1**.

EXHIBIT 17-1 ANA's Principles for Nursing Documentation

Nursing Documentation Principles
Principle 1. Documentation characteristics
Principle 2. Education and training
Principle 3. Policies and procedures
Principle 4. Protection systems
Principle 5. Documentation entries
Principle 6. Standardized terminologies

PRINCIPLE 1. DOCUMENTATION CHARACTERISTICS

High-quality documentation is:

- Accessible
- Accurate, relevant, and consistent

- Auditable
- Clear, concise, and complete
- Legible/readable (particularly in terms of the resolution and related qualities of EHR content as it is displayed on the screens of various devices)
- Thoughtful
- Timely, contemporaneous, and sequential
- Reflective of the nursing process
- Retrievable on a permanent basis in a nursing-specific manner

(continues)

EXHIBIT 17-1   ANA's Principles for Nursing Documentation *(continued)*

PRINCIPLE 2. EDUCATION AND TRAINING

Nurses, in all settings and at all levels of service, must be provided with comprehensive education and training in the technical elements of documentation and the organization's policies and procedures that are related to documentation. This education and training should include staffing issues that take into account the time needed for documentation work to ensure that each nurse is capable of the following:

- Functional and skillful use of the global documentation system
- Competence in the use of the computer and its supporting hardware
- Proficiency in the use of the software systems in which documentation or other relevant patient, nursing and health care reports, documents, and data are captured

PRINCIPLE 3. POLICIES AND PROCEDURES

The nurse must be familiar with all organizational policies and procedures related to documentation and apply these as part of nursing practice. Of particular importance are those policies or procedures on maintaining efficiency in the use of the down time system for documentation when the available electronic systems do not function.

PRINCIPLE 4. PROTECTION SYSTEMS

Protection systems must be designed and built into documentation systems, paper-based or electronic, to provide the following as prescribed by industry standards, governmental mandates, accrediting agencies, and organizational policies and procedures:

- Security of data
- Protection of patient identification
- Confidentiality of patient information
- Confidentiality of clinical professionals' information
- Confidentiality of organizational information

PRINCIPLE 5. DOCUMENTATION ENTRIES

Entries into organization documents or the health record (including but not limited to provider orders) must be:

- Accurate, valid, and complete
- Authenticated; that is, the information is truthful, the author is identified, and nothing has been added or inserted
- Dated and time stamped by the persons who created the entry
- Legible/readable
- Made using standardized terminology, including acronyms and symbols

PRINCIPLE 6. STANDARDIZED TERMINOLOGIES

Because standardized terminologies permit data to be aggregated and analyzed, these terminologies should include the terms that are used to describe the planning, delivery, and evaluation of the nursing care of the patient or client in diverse settings.

Source: From American Nurses Association. (2010). *Principles for nursing documentation.* Silver Spring, MD: Author.

The format and content of nursing documentation have also changed. It is a professional responsibility to document planning, actual care provided, and outcomes. Care coordination and continuity are supported by documentation. With many different staff caring for patients around the clock, it is critical that a clear communication mechanism exists, and this mechanism is documentation. Verbal communication is important, but a written document must be available. Staff can refer to such documentation when other care providers are not available. Documentation serves as a record of the patient's care; it provides data for reimbursement and quality improvement and staff performance; and it supports interprofessional teamwork. Through documentation, outcomes and evaluation of patient care are made clear.

The medical record is a legal document, and as such, rules must be followed when creating and amending it. Once documentation has been created, changes to it must be accompanied by a note indicating who made the change(s) and when (date and time). Only certain staff can document; they must note the date and time on the documentation and include their name and credentials. If there are questions about care or a legal action, such as a malpractice suit, the medical record is the most important evidence. Consequently, medical records need to be saved. A nurse can say that he or she provided certain care, but if it was not documented, then it is as if that care did not occur.

Iyer and Camp (1999, p. 5) listed the following standard critical concerns that pertain to documentation and still apply today, whether a record is paper or electronic:

- The medical record reflects the nursing process.
- The medical record describes the patient's ongoing status from shift to shift (inpatient care) or from patient visit to patient visit (ambulatory care).
- The plan of care and the medical record complement each other.
- The documentation system is designed to facilitate retrieval of information for quality improvement activities and for research.
- The documentation system supports the staffing mix and acuity levels in the current healthcare environment.

The following guidelines (Iyer & Camp, 1999) continue to be important for all who document:

- Do not include opinion, but only objective information in documentation. The nurse does not make subjective comments (e.g., comments about the patient being uncooperative, lazy, or impolite). Nurses document only what they have done and objective data. A nurse would not document another staff member's actions. Supervision of care, however, can be documented.
- Write neatly and legibly. Many HCOs now use computerized documentation, although not all HCOs have moved to an EMR system. If a computerized system is used, typos (typographical errors) may be a problem. Other issues may arise in electronic systems that use a checklist for a particular section of the EMR but do not allow for narrative notes. Nurses and others may be frustrated when they cannot add a narrative note.
- Use correct spelling, grammar, and medical terminology.
- Use authorized abbreviations. Using unapproved abbreviations increases the risk of errors.
- Use graphic records to record specified patient data, such as vital signs and medication administration.
- Record the patient's name on every page (for hard-copy medical records); this should be part of the EMR.
- Follow HCO rules about verbal and telephone orders.
- Transcribe orders carefully; double-check and ask questions if an order is not clear. In computerized systems, orders do not need to

be transcribed; however, this does not mean that there is no risk of an error in an order. All orders need careful review, and if they are not clear, they may require follow-up.

- Document omitted care.
- Document medications and outcomes.
- Document patient noncompliance/nonadherence and the reason(s) for it.
- Document allergies, and use this information to prevent errors and complications.
- Document sites of injections.
- Record all information about intravenous therapy and blood administration.
- Report abnormal laboratory results.
- Document as soon as possible after care is delivered. If documentation is done late, note this in the record. The nurse should not leave blank areas to come back to for later documentation.
- When quoting, use quotation marks and note the person who made the statement.
- When documentation is corrected because of a mistake, follow the HCO policies regarding corrections as per a hard-copy record or electronic record. Medical records are never rewritten.
- Document patient status change.
- When contacting the physician, document the time, date, name of physician, reason for the call, content, physician response, and steps taken after the call. This note should not include subjective analysis of the response such as the physician was rude.

The Joint Commission does not provide details as to what must be in a medical record (the term used by The Joint Commission for this document is *record of care/treatment and services*), but it does provide some guidelines that are required for accreditation (Clark, 2011; The Joint Commission, 2011):

- Content noted by The Joint Commission that needs to be included consists of the patient's name, address, date of birth, name of any legally authorized representative, assessment, diagnosis, clinician notes and actions, signatures and countersignatures as required, dates, details of procedures performed, laboratory reports, medications administered, and treatment plans. This does not mean that other data cannot be included, and other data are typically included. The content listed here is simply the minimum requirement.
- The record should be clear and understandable.
- The record must create a system of communication and an audit trail.
- Storage of documents must be secure and reasonable. For example, the system would consider who has access to records and prevent casual viewing by non-staff. All Medicare storage rules must be followed.
- HIPAA requirements must be followed.

This list applies to hospital medical records. The content is somewhat different for medical records in other types of settings, such as ambulatory care, long-term care, and home care, although some information would be the same. Nurses are not involved in documenting in all these categories because other staff members also have documentation responsibilities.

In 2010, the Joint Commission standard for record of care/treatment and services was one of the top 10 standards with which HCOs were in noncompliance (Clark, 2011). The three major areas where hospitals often did not meet compliance were as follows:

1. Complete and accurate medical record
2. Verbal orders received and recorded by qualified staff
3. Patient assessed and reassessed per defined time frame

Nurses are involved in all three aspects of these documentation standards.

MEANINGFUL USE

The American Recovery and Reinvestment Act of 2009 specifies the following three components of *meaningful use* (HHS & Centers for Medicare and Medicaid Services [CMS], 2014):

- Use of certified EHR in a meaningful manner (e.g., e-prescribing)
- Use of certified EHR technology for electronic exchange of health information to improve quality of health care
- Use of certified EHR technology to submit clinical quality measures (CQM) and other such measures selected by the Secretary of HHS

Meaningful use involves using certified electronic health record technology for the following purposes (HHS & HealthIT.gov, 2014):

- Improve quality, safety, efficiency, and reduce health disparities
- Engage patients and family
- Improve care coordination, and population and public health
- Maintain privacy and security of patient health information

Ultimately, it is hoped that the meaningful use compliance will result in the following benefits:

- Better clinical outcomes
- Improved population health outcomes
- Increased transparency and efficiency
- Empowered individuals
- More robust research data on health systems

Meaningful use identifies specific objectives that eligible professionals and hospitals must achieve to qualify for CMS reimbursement. Given that most hospitals receive CMS reimbursement, there is obviously a strong incentive to follow these requirements. Nurses are also required to consider meaningful use, particularly if they are in leadership positions where decisions about informatics are made.

In response to the legislation passed in July 2010, the Office of the National Coordinator for Health Information Technology and CMS issued new rules identifying criteria that hospitals and eligible providers must meet to be considered meaningful users of health IT (HHS, 2010). Hospitals and eligible providers are not able to receive federal funding related to the EMR initiative unless they meet these requirements; thus a significant amount of funding depends directly on satisfaction of the meaningful use criteria. There are five purposes for establishing these rules:

1. To improve quality, safety, efficiency, and reduce health disparities
2. To engage patients and their families (through electronic communication)
3. To improve care coordination
4. To ensure adequate privacy and security protection for personal health information
5. To improve the health of the population as well as public health—through data collection and analysis of data

All of these purposes are in line with the IOM *Quality Chasm* reports.

A NEED: STANDARDIZED TERMINOLOGY

Health care has expanded in multiple directions and includes the services of many different healthcare providers. Ensuring effective communication among these myriad providers is not always easy. Certainly, there are issues regarding willingness to communicate, lack of time to communicate, and so on, but a critical problem is the lack of a common professional language. For those entering health care, such as nursing students, this is probably a surprising comment. Each healthcare professional area has its own language; there are some common medical terms, but each profession has a specific language that is often not known or understood by other healthcare professionals. "Creating a common language is no small task.

Developing and adhering to distinct profession-specific terms may be a manifestation of professionals' desire to preserve identity, status or control" (IOM, 2003, p. 123). This problem affects all the core competencies and the ability to develop educational experiences that meet the competencies across healthcare professions, such as nursing, medicine, pharmacy, and allied health. It does not just relate to informatics; however, because informatics is dependent on language, the issue of shared language is even more important in NI.

The IOM has recommended that an interprofessional group created by the Department of Health and Human Services develop a common language across health disciplines "on a core set of competencies that includes patient-centered care, interprofessional teams, evidence-based practice, quality improvement, and informatics" (IOM, 2003, p. 124). Accomplishing this feat will require that healthcare professionals be willing to actively work together to achieve this goal. The next major step will then be getting different healthcare professionals to accept a universal language. This will require compromises.

> The data element sets and terminologies are foundational to standardization of nursing documentation and verbal communication that will lead to a reduction in errors and an increase in the quality and continuity of care. It is through standardization of nurse documentation and communication of a patient's care that the many nurses caring for a patient develop a shared understanding of that care. Moreover, the process generates the nursing data needed to develop increasingly more sophisticated decision support tools in the electronic record and to identify and disseminate best nursing practices. (ANA, 2006)

These statements are an example of why developing and accepting a universal language is difficult but necessary. The statements are nursing focused. How to move from this approach and blend with others, such as medicine, is the challenge.

SYSTEMS AND TERMINOLOGIES: INFORMATICS COMPLEXITY

Informatics is not as simple as e-mail and Internet. There are many database systems, terms, and other factors that make this a complex area. The following provides examples to illustrate informatics complexity.

Examples of Systematic Collection of Nursing Care Data or Data Element Sets

- *Nursing Minimum Data Set*: This data set describes patient problems across healthcare settings, different populations, geographic areas, and time. These clinical data also assist in identifying nursing diagnoses, nursing interventions, and nursing-sensitive patient outcomes. In addition, the Nursing Minimum Data Set is useful in assessing resources used in the provision of nursing care. The goal is the ability to link data between HCOs and providers. Data can also be used for research and healthcare policy.

- *Nursing Management Minimum Data Set*: This data set focuses on nursing administrative data elements in all types of settings.

Interface Terminologies

- *Clinical Care Classification*: The clinical classifications software for the *International Classification of Diseases*, 10th revision, Clinical Modification (ICD-10-CM) is a diagnosis and procedure categorization scheme that can be used in many types of projects that analyze data on diagnoses and procedures. The software is based on ICD-10-CM, a uniform and standardized coding system. ICD-10-CM includes more than 13,600 diagnosis codes and 3700 procedure codes (Centers for Disease Control and Prevention [CDC], 2011). Clinical care classification focuses on home care and includes diagnoses, interventions, and outcomes.

- *International Classification of Nursing Practice*: This classification system is a unified nursing language system that applies to all types of nursing care. It is a compositional terminology for nursing practice that facilitates the development of and cross-mapping among local terms and existing terminologies. It includes nursing diagnoses, nursing interventions, and nursing outcomes (International Council of Nurses, 2008).

- *Nursing Intervention Classification and Nursing Outcome Classification*: The North American Nursing Diagnosis Association (NANDA) focuses on nursing diagnoses, Nursing Intervention Classification (NIC) on nursing interventions, and Nursing Outcome Classification (NOC) on nursing outcomes.

- *Omaha System*: The Omaha system is a comprehensive, standardized taxonomy designed to improve practice, documentation, and information management. It includes three components: the problem classification scheme, the intervention scheme, and the problem rating scale for outcomes. When the three components are used together, the Omaha system offers a way to link clinical data to demographic, financial, administrative, and staffing data (Omaha System, 2011). The Omaha system is used in home health care, community health, and public health services.

- *Perioperative Nursing Data Set*: The Perioperative Nursing Data Set is a standardized nursing vocabulary that addresses the perioperative patient experience from preadmission until discharge, including nursing diagnoses, interventions, and outcomes. The Perioperative Nursing Data Set was developed by a specialty organization, the members of the Association of periOperative Registered Nurses, and has been recognized by the ANA as a data set useful for perioperative nursing practice (Association of periOperative Registered Nurses, 2008).

Examples of Multiprofessional Terminologies

- *Logical Observation Identifiers Names and Codes*: This clinical terminology classification is used for laboratory test orders and results. It is one system designated for use in U.S. federal government systems for the electronic exchange of clinical health information (National Library of Medicine, 2008a). This system can be used to collect data about assessments and outcomes for nursing and other healthcare services.

- *Current Procedural Terminology*: This code is used for reimbursement (Larkin, 2008).

- *Systematized Nomenclature of Medicine—Clinical Terms*: This comprehensive clinical terminology is one of several standards approved for use in U.S. federal government systems for the electronic exchange of clinical health information (National Library of Medicine, 2008b). This system is applicable to nursing and other healthcare services and focuses on diagnoses, interventions, and outcomes.

With the increased use of technology for documentation, nursing has been more concerned about two issues (Schwiran & Thede, 2011):

- How to differentiate nursing's contributions to patient care from those of medicine

- How to incorporate descriptions of nursing care into the health record in a manner that is commensurate with its importance to patients' welfare

In a study conducted by Schwiran and Thede (2011), the researchers examined nurses' knowledge of and experience with standardized nursing technologies. The results indicate that most nurses do not have much knowledge of or experience with standardized nursing technologies, such the Nursing Interventions Classification, Nursing Outcomes Classification, and North American Nursing Diagnosis Association. Given the increasing use of informatics in healthcare settings, such a lack of knowledge and experience can hamper nurses' ability to participate actively in informatics.

INFORMATICS: TYPES AND METHODS

For informatics to be effective, three concerns must be addressed. First, the HCO must have effective and easily accessible IT support services. Staff must be able to pick up the telephone and get this support. Failure of the information system has major implications for patient care, so backup systems are critical.

The second critical concern is staff training. This requires resources: financial resources, trainers, and time. Staff need time to attend training, and there must be recognition that it takes time for staff to learn how to use a system.

Incorporation of informatics with any of the methods described next (and others that are not included here) requires a major change in care delivery. Change is stressful for staff, and it needs to be planned, representing the third concern. Trying to implement too many changes at one time can increase staff stress, impact the success of using more informatics in the future, decrease staff motivation to participate, and increase the risk of errors that might impact patient outcomes.

It is not difficult to find nurses who will complain about a hospital's attempt to increase the use of informatics, particularly if it has been badly planned. Often, in these complaints, staff note that the system selected was not effective and that they had no part in the process. Equipment and software can be very costly, and decisions regarding them are critical. Time must be taken to evaluate equipment and software to make sure they meet the needs and demands of the organization and users such as nurses. Examples of current activities in this area are automated dispensing of medications and bar coding; computerized monitoring of adverse events; the use of electronic medical/health records, provider order entry systems, clinical decision support systems, tablets, smartphones, computer-based and reminder systems; accessing patient records at the point of care; prescribing via the Internet; and using nurse call systems, voice mail, the telephone for advice and other services, online support groups for patients and families, the Internet or virtual appointments, and smartphones. These methods are discussed on the following pages.

Automated Dispensing of Medications and Bar Coding

Pharmacies in all types of HCOs are using or moving toward using automatic medication dispensing systems with bar coding. These systems select the medication based on the order and prepare it in single doses for the patient. The bar code is on the packaged dose. This code can then be compared with the bar code on the patient's identification band using a handheld device. Such a system can decrease errors, and it supports all five rights of medication administration:

1. Right drug
2. Right patient
3. Right amount
4. Right route
5. Right time

Bar coding can also be used to collect data about prescribed and administered drugs. Data can then be used for quality improvement and for research. Bar coding systems are expensive to install and maintain, but they can make a difference in reducing errors.

Computerized Monitoring of Adverse Events

Computerized systems that monitor adverse events assist in identifying and monitoring adverse events. Developing and using a database of these events facilitates analysis of data and the development of interventions to decrease adverse events.

Electronic Medical/Health Records

The EMR/EHR is slowly replacing the written medical record for an individual patient while the patient receives care within a specific health-care system. A second type of electronic documentation system is the personal health record (PHR). The PHR is less common than the EMR, but there is hope that it will become standard in the future. The PHR is a computer-based health record for which data are collected over the long term—for a lifetime. With the patient's permission, the healthcare provider can access this record easily to obtain information. To reach this point, there must be agreement on a minimum data set—uniform definitions of data (i.e., standardized language) that would enable all healthcare providers to understand and use the information. There is still much to be done to make this a reality in every HCO, including clinics and medical offices, but the technology is already available.

The electronic medical record (EMR) is a record of the patient's history and assessment, orders, laboratory results, description of medical tests and procedures, and documentation of care provided and outcomes. Care plans are included. Information can be easily input, searched, and reviewed, and reports can be printed. Data can be stored over the long term, which is harder to do with written records: Written records require significant storage space, and they may not be easy to find once archived. In addition, written records can be less readable over time. The hard-copy record is also not always easy to access in a hospital unit. If one person is using the record, others cannot use it. With the EMR, this is not a problem as long as staff can access the computerized record system. EMR systems do require security and backup systems to ensure that data are not lost in the event of a power outage or natural disaster.

The following list developed by Iyer and Camp (1999, pp. 129–130) identifies the projected and current advantages of using EMRs:

- Legible records
- Readily available records
- Improved nursing productivity

- Reduction in record tampering
- Support of nursing process in the system
- Reduction in redundant documentation
- Clinical prompts, reminders, and warnings
- Categorized nursing notes
- Automatically printed reports
- Documentation according to standards of care
- Improved knowledge of outcomes
- Availability of data
- Prevention of medication errors
- Facilitation of cost-defining efforts
- Printed discharge information

EMR documentation may take place at the unit workstation, at a hallway computer station, at the bedside in the hospital, or an examining room in a clinic. Bedside systems are better; they are easy to access when the nurse or other healthcare professional needs information, and point-of-care documentation is enhanced.

The ANA believes that the public has a right to expect that health data and healthcare information will be centered on patient safety and improved outcomes throughout all segments of the healthcare system and the data and information will be accurately and efficiently collected, recorded, protected, stored, utilized, analyzed, and reported. Principles of privacy, confidentiality, and security cannot be compromised as the industry creates and implements interoperable and integrated healthcare information technology systems and solutions to convert from paper-based media for documentation and healthcare records to the newer format of EHRs, including individual personal health record (PHR) products. The ANA strongly supports efforts to further refine the concept and requirements of the patient-centric EHR, including the creation of standards-based electronic health records and supporting infrastructures that promote efficient and effective interprofessional and patient communications and decision-making wherever care is provided. Similar attention must address the secondary uses of data and information to generate knowledge that leads to improved and effective decision tools. All stakeholders, including nurses and patients, must be integral participants in the design, development, implementation, and evaluation phases of the electronic health record. This effort requires the attention and action of nurses, the professional and specialty nursing organizations, and the nursing profession to ensure the EHRs are designed to facilitate and support critical thinking and decision making, such as in the nursing process, and the associated documentation activities. It is ANA's position that the registered nurse must also be involved in the product selection, design, development, implementation, evaluation and improvement of information systems and electronic patient care devices used in patient care setting. (ANA, 2009)*

Provider Order Entry System

The provider order entry system (POES) is included in the EMR, although it can also be a stand-alone system. The healthcare provider inputs orders into this system rather than writing them. One clear advantage of the POES is legibility; written orders are often very difficult to read because handwriting varies, and this has led to many errors. It also takes time to transcribe written physician/provider orders into a form in which the orders can be used. During this process, risk of transcription errors is increased. Typing orders into a computer can also lead to typos, but this is less of a problem than errors with handwritten orders. Clinical decision support systems can be included with the POES. This combination enhances the provider order entry system and can lead to improved care and a decrease in errors.

---

*Integration of EHRs and these information systems into nurses' work environments should improve the safety and quality of patient care without increasing work load or intensity, and should allow more time for interaction with patient and family. Such initiatives must include sufficient and continued investment in the development and maintenance of standardized terminologies that include concepts, terms, and relationships to support nursing practice in every setting, measurement of nurse-sensitive outcomes, and evidence-based practice.

Clinical Decision Support Systems

Clinical decision support systems have led to major changes in healthcare delivery. These systems provide immediate information that can influence clinical decisions. Some of the systems actually intervene when an error is about to be made. For example, when an order for a medication is put into a patient's EMR, the computerized system can indicate that the patient is allergic to that medication by immediately sending an alert, stopping the order. The nurse can also get alerts that the patient is at risk for falls or decubiti. In the past, nurses depended on textbooks or journals that the unit might have to find information, and such searches were not done effectively. Easy electronic access to current information eliminates many problems related to obtaining information when needed. This, too, can improve the quality of care. Evidence-based practice relies heavily on access to evidence-based practice literature, which is most easily accessible via the Internet and databases. As is true for all electronic methods, healthcare professional critical thinking, as well as clinical reasoning and judgment, must still be applied. Errors can still be made with technology. When HIT is used, staff may go on "automatic pilot," assuming that the electronic system will catch errors, which is not always the case.

More research is needed to fully understand the impact of clinical decision support systems on patient outcomes. A study published in 2011 indicated that there was no consistent association between such systems and the quality of care in an investigation that included 3 billion patient visits (Romano & Stafford, 2011). Only one of 20 indicators—diet counseling for high-risk adults—demonstrated significantly better performance when clinical decision support systems were utilized. In contrast, earlier studies had shown that use of the clinical decision support systems improved outcomes. A critique of the 2011 study questions whether its results were influenced by the following factors: (1) Clinical decision support systems rules may have been different in the systems studied; (2) the study focused on medication management, whereas earlier studies were broader; and (3) the study looked at the outcome of a single visit rather than the cumulative effect. More research is needed to better determine the effectiveness of using clinical decision support systems.

Tablets and Smartphones

Tablet computers such as iPads have become hugely popular with the general public. Most mobile telephones now have Internet capability, such as access to the Internet and storage of information; such devices are referred to as smartphones. These phones give users access to information, Internet, e-mail, and text messaging, and, of course, telephone service. Such handheld devices can hold a significant amount of information, serve as a calendar, keep contact information, and are an effective method for transmission of information.

Nurses who use tablets carry information with them and can look up side effects of a medication or any other type of medical information necessary as they provide care. In some cases, the nurse can access EMRs to get to patient information through the tablet. Some textbooks can now be uploaded into tablets, such as pharmacology and clinical laboratory resources. This is useful information for the nurse to have available—it is accessible in seconds at the point of care with this type of HIT. Nurses working outside a structured setting, such as in public health or in home care, may also find this type of system useful for support information and documentation needs (patient information, visit data, and so on); however, they must be very careful to maintain HIPAA regulations. Tablets are used in public health to collect data such as health assessments; these data are stored locally on the tablet and then uploaded to a secure cloud server (i.e., a server that is encrypted to protect personal health information) when the user is back in network/wireless range. Anytime such technology is used, the data must be protected to keep information secure and confidential.

Computer-Based Reminder Systems

Computer-based reminder systems are used to communicate with patients via e-mail to remind them of appointments and screenings and to discuss other health issues. In the future, this method will most likely take the place of telephone calls to remind patients of appointments. This system also must maintain HIPAA regulations. For example, the healthcare provider must ensure that only authorized parties have access to the computer and e-mail data. More narrowly defined, only the patient should have access to the information unless the patient wants the information shared.

Access to Patient Records at the Point of Care

Many hospitals are moving toward providing access to the patient records either in the patient's room or in the hallway via computers. In the future, more nurses will carry small laptops or tablets that allow access to the EMR when needed. This reduces time spent returning to the workstation to get information. Documentation can be completed as soon as care is provided; this reduces errors and improves quality because all care providers know when care has been provided. Point-of-care access decreases the chance that details may be forgotten, documented incorrectly, or not documented at all. In addition, it saves nurses time and eliminates the need to delay documentation. For example, if they do not have this type of immediate access, nurses may document at certain times during the shift such as midmorning or near the end of a shift—a system that can lead to errors, incomplete data in the record if the nurse forgets information, and situations in which other providers need current patient information that has not yet been documented.

Internet Prescriptions

There has been rapid growth in access to prescriptions via the Internet. The medications are then mailed to the patient. The consumer does have to be careful and check the legitimacy of the source to prevent errors.

Nurse Call Systems

Nurse call systems are a form of informatics that is very important in communication within a healthcare system. They allow for improved and efficient communication and are a great improvement on the old method of yelling out for a staff member. Many types of nurse call systems exist, such as pagers, light signals, buzzers, methods that allow patients to talk directly to nurses through a direct audio system that the nurse can easily access, smartphones, miniature label microphones, and locator badges. The goal is to get a message to the right person as soon as possible while maintaining privacy and confidentiality. Doing so can improve care, improve patient satisfaction, reduce errors, and make staff more efficient, preventing the unnecessary work of trying to obtain and share information.

Voice Mail and Texting

Computer-based messaging systems are found in all healthcare settings today so that staff can leave and receive voice messages. Staff and patients can use these systems, often reducing the need for callbacks. Complicated systems can annoy consumers, however, and there is an impersonal quality to this form of communication, though it is part of everyday life today. One has to be very careful about leaving voice mails. Clearly, others can listen to messages, and this can lead to a HIPAA violation.

Telephone for Advice and Other Services

Patient advice systems are used mostly by insurers, although some HCOs and providers provide these services as well. In such systems, nurses use their assessment skills and provide advice to patients who call in with questions. Typically, insurers develop standard protocols that the nurses use for common questions, but nurses must still use professional judgment when providing advice. This type of service should not become "cookbook" care in which there is no consideration of assessment and individual patient needs. Assessment is the key to successful telephone nursing, as it enables providers to identify the interventions required that may or may not be found in the guidelines. Some physician offices have telephone advice services that are manned by a physician in the practice or by a nurse. Pediatric practices are the most common type of practice using this system. Patient advice systems via telephone require clear documentation policies and guidelines that include content related to who is called, when, and for what reason, and the required assessment data and interventions. Telephone advice systems are typically used to answer questions, remind patients of appointments or follow-up needs, and check in on how a patient is doing.

Hospitals are using the telephone to begin the admission process for patients with scheduled admissions. Patients are called before the admission date, asked questions related to required admission information, and told what to expect on admission. Pretesting may be scheduled prior to admission. This saves the hospital time and is more cost-effective, and pretesting can be more convenient for the patient. This method can also identify problems that may impact the needed patient care so that they can be addressed early on.

Online Support Groups for Patients and Families

Online support groups can focus on any problem or disease. Patients and their families can use chat rooms, e-mail, and websites for information sharing. Consumers gain information, education about their health and health needs, and support from others with similar problems. A healthcare provider may or may not be involved. Privacy issues must be discussed with participants, along with the risk of lack of privacy.

Internet or Virtual Appointments

Use of the Internet as a means of increasing accessibility to a physician or advanced practice nurse or to make appointments is increasing. Members of younger generations, as well as some senior citizens, are using the Internet to obtain advice from health professionals. Portable family histories can be maintained in this fashion and passed on to a new primary care provider. Those patients and families who have limited resources—financial, transportation, or insurance—can more affordably receive medical advice in this format. It also keeps some employees from missing work to take a child or other family member to an appointment. Many of these sites link to cellular devices to send an alert of high importance to whoever is on call for virtual hours. This ensures that high-priority questions and requests for advice reach the health professional quickly (Larkin, 2008). These types of services will most likely increase in the future.

As is true with all documentation methods, patient confidentiality must be maintained. Notably, the risk of confidentiality problems increases with use of such technology.

THE FUTURE OF INFORMATICS AND MEDICAL TECHNOLOGY

The future is likely to see major expansion in the use of technology. Some of the possible technological approaches are already being used in some areas. One area that is growing is the use of embodied conversation agents to provide reinforcement of discharge teaching, particularly when there is low health literacy (Paasche-Orlow, 2010). Cutting-edge technology is sometimes hard to believe. Some of the possibilities will be discussed next.

Nanotechnology

Nanotechnology—microscopic technology on the order of one-billionth of a meter—will likely impact the diagnosis and treatment of many diseases and conditions (Gordon, Lutz, Boninger, & Cooper, 2007). Some of the pending technologies are highlighted here:

- Sensing patients' internal drug levels with miniature medical diagnostic tools that circulate in the bloodstreams
- Chemotherapy delivered directly to a tumor site, reducing systemic side effects
- New monitoring devices for the home: a talking pill bottle that lets patients push a button to hear prescription information; bathroom counters that announce whether it is safe to mix two medications; a shower with built-in scales to calculate body mass index; measuring devices in the bathroom to track urine frequency and output and upload these data to a system or care manager; noninvasive blood glucose monitors to eliminate sticks; and sensors to compute blood sugar levels using a multi-wavelength reflective dispersion photometer.

Wearable Computing

A computer can be worn, much as eyeglasses or clothing is worn, and interactions with the user are based on the context of the situation (ANA, 2008). With heads-up displays, embedded sensors in fabrics, unobtrusive input devices, personal wireless local area networks, and a host of other context sensing and communication tools, wearable computers can act as intelligent assistants or data collection and analysis devices. Many of these devices are available now using smart fabrics. Such wearable computer and remote monitoring systems are intertwined with the user's activity so that the technology becomes transparent. Sensors and devices can gather data during the patient's daily routine, providing healthcare providers or researchers with periodic or continuous data on the person's health while he or she is at work, at school, exercising, or sleeping, rather than the current snapshot captured during a typical hospital or clinic visit. A few applications for wearable computing devices include sudden infant death syndrome monitoring for infants; ambulatory cardiac and respiratory monitoring; monitoring of ventilation during exercise; monitoring the activity level of post-stroke patients; monitoring patterns of breathing in asthma; assessment of stress in individuals; arrhythmia detection and control of selected cardiac conditions; and daily activity monitors (Offray Specialty Narrow Fabrics, 2007).

HIPAA: ENSURING CONFIDENTIALITY

The Health Insurance Portability and Accountability Act of 1996 (HIPAA) has had a major impact on healthcare delivery systems and how they communicate. Privacy and confidentiality have long been problematic issues in health care. Because HIPAA focuses on the issue of information and confidentiality, it applies to IT. The law also requires data security and electronic transaction standards. This law was necessary because with the growth of information sharing, it became increasingly evident that existing means of transactions and systems were not ensuring privacy and confidentiality—key elements that had long been part of the healthcare delivery system.

Privacy is the right of a person to have personal information kept private. As discussed, this relates to professional ethics. Privacy restrictions even apply to family members unless the adult patient specifically communicates that it is acceptable for family members to be given information. This cannot be assumed. HIPAA requires that only necessary information be shared among providers, including insurers. Patients may also access their medical records.

Health information cannot be openly shared by healthcare providers—for example, discussing patient information in public places, calling a patient's work or home and leaving a message that reveals information about health or health services, and so on, must not be done. Carrying documents outside an

HCO with patient identifier information is prohibited; this constraint has implications for students who may take notes or have written assignments that include this information. How information is carried in tablets, laptops, or smartphones is also of concern. For example, taking pictures on smartphones in clinical settings is a privacy violation. Many institutions have implemented strict policies about the taking of patient photos even if they are de-identified. As a nurse, you should make sure you know your institution's policy on smartphone use in a clinical setting and follow it.

Development of new technology has been moving so fast that critical prior issues have not always been addressed effectively. The 1996 law, however, requires that staff know the key elements of HIPAA and apply them. As a result, HCOs and healthcare profession schools, such as nursing programs, are required to provide information and training about HIPAA. There are large fines if the law is broken. Patients are informed about HIPAA when they enter the health system; they are given written information and asked to sign documents to indicate that they have been informed. Ensuring that the requirements are met must be incorporated into IT, which has become a major method for communicating health information. With the Internet, it is easy for patients to report HIPAA violations. Violations will be examined, and the provider may have to pay a fee for not following HIPAA regulations.

TELEHEALTH: A GROWING INTERVENTION

Telehealth, or telemedicine, is the use of telecommunications equipment and communications networks for transferring healthcare information between participants at different locations. Telehealth applies telecommunication and computer technologies to the broad spectrum of public health and medicine. This technology offers opportunities to provide care when face-to-face interaction is impossible (such as in home care, in school-based care, and in rural areas) and can be used in a variety of settings and situations as long as the equipment is available. Two-way interactive video is the most effective telehealth method.

> Telenursing refers to the use of telecommunications technology in nursing to enhance patient care. It involves the use of electromagnetic channels (e.g., wire, radio and optical) to transmit voice, data and video communications signals. It is also defined as distance communications, using electrical or optical transmissions, between humans and/or computers. (Skiba, 1998, p. 40)

Issues that arise with telehealth include the cost of equipment and its use; training for staff and for patients if they need to actively use equipment; limited or no insurance coverage for telehealth services; the need for clear policies, procedures, and protocols; privacy and confidentiality of information; and regulatory issues (e.g., a nurse who is located and licensed in one state providing telenursing for a patient in another state where the nurse is not licensed). Telehealth also has implications for international health care because it provides a method for connecting expertise to patients who may need care that is not accessible in their home country.

USE OF THE INTERNET

Nurses use the Internet to obtain information and for communication through e-mail. Patients/consumers are also using the Internet for increasingly more health-related purposes. It can be an excellent source for all types of information, including health and medical information.

When the Internet is used as a source of health information, it is important that nurses evaluate the websites, because they are not all of the same quality. A nurse needs to consider the following factors when evaluating a website:

- The source or sponsor of the website: The most reliable sites are sponsored by the government, academic institutions, healthcare professional organizations, and HCOs.

- Current status of the information: When was it posted or revised?

- Accessibility of the information on the site: Can one find what one needs?

- References provided for content when appropriate.

OTHER BIOMEDICAL AND PATIENT CARE TECHNOLOGIES

Examples of other biomedical and patient care technologies are briefly described in this section.

Remote Telemetry Monitoring

Remote telemetry monitoring technology informs staff when a patient's condition has changed. The patient is placed on a monitor, and signals are sent to staff through a page system. Staff may be informed, for example, of the patient's identity, heart rate, and readout of rhythm without being right next to the patient.

Robotics

The use of robotics in patient care is expected to expand in the future (ANA, 2008). Robots have been used for many years to deliver supplies to patient care areas. Robotics enables remote surgeries and virtual reality surgical procedures. Hand-assist devices help patients regain strength after a stroke ("Robotic Brace," 2007). Robots may provide a remote presence to allow physicians to virtually examine patients by manipulating remote cameras ("Telemedicine Pioneer Helps Physicians," 2007). They are also used for microscopic, minimally invasive surgical procedures. For example, the da Vinci surgical system helps surgeons perform such procedures as mitral valve repairs, hysterectomies, and prostate surgeries (da Vinci Surgery, 2008). In the future, robots may also be used in direct patient care—for instance, to help lift morbidly obese patients.

Genetics and Genomics

Advances in mapping the human genome (genetics), understanding individual DNA, and examining the impact of external factors such as the environment (genomics) will have a dramatic impact on patient care (ANA, 2008). These data, especially once they are integrated into EMRs or PHRs, will lead to advances in customized patient care and medications targeted to individual responses to medications. Care and medication can be precisely customized to patients based on their unique DNA profile and how they have responded to medications and other interventions in the past; this will dramatically change how patients are managed for specific diseases and conditions and extend into the prevention of some diseases. The inherent complexity of customized patient care will demand computerized clinical decision support that reflects individual needs and health history. Predictive disease models based on patients' DNA profiles will emerge as clinicians better understand DNA mapping. These advances have implications for a new model of care and for the informatics nurse's participation in the development of genomic IT solutions. More than ever, patients will need to be partners in this development as part of patient-centered care. Nurses are beginning to collaborate more with bioengineers and informatics experts to develop new products, participate in research using these products, and help to develop implementation and evaluation plans to use with these products.

HIGH-TOUCH CARE VERSUS HIGH-TECH CARE

High-touch care is what most people go into nursing for, but nursing is much more than this today. This chapter describes the growing influence of technology on all segments of health care. This influence will not decrease, but rather will increase in the future. Nurses do need to understand and know how to use technology that is applied to their practice areas. They need to be involved in the development of this technology when possible, and they must be involved in the implementation of the technology. But there are concerns. When we talk through machines, do we lose information and the personal relationship? How can this be prevented so that we are not disconnected from our patients? How can we ensure that the information we are getting is correct and complete? Are people able to communicate fully through some of these other means? It is clear that over time, the public has become increasingly comfortable with informatics, which they are using more and more in their everyday lives. As nursing adopts informatics to an ever greater extent, nurses need to keep in mind the potential for isolation and the need for effective communication, and they must not forget the need for touch and face-to-face communication. When a nurse uses a computer or some type of handheld device asking patient questions and does not look at the patient, this does not engage the patient in the process.

The future will include many more new uses of technology, and change is ongoing. For example, the eICU (e-intensive care unit) is used to monitor patients from afar to improve patient outcomes (Kowalczyk, 2007). In this example a system is attached to four hospitals in Iowa and their ICUs. This system allows intensivists at a remote monitoring center to view patients' vital statistics, electrocardiograms, ventilators, and X-ray and lab results. The eICU includes two-way conference video capability so that patients and staff can interact when required. This type of system has advantages: For example, experts can be located in one place and then consult with multiple locations and staff. This is particularly useful in providing expert medical care for residents in rural and remote areas. There is no reason that this type of system would be limited to physician consultation; it could be used by nurses. For example, a nurse clinical specialist could view data and consult on patient care with nurses in various ICUs. The potential is there for increased access to information and expertise. The other side of this innovation coin is the effect on the touch side of care when the provider is not actually in the room with the patient. It is not clear how this might impact care because these types of systems are very new.

NURSING LEADERSHIP IN INFORMATICS

We are currently at a critical junction for nurses and the IOM informatics competency, with all nurses being called upon to assume more of a leadership role in the expansion of informatics in healthcare. This call to action corresponds to the recommendations in the IOM's *Future of Nursing* report (2011). Ongoing implementation of the Affordable Care Act will lead to further changes in healthcare delivery and more dependence on informatics, and nurse informaticists should be part of the structure that develops and implements greater use of informatics (HIMSS, 2011).

HEALTH IT: THE FUTURE

The IOM report titled *Health IT and Patient Safety: Building Safer Systems for Better Care* (2012) makes a strong statement that health IT is not something separated from care delivery or the providers of care.

> We are at a unique time in health care. Technology—which has the potential to improve quality and safety of care as well as reduce costs—is rapidly evolving, changing the way we deliver health care. At the same time, health care reform is reshaping the health care landscape. As Sir Cyril Chantler of the Kings Fund said, "Medicine used to be simple, ineffective, and relatively safe. Now it is complex, effective, and potentially dangerous." More and more cognitive overload requires a symbiotic relationship between human cognition and computer support. It is this very difficult transition we are facing in ensuring safety in health care. (IOM, 2012, p. ix)

The IOM report highlights patient and family concerns about safety and shared responsibility. These same themes have also been emphasized throughout this text.

CONCLUSION

This chapter has explored the current and future world of healthcare informatics and some aspects of biotechnology. There is much more to this subject than use of e-mail, as the many diverse examples presented in this chapter suggest. The core competency of using informatics is critical for nurses' success in the 21st century. If graduates of the healthcare profession schools cannot understand and use informatics, the safety and quality of the care they provide will be diminished. Communication, coordination, documentation, and care provision (including monitoring and decision making) are linked to informatics. However, each nurse must not get so involved in informatics and technology that the patient as a person is lost—the patient–nurse relationship is an important component of patient-centered care.

DISCUSSION QUESTIONS _____

1. Explain how the core competency "utilize informatics" relates to the other four IOM core competencies.

2. What is informatics, and why is it important in health care and nursing?

3. Describe the certification requirements for an informatics nurse and the role filled by this nurse.

4. Describe four examples of healthcare informatics and implications for nursing.

5. Why is documentation important?

6. Explain how the EMR and PHR can increase quality of care and decrease errors. Provide examples.

7. Discuss issues related to confidentiality and informatics.

REFERENCES

American Nurses Association (ANA). (2006). Nursing practice information infrastructure: Glossary. Retrieved from http://www.nursingworld.org/npii/glossary.htm

American Nurses Association (ANA). (2008). *Nursing informatics: Scope and standards of practice.* Washington, DC: Author.

American Nurses Association (ANA). (2009). *Electronic health record (Position statement).* Silver Spring, MD: Author. Retrieved from http://nursingworld.org/MainMenuCategories/Policy-Advocacy/Positions-and-Resolutions/ANA-Position-Statements/Position-Statements-Alphabetically/Electronic-Health-Record.html

American Nurses Association (ANA). (2010). *ANA's principles for nursing documentation.* Silver Spring, MD: Author.

American Nurses Credentialing Center (ANCC). (2014). Informatics nurse certification exam. Retrieved from http://www.nursecredentialing.org/InformaticsNursing

Appleton, C. (1998). Nursing research: Moving into the clinical setting. *Nursing Management, 29*(6), 43–45.

Association of periOperative Registered Nurses. (2008). Perioperative data set. Retrieved from http://www.aorn.org/Secondary.aspx?id=21100&terms=Perioperative%20data%20set

Bodenheimer, T. (2008). Coordinating care: A perilous journey through the healthcare system. *New England Journal of Medicine, 358,* 1065–1071.

Centers for Disease Control and Prevention (CDC). (2011). International classification of diseases (ICD-10). Retrieved from http://www.cdc.gov/nchs/icd/icd10.htm

Clark, S. (2011). Medical record documentation makes top 10 non-compliance list for first half of 2010. *HIM Connection.* Retrieved from http://www.hcpro.com/CCP-258429-237/Medical-record-documentation-makes-Joint-Commission-top-10-noncompliance-list-for-first-half-of-2010.html

da Vinci Surgery. (2008). Surgery enabled by da Vinci. Retrieved from http://www.davincisurgery.com/davinci-surgery/

Dykes, P., & Collins, S. (2013). Building linkages between nursing care and improved patient outcomes: The role of health information technology. *Online Journal of Issues in Nursing, 18*(3).

Retrieved from http://www.nursingworld.org/MainMenuCategories/ANAMarketplace/ANAPeriodicals/OJIN/TableofContents/Vol-18-2013/No3-Sept-2013/Nursing-Care-and-Improved-Outcomes.html

Englebardt, S., & Nelson, R. (2002). *Healthcare informatics: An interdisciplinary approach.* St. Louis, MO: Mosby-Year Book.

Finkelman, A., & Kenner, C. (2012). *Teaching IOM* (3rd ed.). Silver Spring, MD: American Nurses Association.

Gordon, A., Lutz, G., Boninger, M., & Cooper, R. (2007). Introduction to nanotechnology: Potential applications in physical medicine and rehabilitation. *American Journal of Physical Medicine and Rehabilitation, 86,* 225–241.

Healthcare Information and Management Systems Society (HIMSS). (2011, June 17). Position statement on transforming nursing practice through technology and informatics. http://www.himss.org/library/nursing-informatics/position-statement

Institute of Medicine (IOM). (2003). *Health professions education.* Washington, DC: National Academies Press.

Institute of Medicine (IOM). (2011). *The future of nursing: Leading change, advancing health.* Washington, DC: National Academies Press.

Institute of Medicine (IOM). (2012). *Health IT and patient safety: Building safer systems for better care.* Washington, DC: National Academies Press.

International Council of Nurses (ICN). (2008). International classification for nursing practice (ICNP). Retrieved from http://www.icn.ch/icnp_def.htm

Iyer, P., & Camp, N. (1999). *Nursing documentation.* St. Louis, MO: Mosby.

The Joint Commission. (2011). *Comprehensive accreditation manual for hospitals.* Chicago, IL: Author.

Kowalczyk, L. (2007, November 19). Teletreatment. Monitoring from afar, "eICUs" fill the gap. Retrieved from http://www.boston.com/business/globe/articles/2007/11/19/tele_treatment/

Larkin, H. (2008). Your future chief of staff? *H&HN: Hospitals & Healthcare Networks, 82*(3), 30–34.

National Center for Health Statistics. (2010). More physicians switch to electronic medical record. Retrieved from http://nchspressroom.wordpress.com/2010/04/02/more-physicians-switch-to-electronic-medical-record-use/

National Library of Medicine (NLM). (2008a). Logical observation identifiers names and codes. Retrieved from http://www.nlm.nih.gov/research/umls/loinc_main.html

National Library of Medicine (NLM). (2008b). Unified medical language system: SNOMED clinical terms. Retrieved from http://www.nlm.nih.gov/research/umls/Snomed/snomed_main.html

National Quality Forum (NQF). (2013). Electronic quality measures. Retrieved from http://www.qualityforum.org/Projects/e-g/eMeasures/Electronic_Quality_Measures.aspx

Nelson, R., & Joos, I. (1989, Fall). On language in nursing; from data to wisdom. *PLN Vision*, p. 6.

Offray Specialty Narrow Fabrics. (2007). Smart textiles. Retrieved from http://www.osnf.com/p_smart.html

Omaha System. (2011). The Omaha system: Solving the clinical data-information puzzle. Retrieved from http://www.omahasystem.org

Paasche-Orlow, M. (2010). Usability of conversational agents by patients with inadequate health literacy: Evidence from two clinical trials. *Journal of Health Communication, 15*(suppl 2, special issue), *Health Literacy Research: Current Status and Future Directions*, 197–210.

Richards, J. (2001). Nursing in a digital age. *Nursing Economics, 19*(1), 6–10, 34.

Robotic brace aids stroke recovery. (2007). *Science Daily*. Retrieved from http://www.sciencedaily.com/releases/2007/03/070321105223.htm

Romano, M., & Stafford, R. (2011). Electronic health records and clinical decision support systems: Impact on national ambulatory care quality. *Archives of Internal Medicine, 171*, 897–903.

Schwiran, P., & Thede, L. (2011). Informatics: The standardized nursing terminologies: A national survey of nurses' experiences and attitudes. *Online Journal of Issues in Nursing, 16*(2). Retrieved from http://nursingworld.org/MainMenuCategories/NAMarketplace/ANAPeriodicals/OJIN/Columns/Informatics/Informatics-Participants-Perception-of-Comfort-in-the-Use.html

Skiba, D. J. (1998). Health-oriented telecommunications. In M. J. Ball, K. J. Hannah, S. K. Newbold, & J. V. Douglas (Eds.), *Nursing informatics: Where caring and technology meet* (pp. 40–53). New York, NY: Springer.

Telemedicine pioneer helps physicians on the move stay close to patients. (2007). Retrieved from http://www.cisco.com/?POSITION=SEM&COUNTRY_SITE=us&CAMPAIGN=tomorrowstartshere&CREATIVE=Brand_Cisco+Systems&REFERRING_SITE=Bing&KEYWORD=what+is+cisco+systems_e|mkwid_6dahF5kH|dc_3648159597_0v0xx7y7d0 http://www.hhs.gov/news/press/2013pres/05/20130522a.html

Thompson, D. (2013). U.S. hospitals triple use of electronic health records: Report. Retrieved from http://health.usnews.com/health-news/news/articles/2013/07/08/us-hospitals-triple-use-of-electronic-health-records-report

U.S. Department of Health and Human Services (HHS). (2010). Meaningful use. Retrieved from http://www.hhs.gov/news/imagelibrary/video/2010-07-13_press.html

U.S. Department of Health and Human Services (HHS). (2013). Doctors and hospitals' use of health IT doubles since 2012. Retrieved from http://www.hhs.gov/news/press/2013pres/05/20130522a.html

U.S. Department of Health and Human Services (HHS) & Centers for Medicare and Medicaid Services (CMS). (2014). Meaningful use. Retrieved from http://www.cms.gov/Regulations-and-Guidance/Legislation/EHRIncentivePrograms/Meaningful_Use.html

U.S. Health and Human Services (HHS) & HealthIT.gov. (2014). Meaningful use definition and objectives. Retrieved from http://www.healthit.gov/providers-professionals/meaningful-use-definition-objectives

Theoretical Foundations, Research, and Evidence-Based Practice

The chapters included in Part 4 are not intended to be a summary of major nursing theories or research methods but rather provide a foundation for understanding, critiquing, evaluating, and using theory and research for advanced practice. Theory can provide a framework that encompasses what nurses know, do, and think, and it can guide the advanced practice nurse to know what to ask, what to observe, what to focus on, and what to think about (Chinn & Kramer, 1995).

The terminology and definitions surrounding theory can be confusing for the novice advanced practice nurse to fully understand. Further, scholars of nursing theory do not always agree on the definitions, leading to a lack of clarity in this field of study. As way of introduction to Part 4, the generally agreed-upon definitions of terms that provide the foundation for the chapters in this part are presented here.

What is theory? As with many concepts, a variety of definitions for this term have been proposed, which typically share a common set of characteristics. For our purposes, theories are organized systems that describe, explain, predict, or prescribe phenomenon. They are composed of concepts (constructs or variables) and propositions (hypotheses) that specify the relationships among the concepts. Further theories are substantiated by and derived from established evidence and can be repeatedly confirmed by observation and testing.

Four types of theories are derived from the preceding definition:

1. Descriptive theories describe concepts of a discipline.
2. Explanatory theories explain how the concepts relate to one another.
3. Predictive theories predict the relationships between the concepts of a phenomenon and predict under which conditions it will occur.
4. Prescriptive theories prescribe interventions and the consequences of interventions.

Additionally, four levels of theory can be placed on a continuum ranging from very abstract and broad (metatheory) to very specific and narrow (practice theories):

1. Metatheory is the most abstract and cannot be easily tested. There are no theories labeled as such in nursing. The most commonly cited examples of metatheory are the big bang and evolution.

2. Grand theories define broad perspectives for nursing practice and are less abstract than metatheory is. As such they can be tested. Some of the more well-known nursing theories classified as grand theory are those proposed by Nightingale, Parse, Leininger, Benner, and Henderson. There are many more, however, and a search of the Internet can lead to a long list of nursing grand theories.

3. Middle-range (midrange) theories are moderately abstract and have a limited number of concepts. They can be tested directly. Midrange theories can predict and prescribe nursing interventions and patient outcomes. Many new midrange nursing theories have been proposed over the last two decades. They are often used for both nursing research and practice. Some examples include theories of uncertainty, comfort, pain, social support, and quality of life. A search of the Internet can reveal many nursing middle-range theories useful to the advanced practice nurse.

4. Practice theory traces the outline for practice. Objectives are set and actions are set to meet the objectives.

Another important fundamental understanding of nursing theory is needed before reading the chapters in Part 4. In 1984, Fawcett presented a seminal paper on the metaparadigms of nursing. It is now widely accepted, but not universally, that the metaparadigms for nursing theory are fourfold:

■ Nursing
■ Health
■ Person
■ Environment

Theory, practice, research, and evidence-based practice (EBP) are intimately intertwined. Theory informs practice, just as practice informs theory. Research is used to test the theory but at the same time can be used to develop and refine theory. As nursing goes forward as a discipline, and as consumers and policymakers demand effective, cost-conscious, evidence-based practice, we must understand theory and research and use theories to guide practice, while simultaneously analyzing and critiquing our practice to generate new theories that can be tested by research.

In Chapter 18, the first chapter in Part 4, Rodgers discusses the historical development of nursing as a science and professional discipline and provides an overview of the major principles of epistemology that have influenced the development of theory and nursing science. She also considers emerging trends in nursing knowledge development as it relates to the future of nursing.

In Chapter 19, Kenney provides a foundation from which to appreciate the value and relevance of theory from nursing and other disciplines and application to practice. In Chapter 20, Sultz and Young provide a historical overview of nursing research and highlight the role the Agency for Health Care Policy and Research (AHCPR) has played in the development of clinical practice guidelines. Future trends related to nursing research, including population research, evidence-based practice, and outcomes research, are reviewed. Current opportunities and goals of the National Institute of Nursing Research (NINR) are outlined, with a focus on health promotion, chronic disease management, and reproductive health. It is essential for advanced practice nurses to have a solid foundation in the utilization of EBP guidelines to incorporate research findings into clinical decision making.

In Chapter 21, Milner discusses the historical roots of evidenced-based practice and explores evidenced-based practice models and clinical appraisal tools applicable to advanced practice nursing. The author gives a broad overview of the five elements necessary in the EBP process: (1) formulating an appropriate question, (2) performing an efficient literature search, (3) critically appraising the best available evidence, (4) applying the best evidence to clinical practice, and (5) assessing outcomes of care. A template for implementation of an evidence-based practice project is provided for application to real-life clinical scenarios.

In Chapter 22, the last chapter in Part 4, Tymkow eloquently compares and contrasts clinical scholarship and EBP and the role of the Doctor of Nursing Practice (DNP) to this end. The American Association of Colleges of Nursing (AACN) DNP Essentials document further defines the skills, tools, and methods necessary to implement and support clinical scholarship and EBP as the following: (1) translating research in practice, (2) quality improvement and patient-centered care, (3) evaluation of practice, (4) research methods and technology, (5) participation in collaborative research, and (6) disseminating findings from evidence-based practice.

The AACN recommends separate coursework in research, and an informal survey of DNP and Master of Science in Nursing curricula demonstrates that most often research is done in separate courses in advanced nurse practice programs. Thus it is not the intention of this book to explicate the research process and methods in detail but rather to put the need for health research and nursing research into a broader context so the reader can appreciate how research improves practice and informs decision making.

CHAPTER 18

The Evolution of Nursing Science

Beth L. Rodgers

CHAPTER OBJECTIVES

1. Discuss the historical development of nursing as a science and professional discipline.
2. Describe the major principles of epistemology that have influenced the development of theory and nursing science.
3. Identify emerging trends in nursing knowledge development.

INTRODUCTION

In discussions of nursing, images that commonly come to mind are those of the nurse performing certain acts such as listening to blood pressure sounds, changing a dressing for a wound, assisting someone with ambulation, giving medication, or starting an intravenous line. Undoubtedly, people who have been registered nurses for some time recall their early days in school and the tremendous anticipation of performing the first immunization or urinary catheterization, or the excitement the first time an intravenous catheter was inserted smoothly and successfully.

Nurses who have been engaged in the broad professional role of the registered nurse recognize that there is a great deal more to nursing than the performance of those skills. Nonetheless, when talking about nursing, discussion often turns quite easily to a focus on what nurses *do*—the skills, tasks, and functions that are associated with the actions and behaviors of nurses. Much less common is an emphasis on what nurses *know*—the knowledge base that underlies the performance of those acts—as well as the many more things that nurses do beyond obvious physical functions. No doubt it is much easier to describe the mechanics of listening to breath sounds than it is to describe the detailed thinking that goes into formulating a holistic portrayal of an individual patient for whom those breath sounds are only a small part of his or her scenario.

Nurses engage in a variety of actions that are far subtler than those involving the common skills that are directly observable. For example, they form important working relationships with patients to help them achieve their health and wellness goals; they counsel, educate, guide, facilitate, assess, plan, relate, evaluate, and engage with people as individuals or in groups or communities on a variety of levels consistent with a holistic approach to health concerns and health promotion. Nurses also engage in activities such as arranging for referrals, managing various stages of care, and facilitating access to necessary resources. This list is in no way exhaustive, but it provides some indication of the tremendous number of cognitive activities associated with nursing—activities that, because they lack implements or other tangible equipment, may be recognized less readily by the public. Perhaps even more significant, nurses also are less quick to describe these activities, possibly because of the difficulty associated with articulating the specific thought processes that are essential for effective and appropriate care. Many nurses seem to give themselves less credit than is warranted for the cognitive capabilities and knowledge that go into nursing. When asked why they reacted to a situation in a particular way or what prompted them to intervene, it is not uncommon to hear the nurse say, "I just knew," referring to a gut feeling or intuition as the basis for significant action.

These responses on the part of nurses fail to give credit to the vast amount of knowledge that nurses carry with them every day. It is not the tasks and skills that nurses perform that make them such an indispensable part of health care but rather what they "know." The knowledge of nurses not only lies at the root of competent and effective care but also provides the foundation that makes nurses such important contributors to broader decision making and planning. When nurses argue that they should be involved in committees, on boards, or in other influential positions, and when

they discuss why certain concerns or problems clearly could benefit from nursing involvement, it is the knowledge of nurses that makes these arguments so meaningful. Although nurses often find themselves in a position of needing, or at least wanting, to articulate what is unique about their particular level of preparation, discussion of the knowledge base of nursing can be a challenging undertaking. It is much easier to describe what nurses do than what they know.

THE IMPACT OF THE DOCTOR OF NURSING PRACTICE DEGREE

As nurses have achieved higher levels of education (particularly doctoral degrees), the need to understand the knowledge base of the discipline has become even more imperative. Nurses with doctoral-level education are likely to be perceived as leaders both in the discipline and in the broader community and they should be prepared and willing to assume roles as leaders in a number of contexts. They often are confronted with both the opportunity and the need to explain what constitutes nursing at that level. No doubt this need will persist and it most likely will be greatly expanded as more nurses with Doctor of Nursing Practice (DNP) degrees work within a variety of settings. Not only does the DNP constitute an advanced degree, which surely will grab the interest of the public (whose familiarity with nursing is most likely limited to personal experience with hospital or clinic nurses), but it also is a new degree that carries with it credentials and titles that are not known to the broader public, and perhaps also not well understood within nursing.

At the same time, nurses with the DNP degree are in an important position to serve as leaders in the continuing articulation of the discipline, as well as contributors on multiple levels to the development of the knowledge base for nursing.

All of these factors create a tremendous need for nurses at all levels of preparation to articulate with clarity the nature of nursing knowledge and what nurses are capable of contributing to health in all realms—individual, family, local, community, and global. DNP-prepared nurses have particular responsibility for taking leadership to represent the discipline and profession of nursing well and to identify and discuss the particular expertise and advanced knowledge of the DNP-prepared nurse. In addition, nurses with the DNP degree are prepared and often placed in important positions as essential collaborators in research and innovations that add to the knowledge base of nursing as it continues to develop as a discipline.

SCIENCE AND KNOWLEDGE

Without an understanding of the overall discipline, including the knowledge that underlies the thoughts and actions of the nurse, both practice and research can become isolated, individualistic, situational endeavors. *Science* is the general term used to refer to the knowledge base of a discipline that has been developed rigorously and systematically. The idea of "science" has an interesting history, however, and science was not always the dominant term used to refer to credible knowledge. As evidenced by the writings of Aristotle, for example, and in the work of many others continuing into the nineteenth century, the terms *science* and *knowledge* were used almost interchangeably for much of recorded history. It is only in modern times that science has been recognized as a rather specialized form of knowledge, replete with specific methodologies and means to evaluate credibility. In exploring the underpinnings of nursing work, especially those elements that provide nurses with valuable and trustworthy information as a foundation for practice, it is helpful to look at not just science but the broader realm of nursing knowledge.

The discipline of nursing includes components other than just the knowledge base. Disciplines also involve a human component in that judgments are made about what is acceptable science and what are current priorities. This component necessarily involves the expression of the values embodied in the discipline in regard to what is needed for knowledge development. The human component, what Toulmin (1972) referred to as the "profession," works with and develops the knowledge base of the discipline and develops mechanisms for the sharing of ideas through debate and dialogue, both oral and in the form of publications. Organizations within the discipline provide leadership, whether through societies that have bestowed honors upon esteemed nurses, research organizations that promote the conduct of research and dissemination of results, or specialty organizations that shape practice. Those organizations also have important roles in the ongoing development of nursing as a discipline. Discussion of the science of nursing, or the knowledge base, cannot be carried out without recognition of the context that exists for that knowledge in the discipline. In addition, this nursing context exists within a larger societal context that includes expectations for nurses, as well as standards for what is considered to be knowledge or science, and especially "good" science.

It is easy to identify examples of how knowledge has changed, sometimes rapidly, and just as often in radical ways. Recent discoveries related to genetics are stimulating revolutionary developments in treatment as well as renewed efforts at prevention as that genetic knowledge evolves. Dietary guidelines are evolving as awareness develops that blood lipid profiles are not inextricably linked to dietary intake of fats, with new information being in substantial opposition to prevailing ideology about nutrition and illness. Awareness of the effect of environmental conditions and artificial substances on health and the development of health problems has raised questions in areas that were not given much consideration in the prior germ theory–oriented approach to medicine, questions ranging from food production to vaccination guidelines. In such a context of ever-changing science, often accompanied by competing values and priorities, significant challenges are presented for nurses who not only provide "best practice" in whatever realm they work but also must defend those practices in the face of changing knowledge.

It is clear that context has considerable influence on the discipline of nursing and the development of the corresponding knowledge base. Because of that influence, it is reasonable to look at the evolution of nursing knowledge using a chronological approach; in fact, many aspects of context are associated with historical events and timing. One limitation associated with such a chronology is that it gives the impression that change is linear. That would be quite a naïve view, however. Science is inextricably tied to human behavior and attitudes; given that science is a human enterprise, and multiple stakeholders and influences exist, the development and change of knowledge over time is far from linear. In contrast, the movement of knowledge often involves multiple and simultaneously existing and competing areas of focus influenced by diverse philosophical systems and sets of values.

Nonetheless, early ideas do provide the impetus for later ideas; societal needs and expectations at one period of time eventually lead to other sets of ideas. As such, there is continuity in the progression of ideas, and that continuity provides a useful framework for studying the history of ideas about nursing science. It is important to keep in mind that changes in ideas and emphasis must be considered as an evolutionary process and not necessarily a progression. Progression implies movement toward some specified point or goal, such that it is possible to say that nursing knowledge or science is getting closer to whatever that goal might be. Because of the fluidity of the context of nursing, as well as the context of the greater society, that endpoint or goal must be amenable to change as well. Although the evaluation of progress in regard to knowledge is a difficult task, nurses

can say with certainty and, perhaps, with pride that there have been incredible improvements in educational preparation, in leadership and organization within the discipline, and in the ability to address the changing needs of the people who are the beneficiaries of nursing care. This element of continuity also needs to be examined from the standpoint of ideas about nursing. Nursing, in various forms, has existed, depending on how it is defined, since the beginning of time. Nursing also exists in a global context in spite of the variation that might exist from one setting to the next, even within general geographic regions. It is tempting sometimes to avoid defining nursing, or making clear statements about what nursing "is," because of this variation. However, there are some things that enable all of these disparate situations to be thought of as nursing. In spite of all the differences, there are some things that hold nursing together as a distinct type of knowledge and work; some essence persists across time and contexts and makes it proper to call these things nursing. Leaders and scholars in nursing have the obligation to be able to discuss nursing with others who may have different perceptions of nursing and to be able to articulate to others the nature of nursing and the incredible contributions to human health that can be made by those who are registered nurses.

NURSING AS A DISCIPLINE

In spite of the tremendous contributions of nurses to meeting the healthcare needs of individuals, groups, and populations, and in spite of the pervasiveness of nursing throughout much of history, it can be difficult to delineate clearly what constitutes nursing as a discipline. Problems articulating the nature of the knowledge base of nursing can give the impression that there is not a specific, unique, substance of knowledge or science that underlies the practice of nurses. Such claims might seem absurd to any nurse who has been carrying out acts of nursing for an entire career. While it should be self-evident that nurses cannot act without some base of knowledge—otherwise, their actions would be totally without reason—significant challenges have arisen as they have tried to articulate precisely what constitutes that knowledge base.

This desire to define the knowledge base of nursing has been enhanced by some authors who have argued that it is essential for nursing's continued viability to distinguish its knowledge base from that of other disciplines (Feldman, 1981; Smith & McCarthy, 2010; Visintainer, 1986). While such concerns are not voiced in nursing as frequently today as they were a few decades ago, lingering questions persist about precisely what exemplifies nursing and what reflects or represents some other field of knowledge or inquiry.

To respond to these concerns, unique languages have been created in the form of nursing diagnoses and other taxonomies; research has been conducted rather extensively on intuition and critical thinking, two modes of thinking that are often thought to play a prominent role in nursing. Nurses have focused on the art of nursing and the realm of aesthetics as means other than science to capture the essence of nursing knowledge. These and more themes evident in the evolution of nursing science reflect the ongoing quest by nurse scholars to answer questions about the nature of nursing and, especially, the knowledge base or science that constitutes the discipline.

THE EDUCATION OF NURSES

As noted previously, concern has been expressed in nursing literature, especially during the period of the late 1960s through the late 1980s, about the apparent lack of a unique knowledge base for the discipline. At other times, critics noted a failure to articulate what makes up that unique knowledge. No doubt the history of the development of nursing supports concerns about the existence of a distinct, unique knowledge base in the discipline. Education for nurses has been referred to historically as *training*, a term that was particularly relevant during the apprentice-type model of early nursing preparation. In spite of Florence Nightingale's revolutionizing the preparation of nurses for her day, even well into the twentieth century a substantial portion of the preparation of nurses occurred through on-the-job apprenticeships.

Nurses educated as recently as the 1970s (and sometimes even more recently) may still refer to their preparation as training rather than as education. While these semantics might seem like a minor point, terminology can be quite powerful in terms of its capability to convey unintended messages as well as those desired by the speaker or writer. The term *education* carries a different connotation than does the term *training*; the latter is focused on the ability to perform certain actions, not on the knowledge and understanding that precede reasoned action. In addition to this distinction, the emphasis in early nursing training was placed on selecting the best candidates to be nurses based on personal characteristics that were presumed to be appropriate; the focus was not on the intellectual capacity or aptitude for gaining the knowledge needed to be an effective nurse. A review of conditions for nurse preparation in the early days of the discipline clearly reveals that fortitude and persistence were valued as characteristics essential to successful completion of these preparatory programs. At the same time, rules for nurses mandated subservient behaviors rather than critical thinking.

At the time that nurses began to receive formal education through actual involvement in classroom work and didactic presentations, much of the content of nursing programs was taught by physicians. Programs were associated with hospitals rather than colleges and universities, and the learning of the skills associated with nursing continued to occur primarily by actually doing the work of the nurse. Nursing was not associated closely with academic settings until 1909, when Richard Olding Beard successfully integrated the nursing program into the formal academic structure of the University of Minnesota. This program led to a 3-year diploma and was subsumed under the medical school, yet it was the first instance of nursing education as an official part of a university structure. Yale School of Nursing, which opened in 1924, was the first autonomous school of nursing with its own dean and budget (Kalisch & Kalisch, 1995).

Education at the graduate level developed slowly within the context of academic settings. Master's degrees were available in the early 1930s, yet by 1962 data revealed only 2,472 students pursued the master's degree in nursing; for the period 1961–1962, only 1,098 graduates were enrolled in master's degree programs (U.S. Public Health Service, 1963). Opportunities for doctoral-level education were severely limited in nursing, and nurses who wanted such preparation typically pursued their degrees in the discipline of education rather than nursing per se. The first programs that enabled nurses to pursue doctoral degrees were established in schools of education at Teacher's College, Columbia University, and at New York University, both developed in the 1920s and 1930s.

As nursing evolved as a discipline, recognition of the need for nurses with doctoral-level preparation as researchers grew, yet there was almost no opportunity to obtain such education within the discipline of nursing. In 1962, the U.S. Public Health Service began the Nurse Scientist Program to support advanced education to prepare nurses as researchers. Because of the absence of doctoral programs in the discipline of nursing, nurses who pursued their education as a part of this program had no choice but to receive their education in other fields. As a result, they typically were socialized into those other disciplines, bringing the perspective of physiologists, sociologists, and educators to bear on their ideas about nursing.

Nurses with doctoral preparation in nursing and increased nursing research activity are fairly recent developments. The first doctoral nursing program was established at the University of Pittsburgh in 1954 and was limited to maternal–child health, with a Doctor of Nursing Science (DNS) program being established at Boston University 6 years later in 1960 (Kalisch & Kalisch, 1995). Because many universities did not support doctoral-level preparation in nursing, doctoral programs often had to offer a distinct degree, typically the DNS or DNSc. Journals devoted to nursing research did not emerge until the 1950s, with an additional surge of activity in this area occurring in the 1970s. It is only within the last 30 years or so that a preponderance of people teaching in programs that lead to a doctoral degree in nursing also have had their own doctoral-level preparation in nursing.

Awareness of this historical development in nursing helps to explain the nature of research that has been done and, similarly, the development of the discipline over the last several decades. It is only within the last two or three decades that the individuals conducting research within the field of nursing were likely to have been educated with degrees in nursing and socialized primarily as researchers and scholars in nursing. As a result, there has been an increase in research conducted by nurse investigators with a viewpoint that has been derived from and has reflected a nursing perspective toward the problems addressed by the research.

This brief glimpse into a significant aspect of the history of nursing education makes it easy to see why concerns about borrowed knowledge have had a prominent role in the evolution of nursing as a discipline. This lack of clarity in regard to a unique knowledge base for nursing was compounded by prevailing ideas about the nature of disciplines. Prominent nurse scholars in the 1960s through the late 1970s brought to nursing ideas from education about the nature and structure of disciplines.

DELINEATING THE DISCIPLINE

Underlying all of this historical activity was a variety of theoretical thinking about knowledge in nursing, including nursing as a discipline, the role of theory in nursing, mechanisms for theory development, and, in more recent years, a broad interest in nursing science and its development. In the early stages, attention was focused on the delineation and development of nursing as a discipline, motivated to some extent by the need to demonstrate the unique aspects of nursing. Early efforts were focused particularly on knowledge development consistent with prevailing ideas about the way disciplines were structured. This focus on structure likely was a result of, at least in part, close connections between nursing and the discipline of education, and the structure of disciplines was an area of considerable theoretical interest and emphasis in education, particularly in the 1960s. The premise in the literature that promoted this focus in nursing was that the determination of the nature of nursing as a discipline, including its structure and boundaries, would provide direction for continuing development. Donaldson and Crowley (1978) pointed out the need for work on the discipline of nursing, indicating that such investigation would determine "the essence of nursing research and of the common elements and threads that give coherence to an identifiable body of knowledge" (p. 113).

Invoking ideas about borrowed versus unique knowledge, Donaldson and Crowley (1978) argued that much of the basis for nursing was "tacit rather than explicit" (p. 113), and they emphasized the need to ensure that nursing research was actually research in the discipline of nursing and not merely research that was conducted by nurses. Donaldson and Crowley described a *discipline* as "characterized by a unique perspective, a distinct way of viewing all phenomena, which ultimately defines the limits and nature of its inquiry" (p. 113). Developing nursing knowledge consistent with

this idea of disciplinary structure would make it possible to demonstrate what knowledge was unique to nursing in contrast to knowledge that might be considered borrowed. Donaldson and Crowley's (1978) work was seen as providing some important direction for continuing knowledge to develop what ultimately could be seen as a distinct discipline of nursing.

As part of their work, Donaldson and Crowley (1978) used an approach to disciplines based on the writings of Schwab (1962) to provide guidance for development of the discipline. Schwab (1962) and others who worked in the area of disciplinary structure (Shermis, 1962) argued that disciplines comprised two components: a *substantive structure* and a *syntax*. The content of the discipline constitutes the substantive structure; it includes concepts, theories, and other knowledge, principles, and ideas that make up the knowledge base of the discipline of nursing. Research to develop the discipline, therefore, should focus on content according to this idea of the disciplinary structure. The syntax includes the methods used in inquiry, as well as means to evaluate the value, credibility, or usefulness of inquiry done in the discipline. A general perspective, or worldview, provides the context for the substantive structure and the syntax to be brought together as characteristic of the particular discipline. Overall, these authors argued for the importance of delineating a distinct discipline of nursing, ensuring that the substance of the discipline served as a guide for practice, and establishing clear connections between research, the development of the discipline, and nursing practice.

It is worth noting that the approach to disciplinary structure that was advocated in nursing was that of the natural sciences. While this strategy may seem appropriate, it is important to consider how nursing might have developed differently if an idea relative to social sciences or humanities had been employed. This placement of nursing within the ranks of natural sciences became evident again when the philosophy of science known as *logical positivism* began to influence nursing knowledge development beginning in the 1970s, such that greater use of references in the area of natural, rather than social, sciences (although such works existed within philosophy of science) continues to be found throughout the nursing literature.

THE IDEA OF A "PROFESSIONAL" DISCIPLINE

The focus on disciplines occupied the nursing knowledge literature for some time, providing a framework for discussion of the uniqueness of nursing. This discussion encompassed topics such as the differences between basic and applied sciences, with nursing being held out as distinct from the basic sciences through its focus on application (Donaldson & Crowley, 1978; Johnson, 1959). The notion of applied science as a key aspect of nursing was captured sometimes through the references to nursing as a *professional discipline*. Professional or practice disciplines were thought to have specific characteristics that set them apart from those without a clear practice component. Thus professional disciplines, such as nursing, were viewed as different from the academic disciplines. A unique characteristic of the professional discipline is the delivery of service of some sort by those engaging in practice.

It is easy to argue that all disciplines have individuals who carry out the work of the discipline, who teach its substance, and who contribute to its ongoing development. Anyone who applies the knowledge of a discipline is engaging in practice related to that knowledge. The mere existence of people who engage in practice is not sufficient to differentiate a field from other disciplines whose members lack such a component. Nurses have used the argument that nursing is a "practice discipline" or a "professional discipline" to delineate nursing from other disciplines and to rationalize certain constraints or other challenges that set nursing apart from more traditional disciplines.

However, describing nursing as a practice discipline is misleading because all disciplines have individuals who apply the knowledge. Without such application, there would be no opportunity for testing, studying, enhancing, refining, or sharing the knowledge of the particular discipline. What is important in regard to nursing, however, is that there are social constraints, licensing requirements, and means of public oversight that create a special context for nursing. These aspects are critical to the development of nursing and do require important considerations about the process of knowledge development. These characteristics also translate into specific needs for the nursing knowledge base (Dickoff, James, & Wiedenbach, 1968a, 1968b). Merely referring to nursing as a practice discipline may not draw sufficient attention to these aspects that affect its development. In spite of these social and legal constraints, however, it may not be beneficial to the development of nursing to emphasize these differences. It is not self-evident that nursing as a discipline is sufficiently distinct from other disciplines in its organization and development, and a focus on similarities may bring greater progress to understanding and valuing nursing than a continuing emphasis on differences would. Indeed, failure to recognize the academic basis for nursing practice and the need for ongoing knowledge development may have contributed to the slow acceptance of nursing and valuing of nursing knowledge within university and healthcare settings.

The idea of a discipline having a unique substance, as advanced by scholars in nursing during the 1970s and 1980s, contributed to concerns mentioned previously about whether knowledge can be borrowed. This idea of borrowing knowledge from one discipline to the next does not hold up to further scrutiny. First, for something to be borrowed, it must belong to someone, yet it is not reasonable to think of knowledge as the possession of any one person or group of people. Researchers in the field of psychology may have created much of what is known about stress or behavior change, for example, yet it is clear that there are important connections to physiology, medicine, nursing, and sociology, in addition to other disciplines. Similarly, the members of other disciplines use, expand, critique, revise, and refine what is known on an ongoing basis, often with minimal regard for the origin of the knowledge.

There is some legitimate reason to be concerned about the perspectives that are represented in existing knowledge. To that end, nursing's holistic viewpoint and focus on relationships and contexts could be overlooked if nurses are not involved in the generation of that knowledge. Looked at another way, knowledge developed within other disciplines could fail to address the problems that nurses confront and that are important to their work with their populations of interest. Borrowing and the viability of the discipline of nursing are not the concerns here; rather, there is a legitimate concern that knowledge be generated that addresses the epistemic (knowledge-oriented) needs of nurses.

The idea of borrowed versus unique knowledge may not have much utility or support at this time, yet the need to pay attention to the knowledge base of nursing still has considerable merit. Nurses need to have an understanding of their discipline, particularly nurses who are in positions to help shape that knowledge. Nurses with DNP-level preparation will be in roles that enable them to have a significant influence over which knowledge development activities are pursued, and they should be engaged as members of research teams to ensure that the knowledge generated addresses areas of need. Because of the advanced practice focus of DNP education, DNP-prepared nurses are especially likely to have meaningful interaction with the public—the recipients of care—and, therefore, are in important positions to influence public perceptions of nursing. Understanding the current status of the discipline, and particularly the evolution of nursing to the present day, helps to create an understanding of the discipline that can be shared with others, can guide continuing research, and can shape the individual nurse's own perception of the role of nursing and the area of practice.

The brief mention of nursing history previously points to the continuing emergence of nursing as a discipline with a body of what can be called nursing knowledge. While there are occasional references to nursing as being in an early stage of development, particularly in reference to other disciplines, such a characterization does not do justice to the long history that exists, especially in connection with religious orders or the military, of people providing essential health services to those in need. Human beings have always needed individuals to whom they could turn for support with health and illness situations, whether that support has taken the form of the recommended cures of the day or more long-term care. To the extent that certain humans were identified as being particularly adept at providing such care, nursing has existed. As early as the time of the Crusades (the eleventh century CE), efforts were made to provide a means for placing the work of tending to ill individuals in the hands of those skilled at providing needed care. These early efforts served as a harbinger of nursing that would develop in a more formal sense in later centuries, making it clear that nursing care in some form has been available to people for an exceptionally long period of time. Although the nursing of centuries ago bears little resemblance to the nursing of modern times, it does support the idea that the practice of nursing is not new or embryonic—a characterization occasionally used to describe nursing's state of development. Contemporary nursing involves formal education with complex substantive content reflecting a variety of disciplines, yet integrated into an approach to health and illness situations that represents the special influence of nursing. Arriving at this point in nursing education and practice reflects centuries of ongoing development.

THE EMERGENCE OF NURSING SCIENCE

As emphasis on nursing as a discipline increased, there emerged a concomitant drive to develop what can be referred to as *nursing science*. This emphasis became the specific focus of theory development for nursing and was the primary consideration in the development of the discipline from the 1960s through the 1980s. This section and subsequent sections of this chapter describe the major traditions in epistemology that have influenced the development of theory and nursing science (see **Box 18-1**).

A review of nursing knowledge development over the latter half of the twentieth century shows the steady and profound influence of logical positivism. Logical positivism produced a lasting impact on nursing knowledge development, with one particularly strong example of its influence being extensive theory development activities demonstrated from the late 1960s and into the 1990s. Nurses who received their doctoral-level education in fields other than nursing were influenced by the dominance of this ideology at the time, a factor that helped to ensure its translation to a nursing context. Logical positivism, in fact, was pervasive throughout all of the sciences and has had a lasting impact on broad societal ideas about science and what constitutes appropriate or acceptable scientific activity. Logical positivism no longer occupies the forefront of philosophical thought about science; in fact, Webster, Jacox, and Baldwin (1981) declared it dead in the early 1980s. It is questionable, however, whether any philosophical movement ever dies completely, and there can be no doubt that the influence of logical positivism persists and has had a major role in shaping current ideas about science.

Logical positivism placed great emphasis on the demarcation of science from other forms of knowledge. Science was characterized as developing in a cumulative and linear fashion, with successive studies building on prior research. This process was oriented toward continuously refining and building theory in the quest for parsimonious statements that accurately corresponded with reality. Science, in essence, was seen as a theory-building activity, with the ideal theoretical statements being those that were capable of expression using the rules of logic and mathematics. Theory formed the core of scientific activity, and investigations represented an attempt to further develop, refine, or verify existing theory. With this emphasis on theory, it is easy to see how a discipline that lacked specific theoretical statements and clearly delineated bodies of theory might have been hindered in its efforts to gain recognition as a scientific discipline. If science was a theory-building activity, then nurse scholars suggested that there must be a theoretical foundation for nursing knowledge and practice for the discipline to be considered a science.

BOX 18-1   Epistemologies in Nursing Science Development

Logical positivism	Phenomenological	Feminist
Historicism	Philosophy	Epistemology
Postmodernism	Hermeneutics	

THE THEORY MOVEMENT IN NURSING

Nurse scholars and leaders devoted considerable effort to identifying the core or essence of nursing, to constructing theoretical formulations that would reflect this core, and to promoting further inquiry, as well as theory-based nursing practice. Federal funding was provided during the 1960s to support a series of conferences on theory development. The first conference was held at Case Western Reserve University in 1968; the second was held at the University of Colorado in 1969. Papers and discussion at these conferences clearly revealed the focus on the science of nursing and the influence of the philosophy of logical positivism on such activities during this time. The theoretical activity that took place under this influence amply illustrates the impact of logical positivism and this philosophical movement in the evolution of nursing as a discipline. Early nursing theory development activities, reflected in the work of Orlando (1961), Rogers (1970), Roy (1970, 1971), and others, served as important milestones in the effort to develop a theoretical basis for nursing.

Developing status as a science required not only the identification or development of theory for nursing but also the use of existing theory as a basis for research. Logical positivism, after all, required that scientific activity focus on development and further articulation of theory. Descriptive research—that is, inquiry intended to discover or document events or conditions—did not meet the criteria for science that were espoused by philosophers and the dominant thinking of the period. As a result of this emphasis, the literature of nursing during this time includes a number of articles and ongoing discussion about the necessary connection between theory, research, and practice, with Fawcett's "double helix" metaphor being a particularly poignant example of this focus (Fawcett, 1978, 1985). Writings related to the role of theory in science reflected the tenets of logical positivism; theory development was viewed as a very formal activity with a focus on axioms and propositions in the construction of theory. Reynolds's (1971) *A Primer in Theory Construction* is referenced frequently in the nursing literature of this era and shows the emphasis on the development of formal theory, the importance of concepts being defined in operational terms to show their means of empirical testing, and a focus on quantitative testing of hypotheses derived from the theories. Research with an emphasis on describing situations or phenomena was possibly of some value, but only to the extent that it provided baseline data for further theory development (Fawcett, 1978, p. 60).

Science that was developed according to the tenets of logical positivism represented what is sometimes referred to as *hard science*, yet nurse scholars and leaders in the area of knowledge development encountered considerable difficulty with this philosophy in that a significant amount of nursing was not amenable to this conception of science. In spite of the great strides that were made during this time in developing the scientific and theoretical foundations of nursing, some aspects of nursing just could not fit these specific criteria. Nursing had maintained a long history of being regarded as holistic, humanistic, and relational, with an emphasis on psychological and social aspects of health and wellness as much as physiological and biological aspects. Concepts such as dignity, empathy, presence, and caring could not be forced into the mold of logical positivism without tremendous difficulty and, as nurses readily recognized, without considerable disservice to those crucial aspects of the human condition.

The lack of fit between nursing and prevailing ideas about science left nurses with some difficult choices. One option was for nurses to strive to meet the criteria of science as defined by the logical positivist philosophers. This endeavor would, however, require forcing some elements of nursing knowledge to meet the requirements of the prevailing ideology. Needless to say, this option was akin to the "square peg and round hole" metaphor, and it is debatable whether some of the highly valued aspects of nursing could ever be recast in this fashion without significantly changing their nature.

As a second option, nurses could argue that some components of nursing fit the idea of science, maintaining the logical positivist idea of science, while acknowledging that other aspects did not fit this ideology. Those other aspects are referred to as art: The dogma of nursing as "an art and a science" (Rodgers, 1991) persists throughout the history of modern nursing thought.

As a third option, nurses could accept that the knowledge base of the discipline, in its totality, did not meet the requirements of logical positivism. Carper's (1975, 1978) widely cited work identifying patterns of knowing in nursing addressed some of these concerns, identifying the empirical knowing that is consistent with traditional ideas of science as only one of four types of knowing inherent in nursing. Personal knowing, aesthetic knowing, and ethics were the terms used to label other forms of knowing that she argued were essential in nursing. This schema went beyond the mere separation of knowledge into science and everything else (e.g., art) and emphasized the existence of numerous ways of knowing, all of which are essential to the work of nursing.

THE IMPORTANCE OF EVALUATING PHILOSOPHICAL IDEOLOGY

The fact that nurses largely failed to raise questions about the legitimacy of logical positivism as a useful and acceptable definition of science regardless of discipline is notable. The challenge for nurses should not have been viewed as only the determination of how to adopt and follow a particular line of activity or thought. In the case of logical positivism, nurses could have argued—as some did—that this philosophical approach just was not an acceptable or legitimate approach for nursing. In fact, there

are significant problems with this philosophy regardless of discipline, even for those that seem to be a more reasonable fit with this idea of traditional science.

Although logical positivism was not an appropriate view for the development of the discipline of nursing, looking only at whether this philosophy "fit" nursing (rather than evaluating its merits overall) has two strong detrimental effects. First, it sets nursing apart as different, and not necessarily in a good way, but in a way that indicates nursing cannot, or will not, conform to prevailing standards for science. Second, and particularly significant in the case of logical positivism, it fails to address the crucial question of the legitimacy of the philosophy. Without that challenge, a philosophical tradition can continue to be held as an ideal, and progress in disciplines can be evaluated relative to its major tenets regardless of whether a particular discipline accepts that view. Those who rejected logical positivism as a suitable guide for the development of nursing without assessing the philosophy's inherent value created a situation where nursing could easily be viewed as "different" or as a lesser science than others that appeared to follow prevailing standards. The situation that resulted from this rejection (perpetuated in the argument that nursing is an art and a science) is similar to criticisms that continue to be leveled against qualitative research; in other words, that it is "soft" and fails to meet the criteria of real science.

Trends and paradigm shifts are always occurring, and the critical questions asked by nurses cannot be limited to whether to follow along as viewpoints shift. The most important questions that need to be asked by nurses in regard to the knowledge base involve two things. First, is the latest ideology sound, not just for nursing, but for any discipline? Second, does it enable progress in nursing? In other words, is it an ideology that will help nurse scholars and researchers to make sound moves toward achieving the goals of the discipline? Applying such questions to logical positivism reveals quite quickly that the answer is *no* in regard to both aspects. Indeed, the shortcomings of logical positivism led to its demise as the dominant ideology of science by the mid-1900s.

The ideal put forth by the philosophers of this genre, however, continues to influence expectations and desires in the creation of science in nursing and elsewhere, ideals that persisted long after logical positivism lost its favored status. Science continues to be seen by society at large, as well as in many of the academic disciplines, as a special or unique form of knowledge with greater credibility than other forms of knowledge. Expectations for widespread generalizability of results, for statistical significance as the measure of meaningful results, for theory development as a focus of scientific activity, and for objectivity and a value-free orientation to inquiry continue to shape both the conduct of research and the needs of the public and others who will apply the results of scientific endeavors.

Webster and colleagues (1981) clearly pointed out the effects of "undue adherence to the positions and ideas of the received view" and noted how that perspective "stilted the development of nursing theories" (p. 34). *Truth*, as a criterion for evaluating theory, particularly in the form of correspondence with facts, presented other problems in the logical positivist viewpoint. The correspondence theory requires that phenomena be objectified—that is, measured in some way that is precise, repeatable, rigorous, and, as is evident in any research methods text, a valid measure of the phenomenon being studied. As a result, the phenomenon is believed to be captured successfully through the collection of empirical data.

Although this goal of precision and high validity certainly is an admirable one, it ignores elements of phenomena that can be the source of important information but that are not reducible to means of measurement. With this approach, grief, for example, could

be understood only as "grief as measured by a score on the grief instrument" because that is the only means for assigning numbers to grief to quantify and validate its existence. An individual's description of grief, including its emotional impact, its effect on daily life, and feelings that often are expressed by people using metaphors rather than checklists or Likert scales, could not be included under the heading of scientific.

It is easy to see how social or psychological phenomena are particularly troublesome to study from the perspective of logical positivism, because these phenomena have strong personal or what might be called subjective components. Physiological phenomena, however, are not immune to these difficulties either. Consider, for example, hypertension, measured as the pressure of the blood against vessel walls, or diabetes control, measured with glucose or $HgbA_{1c}$ levels. While these clearly are meaningful measures of these physical phenomena, they do not provide a broad or holistic perspective on how these conditions affect individuals with these diagnoses or what it is like to live with and try to maintain control of these physiological challenges. There are many challenges with the logical positivist philosophy of science. For purposes here, the significant point is to note the barriers to progress in the discipline of nursing that were confronted as a result of the rise in popularity of logical positivism and a staunch adherence to empirical ways of knowing, particularly within the context of a discipline that derives a significant amount of its identity from a holistic approach to human beings. These challenges also led to difficulties with the adoption of logical positivism in other disciplines. In spite of these barriers, however, logical positivism had a profound and lasting role on shaping views of science through the twentieth century and beyond. Specifically, the philosophy created expectations for science in both academic settings and society at large that continue to influence the evaluation of knowledge for its applicability and meaningfulness.

Before moving on to address the changes that have arisen since the logical positivist approach became prominent, it is appropriate to reiterate some important points. Methods and philosophy are linked inextricably: The choice of method that a nurse or any scientist takes in regard to knowledge development has strong philosophical underpinnings that need to be recognized as an inherent part of the science or knowledge development enterprise. These foundations are not always obvious, yet the philosophical position taken by a researcher can be determined by assessing the approach to inquiry that is taken. It also is possible to use similar strategies for inquiry in spite of different philosophical positions.

When a researcher measures some phenomenon, the researcher is indicating that it is possible and appropriate to measure the phenomenon of interest. Yet, one researcher using a quantitative instrument to measure a phenomenon may believe that those measurements reflect true and meaningful data, whereas another may believe that the results are meaningful, but only a piece of a complex human situation, and that the answer to the research question is just one of many possible answers. Logical positivism, for example, undoubtedly leads to a quantitative approach to science, but, conversely, not all quantitative science is necessarily based on logical positivism.

From a philosophical or disciplinary standpoint, it is important to look at assumptions about the nature of reality, truth, the goals and purpose of science, and the criteria that are used for differentiating good science as reflective of the philosophical viewpoint of the researcher or scientist. Those underpinnings are reflected in the methods used, but the methods essentially are tools, and they can be used with perspectives that have some perhaps subtle—but important—variations.

Failure to distinguish method from philosophical underpinnings can lead to wholesale rejection (or, conversely, blind adoption) of alternatives to knowledge development without appropriate thought being given to the choices that are being made. The responses of nurses to various trends as evidenced in the literature of nursing do not always capture this subtle yet important difference. Without that understanding, however, there is a tendency to abandon useful aspects of some approaches to knowledge development or to develop a bandwagon mentality when new trends emerge and either become popular or later are found to be insufficient to meet the needs of the discipline.

As noted earlier, the logical positivist approach to knowledge had significant limitations as a focus for the development of knowledge, especially within the narrower realm of scientific knowledge. As a philosophy of science, it not only presented challenges within the philosophy itself with regard to views of the nature of reality, truth, and the proper goal of science but was also created as a prescriptive view—in other words, a directive dictating how science should be done. In essence, logical positivism was not comprehensive in terms of how science actually was conducted. Prescriptive approaches can be of great value, of course; this point is clearly seen in health care where prescriptions for all sorts of things are intended to set people on a healthier and more productive path, just as a prescriptive view of science could have the same intention. This prescriptive focus likely added to the strength of its influence because it was put forth as a directive for how science should be carried out.

THE SEARCH FOR A NURSING PARADIGM

An obvious problem raised by this prescriptive focus was the fact that it ignored much of how science actually was carried out. An insider view of science would provide great insight into how science worked, not just on the level of particular methods but also in regard to the broader enterprise of science—an enterprise consisting not only of theories and ideas but also of scientists (the people who do the work of science) and the context in which their work takes place. Thomas Kuhn (1970, 1974) provided just such insight into the workings of science and the people who did that work. Because logical positivism was found to be lacking for nursing, Kuhn's views quickly gained the attention of nurses looking for a useful understanding of science.

One of the major shifts presented in Kuhn's writing was the change in the philosophy of science from a focus on product to a focus on process—in other words, the way in which science was done. Kuhn's view of science was organized around the idea that a central paradigm provided a focal point for activity in a discipline. The paradigm served as a disciplinary matrix and included the values and aims inherent in the major substantive content of the discipline. The work of scientists, according to Kuhn, was to articulate this paradigm. Progress, truth, and theory, among other aspects of science, were determined by viewing these developments from the perspective of the paradigm. This was a radically different approach to science than the view of the logical positivist, because it allowed judgments about science to be made relative to a viewpoint—in this case, the disciplinary matrix or paradigm—rather than in reference to an objective reality.

Although there were some limitations to this new perspective, nurses writing during this period gave a great deal of attention to Kuhn's views and argued for the relevance of this philosophical position for knowledge development in nursing. Kuhn's discussion of scientific revolutions and the term *paradigm*, derived from his work, became common features in discussions of nursing as a discipline and, especially, as a science. Writers in nursing during this period ultimately concluded that nursing had a *metaparadigm*, a broader worldview and conceptualization or important elements of the discipline, yet evidence of a paradigm as required by Kuhn was presented as

lacking (Hardy, 1983; Kim, 1989). Kim (1989) identified a number of distinct paradigms that were used in nursing but acknowledged the lack of a single overriding paradigm that would characterize nursing as a discipline in accordance with Kuhn's position.

Interestingly, while logical positivism experienced a relatively long life in nursing, Kuhn's view was quite short-lived in comparison. Nurse leaders and theorists during this time had become more familiar with philosophy and philosophical principles through their advanced education. As a result, there may have been a greater level of sophistication employed in evaluating ideology such as that presented by Kuhn. Limitations of Kuhn's view were quite obvious in nursing and perhaps contributed to acceptance of this tradition being less widespread, as well as shorter in duration in nursing. Although the term *paradigm* still has a prominent place in discussions about science, Kuhn's view overall was supplanted rather quickly by the views of other historicists and the rise of postmodernism, which followed shortly after the popularity of his work faded.

It is important to acknowledge the work of other historicist philosophers and the connection of such ideas to the development of nursing science. Larry Laudan was another noted philosopher of the late 1970s and a historicist whose work received some attention from nurse scholars. Laudan's (1977) philosophy was particularly noteworthy because he provided a view of science that addressed both conceptual and empirical problems in the conduct of science and the determination of progress. In general, Laudan focused on science as a problem-solving activity and assigned some weight to both conceptual and empirical work. Relatively few nurse authors (articles such as Fry [1995] and Tinkle & Beaton [1983] are good examples) described positions in support of Laudan's viewpoint and the practicality of his approach for nursing, and his work, like that of Kuhn, received far less attention than did the positions advocated by the logical positivists. Two significant aspects of the time could have contributed to this lack of attention. First, there was a continuing dominance of logical positivism and its influence on views of science even as historicist viewpoints were being articulated; this entrenched view would not be supplanted easily. Second, the philosophy of postmodernism emerged, developing particularly in the social sciences and then gradually spilling over into a number of other fields. Postmodernism served as a direct counterpoint to the rigidity of logical positivism, its emphasis on foundationalism, and its adherence to a belief in objective reality. This perspective represented quite a radical departure from both positivism and historicism, although it overlooked what might be considered the more moderate or intermediate position presented by historicist philosophers.

CONCEPTUAL PROBLEMS AND CONCEPT DEVELOPMENT

The potential contributions of historicism to nursing knowledge development are evident when reviewing the emphasis placed on concepts during the 1970s and 1980s. Although concepts and conceptual problems received attention during this time, the focus was not totally consistent with a historicist or postmodern perspective; in fact, discussion of concepts during this time had a strong positivist orientation. Concepts were valued primarily as elements of theory or, to use a popular phrase in nursing, as the "building blocks of theory," and not in a broader philosophical sense as ways to reflect, describe, and navigate through existence. Nonetheless, at least some attention was being paid to concepts, an occurrence that stands out in the history of the development of nursing science and points to the significance of concepts within the knowledge base.

Catherine Norris (1982) gave conceptual activity an important emphasis with the publication of a detailed book on concept clarification in nursing. Walker and Avant (1983, 1988) drew on the work of John Wilson (1969) to bring a method of concept analysis to nursing. This method remains popular in nursing and has been used in the analysis or clarification of a wide range of concepts. The text by Walker and Avant (1983, 1988) that addressed a method of concept analysis actually was focused on strategies for theory development in nursing, consistent with that common focus during the time of its initial publication. Content included analysis, synthesis, and derivation in the three categories of concepts, statements, and theories, all discussed as strategies for theory development. Perhaps as a remnant of logical positivism, or perhaps merely as recognition of the role of theory in science, work continued to be focused on theory development through much of the 1990s.

More recent work emphasizing concepts in nursing has been focused on developing useful concepts and resolving conceptual problems without being limited to theory development as the only relevant context for such work. Numerous philosophers addressed the role of concepts in cognition and, to a lesser extent, in science, yet their work has not received much of a reception in nursing. Rodgers (1989) constructed a view of concepts that emphasized concept development, not merely analysis, with analysis being a component of a broader process to generate meaningful and useful concepts. This work was informed by philosophers such as Laudan (1977), Toulmin (1972), Price (1953), and others and was oriented toward providing a solid foundation for conceptual work as part of the development of science and the discipline. Since that time, increased attention has been paid to concept development rather than merely to analysis, or to analysis as a strategy oriented more broadly to the development of useful and effective concepts (Rodgers, 2000a, 2000b; Rodgers & Knafl, 2000). In spite of this development, a great deal of conceptual work in nursing continues to follow the techniques described by Walker and Avant, being empirical in orientation and poorly linked to resolution of conceptual problems. Although sound philosophy and techniques for improving the conceptual base of nursing are readily available, this aspect of knowledge development is not well utilized in nursing. This is an unfortunate situation, because a number of the significant problems regarding nursing knowledge are conceptual in nature rather than empirical. Even for problems that are clinical in nature, clear and sound concepts are needed to ensure that empirical problems are articulated with clarity and relevant variables are understood, defined, and measured appropriately.

There is a need for additional work in concept development because many of the problems that are paramount in nursing are conceptual in nature and because methodological advances in concept development are not well integrated into nursing inquiry. In addition, concepts are important in delineating the identity and scope of the discipline. Consistent with the earlier effort to identify the essence of nursing, fundamental concepts were stipulated as constituting the core of nursing knowledge. Kim (1987), Flaskerud and Halloran (1980), and others identified nursing, person, health, and environment as the key concepts in nursing, with Flaskerud and Halloran referring to the centrality of these concepts as an important area of agreement in nursing. Other writings around this time were consistent with this focus, specifying that these concepts could provide a foundation for theory development in the discipline (Hardy, 1978; Johnson, 1968; Newman, 1972). As noted previously, although work conducted during the 1980s and 1990s reveals attention to the role of concepts in developing the knowledge base, a significant part of this effort, particularly in the early phases, was consistent with the positivist focus on theory development. More recently (Rodgers, 1989, 2000b), concepts have begun to take on a role as significant parts of knowledge outside of theory development. There is a continuing need for attention to concept development that goes beyond the basic level of analysis to modes of inquiry that result in better ways to conceptualize important phenomena in nursing (Rodgers, 2000a, 2000b). The analysis of concepts should not be seen as an endpoint to inquiry; instead, the results of any analysis should be tied to a continuing process of developing knowledge that addresses significant problems in the discipline.

THE POSTMODERN TURN

The historicist tradition (*historicism*) presented a stark contrast to the major tenets of logical positivism. Historicism provided an emphasis on problem solving as evidenced by the work of Laudan (1977), conceptual repertoires as discussed by Toulmin (1972), the notion of science as an enterprise with work conducted by people with their own values and perspectives, and a focus on science as a process rather than the product—all of which prompted questions about appropriate ways of doing and evaluating science. The historicist tradition offered substantial advantages over the rigid requirements placed on science by logical positivism. The potential contributions of historicist philosophy, however, received relatively scant attention in nursing. A review of the literature for nursing knowledge development and nursing science in the 1980s and 1990s reveals few works that address the work of historicist philosophers. This lack of attention likely is related to the development of yet another philosophical tradition, *postmodernism*, which garnered substantial attention in nursing shortly after the peak of historicism.

Postmodernism involves an emphasis on hermeneutics, narrative traditions and discourse, and philosophies of critical social theory and feminism. The emergence of this array of ideologies overshadowed discussions of historicism and quickly became a major focus of interest in nursing. Postmodernism, to many nurse authors at the time, seemed to closely approximate many of the values and purposes of nursing knowledge. This philosophical tradition was based on ideas of relativism, or viewpoints that truths existed on an individual level. This orientation was consistent with a longstanding emphasis in nursing on the whole person and the uniqueness of each individual. Nursing had developed around a focus on individualized care, and postmodernism was wholly consistent with that idea, not only allowing for but requiring recognition of uniqueness related to gender, culture, social status, and other characteristics inherent in the individual. Postmodernism also captured the idea that power differentials present in society are reflected in the healthcare system and interactions with care providers. In contrast to the idea that one single, central, fundamental overarching reality exists, with the purpose of science being to discover that reality, postmodernism was founded on uniqueness, diversity, power structures, and multiple realities as a result of human and social variation. This notion that there is not one single, central truth or story that is applicable to everyone is a defining feature of postmodernism and is referred to as the rejection of metanarrative, overarching narratives that are broadly generalizable.

Feminism, in particular, received a tremendous amount of attention, and it was not uncommon for authors to stipulate that feminism was a natural fit for nursing given that the majority of nurses were female. Feminism provided a clear example of postmodernism and was seen by many nurse leaders as exemplary of the postmodern emphasis on the uniqueness of each individual; the importance of individual realities with their gender, class, social, economic, and other influences; recognition of cultural relativism; and awareness of the role of power differentials in health care as in the rest of society. As a result, postmodernism garnered considerable attention as a good fit as a philosophical system for nursing knowledge development.

Postmodernism represented a radical departure from earlier philosophies dealing with

science and knowledge. As a result of its emergence, new modes of inquiry and new methodologies began to receive attention in nursing. The emphasis on individual beliefs, cultural and social contexts, multiple realities, power differentials, and so on required the development of methods that were able to capture these aspects of existence through research. With such significant philosophical differences, it was clear that traditional scientific principles could not be applied to the study of human beings given their individual and social contexts. At the very least, a pluralistic approach to inquiry would be necessary, balancing the supposedly objective and quantifiable facets with the more personal and individual aspects of human beings. A more extreme form of ideology at the time held that reduction and quantification could be rejected in their entirety and replaced with more holistic traditions of inquiry. Techniques for deconstruction could be applied to language, as well as images, and reveal power differentials and biases implicit in communication. Similarly, narrative or text, including the idea that action constitutes a text as described by Ricoeur (1981, 1984), provided a means to identify precepts, values, hidden meanings, and other contextual elements of experience. During this time there was an increasing emphasis on language and communication, with the development of narrative modes of inquiry that focused on individual story rather than attempts to uncover any form of truth.

Qualitative research began to emerge as a viable option for inquiry in nursing and in other disciplines. Philosophical methods such as phenomenology and hermeneutics had existed for an extended period of time, with hermeneutics having a particularly long history dating back to the early study of biblical texts. In spite of this extensive history, however, these philosophical methods had not been compatible with traditional ideas of science. Acceptance of qualitative research grew slowly and continues to meet resistance in some disciplines and by some researchers even in nursing. Nonetheless, the rise of postmodern philosophy opened the door for, and subsequently fueled rapid growth in, qualitative methodologies to develop knowledge for the discipline. In fact, the popularity of qualitative research grew so quickly that it appeared at times to be a sort of bandwagon, drawing significant attention and support simply because it offered such a stark contrast to the method supported by the quantitative methods of logical positivism. The quality of studies was variable, and there was evidence of some confusion regarding the various specific methods, resulting in awkward piecemeal combinations of different, and sometimes incompatible, methodological traditions. This blending of perspectives and methods was referred to as "method slurring" by Baker, Wuest, and Stern (1992). Over time, an increasing number of publications dealt with aspects of quality in qualitative research, and the initial excitement about qualitative methods gradually evolved to leave a variety of distinct, clear, and highly rigorous approaches for the conduct and the evaluation of such forms of inquiry.

Postmodernism led to the emergence of a particular form of qualitative inquiry referred to as *interpretive approaches*. These approaches focus on experiences as people live them with all their individual interpretations and reactions; consistent with this view is the idea that actions represent values, and an emphasis on the primacy of dialogue and language as means to share realities. As a result, actions, dialogue, and language provide a mechanism for the investigator to gain a greater understanding of those unique realities. Hermeneutical, phenomenological, narrative, and other interpretive approaches have been used to explore a variety of experiences of interest to nurses, including suffering (Steeves, Kahn, & Benoliel, 1990), race and attrition in nursing programs (Jordan, 1996), the care provider–patient relationship (Sundin, Jansson, & Norberg, 2002), and nurses in various roles such as nurse consultant (Walters, 1996).

The philosophy of postmodernism reflects another unique turn in ideas about the development of knowledge by raising significant questions about the presumption of objectivity in the conduct of science. In postmodernism, the separation of what is known from who is doing the knowing no longer exists; moreover, social elements not only have an effect on knowledge but also are viewed as an appropriate focus for inquiry. As noted previously, feminism and feminist epistemology gained considerable attention in relation to the growth of postmodernism. Postmodern philosophy makes it clear that social elements, such as class and gender, are important in regard to knowledge development and, in feminism, the specific emphasis is on gender.

Feminism exists in numerous forms, ranging from a moderate view that gender is important when looking at ways of interacting with the world to a more extreme version that holds gender to be the most important factor in interactions. In the extreme view, political action to counteract the dominant patriarchy is crucial to social progress (Harding, 1986, 1991). Some of the roots of feminism can be traced to historical events in which women were denied what are now considered to be basic social and civil rights.

Adding to this historical origin is a considerable body of research that was biased against women. Kohlberg's (1981) research on moral development, for example, was groundbreaking, but the stages of moral development that were identified, when used in research with female subjects, led to the conclusion that females functioned at a considerably lower level of moral development than their male counterparts did. Subsequent research using a different frame of reference, such as the work conducted by Carol Gilligan (1982), revealed the gender bias inherent in Kohlberg's work. The differences between male subjects and females in regard to development were argued by Gilligan to be not a matter of more or less of something, or one group being more developed than the other, but rather an altogether different way of approaching ethical problem solving. Gilligan's work was foundational in supporting the idea that females have a different frame of reference and a different way of working through ethical problems than males do. Such differences do not equate to higher or lower levels of moral development. Additional work in this area was carried out by Belenky, Clinchy, Goldberger, and Tarule (1986), who interviewed a group of 135 women; their study revealed that women interact with the world and have ways of knowing that appear to be substantially different from how men interact with and know the world.

The recognition of gender differences evident in research, along with the postmodern emphasis on individual realities rather than grand narratives, made it easy to see how feminism could be viewed as a philosophy with a good fit for nursing. In addition, a number of noted scholars in nursing recognized the consistency between a feminist view and the professional status of nurses. History is replete with references to nurses as the handmaidens of the physician, and it is likely that most nurses have heard stories of nurses giving up their chairs or handing over patient charts to the physician whenever he was present (and, of course, in early years, physicians were *he* rather than *she*, as the discipline of medicine demonstrated a similar bias against women). From a political standpoint, then, feminism was seen as offering some potential benefit to a predominantly female profession such as nursing.

Feminist ideology, however, often results in assigning a gender orientation to knowledge, labeling some approaches as distinctly feminine. This can create awkwardness in regard to thinking of knowledge claims as having a particular gender and presenting some views as superior to others based on a gender orientation. Rather than offering a means to overcome problems with bias that are presumed to be present in science, this approach sometimes seems only

to offer yet a different form of bias in knowledge development. Some authors have justified this development, arguing that the masculine, patriarchal orientation is so strong that it is necessary to promote an equally strong feminist orientation as a counterpoint to the male hegemony. Others see feminism as opening the door to more diversity in a broad scope of perspectives that can be considered. Chinn (1989) described nursing as emphasizing wholeness, with any singular perspective—masculine or feminine—being insufficient to accomplish this idea of wholeness in health. According to Chinn, nurses see the world through the lens of integration and wholeness. We cannot conceive of knowing sufficiently in any way nor can we rely on any one way of knowing that disregards another dimension of experience. We know we experience reality in a whole way.

It seems essential that myriad viewpoints be considered in the development of a view that meets the expectations of being holistic and values the uniqueness of individuals. As societies and cultures evolve, the viewpoints to be considered and included in knowledge development have evolved as well, a situation evident in the development of viewpoints based on voices of many unique groups including immigrants and gay, lesbian, and transgendered persons.

The relationship between nursing and feminism as a political movement has been a difficult one in many regards. Historically, men had positions of prominence in nursing because of the association of nursing with the military and with religious orders. In addition, women who in earlier times had worked to advance the professional status of nursing did not always see this work as connected to promoting the status of women in general. The American Nurses Association, for example, was not a supporter of women's right to vote in the early years of the organization. At the same time, as opportunities for women have expanded throughout recent history, there has been a tendency for women in traditionally female occupations to feel disenfranchised for choosing those occupations rather than new ones that have become available to them. The tensions surrounding nurses in relation to feminism as a political movement in nursing, therefore, emanated from both the feminist action side and the nursing professional side.

In spite of political tensions and debates regarding the merits of gender as a specific focus in knowledge development, feminism has had a significant role in the development of nursing knowledge. Leaders in this movement in nursing brought energy to workplace issues that affect both nursing practice and the nursing workforce. Awareness of bias in scientific research—particularly the historical exclusion of women from a large body of medical research—raised questions about the applicability and generalizability of scientific findings to the care of patients. Recognition of the role of gender and science and what Lather (1991) referred to as the failure of traditional science increased awareness of numerous factors in the development of nursing knowledge and the ways in which knowledge is applied in practice.

The postmodern movement, including feminism, led to considerable research in nursing dealing with cultural and unique individual factors and helped to illuminate on a much broader scale the spectrum of human health and illness as lived by real people in their natural social and cultural settings. Through developments consistent with this ideology, meaningful work has been used not only to understand but also to empower people in their interactions related to health and health care. Philosophies of the postmodern, critical social theory, and feminist traditions continue to evolve and stimulate new ideas for research methodology and criteria for evaluating the quality and range of application for research results.

Work remains, however, to explore ideas of postmodernism and the methodologies consistent with these ideas in a context of contemporary science. Prevailing notions of quality and what constitutes science still tend to be consistent with a positivist or logical positivist philosophy. To date, considerable effort has been devoted to articulating standards for evaluating the quality of inquiry in postmodern traditions (Guba & Lincoln, 1989; Hall & Stevens, 1991; Rolfe, 2006), and the rules associated with such work represent a vast departure from traditional notions of science. Reconciling these disparate viewpoints is important so that the merit of each viewpoint is appreciated and the potential usefulness understood. This is an area in which continuing work can develop a cohesive body of nursing knowledge and have that knowledge valued across an array of situations and contexts.

EMERGING TRENDS IN NURSING SCIENCE

The prior examination of developments and trends in the evolution of nursing science provides a glimpse into the progress made in the discipline and attempts to provide a solid foundation for nursing knowledge. Numerous approaches to knowledge relevant to nursing practice have been entertained within the discipline; some were taken as prescriptions for nursing thought, whereas others offered what was considered a closer fit with nursing as it currently exists. While the variety of philosophical approaches and methodologies appears appealing simply because of the diversity of perspectives offered, the plethora of philosophies also places some demands on the nurse in an advanced practice role.

One option for dealing with the myriad approaches that can be appealing to any nurse is to adopt a pluralistic view, or something similar to an *anything goes* attitude. Each era in nursing history has contributed to the development of the discipline of nursing through expansion and articulation of the knowledge base and, concomitantly, a stronger identity for nursing. In addition, each viewpoint has some merits, just as each has limitations. So, why not selectively apply pieces of these traditions, if not the whole tradition, when addressing a problem relevant to nursing? Noted Austrian philosopher Feyerabend (1975) specifically supported an approach allowing for maximum creativity and innovation in the process of knowledge development. Numerous authors in nursing have taken such a position as well, by suggesting that there should be a variety of methods and perspectives from which nurses can choose whatever is appropriate to guide their research or practice (Baker, Norton, Young, & Ward, 1998; Coward, 1990; Schultz, 1987).

Some important considerations must be addressed when adopting an approach such as pluralism, however. The primary issues are *philosophical congruency and incoherence* and *fit* with the values and ontological perspective of the discipline. Philosophical congruency and coherence are evident as concerns when looking at whether different perspectives in nursing are compatible with a philosophical basis. If nursing holds that the human being is holistic and cannot be viewed specifically in terms of parts, the viewpoints that are taken relative to knowledge development need to be consistent on that point. Given this example, positions based on the philosophy of logical positivism are incompatible with views based on postmodernism and critical social theory.

This example also points out the importance of ontological fit with nursing. In this case, the ontological view supports the position that human beings need to be considered on a holistic basis. The human being cannot be both holistic and reducible at the same time, and advocating this position would be inconsistent with nursing's expressed metaphysical position on the nature of the human being. Positions about truth, generalizability, the nature of reality, the nature of facts, the role of the investigator, and the role of ethics and values are fundamental considerations and intrinsic parts of the discipline. There is certainly a need for differing perspectives in the process of knowledge

development, but whatever approaches are taken need to be consistent with the espoused values and worldview held by the discipline at large.

Such a position does not preclude a variety of approaches to developing the knowledge base for nursing. The discipline will benefit most, however, if the use of a variety of means of knowledge development relevant to nursing is based on a consistent philosophical viewpoint that supports such diversity. The purpose of nursing knowledge is to support the work of nurses and provide information critical to both the delivery of effective care and the continuing development of the discipline. These real and practical aims provide an organizing viewpoint for continuing knowledge relevance. Capturing this need for applicable knowledge is the philosophy of *pragmatism* or, a more contemporary variation, *neopragmatism*. The discipline of nursing has paid relatively little attention to this philosophy, although a few articles can be found that have addressed this topic. For example, Rodgers (2005, 2007) advocated a problem-solving approach based on the philosophies of Laudan (1977) and Toulmin (1972) as a way to justify multiple approaches to knowledge development and nursing while still maintaining some consistency and identity for the discipline.

From a philosophical standpoint, a focus on problem solving pertains specifically to epistemic problems in the discipline. The advanced practice nurse with a practice-focused doctoral degree is the ideal person to facilitate this process. The advanced practice nurse has clinical expertise and practical experience that enables the nurse to detect problems that need to be addressed. The DNP-prepared nurse also has sufficient knowledge of processes of inquiry, as well as an understanding of the discipline of nursing, both of which help to ensure that attempts to expand the knowledge base are properly conducted and are relevant to the discipline.

Other developments in nursing have helped to bring some focus and direction to knowledge development in the discipline. During the

1980s and 1990s, a series of conferences was held in the northeastern United States, alternately sponsored by schools of nursing at the University of Rhode Island and Boston College. These conferences served as a vital forum for discussion of ideas about science and knowledge development relevant to the discipline of nursing. After this period of sharing and development, it became apparent to the conference organizers that the next appropriate step would be the development of a consensus statement reflecting crucial areas of agreement about nursing as a discipline. The purpose of the Knowledge Consensus Conference in Boston in 1998 was for the 40 participants "to discuss and synthesize various perspectives on knowledge development related to (1) the nature of the human person, (2) the nature of nursing, (3) the role of nursing theory, and (4) the links of each of these understandings to nursing practice" (*Consensus Statement on Emerging Nursing Knowledge*, 1999, p. 1). The document that resulted from this effort, the *Consensus Statement on Emerging Nursing Knowledge*, served as an important event in the history of contemporary nursing and reflected the values and knowledge that were thought by participants to be essential to the discipline, as well as the practice, of nursing.

The consensus statement was an attempt to move beyond repeated discussion of the nature of nursing and the knowledge base and provide a foundation for continuing focused development of the discipline. What this manifesto provided was a statement of agreed-upon values and perspectives that could provide some cohesiveness among nurses, a reminder of the lens through which nurses see the world and the recipients of their care. A variety of philosophical traditions, modes of inquiry, and research methods may be used to solve epistemic problems in nursing. Keeping in mind the key assumptions and values embedded in the discipline allows plurality in approaches to knowledge development while still supporting a sense of unity in the discipline and the knowledge

that underlies the work of nurses. The consensus statement was disseminated through a website, and there was an opportunity for sharing and continuing dialogue.

THE FUTURE OF NURSING KNOWLEDGE DEVELOPMENT

Predicting the future is an onerous—if not absurd—task. Current trends do lead to future developments, yet precisely how change occurs and which changes may take place along the way are difficult, if not impossible, to predict with accuracy. Preparing for the future in nursing science, then, is more a matter of perspective development than an anticipation of specific occurrences. The future of nursing knowledge development requires nurses to blend philosophical aspects with the emerging social trends and needs in the discipline. It also requires nurses with strong analytical skills to clearly identify problem areas where research is needed, promote awareness of trends within society, as well as within the discipline, and demonstrate the leadership and interpersonal skills to address the needs on all levels.

Along those lines, patterns that reveal potential significance for nursing involvement can be identified. Changes in philosophy, as well as in social context, call for new methods to address pressing issues in nursing. Recognition of the role of culture and social context require increasing development, application, and evaluation of methods effective at capturing those aspects of existence. These changes also require nurses who understand the philosophy and knowledge development enterprises well enough to be able to articulate the value of differing approaches to inquiry. Advanced practice nurses will provide a critical link in this process through their skill and understanding of both the knowledge development and scientific enterprises, as well as the realm of application in practice. Nursing science work without that critical link to practice is likely to fail in meeting the needs of nurses who apply that science on a daily basis. Nurses at levels different from advanced practice need leadership and guidance from advanced practice nurses to offer a few problems suitable for inquiry, as well as to help evaluate and apply new information for evidence-based practice.

Promoting continuing progress in nursing in regard to knowledge development also requires nurses who recognize that the future is something to be constructed as well as anticipated. Perhaps what the future of nursing knowledge development needs most is nurses who have a vision of what nursing can be and who have a commitment and desire to help create that idealized future. Advanced practice nurses will continue to be an essential part of the process of developing the discipline of nursing.

One area in need of increased attention in nursing is that of theory development. Theory often is poorly understood in nursing, with a common misperception being that theory is limited to the work of the grand theorists such as Orem, Johnson, and others. Exposure to theory in nursing programs unfortunately has perpetuated a gross misunderstanding about the role of theory in the knowledge base and in support of the practice of nursing. Ideas of theory need to be expanded beyond these broad narratives about nursing and also beyond the axiomatic and propositional constructions supported by the logical positivists. Theory is merely organized knowledge—knowledge that is connected and structured in such a way as to be slightly abstract, rather than case dependent, and potentially relevant to a variety of situations. Theories exist that can be immensely beneficial to nurses dealing with a wide array of topics commonly encountered in practice. Rather than reject theory development, a position taken by nurses at the 2013 Campaign for Action summit (Future of Nursing: Campaign for Action, 2013), nurses need to recognize the value of theory in regard to providing some organization of knowledge and to focus on theory that is meaningful and useful in practical application. Nurses also need

to recognize that knowledge changes. Just as the history of philosophical views about knowledge has changed over time, knowledge itself can and must change. Nurses need to develop skills that enable thoughtful critique of knowledge, characteristics of flexibility, a spirit of creativity, and a willingness to evaluate and embrace changes in knowledge. Along with this approach, particularly critical for nurses in leadership positions such as those with DNP degrees, nurses need to recognize the vital connection between the knowledge base and the discipline of nursing and look beyond immediate practice implications to promote changes in the discipline and perception of nursing among the public, other health professionals, and nurses. All activities, whether administrative, clinical, or research oriented, should be undertaken with an understanding of the essential connections among the discipline, the knowledge base, and the practice of nursing.

SUMMARY

In this chapter the nonlinear evolution of nursing science was explored in regard to philosophical traditions in epistemology and philosophy of science, specifically logical positivism, historicism, postmodernism, phenomenological philosophy, hermeneutics, and feminist epistemology. Events in the development of nursing as a discipline were examined in light of philosophical change. Emerging trends were presented along with suggestions for continuing development appropriate to the role of the DNP nurse.

DISCUSSION QUESTIONS ⎯⎯⎯⎯⎯

1. Discuss significant historical trends that have shaped the development of nursing knowledge.
2. Which trends in philosophy have influenced the development of nursing science?
3. Describe the role of the advanced practice nurse in the development of nursing science.

4. Given today's heathcare climate, how would you change nursing's value as a discipline and resources to promote knowledge development?

REFERENCES

Baker, C., Norton, S., Young, P., & Ward, S. (1998). An exploration of methodological pluralism in nursing research. *Research in Nursing and Health, 21,* 545–555.

Baker, C., Wuest, J., & Stern, P. N. (1992). Method slurring: The grounded theory/phenomenology example. *Journal of Advanced Nursing, 17,* 1355–1360.

Belenky, M. F., Clinchy, B. M., Goldberger, N. R., & Tarule, J. M. (1986). *Women's ways of knowing: The development of self, voice, and mind.* New York, NY: Basic Books.

Carper, B. A. (1975). *Fundamental patterns of knowing in nursing.* Doctoral dissertation, Teachers College, Columbia University, New York. University Microfilms Cat # 76-7772.

Carper, B. A. (1978). Fundamental patterns of knowing in nursing. *Advances in Nursing Science, 1*(1), 13–23.

Chinn, P. L. (1989). Nursing patterns of knowing and feminist thought. *Nursing and Health Care, 10,* 71–75.

Consensus statement on emerging nursing knowledge: A value-based position paper linking nursing knowledge and practice outcomes. (1999). Nursing Knowledge Consensus Conference, Boston, MA. Retrieved from http://www.bc.edu/bc_org/avp/son/theorist/roy.pdf

Coward, D. D. (1990). Critical multiplism: A research strategy for nursing science. *Image: Journal of Nursing Scholarship, 22,* 163–167.

Dickoff, J., James, P., & Wiedenbach, E. (1968a). Theory in a practice discipline: Part I. Practice-oriented theory. *Nursing Research, 17,* 415–435.

Dickoff, J., James, P., & Wiedenbach, E. (1968b). Theory in a practice discipline: Part II. Practice-oriented theory. *Nursing Research, 17,* 545–554.

Donaldson, S. K., & Crowley, D. M. (1978). The discipline of nursing. *Nursing Outlook, 26*(2), 113–120.

Fawcett, J. (1978). The relationship between theory and research: A double helix. *Advances in Nursing Science, 1*(1), 49–62.

Fawcett, J. (1985). Theory: Basis for the study and practice of nursing education. *Journal of Nursing Education, 24,* 226–229.

Feldman, H. R. (1981). A science of nursing: To be or not to be? *Image: Journal of Nursing Scholarship, 13,* 63–66.

Feyerabend, P. K. (1975). *Against method.* London, UK: Humanities Press.

Flaskerud, J. H., & Halloran, E. J. (1980). Areas of agreement in nursing theory development. *Advances in Nursing Science, 3*(1), 1–7.

Fry, S. T. (1995). Science as problem solving. In A. Omery, C. E. Kasper, & G. G. Page (Eds.), *In search of nursing science* (pp. 72–80). Thousand Oaks, CA: Sage.

Future of Nursing: Campaign for Action. (2013). Top actions we must stop doing. Retrieved from http://campaignforaction.org/resource/top-actions-we-must-stop-doing

Gilligan, C. (1982). *In a different voice: Psychological theory and women's development.* Cambridge, MA: Harvard University Press.

Guba, E. G., & Lincoln, Y. S. (1989). *Fourth generation evaluation.* Newbury Park, CA: Sage.

Hall, J. M., & Stevens, P. E. (1991). Rigor in feminist research. *Advances in Nursing Science, 13*(3), 16–29.

Harding, S. (1986). *The science question in feminism.* Ithaca, NY: Cornell University.

Harding, S. (1991). *Whose science? Whose knowledge?* Ithaca, NY: Cornell University.

Hardy, M. E. (1978). Perspectives on nursing theory. *Advances in Nursing Science, 1*(1), 27–48.

Hardy, M. (1983). Metaparadigms and theory development. In N. L. Chaska (Ed.), *The nursing profession: A time to speak* (pp. 427–437). New York, NY: McGraw-Hill.

Johnson, D. E. (1959). The nature of a science of nursing. *Nursing Outlook, 7,* 291–294.

Johnson, D. E. (1968). Theory in nursing: Borrowed and unique. *Nursing Research, 17,* 206–209.

Jordan, J. D. (1996). Rethinking race and attrition in nursing programs: A hermeneutic inquiry. *Journal of Professional Nursing, 12,* 382–390.

Kalisch, P. A., & Kalisch, B. J. (1995). *The advance of American nursing.* Philadelphia, PA: Lippincott.

Kim, H. S. (1987). Structuring the nursing knowledge system: A typology of four domains. *Scholarly Inquiry for Nursing Practice, 1,* 111–114.

Kim, H. S. (1989). Theoretical thinking in nursing: Problems and prospects. *Recent Advances in Nursing, 24,* 106–122.

Kohlberg, L. (1981). *Essays on moral development.* San Francisco, CA: Harper & Row.

Kuhn, T. S. (1970/1962). *The structure of scientific revolutions* (2nd ed.). Chicago, IL: University of Chicago.

Kuhn, T. S. (1974). Second thoughts on paradigms. In F. Suppe (Ed.), *The structure of scientific theories* (pp. 459–482). Urbana: University of Illinois.

Lather, P. (1991). *Getting smart: Feminist research and pedagogy with/in the postmodern*. New York, NY: Routledge.

Laudan, L. (1977). *Progress and its problems*. Berkeley: University of California Press.

Newman, M. A. (1972). Nursing's theoretical evolution. *Nursing Outlook, 20*, 449–453.

Norris, C. M. (1982). *Concept clarification in nursing*. Rockville, MD: Aspen.

Orlando, I. (1961). *The dynamic nurse–patient relationship*. New York, NY: G. P. Putnam's Sons.

Price, H. H. (1953). *Thinking and experience*. London, UK: Hutchinson House.

Reynolds, P. D. (1971). *A primer in theory construction*. New York, NY: Bobbs-Merrill.

Ricoeur, P. (1981). *Hermeneutics and the human sciences* (J. B. Thompson, Ed. & Trans.). Cambridge, UK: Cambridge University Press.

Ricoeur, P. (1984). *Time and narrative (2 vols.)*. (K. McLaughlin & D. Pellauer, Trans.). Chicago, IL: University of Chicago Press.

Rodgers, B. L. (1989). Concepts, analysis, and the development of knowledge: The evolutionary cycle. *Journal of Advanced Nursing, 14*, 330–335.

Rodgers, B. L. (1991). Deconstructing the dogma in nursing knowledge and practice. *Image: Journal of Nursing Scholarship, 23*, 177–181.

Rodgers, B. L. (2000a). Concept analysis: An evolutionary view. In B. L. Rodgers & K. A. Knafl (Eds.), *Concept development in nursing: Foundations, techniques, and applications* (pp. 77–102). Philadelphia, PA: Saunders.

Rodgers, B. L. (2000b). Philosophical foundations of concept development. In B. L. Rodgers & K. A. Knafl (Eds.), *Concept development in nursing: Foundations, techniques, and applications* (pp. 7–38). Philadelphia, PA: Saunders.

Rodgers, B. L. (2005). *Developing nursing knowledge: Philosophical traditions and influences*. Philadelphia, PA: Lippincott Williams & Wilkins.

Rodgers, B. L. (2007). Knowledge as problem solving. In C. Roy & D. A. Jones (Eds.), *Nursing knowledge development and clinical practice* (pp. 107–117). New York, NY: Springer.

Rodgers, B. L., & Knafl, K. A. (Eds.). (2000). *Concept development in nursing: Foundations, techniques, and applications*. Philadelphia, PA: Saunders.

Rogers, M. E. (1970). *An introduction to the theoretical basis of nursing*. Philadelphia, PA: F. A. Davis.

Rolfe, G. (2006). Judgments without rules: Towards a postmodern ironist concept of research validity. *Nursing Inquiry, 13*(1), 7–15.

Roy, C. (1970). Adaptation: A conceptual framework for nursing. *Nursing Outlook, 18*(3), 42–45.

Roy, C. (1971). Adaptation: A basis for nursing practice. *Nursing Outlook, 19*, 254–257.

Schultz, P. R. (1987). Toward holistic inquiry in nursing: A proposal for synthesis of patterns and methods. *Scholarly Inquiry for Nursing Practice: An International Journal, 1*, 135–146.

Schwab, J. (1962). The concept of the structure of a discipline. *Educational Record, 43*, 197–205.

Shermis, S. (1962). On becoming an intellectual discipline. *Phi Delta Kappan, 44*, 84–86.

Smith, M., & McCarthy, P. M. (2010). Disciplinary knowledge in nursing education: Going beyond the blueprints. *Nursing Outlook, 58*, 44–51.

Steeves, R. H., Kahn, D. L., & Benoliel, J. Q. (1990). Nurses' interpretation of the suffering of their patients. *Western Journal of Nursing Research, 12*, 715–729.

Sundin, K., Jansson, L., & Norberg, A. (2002). Understanding between care providers and patients with stroke and aphasia: A phenomenological hermeneutic inquiry. *Nursing Inquiry, 9*, 93–103.

Tinkle, M. B., & Beaton, J. L. (1983). Toward a new view of science: Implications for nursing research. *Advances in Nursing Science, 5*(2), 27–36.

Toulmin, S. (1972). *Human understanding*. Princeton, NJ: Princeton University Press.

U.S. Public Health Service. (1963). *Toward quality in nursing: Needs and goals*. Washington, DC: Government Printing Office.

Visintainer, M. A. (1986). The nature of knowledge and theory in nursing. *Image: Journal of Nursing Scholarship, 18*, 32–38.

Walker, L. O., & Avant, K. C. (1983). *Strategies for theory construction in nursing*. Norwalk, CT: Appleton & Lange.

Walker, L. O., & Avant, K. C. (1988). *Strategies for theory construction in nursing* (2nd ed.). Norwalk, CT: Appleton & Lange.

Walters, A. J. (1996). Being a clinical nurse consultant: A hermeneutic phenomenological reflection. *International Journal of Nursing Practice, 2*(1), 2–10.

Webster, G., Jacox, A., & Baldwin, B. (1981). Nursing theory and the ghost of the received view. In J. C. McCloskey & H. K. Grace (Eds.), *Current issues in nursing* (pp. 26–35). Boston, MA: Blackwell Scientific.

Wilson, J. (1969). *Thinking with concepts*. New York, NY: Cambridge University Press.

CHAPTER 19

Theory-Based Advanced Nursing Practice

Janet W. Kenney

CHAPTER OBJECTIVES

1. Describe the value and relevance of theory-based nursing for advanced practice nurses.

2. Discuss issues for applying theories in nursing practice.

3. Discuss the structure of nursing knowledge and the transformative process for theory-based practice.

4. Explain the relationship of theory and critical thinking.

5. Discuss the process for selecting and applying appropriate nursing, family, and other disciplines' models and theories to advanced nursing practice.

INTRODUCTION

All professional disciplines are based on their unique knowledge, which is expressed in models and theories that are applied in practice. The focus of nursing knowledge is on humans' health experiences within the context of their environment and the nurse–client relationship. Theory-based nursing practice is the application of various models, theories, and principles from nursing science and the biological, behavioral, medical, and sociocultural disciplines to clinical nursing practice. Conceptual models and theories provide a broad knowledge base to assist nurses in understanding and interpreting the client's complex health situation and in planning nursing actions to achieve desired client outcomes. "Explicit use of conceptual models of nursing and nursing theories to guide nursing practice is the hallmark of professional nursing"; it distinguishes nursing as an autonomous health profession (Fawcett, 1997, p. 212).

This chapter describes the value and relevance of theory-based nursing for advanced practice nurses and discusses some underlying concerns about applying theories in nursing practice. The structure of nursing knowledge and the transformative process for theory-based practice are explained, along with the importance of critical thinking. An overview of various models and theories of nursing, family, and other disciplines is provided. Finally, the process for selecting and applying appropriate models and theories in nursing practice is thoroughly described.

RELEVANCE OF THEORY-BASED PRACTICE IN NURSING

The value of theory-based nursing practice is well documented in numerous books and journal articles. Although many articles illustrate the application of a nursing model or theory to clients with a specific health problem, Alligood (1997b) reviewed the nursing literature and found that about 68% of the articles reflect a medical approach to nursing. She also noted that most nurses described their practice in terms of a specialty area, types of care or health problems, and nursing interventions.

All nurses use knowledge they acquired during their formal education and clinical experience to guide their practice. Some nurse practitioners consistently use models and theories to guide their practice, but most nurses are unaware of existing theories and models or do not know how to apply them. Many nurses are not aware of what knowledge they use or where they learned it; thus, their implicit knowledge tends to be fragmented, diffused, incomplete, and greatly influenced by the medical model (Fawcett, 1997). Although graduate nurse practitioner students learn about nursing models and theories, their education often emphasizes application of medical knowledge as the base for their nursing practice. Thus, the use of medical knowledge and policies of healthcare delivery systems has replaced nursing knowledge and influenced some nurses to become "junior doctors" instead of "senior nurses" (Meleis, 1993).

Theories and models from nursing and behavioral disciplines are used by advanced practice nurses to provide effective, high-quality nursing care. Many nurses believe that use of nursing theories would improve the quality of nursing care but that they do not have sufficient information about them or the opportunity to use them (McKenna, 1997b). According to Meleis (1997), theories improve quality of care by clearly defining the boundaries and goals of nursing assessment, diagnosis, and interventions and by providing continuity and congruency of care. Theory also contributes to more efficient and effective nursing practice and enhances nurses' professional autonomy and accountability. Aggleton and Chalmers (1986) claim that providing nursing care without a theory base is like "practicing in the dark." Kenney (1996) reported that professional nurses can effectively use theories and models from nursing and behavioral disciplines to:

- collect, organize, and classify client data
- understand, analyze, and interpret clients' health situations
- guide formulation of nursing diagnoses
- plan, implement, and evaluate nursing care
- explain nursing actions and interactions with clients
- describe, explain, and sometimes predict clients' responses
- demonstrate responsibility and accountability for nursing actions
- achieve desired outcomes for clients

The healthcare revolution requires that nurses demonstrate efficient, cost-effective, high-quality care within organized delivery systems. "Nursing theory–based practice offers an alternative to the dehumanizing, fragmented, and paternalistic approaches that plague current delivery systems" (Smith, 1994, p. 7). With changes in the current third-party reimbursement systems, nurses will be paid for effective theory-based practice that enhances clients' health and their quality of life. To accomplish this, nurse practitioners must use critical thinking skills combined with theory-based knowledge and clinical expertise to achieve desired client outcomes.

ISSUES RELATED TO THEORY-BASED NURSING PRACTICE

In recent years, the enthusiasm for using nursing models and theories in practice has waned due to criticisms about the theory–practice gap and the lack of relevance to clinical practice. Also, there are philosophical concerns about whether only nursing models should guide practice and whether models and theories of nursing and other disciplines may be integrated in practice. This section discusses some of these issues.

The theory–practice gap refers to the lack of use or inability of nurses to use nursing and other theories in clinical practice. McKenna (1997b) claims that theories are not being used in a systematic way to guide nursing practice, although using theories may improve the quality of care. He believes nurses do not use nursing theories because they do not know about them, understand them, believe in them, know how to apply them, or are not allowed to use them. Professional nursing practice more often reflects the medical or organizational model of care than the application of relevant nursing models or theories.

According to Rogers (1989, p. 114), "Nursing knowledge . . . is often seen as being unscientific, intuitive, and highly subjective." Some nurses believe that conceptual models and theories are too abstract to apply in nursing practice; they do not provide sufficient information to guide nursing judgments, are subject to different interpretations, are incomplete, and lack adequate testing and refinement (Field, 1987; Firlet, 1985). Others argue that some nursing theories were never meant to be directly applied in nursing practice but were intentionally abstract to stimulate thinking, provide new insights, and develop creative ways of viewing nursing (McKenna, 1997b).

As a practice discipline, nursing models and theories should be useful in practice, or their value is questionable. When models and theories are logical and consistent with other validated theories, they may provide the rationale and consequences of nursing actions and lead to predictable client outcomes. Numerous articles and chapters describe application of various models to clinical nursing practice. However, rigorous research studies on how nursing models and theories contribute to desirable nursing actions and client outcomes are lacking.

Another issue is whether only nursing models and theories are appropriate for the discipline, as nursing is an applied science. Most professional nurses are familiar with theories from other disciplines, such as systems theory, family theories, developmental theories, and others; in clinical practice, nurses often combine their nursing and medical knowledge with theories from other disciplines. Some nurse scholars argue that nursing practice must be based on nursing models and theories, as they are consistent with nursing's view of human science and provide the structure for explaining nursing's unique contribution to health care (Cody, 1996; Mitchell, 1992). Because nursing models or theories represent the theorist's unique beliefs about persons, health, and nursing and guide how nurses interact with clients, McKenna (1997b) believes that an eclectic approach, combining theories from nursing and other disciplines, may compromise nursing theories if the concepts are removed from their original context and interwoven with other theories.

In contrast, Meleis (1997) argues that because nurses study other disciplines, nursing theory tends to reflect a broad range of perspectives and premises. Many nursing theorists have incorporated or borrowed theories from other disciplines and then transmuted them to fit within the context of nursing so that their nursing theories comprise shared knowledge used in a distinctive way (Timpson, 1996).

A related issue is whether professional nurses should consistently use only one nursing model or use various models and theories from nursing and other disciplines in their practice. Most professions, like nursing, have multiple theories that represent divergent and unique perspectives about the phenomena of concern to their practice. Within nursing, conceptual models and theories range from broad conceptual models, or grand theories, to specific practice theories. There are advantages and disadvantages to using one or more theories in clinical practice. Depending on the nurse's knowledge and clinical practice area, some nursing models and theories may be more appropriate than others. However, some would argue that use of only one nursing theory limits the nurse's assessment to only those things addressed by the theory, and the nurse may be forced to fit the client situation to the theory.

Others believe that nurses should consider a variety of nursing theories and select the model or theory that best fits the client's health problems. A majority of early nursing theories were based on traditional scientific methods and reflect a reductionistic perspective of humans as passive beings, consisting of elementary parts that respond to external stimuli in a linear, causal, and predictive way (Benner & Wrubel, 1989). Nursing models based on this perspective ultimately dehumanize individuals into disparate parts and systems and lead to fragmented, nonholistic nursing care (Aggleton & Chalmers, 1986). More contemporary nursing models view humans as continuously changing during reciprocal interactions with their environment, thus individual reactions to nursing care are not predictable, nor can they be controlled. However, these newer nursing models are more abstract than earlier models and are less likely to offer specific guidelines for nursing actions. Professional nurses are expected to

develop unique, creative nursing actions suitable for each client's health problem and lifestyle, and theories from other disciplines may be integrated to complement and strengthen some limitations in both early and contemporary nursing models.

Cody (1996) contends that eclecticism, or selecting the best theory from other sources, is not necessarily wrong, but constantly borrowing theories from other disciplines does not contribute to the science of nursing or differentiate nursing from other professions. He believes that nursing practice ought to reflect a coherent, nursing theoretical base to guide practice in specific ways and contribute to the quality of care.

Because professional nurses provide health care for a variety of clients, each of whom is unique yet may have similar health concerns, nurses must use a broad knowledge base from nursing and other disciplines to select and apply relevant models and theories that are congruent with client situations. Health care, based on appropriate nursing models and theories, that integrates appropriate family, behavioral, and developmental theories, is most likely to achieve desired client health outcomes.

STRUCTURE OF NURSING KNOWLEDGE AND PERSPECTIVE TRANSFORMATION

Advanced practice nurses must first understand the structure of nursing knowledge and the process of transforming nursing models and theories into useful perspectives prior to implementing theory-based practice. Fawcett (1995) described the structural hierarchy of nursing knowledge or nursing science. Nursing's metaparadigm, which includes the major concepts of person, health, environment, and nursing, provides the foundation from which nursing philosophies, conceptual models, and theories are derived. Each nurse theorist developed unique definitions of major concepts, based on education, practice, and personal philosophy (values, beliefs, and assumptions) about humans, health, nursing, and environment. The theorist's philosophy also influenced the conceptual model, which describes how the concepts are linked; the model explains the relationships among client–health–nursing situations (Sorrentino, 1991). Conceptual nursing models are usually called "grand theories" because they are broad and abstract and may not provide specific directions for nursing actions. Some nurse theorists have developed midrange or practice theories from their models, which describe specific relationships among the concepts and suggest hypotheses to be tested.

According to Rogers (1989), an individual's personal meaning perspective or conceptual model provides a frame of reference or lens that influences how one perceives, thinks, and behaves in the world, yet most people are not aware of how their perspective influences and affects their view of themselves, others, and their world because underlying beliefs are held in the unconscious mind. In practice, nurses' perceptions, thoughts, feelings, and actions are guided by their personal framework or perspective of nursing, which provides a cognitive structure based on their assumptions, beliefs, and values about nursing (Fawcett, 1995). Many nurses unconsciously use a medical or institutional model as their perspective for organizing care. The prevalent values of such models or perspectives are efficiency, standardized care, rules, and regulations, such as "critical care pathways" (Rogers, 1989). As nurses become aware of the differences between the present and potential possibilities of nursing practice, they experience a cognitive dissonance or discomfort from an awareness of what is versus what could be (Rogers, 1989). Thus, only when nurses experience cognitive dissonance in practice will they change their frame of reference and use nursing models and theories.

For professional nurses to apply conceptual nursing models and theories, a dramatic change, or perspective transformation, must occur (Fawcett, 1995; Rogers, 1989). Perspective transformation is the process of moving from one frame of reference or perspective to another when unresolved dilemmas arise and create dissonance in one's current perspective (Mezirow, 1979). It is a process of critical reflection and analysis of other explanations or perspectives that might resolve the dilemma and explain or guide one's understanding and actions. The process involves gradually acquiring a new perspective that leads to fundamental changes in the way nurses experience, interpret, and understand their world and their relationships with others (Fawcett, 1995).

Fawcett (1995) describes nine phases leading to perspective transformation. Initially, the prevailing stability of the current nursing practice is disrupted when use of a nursing conceptual model or theory-based practice is introduced. Dissonance occurs as nurses consider their own perspective for practice and the challenge of changing to a new conceptual model or theory. Some nurses identify discrepancies between their current practice and how the new model or theory could affect their practice. Confusion may follow as nurses struggle to learn about the model or theory and how to apply it in practice. Nurses often feel anxious, angry, and unable to think during these phases and may grieve the loss of familiar perspectives of nursing. Their former perspective no longer seems useful, yet they have not internalized the new model or theory well enough to use it effectively. While dwelling with uncertainty, nurses acknowledge that their confusion is not due to personal inadequacy, and as their anxiety diminishes, they begin to critically examine former practice methods and explore the possibilities of implementing a new model or theory (Fawcett, 1995; Rogers, 1989).

With the discovery that a new model or theory is coherent and meaningful, synthesis occurs. As ways to apply the new model become clearer, new insights assist nurses to understand the usefulness of the conceptual model or theory in nursing practice (Fawcett, 1995). Resolution occurs as nurses become comfortable using the new model; they may feel a sense of empowerment and view their practice differently. Gradually, nurses consciously change their practice during reconceptualization; they shift from their former patterns to new ways of thinking and acting within the new model or theory. The final phase, return to stability, occurs when nursing practice is clearly based on the new nursing model or theory. Acceptance of a new perspective or paradigm, along with the corresponding assumptions, values, and beliefs, concludes the transformation process.

Models and theories from nursing and other disciplines provide the cognitive structures that guide professional nursing practice. This body of knowledge helps nurses explain what they know and the rationale for their nursing actions that facilitate the client's health (Fawcett, 1997). Theory-based nursing practice depends on the depth of nurses' knowledge of models and theories and their understanding about how to apply them in practice (Alligood, 1997a). Nursing models and theories represent ideal, logical, unique perspectives or maps of the person and health. They provide a structure and systematic approach to examine clients' situations, identify relevant information, interpret data for nursing diagnoses, and plan effective nursing care through critical thinking, reasoning, and decision making (Alligood, 1997a; Mayberry, 1991; Timpson, 1996).

Nurses must use critical thinking skills to apply models and theories to their clients' health concerns. Paul and Nosich's (1991) definition of critical thinking, which follows, is a commonly accepted one.

> Critical thinking is the intellectually disciplined process of actively and skillfully conceptualizing, applying, analyzing, synthesizing, or evaluating information gathered from, or generated by, observation, experience, reflection, reasoning, or communication, as a guide to belief and action. (p. 4)

According to Cradock (1996), it is not what they know that makes nurses advanced practitioners, but how they use what they know. They must make expert clinical decisions based on reflection, complex reasoning, and critical thinking to apply theoretically based knowledge to diverse client situations (Spiracino, 1991). Critical thinking incorporates ideas from both models and theories with clinical experience and provides the structure for unique, creative nursing practice with each client (Alligood, 1997a; Field, 1987; Mayberry, 1991; Sorrentino, 1991). Several nurse authors believe that nursing theories will become the stimuli for reflection and critical thinking, leading to realms for creative expressions in nursing practice (Chinn, 1997; Marks-Moran & Rose, 1997). Theory-based nursing and critical thinking are the foundations of advanced nursing practice (Mitchell, 1992). Specific critical thinking skills for each component of the nursing process are identified in **Table 19-1**.

MODELS AND THEORIES APPLICABLE IN ADVANCED NURSING PRACTICE

Theory-based nursing practice is the creative application of various models, theories, and principles from nursing, medical, behavioral, and humanistic sciences. Models and theories from relevant disciplines provide the knowledge base to understand various aspects of the client's health concerns and guide appropriate nursing management. In advanced nursing practice, the client may be an individual, families, or an aggregate, such as a community or special population. Knowledge of relevant models and theories from nursing and other disciplines enables the nurse to select those that best fit each client. This section provides a brief overview of some nursing, family, community, and other models and theories that may be relevant and useful to nurse practitioners.

TABLE 19-1	Application of Critical Thinking Skills to the Nursing Process

Components and Definitions	Critical Thinking Skills and Activities
Assessment An ongoing process of data collection to determine the client's strengths and health concerns	Collect relevant client data by observation, examination, interview and history, and reviewing the records Distinguish relevant data from irrelevant Distinguish important data from unimportant Validate data with others
Diagnosis The analysis/synthesis of data to identify patterns and compare with norms and models A clear, concise statement of the client's health status and concerns appropriate for nursing intervention	Organize and categorize data into patterns Identify data gaps Recognize patterns and relationships in data Compare patterns with norms and theories Examine own assumptions regarding client's situation Make inferences and judgments of client's health concerns Define the health concern and validate with the client and health team members Describe actual and potential concerns and the etiology of each diagnosis Propose alternative explanations of concerns
Planning Determination of how to assist the client in resolving concerns related to restoration, maintenance, or promotion of health	Identify priority of client's concerns Determine client's desired health outcomes Select appropriate nursing interventions by generalizing principles and theories Transfer knowledge from other sciences Design plan of care with scientific rationale
Implementation Carrying out the plan of care by the client and nurse	Apply knowledge to perform interventions Compare baseline data with changing status Test hypotheses of nursing interventions Update and revise the care plan Collaborate with health team members
Evaluation A systematic, continuous process of comparing the client's response with the desired health outcomes	Compare client's responses with desired health outcomes Use criterion-based tools to evaluate Determine the client's level of progress Revise the plan of care

Nursing Models and Theories

Numerous nursing models and theories have been reported in the literature since the 1950s. Some well-known nurse theorists' works are cited; readers are encouraged to seek other sources for more information about their models and theories. The early nurse theorists' conceptual models focused on individual clients and described nursing goals and activities. Peplau's interpersonal model described a goal-directed, nurse–client interpersonal process to promote the client's personality and living. Orlando's model explained a deliberative nursing approach to understand nurse–patient relationships and the communication process. Hall's core–care–cure model expanded and clarified nursing actions to promote clients' health. Levine's model identified four principles of human conservation to guide nursing activities.

More contemporary nursing theories have been published since 1970, when Rogers introduced her science of unitary man. She described mutually evolving relationships between humans and their environment that are expressed as changing energy fields, patterns, and organization. Orem's self-care model identified requisites for an individual's self-care and specific nursing systems to deliver care according to the client's self-care needs. King designed a systems model that included the individual, family, and society and then developed her theory of goal attainment, which described nurse–patient transactions to achieve the client's goals. Roy's adaptation model identified three types of stimuli that affect a patient's four modes of functioning. She described how the nurse identifies maladaptive behaviors and alters stimuli to enhance the client's adaptation. Paterson and Zderad developed a model of humanistic nursing. Leininger's transcultural nursing model explained differences between universal and cultural-specific views of health and healing, and how nurses can provide culturally congruent health care. According to Watson, nursing is the art and science of human care; nurses engage in transpersonal caring transactions to assist persons to achieve mind–body–soul harmony. Johnson's behavioral systems model focused on nurturing, protecting, and stimulating the individual's seven subsystems to maintain balance and stability. Neuman designed a complex healthcare systems model that identified different types of stressors and levels of defense; nursing actions were based on three levels of prevention. Parse developed a man–living–health theory in which nurses assist individuals to explore their past, present, and future life experiences and to illuminate possible lifestyle choices to enhance their health and lives. Newman's theory of health as expanding consciousness considers disease as part of health and explores time and rhythm pattern recognition with changes in life and health.

Family Models

Although most nursing models were originally designed to focus on individual clients, a few are applicable to families. King views the family as a social system or group of interacting individuals and family health as dynamic life experiences. Roy views the family as part of the client's immediate social environment, whereas Neuman's concept of family is harmonious relationships among family members. These nurse theorists focused on the individual client with the family seen as context. If the family is viewed as the client, the nurse must decide what the model should focus on—family development, interactions and stress, family systems, structure and function, or a combination of these models, such as the Calgary family model.

Family development models are based on the premise that the life cycle of families follows a common sequence of events from marriage through child rearing, retirement, and bereavement. Most are based on the typical nuclear two-parent family and emphasize the stages and adult's responsibilities to accomplish desired goals. Duvall's (1977) model is well known, and Stevenson (1977), a nurse theorist, also designed a family model.

Family interactional models view family members as a unit of interacting personalities within a dynamic life process. These models focus on how members' perceptions and interpretations of themselves and other family members determine their behaviors and actions. Also, these models consider how members' roles affect their interaction with others. Satir's family interaction model is an example. Family stress and coping models, based on the work of Lazarus and Folkman, were developed by Moos and Billings (1982) to identify how the family appraised the situation, dealt with their problems, and handled the resulting emotions. McCubbin and McCubbin (1993) designed the double ABCX model, which examines family life stressors and resources, along with changes that affect their adaptation to health problems and their ability to manage family crises. Curran's (1985) healthy family model identified characteristics of healthy families and common stressors affecting families.

Family systems models view the whole family as greater than and different from the sum of its parts or members. These models focus on the family with a hierarchy of subsystems (mother–father, parent–child) and supersystems in the community (social, occupational, recreational, and religious networks) that interact with the family system. Olson, Russell, and Sprenkle's (1983) model identifies 16 types of family systems based on the premise that a balance must be maintained in family cohesion, so that members do not become too enmeshed or too distant, and on adaptability, wherein too much change creates chaos and too little change leads to rigidity. Communication between family members is the third dimension. The Beavers system model (Beavers & Voeller, 1983) examines the structure, flexibility, and competence of a family and its members. Centripetal families enjoy close family relationships, while centrifugal families seek satisfaction outside the family.

Family structural–functional models view the family as a social system composed of nuclear and extended family members and their social-communicative interactions to achieve family functions. According to Friedman (1992), the structural components include family composition, values, communication patterns, members' roles, and the power structure. Functional components of this model include physical necessities and care; economic, affective, and reproductive behaviors; socialization and placement of family members; and family coping abilities. The structural and functional components are interrelated, and each part is affected by changes in other parts.

A model that combines many of the aforementioned models is the Calgary family model, developed by Wright and Leahey (1994). The major components include the internal and external family structure, similar to Friedman's (1992) model, along with family context, such as race, ethnicity, social class, religion, and environment. Family functions are viewed as instrumental or daily living activities and expressive activities, including communication (emotional, verbal, and behavioral), problem solving, roles, influences, beliefs, and alliances or coalitions. Family developmental stages and tasks, similar to Duvall's (1977), are also part of this comprehensive model.

Any family model may be combined with and complement a nursing model because nursing practice may involve individual clients or families. Nurses with knowledge of various family models are more likely to select the most appropriate and relevant one to meet the family's health concerns.

Community Models

Many community models are useful to nurses, but they differ according to whether community is considered a target population or aggregate or a geographic area. McKay and Segall (1983) described an aggregate model, in which the focus is on a group of individuals who share common characteristics but who may not interact with each other. Shamansky and Pesznecker (1981) identified three interdependent factors that constitute a geographical community: (1) persons who reside in an area; (2) space and time, which includes the community's history and environmental features; and (3) purpose factors that explain functional processes such as government policies, educational services, and forms of communication. The community-as-client model, designed by Anderson, McFarlane, and Helton (1986), combines both the aggregate and geographical community. It addresses the following eight subsystems of the aggregate in the community: physical environment, education, safety and transportation, politics and government, health and social services, communication, economics, and recreation. A community nursing process model was developed by Goeppinger, Lassiter, and Wilcox (1982). It examines the following eight processes in a community: commitment of members, awareness of others' views, articulation of community needs, effective communication within and among members, conflict containment and accommodation, participation in organizations, management of relations with the larger society, and mechanisms to facilitate participant interactions and decision making. Knowledge of several community models facilitates selection of the most appropriate one.

Other Useful Models and Theories

Nurses and theorists in other disciplines have developed many relevant models and theories that are useful in advanced nursing practice. Some of these models include Maslow's hierarchy of needs, Erikson's stages of development, Piaget's cognitive development of children, Pender's (1987) health promotion/disease prevention model, and Loveland-Cherry's (1989) family health promotion model. In addition, there are numerous theories of stress, crises, coping, grief, bereavement, death, and dying developed in psychology and behavioral disciplines. Nurses have transformed some of these

theories to encompass a health–illness context. Nurses who are cognizant of a variety of nursing, family, community, and behavioral models and theories are more likely to select the best-fitting model for their clients.

SELECTION OF RELEVANT MODELS AND THEORIES

This section provides an overview of several nurse scholars' criteria and guidelines for selecting models and theories. Meleis (1997) identified six criteria to guide selection of suitable models and theories for practice. McKenna (1997a) described seven selection criteria based on a review of the literature. Kim (1994) constructed a framework for practice theories with four dimensions to consider in selecting nursing models and theories. Fawcett and associates (1992) suggested that nurses consider three questions to determine the best fit between the client's health concerns and various models and theories. Relevant criteria from these scholars' work were integrated with the author's prior work to delineate five guidelines for selecting appropriate models and theories (Christensen & Kenney, 1996).

Meleis (1997) wrote that selecting models and theories for nursing practice is both a subjective and objective process. She identified the following six criteria for nurses to consider in the selection process:

1. Personal—the nurse's comfort with the theory and congruency with the nurse's own philosophical views of life
2. Mentor—the model or theory learned from a nurse mentor or educator
3. Theorist—the theorist's reputation in the discipline and degree of recognition
4. Literature support—the amount of literature available about the theory and the theory's significance for one's specialty
5. Sociopolitical congruency—the model or theory's acceptability within the nurse's workplace and whether major structural or practice changes are required

6. Utility—the ease with which nurses can understand and apply the model or theory in practice settings

McKenna (1997a) reviewed the literature and identified the following seven criteria for selecting models and theories:

1. The type of client: The client's needs should direct the choice because the theory provides guidelines to achieve the client's goals.
2. Healthcare setting: The type of clinical setting and nursing practice are contextual factors that affect selection of theories.
3. Parsimony/simplicity: Simple and realistic theories are more likely to be understood and applied in practice.
4. Understandability: Nurses must understand a theory if they expect to use it.
5. Origins of the theory: The credibility, prior use, and testing of the theory should also be considered.
6. Paradigms as a basis for choice: Nurses must decide between the totality or simultaneity paradigm, as each provides a different view of clients and nursing actions.
7. Personal values and beliefs: The theory must be congruent with the nurse's own views about humans, health, and nursing.

In her article on practice theories, Kim (1994) defined two dimensions of theories, which include four sets of practice theories relevant to selecting models and theories. One dimension is the target, which addresses both the philosophy of care for the person and the philosophy of therapy for the client's problems. The other dimension is the nurse–agent, which includes two phases—deliberation and enactment. The four sets of practice theories serve to guide nurses in choosing theories that will (1) explain the patient's problems and ideas about therapy for the problems; (2) provide ideas about how the nurse should approach the patient, such as through communication,

caring, or empowerment; (3) explain how to make decisions about appropriate nursing actions for the patient; and (4) explain what happens during enactment of nursing actions. Kim proposed that a science of nursing practice could be developed from this framework.

Fawcett and associates (1992) identified questions to guide nurses' selection of appropriate theories and models. The nurse must understand the differences among various models and theories in nursing and other disciplines to answer these questions. The following three questions will help the nurse identify the most appropriate model:

1. Does the theory or model address the client's problems and health concerns?
2. Are the nursing interventions suggested by the model consistent with the client's expectations for nursing care?
3. Are the goals of nursing actions, based on the model or theory, congruent with the client's desired health outcomes?

These questions help nurses decide which models and theories will assist them to organize the data into patterns, identify other health concerns, and determine congruency of the client's and nurse's view of nursing and health.

The first step toward theory-based nursing practice is the conscious decision to use theories in practice (Fawcett, 1997). The second step is recognizing that use of conceptual nursing models and theories requires a major change in how the nurse thinks about and interacts with clients to alleviate their health concerns. This change, referred to earlier as a perspective transformation, occurs gradually as the nurse discards one framework of practice and learns another perspective. Adopting and applying new models and theories in practice depends on nurses having knowledge of various models and theories and understanding how these models and theories relate to each other (Alligood, 1997a).

GUIDELINES FOR SELECTING MODELS AND THEORIES FOR NURSING PRACTICE

After deciding to implement theory-based nursing practice, the author believes that each nurse must engage in the five steps described here:

1. Consider personal values and beliefs about nursing, clients, health, and environment. Each nurse has a personal frame of reference or perspective of nursing practice, based on his or her conscious or unconscious assumptions, beliefs, and values about nursing. One's perspective of nursing provides a cognitive structure that guides one's perceptions, thoughts, feelings, and nursing actions (Fawcett, 1995). Clarifying one's values and beliefs about clients, health, and nursing practice is necessary before a perspective transformation can occur.

2. Examine the underlying assumptions, values, and beliefs of various nursing models and how the major concepts are defined. After clarifying values and beliefs, the nurse examines the definitions of major concepts in various models and theories to determine whether they are congruent with his or her beliefs (Alligood, 1997a). Nursing models and theories are based on different values and beliefs about the nature of the client's behaviors and abilities, what health and environment are, and what nursing actions facilitate clients' health. Each nursing model and theory provides a unique view for specific nursing practice. Some nursing models reflect a totality paradigm and view humans as having separate biological, social, psychological, and spiritual parts that respond to environmental stimuli or change, and the nurse's role is to facilitate adaptation or equilibrium to maintain health. Other nursing models reflect a simultaneity paradigm and propose that humans are intelligent beings, capable of making informed decisions about their lives, and that they continuously engage in a dynamic, mutual interaction with their environment. In this paradigm, the nurse's role is to guide clients in choosing lifestyles and therapies that are acceptable to them and facilitate their growth and life–health process.

3. Identify several models that are congruent with one's own values and beliefs about nursing, clients, and health. Each nurse must consider whether the theorist's underlying values are congruent with his or her personal values and beliefs about clients, health, and nursing because the theorist's values guide the nurse's critical thinking and reasoning processes (Alligood, 1997a). Models and theories reflect the theorist's views about people and nursing. They directly affect how nurses approach their clients, what information they gather, how that information is processed, what nursing activities are appropriate, and what client outcomes are expected based on the model. For example, some traditional nursing models define the person as a biopsychosocial being who responds to environmental stimuli, and health results from nursing actions that lead to predictable changes. These models would be incongruent with the values and beliefs of contemporary nurses who believe that people are free agents, dynamically interacting with their environment as a whole and capable of making rational decisions, and that the nurse's role is to assist clients to explore various options and choose ones that are acceptable with their values and lifestyle.

4. Identify the similarities and differences in client focus, nursing actions, and client outcomes of these models. Nursing models and theories consist of concepts with specific definitions and statements that describe how the concepts are interrelated. Some propose specific nursing actions and expected client outcomes. The major concepts guide what data are collected during the assessment and how the data are organized to identify and

interpret biobehavioral patterns and determine nursing diagnoses. Nursing models also guide development of the nursing care plans and designate desired outcomes to evaluate. By comparing various models, nurses recognize which ones are congruent with their values and beliefs about nursing and offer the best fit with the client's health concerns.

5. Practice applying the models and theories to clients with different health concerns to determine which ones best fit specific situations and guide nursing actions that will achieve desired client outcomes. The nurse explores specific models in depth and may analyze their usefulness before implementing them. By comparing several models and examining the attributes of the client, the focus of nursing actions, and the proposed outcomes, the nurse will acquire a more in-depth understanding of different models. Each nursing model describes different areas for assessment, unique nursing diagnoses, and specific nursing interventions to assist the client toward health. The nurse must decide which models and theories are most appropriate for each client. Which one offers the best fit for the client's health concerns? Selecting appropriate models and theories for each unique client health situation requires nurses to use their broad knowledge base from various disciplines, critical thinking skills, clinical expertise, and intuition to identify the best fit between the client's health concerns and nursing models (Fawcett et al., 1992).

APPLICATION OF THEORY-BASED NURSING PRACTICE

The choice of theories and models suitable to the client's health concerns occurs during the initial data assessment process. The initial data focus on the client's primary expressed concerns and how they are related to or affect the client's lifestyle and patterns of living. These data assist the nurse in identifying and understanding the client's common and unique patterns. The client's view of health, along with past and present lived experiences and future lifestyle and health concerns, is also considered. Using this information, the nurse considers various models and theories from nursing and other disciplines that are relevant to the client's unique health concerns and congruent with the nurse's own beliefs. Then, the nurse selects those models and other theories that best fit the client's situation and health concerns and will systematically direct nursing practice.

The major concepts of the chosen models and theories guide each component of the nursing process, as shown in **Table 19-2**. The concepts serve as categories to guide additional data collection. They suggest, either directly or indirectly, what information is relevant and should be collected. The models and theories assist the nurse to organize, categorize, and interpret pertinent data that illustrate the client's biobehavioral patterns and identify appropriate nursing diagnoses that are linked to relevant etiological factors.

Nursing and other models and theories guide development of a care plan by suggesting appropriate types of nursing interventions and specific nursing actions. Desired client outcomes are derived from the models and theories and define what changes in the client should be evaluated. For example, if Roy's model is chosen, data about the client's physiological needs, self-concept, role mastery, and interdependence, along with related stimuli, would be collected and used to identify adaptive and maladaptive behavioral patterns. The nurse who uses Orem's self-care model would assess and judge clients' ability to meet their universal and developmental self-care requisites and whether they had any health deviations. From analysis of these data, the nurse would diagnose self-care deficits and determine appropriate nursing plans for partial, compensatory, or health education nursing care. Nursing care plans are

TABLE 19-2 Theory-Based Nursing Practice

Component	Nursing Process Use	Nursing Model Use
Assessment	Describes how to collect data	Guides what data to collect
Diagnosis	Describes how to process data	Guides organizing, categorizing, and interpreting data
	Provides format for nursing diagnosis	Provides concepts for nursing diagnosis
	Describes *how* to plan	Guides *what* to plan
	Facilitates development of care plan unique to client	Designates appropriate types of nursing interventions
Implementation	Describes phases of implementation	Directs model-specific nursing actions
Evaluation	Identifies *how* to evaluate	Guides *what* to evaluate
General	Requires accountability through use of systematic approach to nursing practice	Enhances accountability of theory-based practice
	Process enhances continuity of care	Provides a comprehensive, coherent approach to care of client

based on the model and describe the client's desired outcomes, along with nursing actions to achieve the client's outcomes. Nurses who use Johnson's behavioral systems model would consider ways to nurture, protect, or stimulate the client to facilitate health, whereas the Neuman's healthcare systems model assists the nurse to explore ways to reduce stressors within the three levels of disease prevention.

Some nurses believe that family models complement nursing models and provide a more holistic and comprehensive perspective of clients and their health concerns. Selection of a family model occurs after the nurse gathers preliminary data about the family and identifies its unique and common patterns. Then the nurse decides whether the family as context or family as client would be more appropriate and best fit the client's situation. Also, the nurse's perception and definition of family and health guide the selection of a family model. For example, a pediatric nurse who works in an

outpatient clinic may choose Orem's self-care model to guide care of a 9-year-old child with an ear infection and the mother's treatment of the child. Friedman's family system model may complement Orem's model and enhance understanding of the family's structure and functions. The nurse may also use Erikson's developmental framework to help the mother recognize and encourage her child's normal developmental behaviors. Pain management theories may also be applied to reduce the child's earache.

This example illustrates how nurses examine and judge the value of various models and theories and select those that are most congruent and useful and best fit the client's health concerns and the nurse's perspective of practice. Gradually, nurse practitioners develop an expertise in selecting theories and models that are appropriate and relevant to their client's health concerns and congruent with their own views of advanced practice.

CONCLUSION

This chapter described the importance and value of applying models and theories from nursing and other disciplines in advanced nursing practice. Issues related to the nursing theory–practice gap were discussed, along with concerns about using only one nursing model in practice and about integrating models and theories from other disciplines with nursing models and theories. The structure of nursing knowledge was explained, as was the need for a perspective transformation to occur prior to implementing theory-based nursing practice. Critical thinking, logical reasoning, and creative application of nursing models and theories were emphasized. Different types of nursing, family, community, and other models and theories were discussed. Finally, the process of selecting and applying models and theories was thoroughly described.

In the last few decades, the emergence of nursing models and theories has illuminated several nursing paradigms and explicated their underlying assumptions, beliefs, and values that guide nursing practice. The science of nursing and empirical patterns of knowing are represented by these nursing models and their theories. Application of models and theories from nursing and other disciplines depends on nurses having a broad knowledge base and understanding how models and theories are interrelated. Empowerment of nurses through perspective transformation and the use of nursing models and theories is essential. Nursing models and theories provide the framework for critical thinking within the context of nursing and guide the reasoning that professional nurses need to survive in an era of cost containment and evidence-based practice. Use of models and theories from nursing and related health disciplines enables nurses to demonstrate accountability for their decisions and actions through scientific explanation and provides a coherent approach to theory-based nursing practice.

DISCUSSION QUESTIONS

1. List the reasons to apply nursing, family, and other theories to advanced practice. What are some underlying concerns about applying theories in nursing practice?

2. Based on the review in this chapter of nursing, family, and other disciplines' theories, choose at least one theory to investigate further. Use the five guidelines for selecting models and theories for nursing practice and evaluate the theory's applicability for your current practice. Was the theory applicable or do you need to search for a different one?

3. How does the structure of nursing knowledge relate to nursing's metaparadigms?

4. How can applying theory to practice enhance one's critical thinking skills?

5. What is the process and what are the pitfalls of the process for selecting and applying appropriate nursing, family, and other disciplines' models and theories to advanced nursing practice?

REFERENCES

Aggleton, P. J., & Chalmers, H. (1986). *Nursing models and the nursing process*. Basingstoke, UK: Macmillan.

Alligood, M. R. (1997a). Models and theories: Critical thinking structures. In M. R. Alligood & A. Marriner-Tomey (Eds.), *Nursing theory: Utilization and application* (pp. 31–45). St. Louis, MO: Mosby.

Alligood, M. R. (1997b). Models and theories in nursing practice. In M. R. Alligood & A. Marriner-Tomey (Eds.), *Nursing theory: Utilization and application* (pp. 15–30). St. Louis, MO: Mosby.

Anderson, E. T., McFarlane, J. M., & Helton, A. (1986). Community as client: A model for practice. *Nursing Outlook, 3*(5), 220.

Beavers, W. R., & Voeller, M. N. (1983). Family models: Comparing and contrasting the Olson circumplex model with the Beavers systems model. *Family Process, 22*, 85–98.

Benner, P., & Wrubel, J. (1989). *The primacy of caring.* Menlo Park, CA: Addison-Wesley.

Chinn, P. L. (1997). Why middle-range theory? *Advances in Nursing Science, 19*(3), viii.

Christensen, P. J., & Kenney, J. W. (1996). *Nursing process: Application of conceptual models* (4th ed.). St. Louis, MO: Mosby.

Cody, W. K. (1996). Drowning in eclecticism. *Nursing Science Quarterly, 9*(3), 86–88.

Cradock, S. (1996). The expert nurse: Clinical specialist or advanced practitioner? In G. Rolfe (Ed.), *Closing the theory–practice gap: A new paradigm for nursing.* Oxford, UK: Butterworth-Heinemann.

Curran, D. (1985). *Stress and the healthy family.* Minneapolis, MN: Winston Press.

Duvall, E. M. (1977). *Marriage and family development* (5th ed.). Philadelphia, PA: Lippincott.

Fawcett, J. (1995). Implementing conceptual models in nursing practice. In J. Fawcett (Ed.), *Analysis and evaluation of conceptual models of nursing* (3rd ed.). Philadelphia, PA: F. A. Davis.

Fawcett, J. (1997). Conceptual models of nursing, nursing theories, and nursing practice: Focus on the future. In M. R. Alligood & A. Marriner-Tomey (Eds.), *Nursing theory: Utilization and application* (pp. 211–221). St. Louis, MO: Mosby.

Fawcett, J., Archer, C. L., Becker, D., Brown, K. K., Gann, S., Wong, M. J., & Wurster, A. B. (1992). Guidelines for selecting a conceptual model of nursing: Focus on the individual patient. *Dimensions of Critical Care Nursing, 11*(5), 268–277.

Field, P. A. (1987). The impact of nursing theory on the clinical decision making process. *Journal of Advanced Nursing, 12,* 563–571.

Firlet, S. I. (1985). Nursing theory and nursing practice: Separate or linked? In J. McCloskey & H. K. Grace (Eds.), *Current issues in nursing* (pp. 6–19). Boston, MA: Blackwell Scientific.

Friedman, M. M. (1992). *Family nursing: Theory and practice* (3rd ed.). New York, NY: Appleton & Lange.

Goeppinger, J., Lassiter, P. G., & Wilcox, B. (1982). Community health is community competence. *Nursing Outlook, 30*(8), 464.

Kenney, J. W. (1996). Relevance of theory-based nursing practice. In P. J. Christensen & J. W. Kenney (Eds.), *Nursing process: Application of conceptual models* (4th ed., pp. 1–23). St. Louis, MO: Mosby.

Kim, H. S. (1994). Practice theories in nursing and a science of nursing practice. *Scholarly Inquiry for Nursing Practice: An International Journal, 8*(2), 145–158.

Loveland-Cherry, C. J. (1989). Family health promotion and health protection. In P. Bomar (Ed.), *Nurses and family health promotion: Concepts, assessment, and interventions.* Baltimore, MD: Williams & Wilkins.

Marks-Moran, D., & Rose, P. (Eds.). (1997). *Reconstructing nursing: Beyond art and science.* Philadelphia, PA: Bailliere Tindall.

Mayberry, A. (1991). Merging nursing theories, models, and nursing practice: More than an administrative challenge. *Advances in Nursing Science, 15,* 44.

McCubbin, M. A., & McCubbin, H. I. (1993). Families coping with illness: The resiliency model of family stress, adjustment and adaptation. In C. B. Danielson, B. Hamel-Bissell, & P. Winstead-Fry (Eds.), *Families, health and illness: Perspectives on coping and intervention* (pp. 21–65). St. Louis, MO: Mosby.

McKay, R., & Segall, M. (1983). Methods and models for the aggregate. *Nursing Outlook, 31*(6), 328.

McKenna, H. (1997a). Choosing a theory for practice. In H. McKenna (Ed.), *Nursing theories and models* (pp. 127–157). New York, NY: Routledge.

McKenna, H. (1997b). Applying theories in practice. In H. McKenna (Ed.), *Nursing theories and models* (pp. 158–189). New York, NY: Routledge.

Meleis, A. I. (1993). Nursing research and the Neuman model: Directions for the future. Panel discussion conducted at the Fourth Biennial International Neuman Systems Model Symposium, Rochester, NY.

Meleis, A. I. (1997). *Theoretical nursing: Development and progress* (3rd ed.). Philadelphia, PA: Lippincott.

Mezirow, J. (1979). Perspective transformation. *Adult Education, 28*(3), 100–110.

Mitchell, G. (1992). Specifying the knowledge base of theory in practice. *Nursing Science Quarterly, 5*(1), 6–7.

Moos, R. H., & Billings, A. G. (1982). Conceptualizing and measuring coping resources and processes. In L. Goldberger & S. Breznitz (Eds.), *Handbook of stress.* New York, NY: Free Press.

Olson, D. H., Russell, C. S., & Sprenkle, D. H. (1983). Circumplex models of marital and family systems: VI. Theoretical update. *Family Processes, 22,* 69–83.

Paul, R. W., & Nosich, G. M. (1991). *Proposal for the national assessment of higher-order thinking* (revised version). Washington, DC: U.S. Department of Education Office of Educational Research and Improvement, National Center for Education Statistics.

Pender, N. J. (1987). *Health promotion in nursing practice.* New York, NY: Doubleday.

Rogers, M. E. (1989). Creating a climate for the implementation of a nursing conceptual framework. *Journal of Continuing Education in Nursing, 20*(3), 112–116.

Shamansky, S. L., & Pesznecker, B. (1981). A community is . . . *Nursing Outlook, 29*(3), 182–185.

Smith, M. C. (1994). Beyond the threshold: Nursing practice in the next millennium. *Nursing Science Quarterly, 7*(1), 6–7.

Sorrentino, E. A. (1991). Making theories work for you. *Nursing Administration Quarterly, 15*(3), 54–59.

Spiracino, P. (1991). The reciprocal relationship between practice and theory. *Clinical Nurse Specialist, 5*(3), 138.

Stevenson, J. (1977). *Issues and crises during middlescence.* New York, NY: Appleton-Century-Crofts.

Timpson, J. (1996). Nursing theory: Everything the artist spits is art? *Journal of Advanced Nursing, 23,* 1030–1036.

Wright, L. M., & Leahey, M. (1994). *Nurses and families: A guide to family assessment and intervention* (2nd ed.). Philadelphia, PA: F. A. Davis.

CHAPTER 20

© A-R-T/Shutterstock

Research: How Health Care Advances

Harry A. Sultz and Kristina M. Young

CHAPTER OBJECTIVES

1. Define and recognize the focus of different types of research and how each type contributes to the advancement of knowledge about health and the health care system.

2. Describe the functions and goals of the Agency for Healthcare Research and Quality and how to access information pertinent to advanced nursing practice.

3. Recognize the interface of health research and policy and of research and quality improvement.

4. Discuss future challenges for health care research and the impact they will have on advanced practice nursing.

This chapter explains the focus of different types of research and how each type contributes to the overall advances in health and medicine. In this chapter, health services research, a newer field that addresses the workings of the health care system rather than specific problems of disease or disability, is described. The offices and goals of health services research's major funding source, the federal Agency for Healthcare Research and Quality, are listed. Finally, research into the quality of medical care, the problems being addressed, and the research challenges of the future are discussed.

The last half of the 20th century and early 21st century have seen remarkable growth of scientifically rigorous research in medicine, dentistry, nursing, and other health professions. The change from

FIGURE 20-1 Variations in research focus.

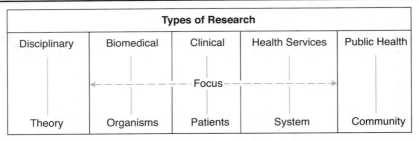

Types of Research				
Disciplinary	Biomedical	Clinical	Health Services	Public Health
		←———————— Focus ————————→		
Theory	Organisms	Patients	System	Community

Source: Aday LA, Lairson DR, Balkrishnan R, et al. *Evaluating the Healthcare System: Effectiveness, Efficiency and Equity.* 3rd ed. Chicago, IL: Health Administration Press; 2004; permission conveyed through Copyright Clearance Center, Inc.

dependence on the clinical impressions of individual physicians and other health care practitioners to reliance on the statistical probability of accurate findings from carefully controlled studies is one of the most important advances in scientific medicine. No longer is health professions' literature filled with subjective anecdotal reports of treatment progress in one or more individual cases. Now readers of peer-reviewed professional journals can monitor the progress of basic science and clinical or technologic discoveries with confidence, knowing that published findings are, with few exceptions, based on research studies that have been rigorously designed and conducted to yield statistically credible results.

In contrast, volumes of reports of medical developments that appear in the popular media are often premature and, depending on the source, may be cause for skepticism. The imprudent publication of inadequately proved or unproved therapies, the sensationalizing of minor scientific advances, and the promotion of fraudulent devices and treatments create unrealistic consumer expectations that often result in disappointments, mistreatment, and costly deceptions.

From both professional and public perspectives, the continuing research yield of new technologies and clinical advances creates ongoing challenges of evaluation, interpretation, and potential applications.

FOCUS OF DIFFERENT TYPES OF RESEARCH

Figure 20-1 illustrates the focus of different types of health care research. There are clear distinctions among researchers in terms of methods and the nature of their subsequent findings. Although the kinds of information derived from each type of research may be different, each knowledge gain is an essential step in the never-ending quest to create a more efficient and effective health care system.[1]

TYPES OF RESEARCH

Research studies conducted by those in professional disciplines fall into several categories. Basic science research is the work of biochemists, physiologists, biologists, pharmacologists, and others concerned with sciences that are fundamental to understanding the growth, development, structure, and function of the human body and its responses to external stimuli. Much of basic science research is at the cellular level and takes place in highly sophisticated laboratories. Other basic research may involve animal or human studies. Whatever its nature, however, basic science research is the essential antecedent of advances in clinical medicine.

Clinical research focuses primarily on the various steps in the process of medical care—the early detection, diagnosis, and treatment of disease or injury; the maintenance of optimal physical, mental, and social functioning; the limitation and rehabilitation of disability; and the palliative care of those who are irreversibly ill. Individuals in all the clinical specialties of medicine, nursing, allied health, and related health professions conduct clinical research, often in collaboration with those in the basic sciences. Much of clinical research is experimental, involving carefully controlled clinical trials of diagnostic or therapeutic procedures, new drugs, or technological developments.

Clinical trials test a new treatment or drug against a prevailing standard of care. If no standard drug exists or if it is too easily identified, a control group receives a placebo or mock drug to minimize subject bias. To reduce bias further, random selection is used to decide which volunteer patients are in the experimental and control groups. In a double-blind study, neither the researchers nor the patients know who is receiving the test drug or treatment until the study is completed and the identifying code revealed.

Research studies have a number of safeguards to protect the safety and rights of volunteer subjects. Studies funded by governmental agencies or foundations are subject to scrutiny by a peer-review committee that judges the scientific merit of the research design and the potential value of the findings. Next, a hospital-based board or an institutional review board (IRB) checks for ethical considerations and patient protections. Finally, volunteer subjects must sign an informed consent form that spells out in clear detail the potential risks or side effects and the expected benefits of their participation. Volunteers must weigh any potential risks against the likelihood that by participating in research they will receive state-of-the-art care and close health monitoring that will contribute to the advancement of science.

Epidemiology

Epidemiology, or population research, is concerned with the distribution and determinants of health, diseases, and injuries in human populations. Much of that research is observational; it is the collection of information about natural phenomena, the characteristics and behaviors of people, aspects of their location or environment, and their exposure to certain circumstances or events.

Observational studies may be descriptive or analytical. Descriptive studies use patient records, interview surveys, various databases, and other information sources to identify those factors and conditions that determine the distribution of health and disease among specific populations. They provide the details or characteristics of diseases or biologic phenomena and the prevalence or magnitude of their occurrences. Descriptive studies are relatively fast and inexpensive and often raise questions or suggest hypotheses to be tested. They are often followed by analytic studies, which test hypotheses and try to explain biologic phenomena by seeking statistical associations between factors that may contribute to a subsequent occurrence and the initial occurrence itself.

Some analytic studies attempt, under naturally occurring circumstances, to observe the differences between two or more populations with different characteristics or behaviors. For example, data about smokers and nonsmokers may be collected to determine the relative risk of a related outcome such as lung cancer, or a cohort study may follow a population over time, as in the case of the Framingham, Massachusetts, study. For years, epidemiologists have been studying a cooperating Framingham population to determine associations between variables such as diet, weight, exercise, and other behaviors and characteristics related to heart disease and other outcomes. These observational studies are valuable in explaining patterns of disease or disease processes and providing information about the association of specific activities or agents with health or disease effects.

Experimental Epidemiology

Observational studies are usually followed by experimental studies. In experimental studies, the investigator actively intervenes by manipulating one variable to see what happens with the other. Although they are the best test of cause and effect, such studies are technically difficult to carry out and often raise ethical issues. Control populations are used to ensure that other nonexperimental variables are not affecting the outcome. Like clinical trials, such studies may raise ethical issues when experiments involve the use of a clinical procedure that may expose the subjects to significant or unknown risk. Ethical questions also are raised when experimental studies require the withholding of some potentially beneficial drug or procedure from individuals in the control group to prove decisively the effectiveness of the drug or procedure.

Other Applications of Epidemiologic Methods

Because the population perspective of epidemiology usually requires the study and analysis of data obtained from or about large-scale population samples, the discipline has developed principles and methods that can be applied to the study of a wide range of problems in several fields. Thus, the concepts and quantitative methods of epidemiology have been used not only to add to the understanding of the etiology of health and disease but also to plan, administer, and evaluate health services; to forecast the health needs of population groups;

to assess the adequacy of the supply of health personnel; and, most recently, to determine the outcomes of specific treatment modalities in a variety of clinical settings.

Advances in statistical theory and the epidemiology of medical care make it possible to analyze and interpret performance data obtained from the large Medicare and other insurance databases. Many of the research findings of seemingly inexplicable geographic variations in the amount and cost of hospital treatments and in the use of a variety of health care services have resulted from the analysis of Medicare claims data and other large health insurance databases.

Health Services Research

Until the last several decades, most research addressed the need to broaden the understanding of health and disease; to find new and more effective means of diagnosis and treatment; and, in effect, to improve the quality and length of life. For the two decades after World War II, supply-side subsidy programs dominated federal health care policy. Like other subsidy programs, Medicare and Medicaid were politically crafted solutions rather than research-based strategies. Nevertheless, these major health care subsidy programs were the driving forces behind the rise of health services research. The continuous collection of cost and utilization data from these programs revealed serious deficiencies in the capability of the health care system to efficiently and effectively deliver the knowledge and skills already at hand. In addition, evidence was growing that the large variations in the kinds and amounts of care delivered for the same health conditions represented unacceptable volumes of inappropriate or questionable care and too much indecision or confusion among clinicians about the best courses of treatment. Health services research was born of the need to improve the efficiency and effectiveness of the health care system and to determine which of the health care treatment options for each health condition produces the best outcomes.

Agency for Healthcare Research and Quality

Beginning with John Wennberg's documenting large differences in the use of medical and surgical procedures among physicians in small geographic areas in the late 1980s, a number of similar studies brought the value of increasingly more costly health care into serious question. Wennberg noted that the rate of surgeries correlated with the number of surgeons in a geographic area and that the number of available hospital beds correlated with the rate of a population's hospitalization rather than with differences among patients.

He found that per capita expenditures for hospitalization in Boston were consistently double those in nearby New Haven.[2-4] Widely varying physician practice patterns provided little direction as to the most appropriate use of even the most common clinical procedures. In addition, adequate outcome measures for specific intervention modalities generally were lacking.

The problem did not escape the attention of the 101st Congress. The development of new knowledge through research has long been held as an appropriate and essential role of the federal government, as evidenced by the establishment and proactive role of the National Institutes of Health (NIH). When it became clear that indecision about the most appropriate and effective ways to diagnose and treat specific medical, dental, and other conditions was contributing to unacceptably large variations in the cost, quality, and outcomes of health care, federal legislation was passed to support the development of clinical guidelines. The Agency for Health Care Policy and Research (AHCPR) was established in 1989 as the successor to the National Center for Health Services Research and Health Care Technology. It became one of eight agencies of the Public Health Service within the Department of Health and Human Services.

AHCPR was responsible for updating and promoting the development and review of clinically relevant guidelines to assist health care practitioners in the prevention, diagnosis, treatment, and management of clinical conditions. The authorizing legislation directed that AHCPR or public and not-for-profit private organizations convene panels of qualified experts. These panels were charged to review the literature that contained the findings of numerous studies of clinical conditions and, after considering the scientific evidence, to recommend clinical guidelines to assist practitioner and patient decisions about appropriate care for specific clinical conditions.[5]

The agency's priority activities included funding two types of research projects: patient outcome research teams and literature synthesis projects or meta-analyses. Both the patient outcome research teams and the smaller literature synthesis projects identified and analyzed patient outcomes associated with alternative practice patterns and recommended changes where appropriate. During its decade-long existence, the AHCPR supported studies that resulted in a prodigious array of publications focused on patient care and clinical decision making, technology assessment, the quality and costs of care, and treatment outcomes. Although no longer directly involved in producing clinical practice guidelines, the agency currently assists private sector groups by supplying them with the scientific evidence they need to develop their own guidelines.

Significant changes occurred in the mandate of AHCPR since its 1989 inception. The agency narrowly escaped the loss of funding and possible elimination in 1996 after incurring the wrath of national organizations of surgeons. In keeping with its original mission, AHCPR had issued clinical guidelines. One such guideline discouraged surgery as a treatment for back pain on the grounds that it provided no better outcomes than more conservative treatments. Organizations of angry surgeons led a lobbying effort that convinced key members of Congress that the agency was exceeding its authority by establishing clinical practice standards without considering the expertise and opinions of the medical specialists involved.[6]

The dispute was resolved when the AHCPR agreed to function as a "science partner" with public and private organizations by assisting in developing knowledge that could be used to improve clinical practice. The agency agreed to produce clinical guidelines that would focus on funding research on medical interventions and analyzing the data that would underlie the development of clinical guidelines.

The Health Care Research and Quality Act of 1999 retitled the AHCPR to the Agency for Healthcare Research and Quality (AHRQ). The mission of AHRQ is to (1) improve the outcomes and quality of health care services, (2) reduce the costs of health care, (3) address patient safety, and (4) broaden effective services through the establishment of a broad base of scientific research that promotes improvements in clinical and health systems practices, including prevention of disease.[7]

While clinical practice guidelines would subsequently be generated by medical specialty and other health care organizations, the AHRQ's role would be to evaluate recommendations made in the clinical practice guidelines to ensure that they were based on a systematic literature review (evidence-based) and were revised for currency on a regular basis.

To date, more than 14,000 such evidence-based clinical practice guidelines that have met the AHRQ's evaluation criteria have been collected in a database, organized by searchable topics, and made available online to health care professionals and the general public at the AHRQ's National Guideline Clearinghouse (http://www.guideline.gov/).

A top priority of the AHRQ is transmitting its sponsored research results and new health information to consumers. In addition to a number of consumer-oriented publications, the agency provides information to the public via the Internet. Its website, http://www.ahrq.gov, offers a robust array of health care information. The AHRQ is now a major collaborating organization of the Patient-Centered Outcomes and Research Institute (PCORI) established by the Affordable Care Act (ACA), which is described later in this chapter.

Health Services Research and Health Policy

Health services research combines the perspectives and methods of epidemiology, sociology, economics, and clinical medicine. Applying the basic concepts of epidemiology and biostatistics, process and outcome measures that reflect the behavioral and economic variables associated with questions of therapeutic effectiveness and cost-benefit are also used. The ability of health services research to address issues of therapeutic effectiveness and cost-benefit during the nation's quest for fiscal exigency has contributed to the field's substantial growth and current value.

The contributions of health services research to health policy are impressive. Major examples include the Wennberg studies of small area variation in medical utilization, the prospective payment system based on diagnosis-related groups,[8,9] research on inappropriate medical procedures,[10] resource-based relative value scale research,[11-13] and the background research that supported the concepts of health maintenance organizations and managed care.

The RAND Health Insurance Experiment,[14,15] one of the largest and longest-running health services research projects ever undertaken, began in 1971 and contributed vast amounts of information on the effects of cost sharing on the provision and outcomes of health services. Participating families were assigned to one of four different fee-for-service plans or to a prepaid group practice. As might have been expected, individuals in the various plans differed significantly in their rate of health care use, with little measurable effect on health outcomes. The Health Insurance Experiment was followed by two large research studies: the Health Services Utilization Study and the Medical Outcomes Study. The findings of both gave impetus to the federal support of outcomes research.[16] Determining the outcomes and effectiveness of different health care interventions aids clinical decision making, reduces costs, and benefits patients.

Quality Improvement

Until the past few years, health care's impressive accomplishments have made it difficult for health care researchers, policy makers, and organizational leaders to publicly acknowledge that poor-quality health care is a major problem within the dynamic and productive biomedical enterprise in the United States. In 1990, after 2 years of study, hearings, and site visits, the Institute of Medicine issued a report that cited widespread overuse of expensive invasive technology, underuse of inexpensive "caring" services, and implementation of error-prone procedures that harmed patients and wasted money.[17,18]

Although these conclusions from this prestigious body were devastating to health care reformers, they were hardly news to health service researchers. For decades, practitioners assumed that quality, like beauty, was in the eye of the beholder and therefore was unmeasurable except in cases of obvious violation of generally accepted standards. The medical and other health care professions had promoted the image of health care as a blend of almost impenetrable, science-based disciplines, leaving the providers of care as the only ones capable of understanding the processes taking place. Thus only physicians could judge the work of other physicians. Such peer review–based assessment has always been difficult for reviewers and limited in effectiveness. Peer review recognizes that only part of medical care is based on factual knowledge. A substantial component of medical decision making is based on clinical judgment. Clinical judgment requires combining consideration of the potential risks and benefits of each physician's internal list of alternatives in making diagnostic and treatment decisions with his or her medical intuition regarding the likelihood of success based on the condition of each patient. Under these complex and often inexplicable circumstances, physicians are repelled by the notion of either judging or being judged by their colleagues.

For these reasons, until recently, quality assurance, whether in hospitals or by regulatory agencies, was focused on identifying only exceptionally poor care. This practice, popularly known as the "bad apple theory," was based on the presumption that the best way to ensure quality was to identify the bad apples or poor performers and remove or rehabilitate them. Thus, during the 1970s and 1980s, quality assurance interventions only followed the detection of undesirable occurrences. For example, flagrant violations of professional standards had to be documented before professional review organizations required physicians to begin quality improvement plans. Physicians were guaranteed due process to dispute the evidence.

Focusing on isolated violations required a great deal of review time to uncover a single case that called for remedial action. In addition, it was an unpleasant duty for reviewers to assign blame to a colleague who might soon be on a committee reviewing their records. Most importantly, such quality inspections represented a method that implicitly defined quality as the absence of mishap. Clinician dislike of quality assurance activities during the 1970s and 1980s was well founded as these processes were professionally offensive and had little constructive impact.

Specifying and striving for excellent care are very recent quality assurance phenomena in the health care arena. Hospitals and other health care organizations that had long focused on peer-review committees, incident reports, and other negative quality-monitoring activities experienced difficulty in transforming to teamwork and higher levels of transparency in quality monitoring and reporting activities.

Health services researchers had known for decades that health care quality was measurable and that excellent, as well as poor, care could be identified and quantified. In 1966, Avedis Donabedian[19] characterized the concept of health care as divided into the components of structure, process, and outcomes and the research paradigm of their assumed linkages, all of which have guided quality-of-care investigators to this day.

Donabedian suggested that the number, kinds, and skills of the providers, as well as the adequacy of their physical resources and the manner in which they perform appropriate procedures, should, in the aggregate, influence the quality of subsequent outcomes. Although today the construct may seem like a statement of the obvious, at the time, attention to structural criteria was the major, if not the only, quality assurance activity in favor. It was generally assumed that properly trained professionals, given adequate resources in properly equipped facilities, performed at acceptable standards of quality. For example, for many years, the Joint Commission on Accreditation of Healthcare Organizations (now known as The Joint Commission) made judgments about the quality of hospitals on the basis of structural standards, such as physical facilities and equipment, ratios of professional staff to patients, and the qualifications of various personnel. Later, it added process components to its structural standards and, most recently, has shifted its evaluation process to focus on care outcomes.

Early landmark quality-of-care studies used implicit and explicit normative or judgmental standards. Implicit standards rely on the internalized judgments of the expert individuals involved in the quality assessment. Explicit standards are those developed and agreed on in advance of the assessment; they minimize the variation and bias that invariably result when judgments are internalized. More current studies judge the appropriateness of hospital admissions and various procedures and, in general, associate specific structural characteristics of the health care system with practice or process variations.

Another method for assessing the quality of health care practices is based on empirical standards. Derived from distributions, averages, ranges, and other measures of data variability, information collected from a number of similar health service providers is compared to identify practices that deviate from the norms. A current popular use of empirical standards is in the patient severity–adjusted hospital performance data collected by health departments and community-based employer and insurer groups to measure and compare both process activities and outcomes. These performance "report cards" are becoming increasingly valuable to the purchasers of care, who rely on an objective method to guide their choices among managed care organizations, health care systems, and group practices. The empirical measures of quality include such variables as the following:

- Timeliness of ambulation
- Compliance with basic nursing care standards
- Average length of stay
- Number of home care referrals
- Number of rehabilitation referrals
- Timeliness of consultation completion
- Timeliness of orders and results
- Patient waiting times by department or area
- Infection rates
- Decubitus rates
- Medication errors
- Patient complaints
- Readmissions within 30 days
- Neonatal and maternal mortalities
- Perioperative mortalities

Normative and empirical standards are both used in studying the quality of health care in the United States. For example, empirical analyses are performed to test or modify normative recommendations. Empirical or actual experience data are collected to confirm performance and outcome improvements after the imposition of clinical guidelines derived from studies using normative standards.

Medical Errors

In 1999, the Institute of Medicine again issued a report on the quality of medical care.[20] Focused on medical errors, the report described mistakes occurring during the course of hospital care as one of the nation's leading causes of death and disability. Citing two major studies estimating that medical errors killed 44,000–98,000 people in U.S. hospitals each year, the Institute of Medicine report was a stunning indictment of the systems of hospital care at that time. The report contained a series of recommendations for improving patient safety in the admittedly high-risk environments of modern hospitals. Among the recommendations was a proposal for establishing a center for patient safety within the AHRQ. The proposed center would establish national safety goals, track progress in improving safety, and invest in research to learn more about preventing mistakes.[20] Congress responded by designating part of the increase in budget for the AHRQ for that purpose.

In 2005, the Patient Safety and Quality Improvement Act was enacted by Congress to establish patient safety organizations (PSOs) to improve the quality and safety of health care delivery by encouraging health care providers and institutions to identify, analyze, and implement prevention strategies to reduce or eliminate risks and hazards associated with the delivery of care to patients and to voluntarily report and share patient safety data without fear of legal discovery. PSOs are overseen by the AHRQ, which also maintains online access to the latest annotated links to patient safety literature and safety news at the Patient Safety Network (PSNet).[21]

Evidence-Based Medicine

Evidence-based medicine is defined as "the systematic application of the best available evidence to the evaluation of options and decisions in clinical practice, management and policy making."[22] Although this statement may appear to be a description of the way physicians and other health care providers have practiced since the inception of scientific medicine, it reflects a concern that the opposite is true. The wide range of variability in clinical practice, the complexity of diagnostic testing and medical decision making, and the difficulty that physicians have in keeping up with the overwhelming volumes of scientific literature suggest that a significant percentage of clinical management decisions are not supported by reliable evidence of effectiveness.

Although it is generally assumed that physicians are reasonably confident that the treatments they give are beneficial, the reality is that medical practice is fraught with uncertainty. In addition, the ethical basis for clinical decision making allows physicians to exercise their preferences for certain medical theories or practices that may or may not have been evaluated to link treatment to benefits.[23]

Proponents of evidence-based medicine propose that if all health services are intended to improve the health status and quality of life of the recipients, then the acid test is whether services, programs, and policies improve health beyond what could be achieved with the same resources by different means or by doing nothing at all. Evidence is the key to accountability. The decisions made by health care providers, administrators, policy makers, patients, and the public need to be based on appropriate, balanced, and high-quality evidence.[24]

The evidence-based approach to assessing the acceptability of research findings considers the evidence from randomized clinical trials involving large numbers of participants to be the most valid. Evidence-based medicine advocates dismiss outcomes research that uses large data files created from claim records, hospital discharges, Medicare, or other sources because the subjects are not randomized. "Outcomes research using claims data is an excellent way of finding out what doctors are doing, but it's a terrible way to find out what doctors should be doing," stated Thomas C. Chalmers, MD, of Harvard School of Public Health, Boston.[22]

In general, most of the investigations reported in the peer-reviewed medical literature have been preliminary tests of innovations and have served science rather than efforts providing guidance to practitioners in clinical practice. Only a small portion of these efforts can survive testing well enough to justify routine clinical application.[24]

The situation has changed rapidly, however. Articles on evidence-based medicine appear frequently in the medical literature.[25] Cost-control pressures that encourage efforts to ensure that therapies have documented patient benefit, growing interest in the quality of patient care, and increasing sophistication on the part of patients concerning the care that they receive have stimulated acceptance of the concepts of evidence-based medical practice.[25]

Outcomes Research and the Patient-Centered Outcomes Research Institute

Given the huge investment in U.S. health care and the inequitable distribution of its services, do the end effects on the health and well-being of patients and populations justify the costs? Insurance companies, state and federal governments, employers, and consumers look to outcomes research for information to help them make better decisions about what kinds of health care should be reimbursed, for whom, and when.

Because outcomes research evaluates results of health care processes in the real world of physicians' offices, hospitals, clinics, and homes,

it contrasts with traditional randomized controlled studies that test the effects of treatments in controlled environments. In addition, the research in usual service settings, or "effectiveness research," differs from controlled clinical trials, or "efficacy research," in the nature of the outcomes measured. Traditionally, studies measured health status, or outcomes, with physiologic measurements—laboratory tests, complication rates, recovery, or survival. To capture health status more adequately, outcomes research measures a patient's functional status and well-being. Satisfaction with care also must complement traditional measures.

Functional status includes three components that assess patients' abilities to function in their own environment:

1. Physical functioning
2. Role functioning—the extent to which health interferes with usual daily activities, such as work or school
3. Social functioning—whether health affects normal social activities, such as visiting friends or participating in group activities

Personal well-being measures describe patients' sense of physical and mental well-being—their mental health or general mood, their personal view of their general health, and their general sense about the quality of their lives. Patient satisfaction measures the patients' views about the services received, including access, convenience, communication, financial coverage, and technical quality.

Outcomes research also uses meta-analyses, a technique to summarize comparable findings from multiple studies. More importantly, however, outcomes research goes beyond determining what works in ideal circumstances to assessing which treatments for specific clinical problems work best in different circumstances. Appropriateness studies are conducted to determine the circumstances in which a procedure should and should not be performed. Even though a procedure is proved to be effective, it is not appropriate for every patient in all circumstances. The frequency of inappropriate clinical interventions is one of the major quality-of-care problems in the system, and research is under way to develop the tools to identify patient preferences when treatment options are available. Although most discussions about appropriateness stress potential cost savings that could be achieved by reducing unnecessary care and overuse of services, outcomes research may be just as likely to uncover underuse of appropriate services.

It is important to recognize that the ultimate value of outcomes research can be measured only by its ability to incorporate the results of its efforts into the health care process. To be effective, the findings of outcomes research must first reach and then change the behaviors of providers, patients, health care institutions, and payers. The endpoint of outcomes research, the clinical practice guidelines intended to assist practitioners and patients in choosing appropriate health care for specific conditions, must be disseminated in acceptable and motivational ways. With the health care industry in a state of rapid change, the need to make appropriate investments in outcomes research became increasingly apparent with the inescapable conclusion that the United States cannot continue to spend almost $3 trillion each year on health care without learning much more about what that investment is buying.[26,27]

The American Recovery and Reinvestment Act (ARRA) of 2009 included $1.1 billion over a period of 2 years to expand "comparative effectiveness research" by the AHRQ and the NIH. The ARRA established a Federal Coordinating Council to recommend research priorities and create a strategic framework for research activities. The Institute of Medicine (IOM) recommended 100 priority research areas for funding by the ARRA and 10 research priority areas. Recommendations from the Federal Coordinating Council and the IOM were released in June 2009, and the ARRA required the secretary of the U.S. Department of Health and Human Services (DHHS) to consider these recommendations in directing research funds.[28,29] The goal of comparative effectiveness research is to enhance healthcare treatment decisions by providing information to consumers, providers, and payers to improve health outcomes by developing and disseminating evidence "on the effectiveness, benefits, and harms of different treatment options. The evidence is generated from research studies that compare drugs, medical devices, tests, surgeries, or ways to deliver health care."[29] Historically, clinical research examined the effectiveness of one method, product, or service at a time. Comparative effectiveness research compares two or more methods for preventing, diagnosing, and treating health conditions, using methods such as practical clinical trials, analyses of insurance claim records, computer modeling, and systematic reviews of literature. Disseminating research findings about the effectiveness of treatments relative to other options in a form that is quickly useable by clinicians, patients, policy makers, health plans, and other payers is key to comparative research effectiveness goals. In addition, "identifying the most effective and efficient interventions has the potential to reduce unnecessary treatments, which may help lower costs."[29,30]

Empowering the Federal Coordinating Council, the ACA of 2010 created the PCORI, a not-for-profit, independent agency dedicated to conducting comparative effectiveness research. The PCORI is governed by a board of directors appointed by the U.S. Government Accountability Office (GAO) and is funded through the Patient-Centered Outcomes Research Trust Fund. The ACA allocated $210 million to PCORI activities for the fiscal years 2010–2012 and a total of $970 million for the years 2013–2019. Support is derived from the general U.S. Treasury fund and fees assessed to Medicare, private health insurance, and self-insured plans.[31]

PATIENT SATISFACTION

As reflected by the strong consumer orientation of the PCORI, patient satisfaction is recognized as an essential component of quality of care. Although the subjective ratings of health care rendered by patients may be based on markedly different criteria from those considered important by health care providers, they capture aspects of care and personal preferences that contribute significantly to perceived quality. It has become increasingly important in the competitive market climate of health care that the providers' characteristics, organization, and system attributes that are important to consumers be identified and monitored. In addition to health care providers' technical and interpersonal skills, patient concerns such as waiting times for appointments, emergency responses, helpfulness and communication of staff, and the facility's appearance contribute to patient evaluations of health services delivery programs and subsequent satisfaction with the quality of care received.

A number of instruments have been devised to measure patient satisfaction with health care, and most insurance plans, hospitals, and other health service facilities and agencies have adopted one or more to assess patient satisfaction regularly. Some, such as the Patient Satisfaction Questionnaire developed at Southern Illinois University School of Medicine, are short, self-administered survey forms. Others, such as the popular patient satisfaction instruments of the Picker Institute of Boston, Massachusetts, may be used as self-administered questionnaires mailed to patients after a health care experience or completed by interviewers during telephone surveys.[32] Whether by mail, direct contact, or telephone interview, questioning patients after a recent health care experience is an effective way to both identify outstanding service personnel and uncover fundamental problems in the quality of care as defined by patients. These activities help promote humane and effective care and are sound marketing techniques for providers.

RESEARCH ETHICS

Since the 1950s, the federal government has invested heavily in biomedical research. The ensuing public–private partnership in health has produced some of the finest medical research in the world. The growth of medical knowledge is unparalleled, and the United States can take well-deserved pride in its research accomplishments.

However, many, if not most, of the sophisticated new technologies have addressed the need to ameliorate the problems of patients who already have a condition or disease. Both the priorities and the profits intrinsic to the U.S. healthcare system have focused on remedial rather than preventive strategies. Only in the case of frightening epidemics, such as that of polio in the 1940s and AIDS in the 1990s, have there been the requisite moral imperatives to adequately fund research efforts that address public health problems. Clearly, much of the funding for medical research has failed to fulfill the generally held belief that the products of taxpayer-supported research should benefit not only the practice of medicine but also the community at large. If its intended goals are achieved, the PCORI will change the research focus to be highly inclusive of all stakeholders with a major voice from health care consumers by involving them in research topic priority determination and identifying the best mechanisms for meaningfully translating findings into clinical settings.[33]

CONFLICTS OF INTEREST IN RESEARCH

The increasing amount of research funding emanating from pharmaceutical and medical device companies is of serious concern. Pharmaceutical companies that pay researchers to design and interpret drug trials have been accused of misrepresenting the results or suppressing unfavorable findings. The conflicts that arise in the testing of new drugs and medical devices and publishing the results deepen as increasing numbers of studies are shifted from academic institutions to commercial research firms.[34]

For example, in 2009 the attorney general of New Jersey issued subpoenas to five prominent medical device makers for failing to disclose financial conflicts of interest among the physicians researching their products. It was learned that physicians who were testing and recommending the use of certain medical devices were being compensated with stock in the companies making those devices.[35]

To compound the problem further, the funding of the U.S. Food and Drug Administration (FDA), which regulates about a fourth of the U.S. economy, has been shifted from the government to the same pharmaceutical companies it is supposed to monitor with damaging effect. Political and pharmaceutical pressures caused the FDA to stray from its science-based public health mandate. For example, the FDA has been sharply criticized for its alleged failure to adequately monitor the risks of widely advertised and commonly used drugs for the treatment of arthritis.[36] The FDA's handling of collected clinical trial data is a major problem. Although the information collected is necessary for FDA approval of a product, once the product is approved, the FDA does not provide the public with a full report of the drug's safety and efficacy. The withheld information falls into the definition of "trade secrets," and the FDA has taken the position that research data are entitled to protection as proprietary information. This explains the number of recent examples of FDA-approved drugs that were later discovered to have major safety risks.[37] Clearly, the FDA must reconsider its position that clinical trial data fall into the classification of trade secrets.

The most egregious violation of professional ethics is found in the growing body of evidence that physicians at some of the most prestigious U.S. medical schools have been attaching their names and reputations to scientific publications ghostwritten by employees of pharmaceutical companies. The publications are intended, of course, to boost the sales of pharmaceutical products.[38] The NIH, which funds much of the nation's medical research, suggests that the universities involved, rather than the government, should address the problem of ghost authorship. Because university administrators find it difficult to censure the prestigious medical faculty at their institutions, the problem remains minimally addressed with no noted measurable decline in frequency in professional biomedical literature.[39]

FUTURE CHALLENGES

Most U.S. health care research has been directed toward improving the health care system's ability to diagnose and treat injury, disease, and disability among those who seek care. Now, largely because of the population focus of health insurers, research studies increasingly focus on identifying and improving the health status of groups of individuals characterized by various sociodemographic and health factors. Research priorities are shifting from an individual patient perspective to a population orientation and toward continuous scrutiny of the efficiency and effectiveness of the care delivered. The ACA and its population-focused initiatives such as the PCORI are providing robust momentum to this continuing change. Experts point out that among the significant challenges to implementing changes promoted by the PCORI will be required alterations in provider behavior, cognitive biases toward rejecting new information, significant realignments of payment incentives, and inadequate resources to disseminate research findings.[40]

Basic science research will continue to contribute to the diagnostic and therapeutic efficacy of health care by adding to the knowledge about the human body and its functions. In small but critically important increments, basic science research will unlock many of the secrets of aging; cell growth regulation; mental degradation; and other mysteries of immunology, genetics, microbiology, and neuroendocrinology. The propensity of medicine to use newly obtained knowledge to alter certain physiologic processes, as in several forms of gene manipulation, will produce new ethical, legal, and clinical issues that then will require further research and adjudication.

Massive databases of gene and protein sequences and structure/function information have made possible a new worldwide research effort called bioinformatics. Bioinformatics research probes those large computer databases to learn more about life's processes in health and disease and to find new or better drugs. It is considered the future of biotechnology.

Of particular interest is research in genomics, the study of genetic material in the chromosomes of specific organisms. The sequencing of the human genome will reshape biology and medicine and lead to significant improvements in the diagnosis of disease and individual responses to drugs.[41]

Similarly, certain advances in clinical medicine and other health disciplines will result in new and disturbing ethical dilemmas. Medical achievements, such as those that permit the maintenance of life in otherwise terminal and unresponsive individuals or the transplantation of organs in short supply that require choosing among recipient candidates when those denied will surely die, generate extremely complex ethical, economic, religious, personal, and professional issues. Thus, much of the basic and clinical research that solves yesterday's problems relating to individual patient care will create new problems to be addressed in the never-ending cycle of discovery, application, and evaluation.

Medical researchers and clinicians are becoming increasingly concerned that U.S. health care is entering a "postantibiotic" era in which bacterial infections will be unaffected by even the most powerful of available antibiotics. Evidence is accumulating that a growing number of microbes, including strains of staphylococcus and streptococcus bacteria, are becoming resistant to common antimicrobials.[42] Staphylococcus bacteria are a major cause of hospital infections. According to the Centers for Disease Control and Prevention, these infections are responsible for about 13% of the 2 million infections that occur in U.S. hospitals each year. Overall, infections result in the deaths of up to 99,000 hospital patients each year.[43]

Although infectious disease epidemiologists and clinical specialists have warned for decades that the misuse and overuse of antibiotics would result in a host of deadly drug-resistant pathogens, neither physicians nor patients took the warnings seriously, with a widespread belief that the development of new antimicrobial drugs would keep medicine a step ahead of bacterial resistance.

Measures have been suggested to help maintain the efficiency of present antibiotic substances, such as limiting their use through "antibiotic stewardship" guideline development and imposing fees on antibiotic use that would cover the estimated cost of resistance inherent in antibiotic use. However, this type of fee-for-use has proved very difficult to calculate and has yet to gain acceptance with policy makers.[44]

Limited development of new antibiotics has failed to keep step with antibiotic resistance; however, scientists now see promising alternatives in bacterial genetics to address antibiotic resistance. Economic incentives to increase the research and development of new antibiotics and a revamping of the drug approval process are some suggested remedies to increase the supply of new antibiotics brought to market.[44]

Health services research will continue to focus on the performance of the health care system as the basis for proposing or evaluating health policy alternatives. It is interdisciplinary, value-laden research concerned with the effectiveness or benefits of care, the efficiency or resource cost of care, and the equity or fairness of the distribution of care. Documenting the influence of financial incentives that affect both patient and provider, understanding the important relationships of socioeconomic status to health and health care, determining the effects of the training and experience of the health care team and the ability of the members to work together, and understanding how these many influences interact are fundamental to improving the quality of care. Reducing the monumental quandaries in medicine and health care about what works well in which situation is the challenge of health services research and the key to a more effective, efficient, and equitable health care system.

Public health research is a related research arena that deserves higher priority and significantly increased political support. If health care is ever to develop a true population perspective rather than an individual patient perspective and to reap the health and economic benefits of preventive rather than only curative medicine, then epidemiology and public health research must be charged with finding ways to better understand and resolve the huge differences in health, health behaviors, health care, and health system effectiveness among communities and the population groups within them. Epidemiology, the core discipline of public health research, can assess the health problems and the provision of health care for the total population rather than just for those who are in contact with health services. Surveillance and monitoring of health conditions and assessing the effect of health care measures on the entire population are important factors in formulating health policy, organizing health services, and allocating limited resources.[45] The strategy for identifying and dealing with real or suspected biologic attacks on citizens of the United States, for example, will depend heavily on the ability of epidemiologists to identify the common source of such outbreaks, the patterns of transmission, and the outcomes of preventive and remedial efforts.

As health care adds to its traditional focus on theories, disease, and individual patient care, the performance of the health care system and the health status of populations, public health, and health services research assume increasing relevance and importance. No matter how well the health care system performs for some of the people, it cannot be fully satisfactory until it can provide a basic level of care for all.

REFERENCES

1. Aday LA, Lairson DR, Balkrishnan R, et al. *Evaluating the Medical Care System: Effectiveness, Efficiency, and Equity*. Ann Arbor, MI: Health Administration Press; 1993.
2. Wennberg JE, Freeman JL, Culp WJ. Are hospital services rationed in New Haven or over-utilized in Boston? *Lancet*. 1987;*1*:1185–1189.
3. Wennberg JE. Which rate is right? *N Engl J Med*. 1986;*314*:310–311.
4. Wennberg JE, Freeman JL, Shelton RM, et al. Hospital use and mortality among Medicare beneficiaries in Boston and New Haven. *N Engl J Med*. 1989;*321*:1168–1173.
5. Agency for Health Care Policy and Research, U.S. Department of Health and Human Services. *AHCPR Program Note*. Rockville, MD: Public Health Service; 1990.
6. Stephenson J. Revitalized AHCPR pursues research on quality. *JAMA*. 1997;*278*:1557.
7. U.S. Department of Health and Human Services, Agency for Healthcare Research and Quality. AHRQ profile. December 2010. Available at http://www.ahrq.gov/cpi/about/profile/index .html. Accessed October 1, 2012.
8. Mills R, Fetter RB, Riedel DC, et al. AUTOGRP: an interactive computer system for the analysis of health care data. *Med Care*. 1976;*14*:603–615.
9. Berki SE. DRGs, incentives, hospitals and physicians. *Health Aff*. 1985;*4*:70–76.
10. Chassin MR, Kosecoff J, Park RE, et al. Does inappropriate use explain geographic variations in the use of health care services? A study of three procedures. *JAMA*. 1987;*258*:2533–2537.
11. Hsiao WC, Stason WB. Toward developing a relative value scale for medical and surgical services. *Health Care Finan Rev*. 1979;*1*:23–28.
12. Hsiao WC, Braun P, Yntema D, et al. Results and policy implications of the resource-based relative value study. *N Engl J Med*. 1988;*319*:881–888.
13. Hsiao WC, Braun P, Yntema D, et al. *A National Study of Resource-Based Relative Value Scale for*

Physician Services: Final Report to the Health Care Financing Administration. Boston, MA: Harvard School of Public Health; 1988.

14. Newhouse JP. A design for a health insurance experiment. *Inquiry.* 1974;*11*:5–27.

15. Newhouse JP, Keeler EB, Phelps CE, et al. The findings of the RAND health insurance experiment—a response to Welch et al. *Med Care.* 1987;*25*:157–179.

16. Newhouse JP. Controlled experimentation as research policy. In: Ginzberg E, Ed. *Health Services Research: Key to Health Policy.* Cambridge, MA: Harvard University Press; 1991:162–194.

17. Lohr KN, The Institute of Medicine. *Medicare: A Strategy for Quality Assurance. Vol. 1.* Washington, DC: National Academy Press; 1990.

18. Surver JD. Striving for quality in health care: an inquiry into policy and practice. *Health Care Manag Rev.* 1992;*17*(4):95–96.

19. Donabedian A. Evaluating the quality of medical care. *Milbank Mem Fund Q.* 1966;*44*:166–206.

20. Kohn LT, Corrigan JM, Donaldson MS. *To Err Is Human: Building a Safer Health System.* Washington, DC: Institute of Medicine; 1999.

21. U.S. Department of Health and Human Services, Agency for Healthcare Research and Quality. Patient safety organization (PSO) program. Available at http://www.pso.ahrq.gov/. Accessed October 1, 2012.

22. Watanabe M. A call for action from the National Forum on Health. *Can Med Assoc J.* 1997;*156*:999–1000. Available at http://www.cmaj.ca/content /156/7/999.full.pdf+html. Accessed October 4, 2012.

23. Marwick C. Federal agency focuses on outcomes research. *JAMA.* 1993;*270*:164–165.

24. Castiel LD. The urge for evidence based knowledge. *J Epidemiol Commun Health.* 2003;*57*:482.

25. Hooker RC. The rise and rise of evidence-based medicine. *Lancet.* 1997;*349*:1329–1330.

26. Reinhardt UE, Hussey PS, Anderson GF. U.S. health care spending in an international context. *Health Aff.* 2004;*23*:10–25.

27. Wayne A. Healthcare spending to reach 20% of U.S. economy by 2021. BloombergBusinessweek. June 13, 2012. Available at http://www .businessweek.com/news/2012-06-13/health-care-spending-to-reach-20-percent-of-u-dot-s-dot-economy-by-2021. Accessed October 1, 2012.

28. Benner JS, Morrison MR, Karnes E, et al. An evaluation of recent federal spending on comparative effectiveness research: priorities, gaps and next steps. *Health Aff.* 2010;*29*:1768–1774.

29. U.S. Department of Health and Human Services, Agency for Healthcare Research and Quality. What is comparative effectiveness research. Available at http://effectivehealthcare.ahrq.gov /index.cfm/what-is-comparative-effectiveness -research1/. Accessed January 8, 2013.

30. Henry J. Kaiser Family Foundation. Explaining health reform: what is comparative effectiveness research? September 29, 2009. Available at http: //www.kff.org/healthreform/7946.cfm. Accessed January 7, 2013.

31. Patient-Centered Outcomes Research Trust Fund. How we're funded. Available at http: //www.pcori.org/content/how-were-funded. Accessed January 8, 2013.

32. Gerteis M, Edgman-Levitan S, Daley J. *Through the Patient's Eyes: Understanding and Promoting Patient-Centered Care.* San Francisco, CA: Jossey-Bass; 1993.

33. Dubois RW, Graff JS. Setting priorities for comparative effectiveness research: from assessing public health benefits to being open with the public. *Health Aff.* 2011;*30*:2236–2240.

34. Walker EP. HHS report slams FDA's conflict of interest oversight. MedPage Today. January 12, 2009. Available at http://www.medpagetoday .com/PublicHealthPolicy/ClinicalTrials/12407. Accessed October 4, 2012.

35. New Jersey Office of the Attorney General. Landmark settlement reached with medical device maker synthes. May 5, 2009. Available at http: //www.nj.gov/oag/newsreleases09/pr20090505a .html. Accessed October 4, 2012.

36. Miller R. FDA hearing to determine arthritis drugs' safety. Health Center Today News. University of Connecticut Health Center. February 16, 2005. Available at http://today.uchc.edu/headlines /2005/feb05/arthritisdrug.html. Accessed October 4, 2012.

37. Bodenheimer T. Uneasy alliance—clinical investigators and the pharmaceutical industry. *N Engl J Med.* 2000;*342*:1516–1544.

38. Singer N. Senator moves to block medical ghostwriting. *New York Times.* August 18, 2009:B1–B2. Available at http://www.nytimes .com/2009/08/19/health/research/19ethics .html?_r=1&scp=1&sq=Ghosts%20in%20the%20 Journals&st=cse. Accessed January 7, 2012.

39. Wislar JS, Flanigan A, Fontanarosa PB, et al. Honorary and ghost authorship in high impact

medical journals: a cross-sectional survey. *BMJ.* 2011;*343*:d6128. Available at http://www .bmj.com/content/343/bmj.d6128. Accessed October 3, 2012.

40. Timbie JW, Schneider EC, Van Busum K, et al. Five reasons that many comparative effectiveness studies fail to change patient care and clinical practice. *Health Aff.* 2012;*31*:2169–2173.

41. Human Genome Project information: medicine and the new genetics. September 2011. Available at http://www.genome.gov/Pages /About/Planning/2011NHGRIStrategicPlan.pdf. Accessed November 1, 2014.

42. Bren L. Battle of the bugs: fighting antibiotic resistance. RxList. 2007. Available at http://www .rxlist.com/script/main/art.asp?articlekey =85705. Accessed October 3, 2012.

43. Klevens MR, Edwards JR, Richards C, et al. Estimating health-care associated infections and deaths in U.S. hospitals, 2002. *Public Health Rep.* 2007;*122*:160–166. Available at http://www .ncbi.nlm.nih.gov/pmc/articles/PMC1820440 /. Accessed October 3, 2012.

44. Höjgård S. Antibiotic resistance—why is the problem so difficult to solve? *Infect Ecol Epidemiol.* 2012:2. doi:10.3402/iee.v2i0.18165. Available at http://www.ncbi.nlm.nih.gov/pmc/articles /PMC3426322/. Accessed October 4, 2012.

45. Ibrahim MA. *Epidemiology and Health Policy.* Gaithersburg, MD: Aspen; 1985.

Evidence-Based Practice

Kerry Milner

CHAPTER OBJECTIVES

1. Discuss the historical roots of evidenced-based practice.
2. Define key assumptions of evidence-based practice in nursing.
3. Explore evidence-based practice models applicable to advanced practice nursing.
4. Develop a searchable question to answer a clinical problem using the PICOT format.
5. Use common bibliographic databases to search for best current evidence.
6. Identify critical appraisal tools for different sources of evidence.

WHAT IS EVIDENCE-BASED PRACTICE?

The concept of evidence-based practice originated in medicine and was first introduced to U.S. healthcare providers in the published literature in a 1992 *Journal of the American Medical Association* article (Ragan & Quincy, 2012). In this article, evidence-based medicine (EBM) was described as deemphasizing tradition, unsystematic clinical experience, and pathology as sufficient grounds for practice decisions, and it was suggested that critical examination of evidence from practice-based studies should underlie clinical decision making (Guyatt et al., 1992). The EBM movement called for physicians to learn the skills of efficient literature searching and the use of formal rules to critically evaluate evidence from the clinical literature.

In the early published definitions of EBM, the areas of foci included identifying, critically appraising, and summarizing best current evidence. However, it became clear that evidence alone was not sufficient to make clinical decisions, so in 2000 the Evidence-Based Medicine Working Group presented the second fundamental principle of EBM. This principle specified that clinical decisions, recommendations, and practice guidelines must not only focus on the best available evidence but also include the values and preferences of the informed patient. Values and preferences refer not only to the patients' perspectives, beliefs, expectations, and goals for life and health but also to the practices individuals use to consider the available options and the relative benefits, harms, costs, and inconveniences of those options (Guyatt et al., 2000).

A similar definition by Canadian medical doctor David Sackett, who is credited with pioneering EBM, emerged around the same time. His definition is as follows:

> The practice of evidence-based medicine means integrating individual clinical expertise with the best available external clinical evidence from systematic research. By individual clinical expertise we mean the proficiency and judgment that individual clinicians acquire through clinical experience and clinical practice. Increased expertise is reflected in many ways, but especially in more effective and efficient diagnosis and in the more thoughtful identification and compassionate use of individual patients' predicaments, rights, and preferences in making clinical decisions about their care. (Sackett, Rosenberg, Gray, Hayes, & Richardson, 1996, p. 71)

While EBM was being written about in U.S. scientific literature, Archie Cochrane, a British epidemiologist and physician, had been vocal about the lack of systematic reviews upon which to base medical practice, so he published a systematic review on care during pregnancy and childbirth. It was so well received that he was granted government funding for the Cochrane Center in 1992 (Cochrane

Collaboration, 2012). The central mission of the Cochrane Collaboration is to promote healthcare decision making throughout the world that is informed by high-quality, timely research evidence. Today the Cochrane Collaboration is an international network of nearly 30,000 people from more than 100 countries helping healthcare providers, policy makers, patients, their advocates, and caregivers make well-informed decisions about health care by preparing, updating, and promoting the accessibility of systematic reviews.

While the United States, Canada, and England were implementing EBM, in Australia, in response to the growing trend of evidence-based health care, the Joanna Briggs Institute was created at the Royal Adelaide Hospital in 1996 to facilitate evidence-based healthcare practice globally (Joanna Briggs Institute, 2014). The institute's original focus was on nursing, and later it changed to incorporating medicine and allied health practitioners. The institute's definition of evidence-based health care is consistent with early definitions of EBM, stating that clinical decisions should be based on best available scientific evidence while recognizing patient preferences, the context of health care, and the judgment of the clinician (Pearson, Wiechula, Court, & Lockwood, 2005).

NURSING AND EBP

Concern about overlooking the patient's values and preferences in the early definition of EBM by Guyatt et al. (1992) prompted nursing to adopt a definition similar to definitions written by Sackett et al. (1996) and the Joanna Briggs Institute. In 2000, Ingersoll (2000) articulated the following definition of evidence-based practice (EBP) for nursing:

> Evidence-based nursing practice is the conscientious, explicit, and judicious use of theory-derived, research-based information in making decisions about care delivery to individuals or groups of patients and in consideration of individual needs and preferences. (p. 154)

Unique to this EBP definition was the inclusion of the use of theory as well as evidence when making clinical practice decisions. Leaders in nursing believed that theory and clinical research should be the basis for evidence-based nursing instead of ritual, isolated, and unsystematic clinical experiences, ungrounded opinion, and tradition (Fain, 2009; Ingersoll, 2000). The goal of EBP is to promote effective nursing practice, efficient care, and improved outcomes for patients, as well as to provide the best available evidence for clinical, administrative, and educational decision making (Newhouse, Dearholt, Poe, Pugh, & White, 2007b). Key assumptions of EBP in nursing practice include the following:

1. Nursing is both a science and an applied profession.
2. Knowledge is important to professional practice, and there are limits to knowledge that must be identified.
3. Not all evidence is created equal, and there is a need to use the best available evidence.
4. Evidence-based practice contributes to improved outcomes.

Two educators and researchers in nursing, Melnyk and Fineout-Overholt (2011), define EBP using Sackett's definition as a platform and identify seven steps in the EBP process:

1. Cultivate a spirit of inquiry.
2. Ask a burning clinical question in PICOT (P = population; I = intervention; C = comparison; O = outcome; T = time) format.
3. Search for and collect the most relevant best evidence.
4. Critically appraise the evidence.
5. Integrate the best evidence with one's clinical expertise and patient preferences and values when making a practice decision or change.
6. Evaluate the outcomes of the practice decision or change based on evidence.
7. Disseminate the outcomes of the EBP decision or change.

All of these steps are vital to the effective implementation and integration of EBP in clinical settings.

Evidence-based practice for nursing is not EBM because it is imperative that many sources of evidence are critically appraised when making practice decisions. While randomized controlled trials or systematic reviews may provide the most rigorous scientific evidence for EBM, that evidence may not be applicable to nursing and patient care, which requires a holistic approach and a broad range of methodologies as the basis for care (Houser & Oman, 2011). No one research design is better than another when evaluating evidence on effective nursing practices, and appropriate clinical decision making can only be achieved by using several sources of evidence (DiCensco & Cullum, 1998; Rycroft-Malone, Seers, Titchen, Kitson, & McCormack, 2004).

A newer term in the nursing literature that further defines evidence in health care is *practice-based evidence* (Leeman & Sandelowski, 2012). Practice-based evidence includes "evidence concerning the contexts, experiences, and practices of healthcare providers working in real-world practice settings" (Leeman & Sandelowski, 2012, p. 171), and the use of qualitative methodologies play an essential role in creating more practice-based evidence in the evidence base for nursing practice used for clinical decision making.

Missing from the earlier definitions of EBM and EBP is clinical decision making related to available resources. The reality is that there is a limited amount of healthcare dollars. Therefore, when making evidence-based clinical decisions, nurses and other healthcare professionals must also weigh the cost of benefit, cost of harm, and cost to the system when providing evidence-based care (Hopp & Rittenmeyer, 2012).

Evidence-based practice is not unique to nursing. It is clear from the inception of EBM and EBP that all healthcare disciplines should be making decisions based on the best available evidence, clinical expertise, patient values and preferences, and available resources.

Why Should NPs Use EBP?

If you were diagnosed with breast cancer and were faced with the decision of whether to have a lumpectomy versus mastectomy and chemotherapy versus radiation, would you want your nurse practitioner (NP) to give you the best and latest information on treatment options and the risks and benefits associated with each treatment from randomized controlled trials (RCTs) or systematic reviews including patients with the same diagnosis and similar personal characteristics? Would you want to know about how others with your type of cancer coped with the treatment based on evidence from well-designed descriptive or qualitative studies?

There are many reasons why NPs should practice using EBP. First and foremost, as their basis of patient care, NPs should integrate research evidence with clinical evidence and patient values while considering available resources in order to provide the best care. Nurse practitioners should use the EBP paradigm to promote optimal patient outcomes, stimulate innovation in clinical practice, and promote the value of the nursing profession in the healthcare system (DeBourgh, 2001). In today's complex and dynamic patient-care environment, nursing practice informed by the best evidence is vital to realizing healthcare improvements and cost savings (Newhouse et al., 2007b). The role of the NP has expanded over the years to include a wider scope of practice in many states, thus prompting the need for all NPs to acquire EBP skills and use best current evidence for clinical decision making (Facchiano & Snyder, 2012a). Nurse practitioners need to practice using EBP because studies have shown that patient care outcomes are substantially improved when

health care is based on well-designed studies rather than relying on tradition and clinical expertise alone (Houser & Oman, 2011; Leufer & Cleary-Holdforth, 2009).

Existing practices based on tradition or clinical expertise may be harming patients. It is unethical to continue using untested interventions. Nurse practitioners need to use and understand the EBP process so they can take a lead role in facilitating the evaluation of evidence to develop EBP guidelines, form EBP teams, identify practices and systems that need study, and collaborate with nurse scientists to initiate research (Houser, 2015).

HOW TO TRANSLATE EBP INTO PRACTICE

Many EBP models exist that help to guide healthcare systems and their clinicians with implementing EBP policies, protocols, and guidelines. It is important for organizations or healthcare systems to have EBP models that assist clinicians with translating research evidence into the practice setting. A central goal of these EBP models is to speed up the transfer of new knowledge into practice, because in the past this has taken years. Use of a model provides an organized approach to EBP implementation and can maximize use of nursing time and resources (Gawlinski & Rutledge, 2008). There are several EBP models that help with translating research into practice. Common aspects of these models include the EBP process that identifies problems and practice questions and reviews latest evidence, existing clinical practices and practice guidelines, and other data specific to quality indicators in that setting. No one model of EBP exists that meets the needs of all nursing environments. For the purposes of this chapter, some of the more popular models are described in **Table 21-1**.

TABLE 21-1	Evidence-Based Practice Models

Model	Description	Processes
ACE Star (Stevens, 2004)	EBP framework for systematically putting EBP processes into operation	1. Knowledge discovery 2. Evidence summary 3. Translation into practice recommendations 4. Integration into practice 5. Evaluation
Advancing Research and Clinical Practice through Close Collaboration Model (ARCC Model) (Melnyk & Fineout-Overholt, 2011)	Provides healthcare systems with a guide for implementation and sustainability of EBP to achieve quality outcomes	1. Assessment of organizational culture and readiness for EBP 2. Identification of strengths and major barriers 3. Development and use of EBP mentors 4. EBP implementation
John's Hopkins Nursing Evidence-Based Practice Model (Newhouse et al., 2007a)	Assists nurses at the bedside in translating evidence to clinical, administrative, and educational practice	1. Practice question 2. Evidence 3. Translation
Iowa Model of Evidence-Based Practice to Promote Quality Care (Titler et al., 2001)	A guide for nurses and clinicians in making decisions about day-to-day practices that affect patient outcomes	1. Identify type of organizational trigger: problem or knowledge focused 2. Form a team 3. Gather and critically appraise evidence 4. Assess if sufficient evidence 5. Pilot practice change or conduct research 6. Evaluate pilot practice change 7. Institute practice change
Promoting Action on Research Implementation in Health Services Framework (PARIHS Framework) (Kitson, Harvey, & McCormack, 1998)	Provides healthcare systems a framework for how research findings can be successfully implemented into practice with equal recognition of level of evidence, the context into which the evidence is being implemented, and the method of facilitating the change	1. Critical appraisal of evidence 2. Gain understanding of practice area where change will happen 3. Create a strategic plan for practice change 4. Successful implementation is a function of evidence, context, and facilitation

(continues)

TABLE 21-1	Evidence-Based Practice Models *(continued)*

Model	Description	Processes
Model for EBP Change (Rosswurm & Larrabee, 1999)	Model for translating EBP into healthcare organization	1. Assess the need for change in practice 2. Locate the best evidence 3. Critically analyze the evidence 4. Design practice change 5. Implement and evaluate change in practice 6. Integrate and maintain change in practice
Transdisciplinary Model of EBP (Newhouse & Spring, 2010)	Interdisciplinary EBP model to accelerate the translation of EBP across disciplines	1. Primary researcher 2. Systematic reviewer 3. Practitioner
Trinity Evidence-Based Practice Model (Vratney & Shriver, 2007)	A conceptual model for EBP that addresses how to overcome barriers to implementation; a guide for growing EBP in your organization while weeding out barriers	1. Breaking ground 2. Planting seeds 3. Sprouting up 4. Showering of education 5. Heating things up 6. Branching out 7. Bearing fruit

The ACE Star model, ARCC, PARIHS, EBP Model for Change, and Trinity EBP model are all models or frameworks for systematically putting the EBP process into operation within a healthcare system. The Johns Hopkins Nursing EBP Model and the Iowa Model of Evidence-Based Practice to Promote Quality Care are geared toward clinical decision making at the bedside. The goal of the Transdisciplinary Model of EBP is to accelerate the translation of the EBP process across disciplines within an organization. In summary, there are many models and frameworks that nurse leaders can choose to help guide and integrate EBP into their healthcare system.

Developing a Searchable Question

Before you can find the best current evidence for clinical decision making, you must identify a clinical problem and translate it into a searchable, answerable question. The PICOT method is a widely accepted format for creating clinical questions. Melnyk and Fineout-Overholt (2011) have developed question templates for asking PICOT questions in nursing based on the type of clinical problem (e.g., intervention/therapy, prevention, diagnosis) (see **Figure 21-1**).

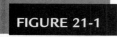

FIGURE 21-1   PICOT definition and questions.

The definition of PICOT is as follows:

P: Population/disease (age, gender, ethnicity, with a certain disorder)
I: Intervention or variable of interest (therapy, exposure to a disease, risk behavior, prognostic factor)
C: Comparison: (alternate therapy, placebo or usual practice, absence of risk factor)
O: Outcome: (risk of disease, accuracy of a diagnosis, rate of occurrence of adverse outcome)
T: Time: The time it takes to demonstrate an outcome (time it takes for the intervention to achieve an outcome or time populations are observed for outcome)

The templates for PICOT questions based on the type of clinical problem are as follows:

Intervention/therapy query:
In _____(P), how does _____(I) compare to _____(C) affect _____(O) within _____(T)?

Prevention query:
For _____ (P), does the use of _____ (I) reduce the future risk of _____ (O) compared with _____ (C)?

Prognosis/prediction query:
In _____(P), how does _____(I) compare to _____(C) influence/predict _____(O) over _____(T)?

Diagnosis or diagnostic test query:
In _____(P), are/is _____(I) compared with _____(C) more accurate in diagnosing _____(O)?

Etiology query:
Are _____(P) who have _____(I), compared with those without _____ (C), at _____risk for/of _____(O) over _____(T)?

Meaning query:
How do _____(P) with _____(I) perceive _____(O) during _____(T)?

Source: Melnyk, B., & Fineout-Overholt, E. (2010). *Evidence-based practice in nursing and healthcare*. Philadelphia, PA: Lippincott Williams & Wilkins. Reprinted by permission of Lippincott Williams & Wilkins.

PICOT Question Using Prevention Template

The clinical scenario involves a 72-year-old Hispanic female who is an Arizona winter visitor and is being seen at a routine office visit for recent hospitalization of congestive heart failure, her third one this year. As her NP, you wonder what other treatment modalities (e.g., telemedicine) may decrease readmissions, lead to better treatment compliance, and augment the existing provider–client relationship.

(continues)

PICOT Question Using Prevention Template *(continued)*

Population: Hospitalized adults with congestive heart failure

Intervention: Telemedicine

Comparison: Routine office visit

Outcome: Decrease readmission to hospital

Time: 1-year period

In adults hospitalized with congestive heart failure, does telemedicine compared to standard care (routine office visits) decrease readmission to the hospital for congestive heart failure over 1 year? (Facchiano and Snyder, 2012a)

PICOT Question Using Therapy Template

The clinical scenario involves you working as an NP in an urgent care late one night when a 2-year-old child presents with a 3-day history of rhinorrhea, cough, sneezing, nasal congestion, and no fever. Her 19-year-old mother is requesting an antibiotic. As her NP, you believe this is a viral nasopharyngitis, which does not require an antibiotic at this time, and you want to discuss antibiotic use with the child's mother. The PICOT question would be the following: In children between the ages of 2 and 5 with upper respiratory infections (P), does the use of an antibiotic (I) compared to no antibiotic (C) shorten the duration of the upper respiratory infection or illness (O)? (Facchiano & Snyder, 2012a)

SEARCHING DATABASES FOR BEST CURRENT EVIDENCE

Successful searching for the best current evidence after developing a PICOT question is the next step in the EBP process. Melnyk and Fineout-Overholt (2011) identified eight steps for an efficient search:

1. Begin with a PICOT question and the key words (e.g., P = hospitalized adult with congestive heart failure, I = telemedicine, C = routine office visit, O = readmission, T = 1 year) that will be used for the search.

2. Establish inclusion and exclusion criteria before searching (e.g., studies published in last 5 years).

3. Use controlled vocabulary headings when available (e.g., MeSH).

4. Expand search using explode option.

5. Use tools to limit the search so the topic of interest is the main point of article.

6. Combine searches generated from PICOT key words.

7. Limit final search results with meaningful limits, such as year, type of study, age, gender, and language.

8. Organize studies in a meaningful way using a matrix.

Bibliographic databases commonly used for searches by NPs include the Cochrane Library, Cumulative Index to Nursing and Allied

Health Literature (CINAHL), Medical Literature Online (MEDLINE), PubMed, the Joanna Briggs Institute Library, National Guideline Clearinghouse, and Embase. Several of these databases require a subscription fee. **Table 21-2** lists many databases that are useful for finding evidence on clinical problems, a description of the evidence that can be found, their website addresses, and whether they require a fee to access. In the following paragraphs some of the more popular databases are described in more detail.

The Cochrane Library is a collection of seven databases that may be used to find best current evidence in health care. The most popular database is the Cochrane Database of Systematic Reviews. This database contains systematic reviews of primary research in human health care and health policy. This database is maintained by the Cochrane Working Group, and their reviews are held to the highest scientific standards. Abstracts of reviews are available free of charge from the Cochrane website; however, full reviews are available by subscription. The Cochrane Database of Systematic Reviews is found online at http://www.cochrane.org/cochrane-reviews.

The CINAHL database produced by EBSCO Information Systems has more than 2.6 million records and provides indexing to more than 3,000 journals from nursing and allied health fields. In addition to journals, this database has publications from the National League for Nursing and American Nurses Association, references to healthcare books, nursing dissertations, legal cases, clinical innovations, critical paths, drug records, evidence-based care sheets, research instruments, and clinical trials. To access this database you need a subscription. You can access this database online at http://www.ebscohost.com/biomedical-libraries/the-cinahl-database.

The MEDLINE database is provided by the National Library of Medicine and is widely known as the premier source for bibliographic

and abstract coverage of biomedical literature. It has indices that reference more than 5,000 journals, and it includes at least 300 journals specific to nursing. PubMed is the National Library of Medicine's Web interface, through which MEDLINE can be accessed for free. PubMed has free tutorials on how to conduct searches. Abstracts are free as are some full text articles; otherwise, a fee is charged to retrieve full-text articles. A guide of MEDLINE and PubMed resources can be found at http://www.nlm.nih.gov/bsd/pmresources.html.

The Joanna Briggs Institute is an international collaboration involving nursing, medical, and allied health researchers, clinicians, academics, and quality managers across 40 countries around the world. The Joanna Briggs Institute connects healthcare professionals with the best available international evidence at the point of care. It offers systematic reviews, best practice information sheets, and critical appraisal tools. Some information is free, but most information is accessed by paying a fee. You can find out more about the Joanna Briggs Institute at http://www.joannabriggs.org/about.html.

The National Guideline Clearinghouse is a search engine for finding clinical practice guidelines. This database is available free of charge from the Agency for Healthcare Research and Quality and is a mechanism for obtaining objective, detailed information on clinical practice guidelines from all over the world. Guidelines can be searched using medical subject headings (MeSH) or by disease/condition, treatment/intervention, or health services administration. You can also sign up for email alerts about topics of interest. You can access the National Guideline Clearinghouse and browse by topic here: http://guideline.gov/browse/by-topic.aspx.

Embase (http://www.embase.com) is a subscription-based international biomedical and pharmaceutical database that includes more than 24 million indexed records and 7,600 peer-reviewed journals. All MEDLINE records

TABLE 21-2 Sources of Evidence

Name of Source	Type of Evidence	Access	Fee
ACP Smart Medicine (American College of Physicians—Physicians Information & Education Resource)	Includes guidelines and recommendations based on all levels of medical evidence including RCTs, cohort and observational studies, case reports, and expert opinions	http://www .acponline.org /clinical_ information /smart_medicine	ACP member /fee
Agency for Healthcare Research and Quality (AHRQ)	Clinical Information Effectiveness: ■ Evidence-based practice ■ Outcomes and effectiveness ■ Technology assessments Guidelines: ■ Preventive services ■ Clinical practice guidelines ■ National Guideline Clearinghouse	http://www.ahrq .gov	Free
Cochrane Collaboration	Cochrane Reviews	http://www .cochrane.org	Free abstract Subscription for full text
Center for Evidence-Based Medicine (Oxford)	Conferences, workshops, and EBM tools for how to access, appraise, and use evidence	http://www.cebm .net	Some free, some fee to access
Clinical Evidence	Database of best available evidence on common clinical interventions	http:// clinicalevidence. bmj.com	Subscription
CINAHL Plus with Full Text	Comprehensive nursing and allied health research database, providing full text for more than 770 journals Evidence-based care sheets	http://www .ebscohost.com /academic /cinahl-plus -with-full-text	Subscription
DARE: Database of Abstract Reviews of Effects	Contains 15,000 abstracts of systematic reviews	http://site.ovid .com/products /ovidguide /daredb.htm	Subscription
EBN Online, Evidence-Based Nursing	Electronic journal providing EBN	http://ebn.bmj .com	Subscription

(continues)

TABLE 21-2	**Sources of Evidence** *(continued)*		
Name of Source	**Type of Evidence**	**Access**	**Fee**
Embase	Core strengths of Embase include coverage and in-depth indexing of the drug-related and clinical literature, with a particular focus on comprehensive indexing of adverse drug reactions; emphasis on evidence-based medicine (EBM) indexing, including systematic reviews and coverage and indexing of journals and articles relevant to the development and use of medical devices	http://www.embase.com	Subscription
Joanna Briggs Institute	Reliable evidence for health professionals to use to inform their clinical decision making; tools for how to access, appraise, and use evidence	http://joannabriggs.org/jbi-education.html	Subscription
National Guideline Clearinghouse	A comprehensive free database of evidence-based clinical practice guidelines and related documents, an initiative of the Agency for Healthcare Research and Quality (AHRQ); browse the database by condition or treatment/intervention	http://www.guideline.gov	Free
NICE: National Institutes of Health and Clinical Excellence	NICE develops evidence-based clinical guidelines on the most effective ways to diagnose, treat, and prevent disease and ill health; also have patient-friendly versions of guidelines to help educate and empower patients, caregivers, and the public to take an active role in managing their conditions	http://www.nice.org.uk	Free
PubMed/MEDLINE/NLM	Provides free access to Medline and the NLM database of indexed citations and original abstracts in medicine, nursing, and health care; search tutorials; evidence-based medical reviews (EBMR)	http://www.ncbi.nlm.nih.gov/pubmed	Free abstracts Some free articles Subscription for full text

(continues)

TABLE 21-2	Sources of Evidence *(continued)*

Name of Source	Type of Evidence	Access	Fee
RePORT	Access to reports, data, and analyses of NIH research activities and the results of NIH-supported research	http://report.nih.gov	Free
Turning Research into Practice (TRIP) Database: For Evidence-Based Medicine	Meta-search engine for evidence-based healthcare topics; searches hundreds of EBM and EBN websites that contain synopses, clinical answers, textbook information, clinical calculators, systematic reviews, and guidelines	http://www.tripdatabase.com	Free
UpToDate	Clinical decision support system that combines the most recent evidence with the experience of expert clinicians	http://www.uptodate.com	Subscription
Worldviews on Evidence-Based Nursing	Evidence-based review journal	http://onlinelibrary.wiley.com/journal/10.1111/(ISSN)1741-6787	Subscription

produced by the National Library of Medicine are included, as well more than 5 million records not covered on MEDLINE. Embase has in-depth indexing of the drug-related and clinical literature, with a particular focus on comprehensive indexing of adverse drug reactions, systematic reviews, and development and use of medical devices.

Busy NPs with limited resources or limited time should start their search in PubMed because it is a free database that can be accessed via the Internet from any mobile device (Facchiano & Snyder, 2012b). Natural language or key words can be used for the search by typing in words from your PICOT question (e.g., *congestive heart failure*). Searches may also be done using controlled vocabulary called medical subject headings (MeSH). In PubMed, when you type in key words or

natural language you will automatically get MeSH, and you can click on these words and continue the search with these words. You can use built-in filters within PubMed to further refine the search. One example is the clinical queries filter that extracts evidence based on the best study design to answer that PICOT question. Boolean operators include *AND*, *OR*, and *NOT*. They can link key words and further define the search, such as *congestive heart failure and hospitalized adult*. Searches can be further defined using the limit feature. This feature includes many categories such as age, gender, English language, year of publication, and humans or animals. It is important to become familiar with how to do searches efficiently. PubMed offers free tutorials on how to search the database that can be accessed via the homepage.

WHAT COUNTS AS EVIDENCE?

Nurse practitioners use a variety of sources of evidence to make clinical decisions regarding diagnoses, treatments, and interventions on a daily basis. What is important to remember is that not all evidence is equally rigorous. Evidence from a textbook, colleague, or single journal article is not the same as evidence from a systematic review of randomized controlled trials that answers a particular research question. It is important to know that hierarchies for grading evidence vary between organizations or healthcare systems. In most hierarchies meta-analysis of systematic reviews is considered the highest level of evidence, with expert opinion being the lowest. In this section, select evidence hierarchies from different organizations in nursing and medicine will be described.

Melnyk and Fineout-Overholt (2011) established one of the earliest hierarchies of grading evidence in nursing to be used when critically appraising studies (**Table 21-3**). In this hierarchy, systematic reviews or meta-analysis of randomized controlled trials or clinical guidelines based on systematic reviews are the strongest levels of evidence. Expert opinion is the weakest level of evidence.

The American Association of Critical Care Nurses (AACN) created a new evidence-leveling system for all their publications, outlined in **Table 21-4** (Armola et al., 2009). The AACN's system is unique in that it includes meta-analysis of multiple controlled trials or meta-synthesis of qualitative studies in the highest level of evidence and manufacturer's recommendations in the lowest level of evidence. All new and revised AACN resources will include the new evidence-leveling system so practitioners have a reliable guide to determine the strongest evidence.

The Oxford Centre for Evidence-Based Medicine (OCEBM) 2011 Levels of Evidence is a hierarchy of evidences described in **Table 21-5**. The OCEBM hierarchy of evidences was designed to help busy clinicians, researchers, or patients find the best evidence. It is based on a series of questions in the areas of diagnosis, prognosis, treatment benefits, treatment harms, or screening. A clinician who needs to find the best evidence for

TABLE 21-3	Levels of Evidence Based on Research Design

Level	Evidence Type
1	Systematic review of randomized trials
	Meta-analysis of randomized trials
	Systematic review of nonrandomized trials
2	One or more randomized trials
3	Single nonrandomized trial
4	Systematic review of correlation/observational studies
5	Single case-control or cohort study
6	Systematic review of descriptive and qualitative studies
7	Single descriptive or qualitative study
8	Expert opinion

Source: Melnyk, B., & Fineout-Overholt, E. (2010). *Evidence-based practice in nursing & healthcare.* Philadelphia, PA: Lippincott Williams & Wilkins. Reprinted by permission of Lippincott Williams & Wilkins.

TABLE 21-4   AACN New Evidence-Leveling System

Level	Evidence Type
A	Meta-analysis of multiple controlled studies or meta-synthesis of qualitative studies with results that consistently support specific action, intervention, or treatment
B	Well-designed controlled studies, both randomized and nonrandomized, with results that consistently support a specific action, intervention, or treatment
C	Qualitative studies, descriptive or correlational studies, integrative reviews, systematic reviews, or randomized controlled trials with inconsistent results
D	Peer-reviewed professional organizational standards, with clinical studies to support recommendations
E	Theory-based evidence from expert opinion or multiple case reports
M	Manufacturers' recommendations only

Source: Armola, R. R., Bourgault, A. M., Halm, M. A., Board, R. M., Bucher, L., Harrington, L., . . . Medina, J. (2009). AACN levels of evidence: What's new? © AACN. *Critical Care Nurse*, *29*(4), 70–73. Reprinted by permission.

TABLE 21-5   OCEBM Levels of Evidence

Type of Question	Level of Evidence
Intervention	
Diagnostic or diagnostic test	1. Systematic review/meta-analysis (i.e., synthesis) of RCTs 2. RCTs 3. Nonrandomized controlled trials 4. Cohort study or case-control studies 5. Meta-synthesis of qualitative or descriptive studies 6. Qualitative or descriptive single studies 7. Expert opinion
Prognosis/prediction or etiology	1. Synthesis of cohort study or case-control studies 2. Single cohort study or case-control studies 3. Meta-synthesis of qualitative or descriptive studies 4. Single qualitative or descriptive studies 5. Expert opinion
Meaning	1. Meta-synthesis of qualitative or descriptive studies 2. Single qualitative studies 3. Synthesis of descriptive studies 4. Expert opinion

Source: OCEBM Levels of Evidence Working Group, 2011. Reprinted by permission.

a treatment benefits-and-harms clinical query should look for systematic reviews of randomized trials first because they usually provide the most reliable answers. If no evidence is found, the search should continue with individual randomized trials, and so on down the OCEBM Levels of Evidence table (OCEBM Levels of Evidence Working Group, 2011).

In summary, it is important for NPs to use the highest level of evidence available to make clinical decisions and to use an existing hierarchy of evidence to rate the evidence level. However, highest levels of evidence such as meta-analyses or systematic reviews of RCTs may not always be available in the literature, and this should be considered when making clinical decisions.

CRITICAL APPRAISAL OF EVIDENCE

Critical appraisal of evidence is an important step in the EBP process that comes after the search for best current evidence. Publication of research studies and other types of evidence does not guarantee quality, value, or applicability to clinical practice. Clinicians must have strong research literacy, including knowledge of research methods and the skills to critically appraise sources of evidence.

In EBP, evidence sources may include quantitative or qualitative research studies or reviews, clinical expertise, and patient preferences and values. Many types of critical appraisal tools ask specific questions based on a particular research methodology or design. It is important to pick the correct critical appraisal tool based on research methodology or design of the study you are critically appraising. Regardless of which tool is selected, it is important to remember that the goal of critical appraisal is to identify strengths and weaknesses of the evidence, weigh strengths and weaknesses within the clinical context, including patient values and preferences, and make a judgment as to whether the evidence will help the patients in your care.

Several critical appraisal tools that NPs can use to generate appropriate critical questions and make a determination regarding the quality of the evidence are described in **Table 21-6**.

TABLE 21-6　Critical Appraisal Tools for Different Sources of Evidence

Author	Tool	Research Method	Access
Johns Hopkins Nursing Evidence-Based Practice Research Evidence Appraisal	Research appraisal questions organized by research design	RCTs Meta-analysis of RCTs Quasi-experimental Nonexperimental Qualitative Meta-synthesis of qualitative studies	Newhouse, R. P., Dearholt, S., Poe, S., Pugh, L. C., & White, K. (2007a). *Johns Hopkins evidence-based practice model and guideline.* Indianapolis, IN: Sigma Theta Tau International.
Melnyk and Fineout-Overholt	Rapid Critical Appraisal (RCA) Checklist; method specific	Case-control Cohort RCTs Systematic reviews Qualitative	Melnyk, B. M., & Fineout-Overholt, E. (2011). *Evidence-based practice in nursing and health care: A guide to best practice second edition.* Philadelphia, PA: Lippincott Williams & Wilkins.

(continues)

TABLE 21-6 Critical Appraisal Tools for Different Sources of Evidence *(continued)*

Author	Tool	Research Method	Access
Fain	Research Appraisal Checklist	All types of research methods	Fain, J. (2009). *Reading, understanding, and applying nursing research* (3rd ed.). Philadelphia, PA: F. A. Davis.
Joanna Briggs Institute	RAPid Critical Appraisal Program (RAPCAP)	Prognostic studies Intervention studies Risk studies Cost studies Qualitative studies Systematic reviews Diagnostic studies	http://connect.jbiconnectplus.org/Appraise.aspx
Centre for Evidence-Based Medicine	Critical Appraisal Sheets	Systematic Prognostic Diagnostic RCT Educational prescription	http://www.cebm.net/index.aspx?o=1157
Solutions for Public Health Critical Appraisal Skills Programme	CASP critical appraisal checklists	Systematic reviews RCTs Qualitative research Economic evaluation studies Cohort studies Case-control studies Diagnostic studies Clinical prediction rule	http://www.casp-uk.net
Craig Hospital, Englewood, CO	Appraisal support tool in the form of a bookmark	All types of research methods	(See Figure 21-2.)
Critical Appraisal Tools for Clinical Guidelines			
U.S. Preventive Services Task Force (USPSTF)	Recommendation grades and suggestions	Clinical practice guidelines	http://www.uspreventiveservicestaskforce.org

(continues)

TABLE 21-6	Critical Appraisal Tools for Different Sources of Evidence *(continued)*		
Author	**Tool**	**Research Method**	**Access**
The Agree Collaboration	AGREE II Instrument	Clinical practice guidelines	http://www.agreetrust.org
The International Centre for Allied Health Evidence (iCAHE), UniSA, Australia	iCAHE	Clinical guideline checklist	http://www.unisa.edu.au /Research/Sansom-Institute-for -Health-Research /Research-at-the-Sansom /Research-Concentrations /Allied-Health-Evidence /Resources/CAT /#Clinical-Guidelines
Melnyk and Fineout-Overholt	RCA for Evidence-Based Guidelines	Clinical guideline checklist	Melnyk, B. M., & Fineout-Overholt, E. (2011). *Evidence-based practice in nursing and health care: A guide to best practice* (2nd ed.). Philadelphia, PA: Lippincott Williams & Wilkins.

The main purpose of these tools is to provide a means for clinicians to rapidly appraise evidence and quickly determine whether the evidence is valid and applicable to practice. The Johns Hopkins Nursing EBP Model, Melnyk and Fineout-Overholt (2011), the Joanna Briggs Institute, Oxford England Centre for Evidence-Based Medicine, and Solutions for Public Health have developed separate checklists based on research design. A general critical appraisal checklist has been developed by Craig Hospital in Colorado and Fain (2009). Craig Hospital made their checklist into a bookmark that nurses can easily carry in their pocket and use as a quick guide when reading research (**Figure 21-2**). The Fain (2009) checklist can be obtained on a disc; clinicians answer a series of questions, and a score is calculated—the higher the score, the stronger the level of evidence.

Nurse practitioners should be able to rapidly appraise the strength of clinical practice guidelines and the quality of evidence used to create the guidelines. Guidelines should be critically appraised in terms of validity, usefulness, when last updated, and clinical context, including environment and patient values and preferences. Rapid critical appraisal checklists for clinical practice guidelines have been developed by Melnyk and Fineout-Overholt (2011), the AGREE Collaboration, and the International Center for Allied Health Evidence (iCAHE). Table 21-6 contains a listing of the tools for appraising clinical guidelines and the websites where they can be accessed.

The AGREE II tool is a refinement of the original AGREE instrument released in 2003 (Brouwers et al., 2010). The AGREE II tool is both valid and reliable with 23 items organized into the original domains of scope and purpose, stakeholder involvement, rigor of development, clarity of presentation, applicability, and editorial independence. Each of

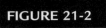

FIGURE 21-2 Craig Hospital critical appraisal tool.

Credibility: • Authors' credentials • Credibility of publication • No evidence of conflict of interest	**Level I evidence:** Multiple studies reported as meta-analysis, systematic review, or integrative review, or an evidence-based practice guideline Well-designed studies with large sample sizes or large effect sizes
Validity: • Research question has PICO elements (below) • Clear design matches the question • Extraneous variables controlled • Instrument reliability and validity (> 0.7) • Sampling procedure (key: randomness) • Sample size/power (> 80%) • Results reported clearly • Evidence of significance (P < .05)	**Level II evidence:** Evidence from at least one well-designed randomized trial Single randomized trials with small samples Single studies with small to moderate effect sizes
Generalizability: • Sample represents similar patients • Setting is similar	**Level III evidence:** IIIA: Evidence from well-designed trials without randomization IIIB: Evidence from studies of intact groups Ex post facto and causal-comparative studies Case/control or cohort studies
Elements of research question: P: Population I: Intervention or trait of interest C: Comparison group or time O: Outcome of interest	
Evaluating a research opportunity: F: Feasible I: Interesting N: Novel E: Ethical R: Relevant	IIIC: Evidence obtained from time series with and without an intervention Single experimental or quasi-experimental studies with dramatic effect sizes
Linking evidence to practice: Level I: Required Level II: Recommended Level III: Recommended Level IV: Optional	**Level IV evidence:** Evidence from expert panels Systematic reviews of descriptive studies Case series and uncontrolled studies

Source: Journal Club Critique Book Mark. Research/EBP/Quality Committee, Craig Hospital, Englewood, CO. Used with permission.

the 23 items focuses on an area of practice guideline quality. The AGREE II also includes two overall guideline assessment items where the appraiser rates the overall quality of the practice guideline and makes a determination of whether or not to use the practice guideline (see **Table 21-7**).

The iCAHE guideline checklist provides clinicians with a quick way of appraising the quality of a clinical guideline. It consists of

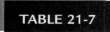

TABLE 21-7   AGREE II Instrument

Scope and Purpose

The overall objective(s) of the guideline is (are) specifically described.

The health question(s) covered by the guideline is (are) specifically described.

The population (patients, public, etc.) to whom the guideline is meant to apply is specifically described.

Stakeholder Involvement

The guideline development group includes individuals from all relevant professional groups.

The views and preferences of the target population (patients, public, etc.) have been sought.

The target users of the guideline are clearly defined.

Rigor of Development

Systematic methods were used to search for evidence.

The criteria for selecting the evidence are clearly described.

The strengths and limitations of the body of evidence are clearly described.

The methods for formulating the recommendations are clearly described.

The health benefits, side effects, and risks have been considered in formulating the recommendations.

There is an explicit link between the recommendations and the supporting evidence.

The guideline has been externally reviewed by experts prior to its publication.

A procedure for updating the guideline is provided.

Clarity of Presentation

The recommendations are specific and unambiguous.

The different options for management of the condition or health issue are clearly presented.

Key recommendations are easily identifiable.

Applicability

The guideline describes facilitators and barriers to its application.

The guideline provides advice and/or tools on how the recommendations can be put into practice.

The potential resource implications of applying the recommendations have been considered.

The guideline presents monitoring and/or auditing criteria.

Editorial Independence

The views of the funding body have not influenced the content of the guideline.

Competing interests of guideline development group members have been recorded and addressed.

Overall Guideline Assessment

Rate overall quality of guideline.

I would recommend this guideline for use.

14 questions and can be used either as a checklist or a total score (see **Table 21-8**). Questions are organized into six areas: availability, dates, underlying evidence, guideline developers, guideline purpose and users, and ease of use.

Grading recommendation systems have been created to assist the clinician with evaluating the strength of recommendations and quality of underlying evidence that the clinical guideline is based upon. The strength of a recommendation reflects the extent to which the clinician can be confident that the clinical

guideline has the desired effect rather than the undesired effect (Guyatt et al., 2008). A systematic approach in the grading of recommendations is important in order to cut down on bias and aid in the interpretation of clinical guidelines developed by experts. Two examples of grading systems are the United States Preventative Services Task Force (USPSTF) and the GRADE approach that is used by clinical decision-making systems like UpToDate.

The USPSTF grading system is displayed in **Table 21-9**. In this system Grade A is the

TABLE 21-8	The iCAHE Guideline Checklist for Critical Appraisal of Clinical Guidelines

Availability

Is the guideline readily available in full text?

Does the guideline provide a complete reference list?

Does the guideline provide a summary of its recommendations?

Dates

Is there a date of completion available?

Does the guideline provide an anticipated review date?

Does the guideline provide dates for when literature was included?

Underlying evidence

Does the guideline provide an outline of the strategy they used to find underlying evidence?

Does the guideline use a hierarchy to rank the quality of the underlying evidence?

Does the guideline appraise the quality of the evidence that underpins its recommendations?

Does the guideline link the hierarchy and quality of underlying evidence to each recommendation?

Guideline developers

Are the developers of the guideline clearly stated?

Do the qualifications and expertise of the guideline developer(s) link with the purpose of the guideline and its end users?

Guideline purpose and users

Are the purpose and target users of the guideline stated?

Ease of use

Is the guideline readable and easy to navigate?

Source: iCAHE Guideline Checklist. International Centre for Allied Health Evidence (iCAHE). http://unisa.edu.au/cahe

TABLE 21-9	USPSTF Task Force Recommendation Grades and Suggestions

Grade	Grade Definitions	Suggestions for Practice
A	The USPSTF recommends the service. There is high certainty that the net benefit is substantial.	Offer or provide this service.
B	The USPSTF recommends the service. There is high certainty that the net benefit is moderate or there is moderate certainty that the net benefit is moderate to substantial.	Offer or provide this service.
C	*Note: The following statement is undergoing revision.* Clinicians may provide this service to selected patients depending on individual circumstances. However, for most individuals without signs or symptoms, there is likely to be only a small benefit from this service.	Offer or provide this service only if other considerations support offering or providing the service in an individual patient.
D	The USPSTF recommends against the service. There is moderate or high certainty that the service has no net benefit or that the harms outweigh the benefits.	Discourage the use of this service.
I Statement	The USPSTF concludes that the current evidence is insufficient to assess the balance of benefits and harms of the service. Evidence is lacking, of poor quality, or conflicting, and the balance of benefits and harms cannot be determined.	Read the clinical considerations section of USPSTF Recommendation Statement. If the service is offered, patients should understand the uncertainty about the balance of benefits and harms.

Source: USPSTF Task Force. (2013, February). Grade definitions. Retrieved from http://www.uspreventiveservicestaskforce .org/uspstf/grades.htm. The USPSTF, AHRQ, or U.S. Department of Health and Human Services endorsement of such derivative products may not be stated or implied.

strongest recommendation, and clinicians should offer this service to their patients. Grade D is the weakest recommendation, and clinicians should not provide this service to patients. There is an additional recommendation of Grade I, which means clinicians should proceed with caution, and patients who want the service need to be aware of the uncertainty of the benefits and harms. Clinicians can visit the website and access free clinical guidelines for many clinical categories (e.g., cancer, heart and vascular diseases, mental health conditions).

The guidelines are created by rigorously evaluating clinical research and assessing the merits of preventive measures, including screening tests, counseling, immunizations, and preventive medications. The USPSTF provides a grade for each clinical guideline.

In the GRADE approach, recommendations are classified as strong or weak, according to the balance between desirable effects (health benefits, less burden, cost savings) versus undesirable effects (harms, more burdens, costs). A strong recommendation means that the most informed patients would choose the recommended management, and clinicians can recommend the intervention to patients. Weak recommendations mean the intervention has too many undesirable consequences (Guyatt et al., 2008). The GRADE approach also includes quality of evidence and patient preferences. UpToDate, a clinical decision system, uses the GRADE approach (see **Table 21-10**). In this system, a grade of 1A means a strong recommendation to use this intervention and the guideline has high-quality evidence backing it. Conversely, a grade of 2C means a weak recommendation with low-quality evidence, and other options should be explored.

TABLE 21-10	UpToDate Grading System for Clinical Practice Recommendations

Grade of Recommendation	Clarity of Risk/Benefit	Quality of Supporting Evidence	Implications
1A Strong recommendation, high-quality evidence	Benefits clearly outweigh risks and burdens, or vice versa.	Consistent evidence from well-performed randomized controlled trials or overwhelming evidence of some other form. Further research is unlikely to change our confidence in the estimate of benefit and risk.	Strong recommendation, can apply to most patients in most circumstances without reservation. Clinicians should follow a strong recommendation unless a clear and compelling rationale for an alternative approach is present.
1B Strong recommendation, moderate-quality evidence	Benefits clearly outweigh risks and burdens, or vice versa.	Evidence from randomized controlled trials with important limitations (inconsistent results, methodologic flaws, indirect or imprecise), or very strong evidence of some other research design. Further research (if performed) is likely to have an impact on our confidence in the estimate of benefit and risk and may change the estimate.	Strong recommendation and applies to most patients. Clinicians should follow a strong recommendation unless a clear and compelling rationale for an alternative approach is present.
1C Strong recommendation, low-quality evidence	Benefits appear to outweigh risks and burdens, or vice versa.	Evidence from observational studies, unsystematic clinical experience, or from randomized, controlled trials with serious flaws. Any estimate of effect is uncertain.	Strong recommendation, and applies to most patients. Some of the evidence base supporting the recommendation is, however, of low quality.

(continues)

| TABLE 21-10 | | UpToDate Grading System for Clinical Practice Recommendations *(continued)* |

Grade of Recommendation	Clarity of Risk/Benefit	Quality of Supporting Evidence	Implications
2B Weak recommendation, moderate-quality evidence	Benefits closely balanced with risks and burdens, some uncertainty in the estimates of benefits, risks, and burdens.	Evidence from randomized, controlled trials with important limitations (inconsistent results, methodologic flaws, indirect or imprecise), or very strong evidence of some other research design. Further research (if performed) is likely to have an impact on our confidence in the estimate of benefit and risk and may change the estimate.	Weak recommendation, alternative approaches likely to be better for some patients under some circumstances.
2C Weak recommendation, low-quality evidence	Uncertainty in the estimates of benefits, risks, and burdens; benefits may be closely balanced with risks and burdens.	Evidence from observational studies, unsystematic clinical experience, or from randomized controlled trials with serious flaws. Any estimate of effect is uncertain.	Very weak recommendation; other alternatives may be equally reasonable.

Source: Reproduced with permission from: UpToDate, Post TW (Ed), UpToDate, Waltham, MA, and GRADE (http://www.gradeworkinggroup.org). Copyright © 2014 UpToDate, Inc. For more information visit www.uptodate.com and www.gradeworkinggroup.org.

EVIDENCE SYNTHESIS

As noted early in this chapter, the EBP process begins with a clinical question using the PICOT format. The next step is identification of a search strategy that is most likely to uncover relevant studies. Once the relevant studies are collected, a critical appraisal tool or a critical appraisal method should be used to appraise the evidence from each study. The next step is to assign a level of evidence designation or grade to each study using one of the many levels of evidence hierarchies or grading systems if it is a clinical guideline. The next step is to organize all the important pieces of each study in a meaningful way, and this can be done by using an evidence table. Using Word or Excel software, you may create an entry for each study by using a summary of evidence table (**Table 21-11**) and filling in each column with the appropriate information. **Table 21-12** is an evidence evaluation table created by Facchiano and Snyder (2012c), and it incorporates the PICOT format. The underlying concept is to choose a table format that will help you organize evidence from studies in the most efficient manner.

TABLE 21-11 Summary of Evidence Table

Citation	Level of Evidence	Theo-retical Framework	Study Design	Country	Sample Character-istics/Size Setting	Major Variables	Scales/ Instrument	Results/ Findings	Implica-tions/ Conclu-sions
Study 1 Author, Year, Title	Assign a value using one of the level-of-evidence systems	Theoretical basis for study	Indicate the design and briefly describe what was done in the study	Country in which study takes place	Sampling method, character-istics of sample/ setting, number of sub-jects, and attri-tion rate (explain why)	Indepen-dent and depen-dent variables	What scales were used to mea-sure the outcome variables, such as name of scale, author, reliability and validity info (e.g., Cronbach's alpha)	Statistical findings	Strengths and limi-tations of the study Feasibility of use in your practice
Study 2, etc.									

TABLE 21-12 Evidence Summary Table for Randomized or Nonrandomized Trials

Citation	Funding Source	Level of Evidence	Purpose/ Research Design	Intervention/ Comparison Group Results	Strengths/ Weaknesses	Worth to Practice
Authors and title	*Funding agency, note any conflicts*	*Use level-of-evidence table from this chapter*	*Number of subjects invited to participate, attrition rate, trial length*	*Describe intervention group and comparison group*	*Critically appraise study using appropriate critical appraisal tool*	*Clinical significance*
Study 1						
Study 2						

TABLE 21-13	Evidence Synthesis		
Citation	Major Strengths	Major Weaknesses	Level of Evidence
Study 1 Author, Year			
Study 2			

The next step in the EBP process after organizing studies in a meaningful way using a matrix involves synthesis of the evidence from the individual studies. This can be done using an evidence synthesis table (**Table 21-13**). Depending on the study characteristics that you want to focus on in the synthesis, the ultimate purpose of the evidence synthesis table is to display how the studies are different and how they are alike. Sometimes the evidence synthesis table reveals lots of strong evidence and supports a practice change, or there may be no evidence or very weak evidence available, and you find that you may need to conduct your own study in order to gather evidence.

In summary, this is a three-step process that includes a summary of evidence (matrix); judgments about your evidence (LOE); and conclusions made from comparisons of the different evidence you have gathered based on characteristics that are important to your inquiry (PICOT question). Some characteristics that may drive your evidence synthesis are such issues as the clinical problem that prompted the search for evidence; variations in methodologies among the sources of evidence such as design, sampling, subjects, measures (scales/instruments), or analysis; conflicting findings among evidence; or missing or inadequate inquiries in the evidence.

CRITICAL APPRAISAL OF A SINGLE INTERVENTION STUDY

It is probable as an NP that you will hear about results from a single randomized clinical trial and ask, "Should I incorporate these findings into my practice?" To answer this question you should follow the EBP process from the critical appraisal step. Read the study abstract to assess whether the study is relevant to your practice and patients in your practice. If the clinical problem is one you encounter frequently, then you should read the whole article to determine whether the treatment is feasible given the resources in your practice (Kania-Lachance, Best, McDonah, & Ghosh, 2006). The next step is to determine the effect of the treatment and weigh the risks versus the benefits. This can be done by looking at number needed to treat (NNT) and absolute relative risk, otherwise known as the effect size. The absolute risk reduction (ARR) compares the event rate in the treatment group to the event rate in the control group. If a study found 80% of patients in the treatment group improved and 20% of patients in the control group improved, the ARR would be 80% − 20% = 60%. The NNT is calculated by dividing 100 by the ARR: 100 / 60 = 1.6; so, for every two patients exposed to the treatment, one will benefit. After validating the findings from the study, the last step is to determine whether patients in your practice mirror the patients described in the study. If this were a real-life example and your patients' values and preferences were open to the treatment, costs were low, and the treatment could be easily adopted into your setting, then you would adopt this new treatment.

BARRIERS TO EBP

There are a variety of reasons that EBP has not been adopted as a standard nursing practice. Houser and Oman (2011) identified three categories associated with barriers to using evidence in clinical practice. The first category includes limitations in EBP systems caused by an overwhelming amount of evidence and sometimes contradictory findings in the research. The second category is human factors that create barriers. These factors include lack of knowledge about EBP and skills needed to conduct EBP, nurses' negative attitudes toward research and evidence-based care, nurses' perception that research is only for medicine and is a cookbook approach, and patient expectations. The last category is the lack of organizational systems or infrastructure to support clinicians using EBP. Causes for barriers in this category include lack of authority for clinicians to make changes in practice, peer emphasis on practicing the way they always have practiced, lack of time during the workday, lack of administrative support or incentives, and conflicting priorities between unit work and research.

These barriers may seem overwhelming; however, all healthcare-related disciplines are becoming evidence based, and professional organizations, accrediting bodies, insurers, and third-party payers are requiring nurses to use evidence to support clinical practices and decision making. Therefore, organizations need to address these barriers and put systems in place to support EBP.

SUMMARY

Evidence-based nursing practice is the conscientious, explicit, and judicious use of theory-derived, research-based information in making decisions about care delivery to individuals or groups of patients and considers individual needs and preferences. It is vital to a practice-based profession such as nursing to use the best current evidence when making clinical practice decisions. All types of research methodologies are important when gathering and appraising evidence for making practice decisions within the discipline of nursing. There are several steps in the EBP process, beginning with fostering a spirit of inquiry, asking the right clinical question in a PICOT format, finding the best current evidence, critically appraising the evidence, and integrating the synthesis of evidence with patient values and preferences. (See the following boxed text.) Best current evidence can be found in many web-based electronic databases, such as the Cochrane Database of Systematic Reviews. There are several databases for clinical practice guidelines, including the National Guideline Clearinghouse and American College of Physicians ACP Smart Medicine. General quantitative or qualitative tools or checklists specific to study design type exist to assist clinicians with rapidly appraising evidence. There are also tools to help clinicians critically appraise clinical practice guidelines. Different systems exist for grading the level of evidence based on study design. Once the evidence is appraised and synthesized, clinicians need to incorporate patient values and preferences and make a clinical practice decision. Once the clinical practice guideline or practice decision is in place, NPs should evaluate how the practice is working.

TEMPLATE FOR EBP PROJECT

Identify Clinical Problem and Stakeholders

- Identify and describe a practice-based problem (e.g., clinical, administrative, or education).
- Identify the stakeholders. Who is this important to? Include a brief overview addressing who, what, when, why, where, and how. Analyze appropriate client needs and healthcare goals, staff needs and goals (include all appropriate members of the healthcare team), and healthcare delivery system concerns that are affected by the project.

(continued)

- Give the rationale for choosing this problem.
- Discuss how the project fits with the mission of the organization or healthcare system strategic plan.
- Does the organization or healthcare system follow an EBP model? If yes, describe.
- Discuss in a broader context how the project relates to local—and to global—healthcare trends, systems, policy, professional standards, clinical practice guidelines, and so on.
- Include the central phenomena, concepts, or variables under study.
- Identify an EBP mentor.
- Discuss with whom on the interdisciplinary team you will be collaborating.
- Write PICOT questions using one of the templates from this chapter.

Find the Evidence and Critically Appraise It

- Conduct a literature search using appropriate databases and key words from your PICOT question or MeSH triggered from PICOT key words. Identify filters and search limits. Save your search history. Retain studies that meet inclusion criteria.
- Consult with a librarian regarding optimal search techniques.
- Critically appraise evidence from your search results using an appropriate critical appraisal checklist.
- For clinical practice guidelines, note the grading system used to evaluate the strength of evidence.
- Organize individual study, review, or guideline data into a matrix format using one of the templates in this chapter.
- Consult with your EBP mentor to discuss how completely your summary of evidence table answers the PICOT question.
- Based on your EBP mentor's feedback, you may need to search for more evidence or refine your search.
- Summarize the evidence in an evidence synthesis table using a template from this chapter.

Plan and Implement Practice Change

- Write out your project protocol.
- State the outcomes for the proposed project in specific, measurable terms.
- State and sequence objectives in terms of specific resources, time lines, strategies, and responsible parties for each outcome.
- Define baseline data collection sources, methods, and measures.
- Define the design, sampling methods, data collection procedures, and data analysis.
- Consult with your EBP mentor for feedback on the project protocol.
- Obtain IRB approval if appropriate.
- Implement your EBP project.

Results

- Report results of project evaluation to stakeholders.
- If the organization or healthcare system has a venue for dissemination of project results, obtain a date to present findings. Otherwise, consult with your EBP mentor about the best venue for presenting your project results.

Conclusions

- Review project progress, lessons learned, and new questions generated from the EBP process.
- If applicable, consult with your EBP mentor about new questions.

DISCUSSION QUESTIONS

1. Explain the steps of the EBP process.
2. Develop a checklist that you can use in clinical practice to create a searchable question, and identify the databases that will be most useful for finding evidence.
3. Sign up for clinical practice alerts from the TRIP database in your specialty area.
4. Think about a patient problem you have had in the clinical setting and answer the following:
   a. What formal structures were in place to help you address the problem?
   b. How did you use evidence to investigate the problem?
   c. Did you have time to search for evidence? If no, what were the barriers?
   d. What databases did you access for evidence and why?
5. Go to http://www.guideline.gov and search for chronic pain management clinical practice guidelines. Compare and contrast two guidelines.

REFERENCES

American Association of Critical-Care Nurses (AACN). (2012). AACN practice alerts. Retrieved from http://www.aacn.org/practicealerts

Armola, R. R., Bourgault, A. M., Halm, M. A., Board, R. M., Bucher, L., Harrington, L., . . . Medina, J. (2009). AACN levels of evidence: What's new? *Critical Care Nurse, 29*(4), 70–73. Retrieved from http://ccn.aacnjournals.org/content/29/4/70.full

Brouwers, M., Kho, M. E., Browman, G. P., Burgers, J. S., Cluzeau, F., Feder, G., . . . Zitzelsberger, L., for the AGREE Next Steps Consortium. (2010). AGREE II: Advancing guideline development, reporting and evaluation in healthcare. *Canadian Medical Association Journal.* doi:10.1503/cmaj.090449

Cochrane Collaboration. (2012). Our principles. Retrieved from http://www.cochrane.org/about-us/our-principles

DeBourgh, G. A. (2001). Champions for evidence-based practice: A critical role for advanced practice nurses. *AACN Clinical Issues, 12*(4), 491–508.

DiCensco, A., & Cullum, N. (1998). Implementing evidence-based nursing: Some misconceptions. *Evidence-Based Nursing Journal, 1*(2), 38–40.

Facchiano, L., & Snyder, C. H. (2012a). Evidence-based practice for the busy nurse practitioner: Part one: Relevance to clinical practice and clinical inquiry process. *Journal of the American Academy of Nurse Practitioners, 24*(10), 579–586.

Facchiano, L., & Snyder, C. H. (2012b). Evidence-based practice for the busy nurse practitioner: Part two: Searching for the best evidence for clinical queries. *Journal of the American Academy of Nurse Practitioners, 24*(11), 640–648.

Facchiano, L., & Snyder, C. H. (2012c). Evidence-based practice for the busy nurse practitioner: Part four:

Putting it all together. *Journal of the American Academy of Nurse Practitioners, 25*(1), 24–31.

Fain, J. (2009). *Reading, understanding, and applying nursing research* (3rd ed.). Philadelphia, PA: F. A. Davis.

Gawlinski, A., & Rutledge, D. (2008). Selecting a model for evidence-based practice changes: A practical approach. *AACN Advances in Critical Care, 19*(3), 291–300.

Guyatt, G., Cairns, D. C., Cook, D., Haynes, B., Hirsh, J., Irvine, J., . . . Tugwell, P. (1992). Evidence-based medicine: A new approach to teaching the practice of medicine. *Journal of the American Medical Association, 268*(17), 2420–2425.

Guyatt, G. H., Haynes, R. B., Jaeschke, R. Z., Cook, D. J., Green, L., Naylor, C. D., . . . Richardson, W. S. (2000). Users' Guides to the Medical Literature: XXV. Evidence-based medicine: Principles for applying the Users' Guides to patient care. Evidence-Based Medicine Working Group. *Journal of the American Medical Association, 284*(10), 1290–1296.

Guyatt, G., Oxman, A., Vist, G., Kunz, R., Falck-Ytter, Y., Alonso-Coello, P., . . . GRADE Working Group. (2008). GRADE: An emerging consensus on rating quality of evidence and strength of recommendations. *BMJ* (Clinical Research Ed.), *336*(7650), 924–926.

Hopp, L., & Rittenmeyer, L. (2012). *Introduction to evidence-based practice: A guide for nursing.* Philadelphia, PA: F. A. Davis.

Houser, J. (2015). *Nursing research: Reading, using, and creating evidence* (3rd ed.). Burlington, MA: Jones & Bartlett.

Houser, J., & Oman, K. S. (2011). *Evidence-based practice: An implementation guide for healthcare organizations.* Burlington, MA: Jones & Bartlett.

Ingersoll, G. L. (2000). Evidence-based nursing: What it is and what it isn't. *Nursing Outlook, 48*(4), 151–152.

International Centre for Allied Health Evidence. *iCAHE Guideline Quality Checklist.* Retrieved from http://www.unisa.edu.au/Global/Health/Sansom/Documents/iCAHE/iCAHE%20Guideline%20Quality%20Checklist.pdf

Joanna Briggs Institute. (2014). About us. Retrieved from http://www.joannabriggs.org/about.html

Kania-Lachance, D. M., Best, P. J. M., McDonah, M. R., & Ghosh, A. K. (2006). Evidence-based practice and the nurse practitioner. *Nurse Practitioner, 31*(10), 46–54.

Kitson, A., Harvey, G., & McCormack, B. (1998). Enabling the implementation of evidence based practice: A conceptual framework. *Quality in Health Care, 7*(3), 149–158.

Leeman, J., & Sandelowski, M. (2012). Practice-based evidence and qualitative inquiry. *Journal of Nursing Scholarship, 44*(2), 171–179.

Leufer, T., & Cleary-Holdforth, J. (2009). Evidence-based practice: Improving patient outcomes. *Nursing Standard, 23*(32), 35–39.

Melnyk, B., & Fineout-Overholt, E. (2010). *Evidence-based practice in nursing and healthcare.* Philadelphia, PA: Lippincott Williams & Wilkins.

Melnyk, B. M., & Fineout-Overholt, E. (2011). *Evidence-based practice in nursing and health care: A guide to best practice* (2nd ed.). Philadelphia, PA: Lippincott Williams & Wilkins.

Newhouse, R. P., Dearholt, S., Poe, S., Pugh, L. C., & White, K. (2007a). *Johns Hopkins evidence-based practice model and guideline.* Indianapolis, IN: Sigma Theta Tau International.

Newhouse, R. P., Dearholt, S., Poe, S., Pugh, L. C., & White, K. M. (2007b). Organizational change strategies for evidence-based practice. *Journal of Nursing Administration, 37*(12), 552–557.

Newhouse, R. P., & Spring, B. (2010). Interdisciplinary evidence-based practice: Moving from silos to synergy. *Nursing Outlook, 58*(6), 309–317.

OCEBM Levels of Evidence Working Group. (2011). The Oxford 2011 levels of evidence. Oxford Centre for Evidence-Based Medicine. Retrieved from http://www.cebm.net/index.aspx?o=5653

Pearson, A., Wiechula, R., Court, A., & Lockwood, C. (2005). The JBI model of evidence-based healthcare. *International Journal of Evidence-Based Healthcare, 3*(8), 207–215.

Ragan, P., & Quincy, B. (2012). Evidence-based medication: Its roots and its fruits. *Journal of Physician Assistant Education, 23*(1).

Rosswurm, M. A., & Larrabee, J. H. (1999). A model for change to evidence-based practice. *Sigma Theta Tau International, 31*(4), 317–322.

Rycroft-Malone, J., Seers, K., Titchen, A., Kitson, A., & McCormack, B. (2004). What counts as evidence in evidence-based practice? *Journal of Advanced Nursing, 47*(1), 81–90.

Sackett, D. L., Rosenberg, W. M., Gray, J. A., Hayes, R. B., & Richardson, W. S. (1996). Evidence-based medicine: What it is and what it isn't. *British Medical Journal, 312*(7023), 71–72.

Satterfield, J. M., Spring, B., Ross, B. C., Mullen, E. J., Newhouse, R. P., Walker, B. B., & Whitlock, E. P. (2009). Toward a transdisciplinary model of evidence-based practice. *Milbank Quarterly, 87*(2), 368–390.

Stevens, K. R. (2004). *ACE star model of EBP: Knowledge transformation*. San Antonio, TX: Academic Center for Evidence-Based Practice. Retrieved from http://www.acestar.uthscsa.edu

Titler, M. G., Kleiber, C., Steelman, V. J., Rakel, B. A., Budreau, G., Everett L. Q., . . . Goode, C. J. (2001). The Iowa model of evidence-based practice to promote quality care. *Critical Care Nursing Clinics North America, 13*, 497–509.

UpToDate. (n.d.). Grading guide. Retrieved from http://www.uptodate.com/home/grading-guide

U.S. Department of Health and Human Services, Agency for Healthcare Research and Quality (AHRQ). (2002). Systems to rate the strength of scientific evidence. Retrieved from http://archive.ahrq.gov/clinic/epcsums/strengthsum.htm

U.S. Preventive Services Task Force. (2013, February). Grade definitions. Retrieved from http://www.uspreventiveservicestaskforce.org/uspstf/grades.htm

Vratny, A., & Shriver, D. (2007). A conceptual mode for growing evidence-based practice. *Nursing Administration Quarterly, 31*(2), 162–170.

CHAPTER 22

Clinical Scholarship and Evidence-Based Practice

Catherine Tymkow

True scholarship consists in knowing not what things exist, but what they mean; it is not memory, but judgment.

—James Russell Lowell

CHAPTER OBJECTIVES

1. Differentiate between the concepts of clinical scholarship and evidence-based practice.
2. Analyze the hierarchy for evaluating evidence in clinical practice.
3. Identify the different types of research evidence.
4. Explore the steps in the research process.
5. Review methods for critical appraisal of clinical practice guidelines.
6. Discuss approaches for disseminating findings from evidence-based practice.

INTRODUCTION

Any discussion of scholarship and evidence-based practice and the Doctor of Nursing Practice (DNP) role must first begin with some essential questions. These include questions as basic as the following: What is scholarship? Are evidence-based practice and clinical scholarship the same thing? How does clinical scholarship differ from the traditional definition of scholarship? Why do we need nursing scholars in practice settings? What is the role of the DNP in clinical scholarship? What are the knowledge resources, tools, and methods necessary to implement and support clinical scholarship and evidence-based practice?

These questions are important ones to consider as healthcare organizations and schools of nursing redefine and expand nurses' roles. If nursing is to maintain a full partnership with medicine in the delivery of health care, the education of nurse leaders and nurses in advanced practice roles must be at a comparable level with other doctorally prepared healthcare practitioners such as MDs, PharmDs, and PsyDs. The merging of nursing leadership skills, evidence-based decision making, and expert clinical care will ensure that nursing has a strong and credible presence in an ever-changing and complex healthcare system. In a presentation by President Faye Raines to the American Association of Colleges of Nursing (AACN), the leader noted that "the DNP degree more accurately reflects current clinical competencies and includes preparation for the changing healthcare system" (Raines, 2010).

The Doctor of Nursing Practice degree is a terminal practice degree and is now considered by many healthcare organizations as the preferred degree for nursing leaders involved in the delivery and organization of clinical care and healthcare systems. To meet this need, many new DNP programs have opened or are planning to open. In a recent survey, the AACN reported that 161 DNP programs are in the planning stages (American Association of Colleges of Nursing [AACN], 2010). In this survey, which had a response rate of 99.2%, 660 DNP-prepared nurses reportedly graduated from 119 programs. The DNP academic preparation, with a strong curricular base in advanced practice principles, experiential learning, intra- and interprofessional collaboration, and application of the best clinical research evidence, can best fulfill nursing's goals for leadership in practice and clinical education. In addition, clinical scholarship, including critical inquiry, analysis, synthesis, creativity, and research, must be a distinguishing feature of the DNP's role and expertise.

The purpose of this chapter is to define and explore the meaning of clinical scholarship, to distinguish evidence-based practice from other forms of scholarly activity, to describe the unique role of the DNP in scholarship, and to provide an overview of the language, methodological tools, strategies, and thought processes that are necessary to ensure that nursing's scholarship is useful, significant, and of the highest quality. Entire books are dedicated to research processes, methodologies, and evidence-based practice. This is not the intent of this chapter; rather, it is to explore the concepts, provide resources, and whet the reader's appetite for more in-depth information on the topic.

WHAT IS CLINICAL SCHOLARSHIP?

In Sigma Theta Tau International's (1999) *Clinical Scholarship Resource Paper*, Melanie Dreher (Sigma Theta Tau International Clinical Scholarship Task Force, 1999), chair of the task force, wrote that "clinical scholarship is about inquiry and implies a willingness to scrutinize our practice" (p. 26). Also, "clinical scholarship is not clinical proficiency, . . . unless we are questioning the reason for its use in the first place . . .; and neither is it clinical research, although it is informed by and inspires research" (p. 26). Finally, she noted that "clinical scholarship is an intellectual process. . . . It includes challenging traditional nursing interventions, testing our ideas, predicting outcomes, and explaining both patterns and exceptions. In addition to observation, analysis, and synthesis, clinical scholarship includes application and dissemination, all of which result in a new understanding of nursing phenomena and the development of new knowledge" (p. 26).

The American Association of Colleges of Nursing's (AACN) *Position Statement on Defining Scholarship for the Discipline of Nursing* (1999) defined scholarship as "those activities that systematically advance the teaching, research, and practice of nursing through rigorous inquiry that: 1) is significant to the profession, 2) is creative, 3) can be documented, 4) can be replicated or elaborated, and 5) can be peer-reviewed through various methods" (p. 1). Citing the work of Schulman (1993), the National Organization of Nurse Practitioner Faculties NONPF, 2005) noted further that practice, to be considered scholarship, "must be public, susceptible to critical review and evaluation, and accessible for exchange and use of other members of one's scholarly community" (p. 6).

These definitions are congruent with the evolving definition of scholarship in academia since Boyer's (1990, 1997) groundbreaking work, *Scholarship Reconsidered: Priorities of the Professoriate*. Ernest L. Boyer was an American educator, chancellor, and president of the Carnegie Foundation for the Advancement of Teaching (Carnegie Foundation for the Advancement of Teaching, 1996). Since the publication of *Scholarship Reconsidered* (1990), a new and expanded role for scholarship has emerged in academia that makes the previously mentioned definitions of scholarship more compatible with the goals and processes of practice disciplines. The traditional definition of scholarship in academia did not account for the nuances and rigors of clinical practice knowledge and its application for problem solving and interactive, human engagement (AACN, 2006). Boyer's model (1990, 1997), however, is well suited to scholarship in nursing practice. In Boyer's view, scholarship is not linear; rather, there is a constant, reciprocal, iterative relationship between each of its four aspects. It embraces the concepts of discovery (building new knowledge through research and careful inquiry to refine existing knowledge), integration (interpreting knowledge through dissemination in various forms), application (using knowledge for problem solving, service, and growth), and teaching (developing and testing instructional materials to advance learning, including the formation and sustaining of an engaging environment for learning between teacher and student) (Boyer, 1990, 1997; Stull & Lanz, 2005).

The AACN's *Essentials of Doctoral Education for Advanced Nursing Practice* (2006) embodies much of Boyer's criteria in the specification of the eight core essentials and specialty-focused competencies as the basic underpinnings to be integrated into the Doctor of Nursing Practice curriculum (AACN, 2006). Essential 3 of the core elements is "clinical scholarship and analytic methods for evidence-based practice" (AACN, 2006). In this document, the authors stated that "scholarship and research are the hallmarks of doctoral education" (p. 11) and, further, that "research doctorates are designed to prepare graduates with the research skills necessary to discover new knowledge in the discipline. However, DNPs engaged in advanced nursing practice provide leadership for evidence-based practice. This requires competence in knowledge development activities such as the translation of research in practice, the evaluation of practice, activities aimed at improving the reliability of health care practice and outcomes, and participation in collaborative research" (DePalma & McGuire, as cited in AACN, 2006, p. 11). Therefore, DNP programs focus on the translation of new science, its application, and its evaluation. In addition, DNP graduates generate evidence to guide practice.

More recently, the idea that only those with research doctorates (PhD, DNS, and DNSc) should conduct "discovery" research for generating new knowledge has been challenged (Ironside, 2006; Reed & Shear, 2004; Webber, 2008). Webber asserted that level-appropriate research should be promoted from the baccalaureate through doctoral level because "everyday practice involves daily interaction with an informed public, interpreting the most updated research that is available with the click of a mouse, and identifying phenomena unique to the practice. The only missing piece is the skills necessary to investigate the phenomenon" (p. 468).

As DNP programs have proliferated, the curriculum has evolved to include more focus on research translation and evidence-based practice. An Internet review of the curricula from several national DNP programs indicates that growing numbers of schools are adding courses such as Theory, Research Methods, Discovery and Utilization of Evidence-Based Care, and Translating Evidence into Practice so that graduates have the skills needed to participate in whatever level of research is appropriate to their setting and scholarship goals.

EVIDENCE-BASED PRACTICE AND CLINICAL SCHOLARSHIP: ARE THEY THE SAME?

Scholarship is an evolutionary process that raises the level of the profession through participation in the generation of new knowledge and through scientific and social exchange. "The difference between evidence based nursing practice and scholarship or applied nursing research is that evidence based practice is practice driven" (French, 1999, p. 77). Whereas scholarship was often viewed by many practicing professionals as an add-on, optional activity, evidence-based practice has become a necessity in our current information-based technological age. Computers have given everyone access to both good and bad information. The defining feature of evidence-based practice is the linking of current research findings with patients' conditions, values, and circumstances. In addition, it involves "the conscientious, explicit, and judicious use of current best evidence for making decisions about the care of individuals" (Sackett, Richardson, Rosenberg, & Haynes, 1997, p. 2). Nursing's unique addition to this process must offer a more holistic approach that adds artful practice and ethical standards to the empirics of evidence (Fawcett, Watson, Neuman, Hinton Walker, & Fitzpatrick, 2001).

The work of clinical scholars has increased during the past two decades. A review of nursing articles published from 1986 to 2011 in the Cumulative Index to Nursing and Allied Health Literature (CINAHL) database resulted in 131 published articles with clinical scholarship as the focus. When "evidence-based practice" was added to the search terms, an additional 16 articles were found. When "evidence-based practice" alone was used as the search term, the search returned 31,148 articles published between 1999 and 2010. Although not all of the latter were nursing articles, 1,729 articles, or nearly half, were nursing-focused articles.

Holleman, Eliens, van Vliet, and van Acterburg (2006) extensively reviewed six databases, including CINAHL, PubMed, Scirus, Invert, Google, and the Cochrane databases, focusing on the years between 1993 and 2004. In their meta-analysis of the literature on promotion of evidence-based practice (EBP) and professional nursing associations, the authors found 179 articles that addressed EBP activities. Of the 179 articles, 47 dealt with EBP as structural measures (policy, role, quality indicators), 103 as competence and attitude-oriented (journals, conferences, workshops, research committees, etc.), and only 29 as behavior-oriented (care models, guidelines). The increase in EBP articles shows the growing interest and use of evidence to guide practice. Despite this progress, significant gaps remain in nursing science discovery and application or implementation in practice. The Doctor of Nursing Practice degree is intended to bridge this gap (McCloskey, 2008).

The principles of EBP were an outgrowth of the work of Dr. Archie Cochrane, a British epidemiologist who criticized the medical profession for not using evidence from randomized clinical trials as a basis for clinical care. He believed that the evidence from these trials should be systematically reviewed and constantly updated to afford patients the best quality care (Cochrane Collaboration, 2004). Evidence-based practice includes an emphasis on the efficacy of treatments or interventions based on the results of experimental comparison between untreated control groups, treatments, or both. The core principles include (1) formulating the clinical question; (2) identifying the most relevant articles, research, and other best

TABLE 22-1	Hierarchy for Evaluating Evidence for Practice
Level 1 (strongest)	Systematic reviews/meta-analysis of all randomized controlled trials (RCTs); clinical practice guidelines based on RCT data
Level 2	Evidence from one or more RCTs
Level 3	Evidence from a controlled trial; no randomization
Level 4	Case-control or cohort studies
Level 5	Systematic reviews of descriptive/qualitative studies
Level 6	Single descriptive or qualitative study
Level 7 (weakest)	Opinions of authorities/experts

Note: All levels assume a well-designed study.

evidence; (3) critically evaluating the evidence; (4) integrating and applying the evidence; and (5) reevaluating the application of evidence and making necessary changes. **Table 22-1** presents the hierarchy of evidence for practice.

That the definition of "evidence-based practice" has been adapted to include provisions for the provider's experience and the patient's values in making the ultimate clinical care decisions is in keeping with James Russell Lowell's (1819–1891) definition of scholarship: "True scholarship consists in knowing not what things exist, but what they mean; it is not memory, but judgment" (Lowell, n.d.). Although Lowell was not a healthcare professional, his definition is applicable to advanced nursing practice. It is through the incorporation of intuition, observation, theory, research, intelligent analysis, and judgment based on the data that nurses provide care that is truly individualized, reflective, and evidence based. With an increased knowledge of the theory and the tools necessary to critique and translate research into practice, the DNP-prepared nurse is in a prime position to affect the delivery of care and to aggregate and translate evidence that can be disseminated to improve overall care and outcomes in myriad clinical areas.

The translation and dissemination of clinical knowledge are cores of clinical scholarship.

WHAT IS THE ROLE OF THE DOCTOR OF NURSING PRACTICE DEGREE IN CLINICAL SCHOLARSHIP?

In advanced practice, scholarship should be integrated with practice as a purposeful, systematic, and conscious endeavor. The emphasis is on inquiry, outcomes, and evidence to support practice (Sigma Theta Tau International Clinical Scholarship Task Force, 1999). Because of their education, advanced practice nurses (APNs), particularly DNP-prepared nurses, are expected to have mastery of essential information so that the teaching of staff, patients, and communities becomes a key function of the role. The dynamic nature of health care requires that DNP-prepared nurses be up-to-date on new information and that they be able to discern nuances in research findings so as to translate those findings in understandable ways that improve care and practice. This requires constant critique and integration and synthesis of new information from various sources into formats that can be disseminated to patients, colleagues, and others.

What distinguishes the role of the DNP-prepared nurse from other advanced practice degree holders? The answer is not a simple one; the difference is, in fact, a combination of knowledge, expert skill, and the integration of *best* research to advance the practice and the profession. This skill comes from additional formal education, experience, and the translation, application, and evaluation of research in practice. Although most practicing nurses are exposed to "research" and "evidence" in practice, the DNP must not only embrace the process but also implement the findings in ways that ultimately change or, at least, improve practice and outcomes. Scholarship is the dissemination of those findings in publications, presentations, and Internet offerings that can be used by others. As envisioned in the *Essentials of Doctoral Education for Advanced Nursing Practice* (AACN, 2006), the DNP program prepares graduates to:

1. Use analytical methods to critically appraise existing literature and other evidence relevant to practice.

2. Lead the evaluation of evidence (existing literature, research findings, and other data) to determine and implement the best evidence for practice.

3. Design and implement processes to evaluate outcomes of practice, practice patterns, and systems of care within a practice setting, healthcare organization, or community against national benchmarks to determine variances in practice outcomes and population trends.

4. Design, direct, and evaluate quality improvement methodologies to promote safe, timely, effective, efficient, equitable, and patient-centered care.

5. Evaluate practice patterns against national benchmarks to determine variances in clinical outcomes and population trends.

6. Apply relevant findings to develop practice guidelines and improve practice and the practice environment.

7. Inform and guide the design of databases that generate meaningful evidence for nursing practice.

8. Use information technology and research methods appropriately to:
   - Collect appropriate and accurate data to generate evidence for nursing practice
   - Inform and guide the design of databases that generate meaningful evidence for nursing practice
   - Analyze data from clinical practice
   - Design evidence-based interventions
   - Predict and analyze outcomes
   - Examine patterns of behavior and outcomes
   - Identify gaps in evidence for practice

9. Function as a practice specialist/consultant in collaborative knowledge-generating research.

10. Disseminate findings from evidence-based practice to improve healthcare outcomes.

These objectives encompass the essential skills, tools, and methods necessary to implement and support clinical scholarship and evidence-based practice. They can be distilled into six categories: (1) translating research in practice, (2) quality improvement and patient-centered care, (3) evaluation of practice, (4) research methods and technology, (5) participation in collaborative research, and (6) disseminating findings from evidence-based practice. Each of these areas is discussed in the following sections.

TRANSLATING RESEARCH IN PRACTICE

The use of evidence to support clinical practice is not a new phenomenon. Medical professionals have relied on data from science, empirical observation, case reviews, and other means for centuries (Monico, Moore, & Calise, 2005). However, as electronic access to sources of data has increased, the amount of evidence now available as a basis for clinical practice has become overwhelming.

The key to making best-practice decisions is using the best-quality evidence, evidence that is scientifically based and that has been replicated with success in repeated research and application. Although critical appraisal of research for use in practice is an important aspect of evidence-based practice, it is not the only criterion. Unfortunately, many lack the knowledge and skills on which to base their practice decisions (Pravikoff, Tanner, & Pierce, 2005). Melnyk and Fineout-Overholt (2005) specified three primary knowledge sources for EBP: valid research evidence, clinical expertise, and patient choice. Currently, evidence generated from large-scale randomized controlled trials is considered the gold standard for application in interventions (Fawcett & Garrity, 2009). Depending on the clinical situation and the patient's personal preference, other sources of evidence may be appropriate, including meta-analyses of all relevant randomized controlled trials; EBP guidelines from systematic reviews of randomized controlled trials, case-control studies, or cohort studies; expert opinion; and nursing theory (Fawcett & Garrity, 2009; Melnyk & Fineout-Overholt, 2005).

To understand research evidence that may be used in practice, the following sections on qualitative and quantitative research offer a brief description of the processes and questions to be considered in the evaluation of such research. Exhaustive coverage of every research method is beyond the scope of this chapter. However, the definitions, discussion, and examples are meant to illustrate how different types of research might be applied or used in practice and how their rigor and adequacy as evidence for practice should be evaluated.

UNDERSTANDING, DISTINGUISHING, AND EVALUATING TYPES OF RESEARCH EVIDENCE

Qualitative Research Evidence

Qualitative research is based on four levels of understanding:

1. What is the nature of reality? (Ontology)
2. What constitutes knowledge? (Epistemology)
3. How can we understand reality? (Methodology)
4. How can we collect the evidence? (Methods) (Porter, 1996, as cited in Maggs-Rapport, 2001)

Types of Qualitative Research Studies

Qualitative research is important in that it allows the nurse to consider the context of a situation while connecting with patients and noting individual differences. In addition, it permits nursing's unique perspective to be valued and considered critically when making clinical decisions. In her discussion of qualitative research and evidence-based nursing, Zuzelo (2007) proposed that "nursing needs to ensure that qualitative research is as much a part of the considered evidence as quantitative evidence is" (p. 484).

There are several kinds of qualitative research studies, including critical social theory, ethnographic studies, grounded theory research, historical research, phenomenological studies, and philosophical inquiry. Each of these methods is discussed briefly so as to provide an overview of the scope and potential uses of qualitative evidence and to provide a basis for evaluating the use of qualitative studies as causes of changes in practice.

Critical Social Theory

Critical social theory uses multiple research methods as a basis for promoting change in areas where power imbalances exist (Burns & Grove, 2009). According to Horkheimer (1895–1973), Marcuse (1898–1979), Adorno (1903–1969), and Habermas (1929–), critical social theory is based on the belief that individuals should seek freedom from domination (Maggs-Rapport, 2001). Habermas, particularly, believed that people must understand the nature of "constraining circumstances" before they can be liberated from them (Maggs-Rapport, 2001).

Another critical social theorist, Giddens (1982, as cited in Maggs-Rapport, 2001), believed that we can understand why people act in certain ways only if we can appreciate the meanings of their actions.

The DNP might use data from critical social theory to identify meaning or patterns of concern where certain societal cultural norms exist in the form of barriers that affect particularly vulnerable populations such as elderly persons, incarcerated persons, abused women, and chronically ill persons. Analysis would necessarily include an examination of the underlying conditions, a critique of the social phenomena, and the discovery and revelation of the social and political injustices embedded in the experience of the population in question that could lead toward removal of barriers (Maggs-Rapport, 2001).

Ethnographic Research

Ethnographic research is used to describe the nature or characteristics of a culture to gain insight into the lifeways or behaviors of a group. Distinguishing features are immerged in the participant's way of life (Polit & Hungler, 1997), and the information gathered speaks for itself rather than being interpreted or explored for additional meanings (Maggs-Rapport, 2001). Field notes based on researcher observations over time describe daily interactions with subjects.

In one ethnographic study, Kovarsky (2008) compared clients' and families' personal experiences of outcomes and interventions with written professional discourse, technical reports, and other conceptualizations of evidence in practice. Unfortunately, the author noted that "the dismissal of subjective, phenomenally oriented information has functioned to marginalize and silence voices . . . of clients when constituting proof of effectiveness," and further, "the current

version of EBP needs to be reformulated to include subjective voices from the life-worlds of clients as a form of evidence" (Kovarsky, 2008, p. 47). As one example of an ethnographic approach, Kovarsky proposed the personal experience narrative as a measure of qualitative outcomes and intervention analysis (Kovarsky, 2008, p. 48). Citing a study by Simmons-Mackie and Damico (2001), Kovarsky described an ethnographic interview with a patient experiencing poststroke aphasia. These statements support an altered level of life activity that cannot totally be accounted for or appreciated in objective technical descriptions of outcomes of disease processes and their sequelae.

The ethnographic narrative is a method of subjective evidence gathering that can enhance the specificity and richness of other research methodologies, including evidence gained from logical positivist approaches such as randomized controlled trials. In particular, DNPs in public health or community health could use this method in conjunction with other, more traditional, forms of evidence to gain a better real-world understanding of the populations they serve.

Grounded Theory Research

Grounded theory research is focused on the influence of interactional processes (identification, description, and explanation) between individuals, families, or groups within a social context (Strauss & Corbin, 1994). It is an observational method used to study problems in social settings that are "grounded" in the data obtained from those observations (Burns & Grove, 2009; Glaser & Strauss, 1967). Grounded theory is an applicable framework for study of myriad contexts, situations, and settings because it bridges the gap between empirical observation and the generation of theory by providing a structured method of sampling procedures and coding observations for explaining social phenomena or generating new theory (Annells, 1996; Barnes, 1996; Glaser & Strauss, 1967; Hammersley, 1989).

For example, a study of the implementation of evidence-based nursing in Iran (Adib-Hajbaghery, 2007) sought to distinguish factors influencing the implementation of evidence-based practice in Eastern countries (versus Western countries), particularly Iran. A brief description of this study using the grounded theory approach is presented here. Data collection consisted of purposive sampling of 21 nurses (nine staff and six head nurses in differing clinical settings) with experience in nursing greater than 5 years. An interview questionnaire consisted of open-ended questions, such as "What is the basis of care you give your patients?" (p. 568), "In your opinion, what is the basis of evidence based nursing?" (p. 568), and "Can you describe some instances in which you used scientific evidence in nursing?" (p. 568). "Issues were clarified and interviews were audiotaped, transcribed verbatim and analyzed consecutively" (Adib-Hajbaghery, 2007, p. 568). A total of 36 hours of observations and interviews were carried out concurrently and involved observations of those interviewed and others working on the units. According to the procedure identified by Strauss and Corbin (1998), each interview was analyzed before the subsequent interview took place, and the results were coded in three ways: open coding (breaking down, examining, comparing, conceptualizing, and categorizing), axial coding (putting data back together in new ways by linking codes to contexts, consequences, and patterns of interactions), and selective coding (identifying core categories and systematically relating and validating relationships) (Adib-Hajbaghery, 2007). To confirm the credibility of the data, participants were given a full transcript of their responses and a list of codes and themes to determine whether the codes and themes matched their responses. To establish validity, two peer researchers also checked codes and themes using the same procedure as the researcher. The results were that two main categories emerged from the research: (1) the meaning of evidence-based nursing (EBN); and (2) factors in implementation of EBN, including the themes of possessing professional knowledge and experience, having opportunity and time, becoming accustomed, self-confidence, the process of nursing education, and the work environment and its expectations (Adib-Hajbaghery, 2007).

The process and results of grounded theory research and analysis provide rich data for application in practice when paired with evidence from other sources. This is especially true when there is little clinical trial evidence to support the affective dimension of care or practice.

Historical Research

Historical research is a description or analysis of events that have shaped a discipline. Although historical research may not be used directly in practice, it provides the foundation for examination of the discipline and for providing future directions (Burns & Grove; 2009; Fitzpatrick & Munhall, 2001). Often history is handed down in written documents. The Library of Congress's (n.d.) American Memory Collection has original writings, newspaper clippings, photos, and other documents that provide a realistic account of the influence and actions of famous women in history, including nursing leaders. Pictures and other documents showcase the original work of early nurse leaders such as Lavinia Dock (1858–1956), Margaret Sanger (1879–1966), Clara Barton (1821–1912), and Mary Breckinridge (1881–1965), which provides a basis for advanced nursing practice and can be used by DNPs in education to provide a historical perspective for practice.

Another source of historical research is oral history. Using both written documents and oral history, Libster and McNeil (2009) traced the history and meaning of a religious tradition of care of the sick and poor by the Sisters of Charity. Wall, Edwards, and Porter (2007) used oral history and a method of textual analysis to determine how retired nurses made sense of their educational experiences. Decker and Iphofen (2005) described a method of oral history research to discover knowledge about, and change within, a profession, particularly as it relates to evidence-based practice. Tropello (2000) used oral history technique in her dissertation, *Origins of the Nurse Practitioner Movement: An Oral History*. The purpose was to gain a better understanding of current advanced nursing practice roles through an exploration of the original movement. Eight participants in the original movement were the primary sources, and the information obtained and transcribed from taped interviews was enhanced by supportive papers, correspondence, and other documents, including secondary sources. One conclusion of the study was that the politics of the 1960s, which emphasized greater freedoms for women and a focus on social programs, helped alleviate healthcare manpower shortages (Tropello, 2000). This movement has paved the way for additional professionalization in nursing, including the evolution of the Doctor of Nursing Practice curriculum. Started as a research project, it became part of the core curriculum under the continuing education division of the School of Nursing at the University of Colorado. The program used a nursing–physician team approach to aid families with limited access to primary providers (Tropello, 2000).

For DNP-prepared nurses to prescribe their future, they must have a clear understanding of and appreciation for their history so that they can build on and shape evidence-based practice in ways that preserve the essence of nursing. The National League of Nursing and Sigma Theta Tau have excellent historical resources.

Several of the audiotapes, videotapes, and other historical resources produced by these and other nurse theorists whose original work and theory development continue to provide frameworks for advancing nursing practice were referenced by Allen (1996) in a special report, *Celebrating Nursing History: What to Keep*.

Phenomenological Research

The aim of a *phenomenological (hermeneutic) study* is to understand a phenomenon through the recognition of its meaning. Researchers explore an experience as it is lived by the participants in the study. The phenomenon of interest may include any number of experiences, such as death, divorce, pain, or cancer. The researcher collects data and interprets the experiences as they are lived (Burns & Grove, 2009). Phenomenology focuses on revealing meaning of an experience or occurrence to discern the real truth of a phenomenon rather than arguing a point or developing abstract theory (Hallet, 1995) One example of a phenomenological study by Marineau (2005) involved perceptions of telehealth support by an advanced practice nurse for patients discharged from the hospital with acute infections. Because empirical data were insufficient in patients who had previously been enrolled in a quantitative pilot study of telehealth, eidetic phenomenology, which compares variations in imagination after an event to capture patients' lived experiences after discharge, was used. Theme categories were initial response, engaging in care, and experiencing the downside. Of the 10 participants in the trial, only one had a negative experience. The study was seen as useful in adding to the understanding of the transitional process of care (Marineau, 2005).

In another phenomenological approach, Maggs-Rapport (2001) used van Manen's (1990) social scientific approach to look at women's immediate response to the phenomenon of egg sharing (donation of one woman's eggs to another woman) after consultation with a clinician and their lived experiences of egg sharing in return for free fertility treatment. The in-depth open-ended interviews of this technique established a conversational relationship about the meaning of the experience and produced a narrative that "enriches the understanding of the phenomena" (Maggs-Rapport, 2001). Before each description can be transformed into phenomenological language, meaning units must be made of each description (Giorgi, 2000). However, only a small number of descriptions are necessary for the nature of the phenomenon to become apparent (Giorgi, 2000; van Manen, 1990).

More recent studies that utilized the phenomenological approach in advanced practice include studies about the needs of patients and families living with severe brain injury (Bond, Draeger, Mandleco, & Donnelly, 2003); advanced nursing practice in rural areas (Conger & Plager, 2008); the meaning of U.S. childbirth for Mexican immigrant women (Imberg, 2008); the meaning of desire for euthanasia (Mak, 2003); how family practice physicians, nurse practitioners, and physician assistants incorporate spiritual care into practice (Tanyi, McKenzie, & Chapek, 2009); the leadership and management role of the DNP in the care of older persons in the United States (Stoekel, 2010); sociophenomenology and conversation analysis; and interpreting video life-world healthcare interactions (Bickerton, Procter, Johnson, & Medina, 2011). Phenomenological techniques with a strong nursing orientation include those of Crotty (1996) and Munhall (1994, 2007). Phenomenological studies contribute to the evidence base by enhancing our understanding of the true meaning of patients' experiences and the broader dimensions of a problem, thus aiding in a more holistic perspective in practice.

Philosophical Inquiry

Philosophical inquiry is used to explore the nature of knowledge, values, meaning, and ethical factors related to a question of interest. Although philosophical inquiry is related to theory, it is not the same as theory, which is more specific and concrete (Pesut & Johnson, 2007). Citing Edwards (2001), Pesut and Johnson (2007) described three "strands" that compose philosophical inquiry: (1) philosophical presupposition, which involves identifying and analyzing presuppositions in nursing (an example might be a concept analysis of nursing practice or advanced practice); (2) philosophical problems, such as what constitutes knowing in a particular situation, or ethical analyses, such as the ethics of caring in situations where nurses' and patients' values conflict; and (3) scholarship, in which nurse theorists' works are examined from a philosophical perspective. In this case, as noted by Burns and Grove (2009), the researcher would "conduct an extensive search of the literature, examine conceptual meaning, pose questions and propose answers including the implications for those answers" (p. 26).

In a practical application of philosophical inquiry, Dorn (2004) described a model, caring-healing inquiry for holistic nursing practice, to guide nursing research and quality improvement in a tertiary hospital. The model, which integrated the values of the hospital, provided the basis for nurses to describe their contributions to care through research and practice improvement. In a partnership between a hospital and university nursing program, a nursing research committee was formed, composed mostly of APNs. The group served as an advisory group for program planning and development. The nurse-researcher faculty member facilitated the work of the committee and provided staff development in research and clinical innovation. Knowledge about the process of philosophical inquiry and a focus on value analysis, as demonstrated in these examples, provide DNP-prepared nurses with a basis for facilitating ethical decision making in practice.

Evaluating Qualitative Research Evidence

What are the evaluative questions? Regardless of the type of research design, the general criteria for evaluation of qualitative studies are as follows (Gifford, Davies, Edwards, Griffin, & Lybanon, 2007; Patton, 1990; Russell & Gregory, 2003):

1. *Question, purpose, and context:* Is the research question clear, the primary purpose and the focus of the study stated, and the context described?

2. *Design:* Was the design appropriate, were the units of analysis and sampling strategy described, and are the sampling criteria clear?

3. *Data collection:* What types of data were collected? Were data collection processes systematic and adequately described? How were logistical issues addressed?

4. *Data analysis:* Was data analysis systematic and rigorous? What controls were in place? What analytical approach or approaches were used? How were validity and confidence in the findings established?

5. *Results:* Were results surprising, interesting, or suspect? Were conclusions supported by data and explanation (theory)? Were the authors' positions clearly stated?

6. *Ethical issues:* How were ethical issues and confidentiality addressed?

7. *Implications:* What is the worth/relevance to knowledge and practice?

Qualitative research questions and methods provide an avenue for truly knowing patients and practicing both the "art" and "science" of nursing. These are the hallmarks of nursing that nurses at every level must retain and that DNP-prepared nurses must foster as role models to ensure that "best practice" does not exclude the best of nursing's perspective.

Quantitative Research Evidence

Steps in the Quantitative Research Process

Two important aspects of any quantitative research project is that the project builds on prior results or evidence and provides a basis for future research and discovery (Burns & Grove, 2009). **Figure 22-1** shows the steps in the quantitative research process.

The *research problem* is often derived because there is a gap in knowledge that needs to be addressed or described. Research problems or questions often arise from direct observations made in practice. The *purpose* of the study is to address the problem. To better understand the problem, an extensive *literature review* must be done in order to develop an understanding of the nature and scope of the problem and to determine what research has already been done. A framework, map, or theoretical base made up of concepts is developed to provide structure and help the researcher make sense of the findings. The *research objectives, questions,* or *hypotheses* set the study limits in terms of who will be studied, what question(s) will be addressed, and what relationships among variables exist.

The remaining steps are to define the variables in conceptual terms (theoretical meaning) and operational terms (how the variables will be measured or manipulated); explain assumptions (those things we take for granted to be true, whether proven or not); and identify study limitations (any issue within the study that serves to limit a study's generalizability beyond the population or sample studied). Limitations may be weaknesses in the study itself or in the theoretical basis.

Categories and Selection of a Design

Quantitative research may be categorized as experimental, quasi-experimental, or nonexperimental (descriptive or correlational). Quantitative research may be either basic research (as in laboratory studies) or applied (as in clinical research). In an experimental or quasi-experimental study,

FIGURE 22-1 The quantitative research process.

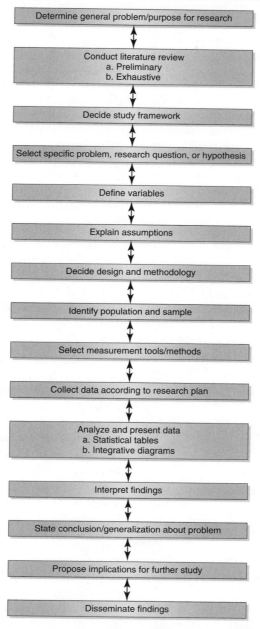

Source: This article was published in *The practice of nursing research, appraisal, synthesis, and generation of evidence,* 6e, Burns, N. & Grove, S. K., p. 37, Copyright Elsvier Saunders 2009. Used with permission.

the researcher actively manipulates the independent variable (treatment or intervention) to see the effect on the dependent variable. In an experimental study, the variables and the setting are highly controlled. In a nonexperimental design, the researcher may simply want to describe or explain a phenomenon or predict a relationship (Burns & Grove, 2009).

Quantitative designs may also be retrospective (the proposed cause and effect have already occurred), prospective (the cause, but not the effect, has occurred), cross-sectional (examines groups in various stages of development), or longitudinal (the same subjects are studied over a period of time). None of the categories are mutually exclusive (Schmidt & Brown, 2009).

The Population and Sample

The *population* is everyone or everything that meets the criteria for inclusion. The criteria for inclusion may be narrow or broad, depending on the size and scope of the study and the specific research question to be addressed. The *sample* is a subset of the population and the process for how the subset will be selected. This may be random (all have a better than zero chance of selection), nonrandom (convenience), cross-sectional (groups studied over time), or stratified (divided to ensure representation from groups when some variables are known). Often the population and the sample are determined by the method and how accessible the population is to the researcher (Burns & Grove, 2009).

Measurement Instruments

Measurement instruments are tools used by the researcher to answer the operational questions posed in research studies. These tools may be questionnaires, tests, indicators of health status, and a variety of other measurement techniques.

Data Collection, Analysis, and Interpretation

Most data collected in quantitative research studies are coded numerically so that they can be systematically analyzed and interpreted

through the use of statistics. A plan for data collection and analysis is an important part of the research process and is crucial to meaningful interpretation of results. Interpretation involves "1) examining the results from data, 2) exploring the significance of findings, 3) forming conclusions, 4) generalizing the data, 5) considering the implications for further study, and 6) suggesting further studies" (Burns & Grove, 2005, p. 45). Once interpreted, the researcher synthesizes and reports implications for further study, practice, or both.

This cursory overview of the research process provides the basis for evaluating evidence from research. The reader is referred to a research text for a complete discussion of definitions and the various designs, analyses, and implementation processes.

Evaluating Quantitative Evidence

When a quantitative study is appraised for use in practice, three questions are generally considered: Is the study valid? Is the study reliable? Is the study applicable in the identified case?

Is the Study Valid? Specifically, were the methods used scientifically sound? Are the independent (manipulated variable) and dependent variables (observed result) clearly identified? Is the study free from bias or confounding variables?

Bias is a standard point of view or personal prejudice, especially when there is a tendency "to affect unduly or unfairly, or to impose a steady negative potential upon," according to *Funk & Wagnalls*. It is an influence or action that distorts or "slants findings away from the expected" (Burns & Grove, 2009, p. 220). In research, bias may occur when participants' characteristics specifically differ from those of the population (Burns & Grove, 2005). This is always possible because volunteers are used for samples. It is less likely to occur, however, if the sampling strategy is well planned and followed and there is random assignment to groups. Bias may also occur if the instruments or measurement tools are faulty or the data or statistics are inaccurate.

Selection Bias When a researcher decides to prospectively compare two types of strategies for educating nursing students, such as online instruction and traditional classroom instruction, *selection bias* may occur if the students are allowed to select which group they enter. Students who select online teaching may be very different from those who choose the traditional classroom experience. Random assignment to the groups minimizes the risk of selection bias.

Gender Bias Another form of bias is *gender bias*. Gender bias occurs in research when one gender, more than the other, is used to study research interventions. Timmerman (1999) outlined a procedure for ensuring that research decisions avoid gender bias. The procedure in-

cludes critically analyzing the literature, testing gender-specific differences, and identifying researchers' personal biases. The following example of binge-eating behaviors between men and women illustrates the point. Timmerman (1999), citing Hawkins and Clement (1984) and Spitzer et al. (1992), stated, "We know that men tend to binge less frequently, consume less during binges and are less distressed by their binge eating behavior than women" (p. 642). And, "In this case, the literature provides justification for either separately studying binge eating behavior in men and women, or, if the sample has both men and women, analyzing the data separately for men and women" (Timmerman, 1999, p. 642). **Table 22-2** lists some gender-based studies. Additional gender-based studies can be found online through the Office on Women's Health of the U.S. Department of Health and Human Services.

TABLE 22-2	Gender-Based Studies
Celik, Lagro-Janssen, Widdershoven, & Abma (2011)	Bringing gender sensitivity into healthcare practice: A systematic review
Diaz-Granados et al. (2011)	Monitoring gender equality in health using gender-sensitive indicators: A cross-national study
Doster, Purdum, Martin, Goven, & Moorefield (2009)	Gender differences, anger expression, and cardiovascular risk
Dunlop & Beauchamp (2011)	En-gendering choice: Preferences for exercising in gender-segregated and gender-integrated groups and consideration of overweight status
Luttik, Jaarsma, Lesman, Sanderman, & Hagedoorn (2009)	Quality of life in partners of people with congestive heart failure: Gender and involvement in care
Masharani, Goldfine, & Youngren (2009)	Influence of gender on the relationship between insulin sensitivity, adiposity, and plasma lipids in lean nondiabetic subjects
McCollum, Hansen, Lu, & Sullivan (2005)	Self-care differences in men and women with diabetes
Reeves et al. (2009)	Quality of care in women with ischemic stroke in the GWTG program

Confounding Variables If occurs when a third variable, either known or unknown, produces the relationship with the outcome instead of the research intervention itself. Or, stated differently, confounding may occur when comparing two groups that may be different in additional ways from the treatment being studied (Leedy & Ormrod, 2010). Randomizing participants to either the intervention or study group helps to eliminate the possibility of confusion because there is an equal chance that extraneous variables will appear equally in both groups, thus minimizing the confounding effect.

One type of confounder is the effect of *history*. The history effect occurs when an event outside the researcher's control occurs at the same time as, or during, the period of the intervention. For example, in a study of patients with hypertension, a researcher was interested in the impact of a low-salt diet on hypertension levels. A baseline blood pressure was taken; patients were then started on the low-salt diet. However, during the study period, some of these same patients also began a rigorous exercise routine, whereas others did not. In this case, the intervening exercise program would make it difficult to attribute the outcome solely to the effect of the intervention. Adding a control group whose members adhered to a low-salt diet and exercise routine or using statistical tests to control for this confounding variable would minimize the threat to validity in this study.

In another example of confounding, a researcher was interested in comparing lung cancer and smoking incidence in various regions of the country. In this study, a particular region was seen to have a significantly higher rate of lung cancer death among smokers (15 times higher) than did other regions of the country. The confounding factor was that these smokers had also worked in asbestos coal mines for many years. When the researchers controlled for the variable of working with asbestos by removing the confounder, the rate of cancer due to smoking was nearly the same as that in other regions of the country. **Figure 22-2** shows the

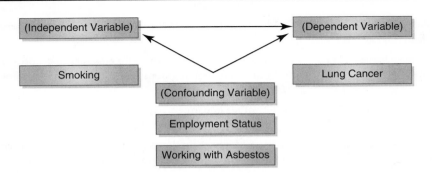

| **FIGURE 22-2** | Interrelationships among smoking, working in an asbestos coal mine, and risk for lung cancer in a cohort/case-control study. |

(Independent Variable) → (Dependent Variable)

Smoking

Lung Cancer

(Confounding Variable)

Employment Status

Working with Asbestos

Source: Varkevisser, C.; Pathmanathan, I.; Brownlee, A. 2003. Designing and Conducting Health Systems Research Projects: Volume 2: Data Analyses and Report Writing. International Development Research Centre, Ottowa, ON, Canada. http://www.idrc.ca/EN/Resources/Publications/Pages/IDRCBookDe tails.aspx?PublicationID=208. Used with permission of IDRC Canada.

relationship among the independent variable (smoking) and confounding variable (working in an asbestos coal mine) in relationship to the dependent variable (lung cancer) (International Development Research Centre, 2009).

Is the Study Reliable?

The reliability of a study is based on questions such as the following: Does the instrument or test measure what it is supposed to measure? Does it do this consistently? Do the items on the instrument consistently measure the same characteristic? How much consistency is there between raters? (Burns & Grove, 2009; Fain, 2009). Reliability is measured through the use of a reliability coefficient (r) and ranges from 0.00 (lowest) to 1.00 (highest). Therefore, the closer a reliability score is to 1.00, the higher the reliability. In most cases, a coefficient of 0.80 or higher is considered acceptable if the instrument has already been tested and has been used frequently. If an instrument is new, a reliability coefficient of 0.70 may be acceptable depending on the purpose of the study (Griffin-Sobel, 2003). Reliability also focuses on stability (test–retest reliability—whether an instrument yields the same results for the same two people on two different occasions), homogeneity (internal consistency—the extent to which all of the items within a single instrument yield similar results), and equivalence (interrater reliability—the extent to which two or more individuals evaluating the same product or performance give identical judgments) (Fain, 2009; Leedy & Ormrod, 2010).

A simple example of reliability is seen in the selection of timing devices used in sports events. Timing devices must work consistently each and every time so that competitors are ensured an equal chance of winning. An example of interrater reliability is that of a classroom situation in which two evaluators are trained to use the same tool with a Likert scale to measure student performance on oral presentations.

Are the Results of the Study Applicable in the Identified Case?

Once the science of a study has been appraised and the reliability of results assessed, the next important questions are: Do the results apply to the case of interest? Are the populations in the study and in the proposed population for application similar? If the populations studied are not similar, the significance of results in the study has little value for real-life implementation in a given clinical situation.

Is the effect size sufficient so that application of the study intervention will make a significant difference? The *effect size* is calculated by determining the mean difference between two groups (intervention and control) and dividing by the standard deviation. It is not the same as the statistical significance, but rather is the size of the difference between two groups. The effect size is often used in meta-analysis for combining and comparing estimates from different studies in order to determine the effectiveness of an intervention. "An effect size is exactly equivalent to the Z-score of a normal standard deviation. For example an effect size of 0.8 means that the score of the average person in the experimental group is 0.8 standard deviations above the average person in the control group, and hence exceeds the scores of 79% of the control group" (Coe, 2002, p. 2.). Thus,

$$\text{Effect size} = \frac{\text{Mean of experimental group} - \text{Mean of control group}}{\text{Standard deviation}}$$

Generally, in evaluating any quantitative study, additional questions include the following: Why was the study done? How was the sample size decided? How were the data analyzed? Were there any surprises or unexpected events that occurred during the study? How do the results of this study compare with others? (Melnyk & Fineout-Overholt, 2005).

TABLE 22-3	Clinical Statistical Measures

Clinical Statistic	Description
Odds ratio (OR)	The odds of risk for a person in the experimental group having an adverse outcome compared with a person in the control group. An odds ratio of 1 means the event is equally likely in both groups. An odds ratio greater than 1 means the event is more likely in the intervention group than in the control group. An odds ratio less than 1 means the event is less likely in the intervention group than in the control group. Used most in case-control and retrospective studies.
Relative risk ratio (RR)	The risk of an outcome in the intervention/treatment group (Y) compared to the control group (X). $RR = Y / X$. A relative risk of 1 means there is no difference between the two groups. A relative risk of less than 1 means a smaller potential for the effect to occur in the intervention group than in the control group. Used most in randomized controlled trials and cohort studies.
Relative risk reduction (RRR)	The percentage of reduction in the treatment group (Y) compared with the control group (X). $RRR = 1 - Y / X \times 100\%$.
Absolute risk reduction (ARR)	The difference in risk between the control group (X) and the intervention group (Y). $ARR = X - Y$.
Number needed to treat (NNT)	The number of patients that must be treated over a given period of time to prevent one adverse outcome. $NNT = 1 / (X - Y)$.

Source: Long, C. O. (2009). Adapted from Weighing in on the evidence. In N. A. Schmidt & J. M. Brown (Eds.), *Evidence-based practice for nurses.* Sudbury, MA: Jones and Bartlett, p. 323.

The standard of care for practice is increasingly based on scientific evidence. Finding the most current research based on well-conducted clinical trials is an important first step. But how do we evaluate that evidence in practice? Several statistical measures help in the evaluation of study results. **Table 22-3** briefly describes some commonly used statistical tests. An excellent guide to biostatistics is also available from on *MedPage Today* online (Israni, 2007).

What happens if the evidence conflicts with patients' values and preferences? What if our own experience conflicts with the evidence? The key is that the evidence must be relevant to the problem and tested through application.

In addition, some scholars (Fawcett et al., 2001; Kitson, Harvey, & McCormack, 1998; Rycroft-Malone et al., 2004) insisted that evidence as defined by medicine is too narrowly focused and does not recognize the complexities of nursing practice. They recommended that the definition include the influence of context in the application of evidence (Scott-Findley & Pollack, 2004). This would include findings from qualitative research.

Regardless of the definition, however, once evidence is implemented, the results must be evaluated. Did the evidence support better decision making? Was the patient's care improved? In what ways were care or outcomes improved? If they were not improved, why not? (Melnyk & Fineout-Overholt, 2005).

DETERMINING AND IMPLEMENTING THE BEST EVIDENCE FOR PRACTICE

A distinguishing feature of evidence-based nursing is that nurses treat and work *with* patients rather than "work on them" (McSherry, 2002). In addition, nursing's approach is more holistic so that "effectiveness of treatment" is but one indicator; cost-effectiveness and patient acceptability also matter (McSherry, 2002). According to the Agency for Healthcare Research and Quality (AHRQ, 2002, as cited in Melnyk & Fineout-Overholt, 2005), three benchmark domains must be considered when evaluating evidence: quality, quantity, and consistency. *Quality* refers to the absence of biases due to errors in selection, measurement, and confounding biases (internal validity). *Quantity* refers to the number of relevant, related studies; total sample size across studies; size of the treatment effect; and relative risk or odds ratio strength (causality). *Consistency* refers to the similarity of findings across multiple studies regardless of differences in study design. These considerations make it essential that all types of evidence be considered when delivering individual care and implementing systems of care. Based on these domains of evidence, a critical appraisal of types of studies can be facilitated and evaluated to determine the best approach for practice.

QUALITY IMPROVEMENT AND PATIENT-CENTERED CARE

In patient care, a process that facilitates continuous improvement is central to an environment that produces changes in practice, is patient centered and focused on care, and is both evidence based and of high quality. The process must be based on a commitment by all those involved to change practice, and this commitment must be made in advance so that the research findings are applied early on in the

process (French, 1999). As changes are made, they must be continuously evaluated for their impact on care and care systems. The EBP process is consistent with total quality improvement, and often the same resources can be used for both processes.

The steps in the quality management, monitoring, and evaluation processes are based on the work of William Edwards Deming, an American author, professor, statistician, and consultant best known for his work in improving manufacturing production efficiency during World War II. Deming believed that quality is based on continuous improvement of processes and that when work is focused on quality, costs decrease over time (Deming, 1986).

As an APN, the DNP-prepared nurse must be constantly attuned to and knowledgeable about changes in practice to ensure that current best practice is maintained within the context of empirical evidence and patients' preferences.

CONCEPTUAL FRAMEWORKS FOR EVIDENCE AND PRACTICE CHANGE

Two conceptual frameworks that help in the promotion and translation of evidence into practice are the PARIHS (promoting action on research implementation in health services) model (Rycroft-Malone et al., 2002) and the AGREE (appraisal of guidelines for research and evaluation) model (AGREE Collaboration, 2001). The PARIHS model, which is based on the work of Kitson et al. (1998), suggests that the integration of evidence is based on three factors: the nature of the evidence, the context of the desired change, and the mechanism of facilitating change. This evidence, and its translation for practice, includes practice guidelines and other forms of evidence specific to patient outcomes. The use of randomized controlled trials was central to implementation of this model. The model was revised by Rycroft-Malone et al. (2002) to include research information, clinical experience, and patient choice. In the new conceptualization, which involves continuous improvement of patient care through evidence-based nursing, there was recognition of a need for different types of evidence to answer some clinical questions. Evidence based on one's "professional craft" or experience was part of the evidence contribution (Rycroft-Malone et al., 2004).

Further work by Doran and Sidani (2007) identified gaps in the PARIHS model that led to an intervention framework that specifically addressed indicators for evaluating nursing services, systems, performance measures, and feedback to design and evaluate practice change. The intervention framework incorporates the work of Batalden and Stoltz (1993) and

Batalden, Nelson, and Roberts (1994), which identified four categories of information in making care improvements. This information included "clinical (e.g. signs and symptoms), functional (e.g. activities of daily living), satisfaction (e.g. perceived benefit of care) and cost (i.e. both direct and indirect cost to the health care system and the patient)" (Doran & Sidani, 2007, p. 5). **Figure 22-3** depicts Doran and Sidhani's (2007) outcomes-focused knowledge translation intervention framework.

The purpose of the AGREE instrument, as defined by the collaborators, "is to provide a framework for assessing the quality of clinical practice guidelines" (AGREE Collaboration,

FIGURE 22-3 Outcomes-focused knowledge translation intervention framework.

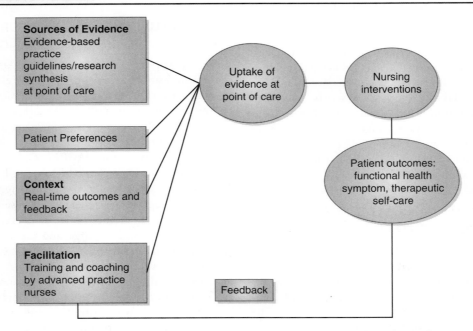

Source: Modified from Doran, D. M., & Sidhani, S. (2007). Outcomes-focused knowledge translation: A frame-work for knowledge translation and patient outcome improvement. *Worldviews on Evidence-Based Nursing, 4*(1), 3–13.

2001, p. 2). Further, "by quality . . . we mean the confidence that the potential biases of guideline development have been addressed adequately and that the recommendations are both internally and externally valid, and are feasible for practice. This process involves taking into account the benefits, harms and costs of the recommendations, as well as the practical issues attached to them. Therefore, the assessment includes the judgments about the methods used for developing the guidelines, the content of the final recommendations, and the factors linked to their uptake" (p. 2). The AGREE instrument consists of 23 items organized in 6 domains: scope and purpose (items 1–3), stakeholder involvement (items 4–7), rigor of development (items 8–14), clarity and presentation (items 15–18), applicability (items 19–21), and editorial independence (items 22–23). The complete instrument and user guide are available for download on the Internet.

The nursing faculty at one family nurse practitioner program, the Lienhard School of Nursing at Pace University, used the AGREE instrument to teach family nurse practitioner students how to critically appraise clinical practice guidelines (Singleton & Levin, 2008). In this program, students practice critiquing single studies, systematic reviews, and clinical practice guidelines. **Tables 22-4** and **22-5** present an exemplar of a learning activity using the AGREE instrument.

The Johns Hopkins model is another evidence-based model, which was developed as a collaborative effort between Johns Hopkins Hospital and the Johns Hopkins School of Nursing. The model is explained in six sections. Section I introduces the concept, the evolution of EBP, and the role of critical thinking in EBP. Section II describes the components of the model. The model uses the PET process (practice question, evidence, and translation).

TABLE 22-4 Learning Activity for the Critical Appraisal of Clinical Practice Guidelines

Steps

1. Preparatory reading:

Slutsky, J. (2005). Using evidence-based practice guidelines: Tools for improving practice. In B. M. Melnyk & E. Fineout-Overholt (Eds.), *Evidence-based practice in nursing and healthcare: A guide to best practice* (pp. 221–227). Philadelphia, PA: Lippincott Williams & Wilkins.

2. Focus for assignment:

Academy of Breastfeeding Medicine. (2004). *Breastfeeding the near term infant (35–37 weeks gestation)*. New Rochelle, NY: Academy of Breastfeeding Medicine.

3. Work in teams.

4. Obtain the guideline.

5. Use the AGREE instrument to critically appraise the guideline.

6. Report back.

Source: Reprinted with permission from SLACK Incorporated: Singleton, J., & Levin, R. (2008). Strategies for learning evidence-based practice: Critically appraising clinical practice guidelines. *Journal of Nursing Education, 47*(8), 380–383.

TABLE 22-5	**Sample Domain and Items from the AGREE Instrument for Critical Appraisal of Clinical Practice Guidelines, with Rating Scale**

Scope and Purpose

The overall objective(s) of the guideline is (are) specifically described.

The clinical question(s) covered by the guideline is (are) specifically described.

The patients to whom the guideline(s) is (are) meant to apply are specifically described.

Rating Scale

Strongly agree 4 3 2 1 Strongly disagree

Source: Reprinted with permission from SLACK Incorporated: Singleton, J., & Levin, R. (2008). Strategies for learning evidence-based practice: Critically appraising clinical practice guidelines. *Journal of Nursing Education, 47*(8), 380–383.

Section III further explores the PET process in developing EBP projects. Section IV describes the environment necessary for the success of EBP. Section V provides examples of EBP projects. Section VI contains tools used for EBP at Johns Hopkins. A table of contents and sample, including levels of evidence from the model and guidelines, can be downloaded from the Nursing Knowledge International website.

The model and guidelines have "leveled objectives" for nursing students at the baccalaureate, graduate, and doctoral levels. At the doctoral level, the focus is on reviewing, rating, synthesizing, evaluating, and translating evidence at an advanced level (Newhouse, Dearholt, Poe, Pugh, & White, 2008). An example of one evidence-based project, developed by the Neuroscience Nursing Practice Committee, is a question related to the correct procedure for establishing nasogastric tube placement in adult patients. Using the PICO (patient, intervention, comparison, and outcomes) format and levels of evidence, the existing protocol that required insufflations of air was discontinued. A table of the process and levels of evidence is shown in the Johns Hopkins model instructor's guide (Newhouse et al., 2008), available on the Internet.

DESIGNING AND IMPLEMENTING PROCESSES TO EVALUATE OUTCOMES OF PRACTICE AND SYSTEMS OF CARE

As nursing moves practice decisions from those based on tradition to those based on empirical evidence, the APN, particularly the DNP, is in the best position to effect and assess change within the clinical setting. Why? Evidence-based practice and quality management are both practice-driven processes (French, 1999). Each is informed by experience and outcomes that can be directly seen and measured. In most cases, the observations that arise during daily practice provide the basis for questions, which can be empirically tested and their results implemented and evaluated. The findings of previous research studies can be replicated in a variety of settings with resources that are already in place.

The curriculum of Doctor of Nursing Practice programs includes specialty-focused competencies delineated by specialty nursing organizations, and the core essentials include courses and application experiences in research methods and statistical analysis (AACN, 2006). This education, coupled with advanced clinical knowledge, provides the DNP-prepared nurse with the requisites necessary to design and collaborate in studies that can make a practical difference in the delivery of clinical care (French, 1999; Reavy & Tavernier, 2008). **Table 22-6** lists some examples of clinical studies concerning advanced practice nursing interventions and outcomes, as well as studies or interventions designed by DNP-prepared nurses.

TABLE 22-6 Selected DNP Scholarly Publications: Evidence-Based Research Interventions and Outcomes

Author/Year	Design, Sample, Setting	Framework/ Intervention/ Measures	Goal/Aim	Outcomes/ Findings
Santucci, S. (2011)	EBP; community needs assessment and gap analysis; convenience sample of 50 adults; underserved southeastern U.S. community.	Health Belief Model with prevention constructs. Policy change in Community Rapid Testing Program to allow referral of HIV-positive patients to hospital-based ID clinic for follow-up and prevention; data on system change variables—e.g., tests/ results, referrals—were entered weekly in database.	Close gap to secondary prevention service to decrease HIV morbidity, mortality, and transmission.	New system for expedited care to marginalized groups; change decreased time to test results/referral for treatment from 6–8 weeks to 1–2 weeks.
Graling, P. R. (2011)	EBP; quality improvement N = 283 surgical care providers (2009); N = 287 (2010) at large university hospital.	Framework for Knowledge Transfer of Patient Safety (AHRQ); Universal Protocol (The Joint Commission, 2009); Attitude Questionnaire (Self-Assessment Questionnaire); team education; implementation of safety checklist.	Enhance perioperative teamwork; decrease safety events; improve compliance with Universal Protocol (The Joint Commission, 2009).	Statistically significant differences were found in safety climate and working differences overall; safety events decreased by 50%; compliance with the safety checklist increased in 2010, but could not be compared with 2009 because the checklist changed; resources have now been allocated for perioperative safety initiatives.

(continues)

| | | **TABLE 22-6** | Selected DNP Scholarly Publications: Evidence-Based Research Interventions and Outcomes *(continued)* | |

Author/Year	Design, Sample, Setting	Framework/ Intervention/ Measures	Goal/Aim	Outcomes/ Findings
Chism, L. A. (2009)	Descriptive-correlational. *N* = 223 graduate and undergraduate nursing students; convenience sample.	Chism's Middle Range Theory of Spiritual Empathy; do empirical data support the theory that relates nurses' spiritual care perspectives to expressions of spiritual empathy? Measures were Spiritual Care Perspectives scale; expression of spiritual empathy scales 1 and 2; demographic worksheet.	Explore relationships among demographic variables, spiritual care, and levels of spiritual empathy; determine extent to which nursing students' spiritual care perspectives influenced expression of empathy after controlling for demographic variables.	Church attendance, gender, and religious affiliation showed small/ significant correlation with nursing students' attitudes about spiritual care. Considering oneself spiritual showed moderately strong positive relationship with nursing students' attitudes about spiritual care. Study limitations were described; implications for educational programs for nursing students were discussed.
Andrews (2008)	Case study. Rare disease diagnosis: pheochromocytoma genetics, 40 y.o. African American male with refractory hypertension presenting to ER.	Holistic evidence-based approach to clinical history taking and evaluation for correct diagnosis.	Lab tests, assessment of diagnostic clues and probability characteristics, genetic pedigree analysis.	B/P management; surgical intervention; genetic testing. Advanced practice nurses' well-honed evidence-based approach and interview skills allow them to play a pivotal role in exploration, diagnosis, and management of this type of complex situation.

| | | **TABLE 22-6** | **Selected DNP Scholarly Publications: Evidence-Based Research Interventions and Outcomes** *(continued)* | |

Author/Year	Design, Sample, Setting	Framework/ Intervention/ Measures	Goal/Aim	Outcomes/ Findings
Doyle-Lindrud (2008)	Case study. Gestational breast cancer; 33 y.o. Asian female with breast lump and positive pregnancy test. Outpatient cancer center.	Health history and examination; health promotion; anticipatory guidance; collaborative approach to care; chronic disease management.	Lab tests; radiology; long-term follow-up care; psychosocial care; chronic care management.	The DNP elements of doctoral competency were illustrated in the evaluation, collaboration, anticipatory planning, and disease management of care in this complex situation.
Dohrn, J. (2008)	Case study. HIV treatment for pregnant women, rural Eastern Cape, South Africa, with 30–35% HIV prevalence and less than half of facilities providing prevention interventions. Pregnant women enter antenatal care after 24 weeks.	Design of midwifery model of care; interviews; observations; self-assessment of skills and capacity to deliver HIV care.	Voluntary testing and counseling; mother-to-child prevention intervention; antiretroviral treatment; peer counseling; community worker outreach; fast-tracking for antiretroviral therapy; maternity nurse training; anticipatory counseling; early postpartum care/education; midwife training; nurse mentoring; communication between nurses and MDs; strengthen community worker role.	Study resulted in consensus on model of care for HIV-infected women that included HIV prevention, testing, and management. This model has the potential to impact qualitatively and quantitatively the health of South Africans by decreasing the number of infants born with HIV and decreasing maternal mortality, aiding orphans and quality of life.

The Essentials of Doctoral Education for Advanced Nursing Practice (AACN, 2006) states that "DNP graduates must understand principles of practice management, including conceptual and practice strategies for balancing productivity and quality care" (p. 4). In addition, "they must be able to assess the impact of clinical policies and procedures on meeting the health needs of the patient populations with whom they practice" (p. 4). Also, "they must be proficient in quality improvement strategies and in creating and sustaining changes at the organizational and policy levels" (p. 4).

QUALITY IMPROVEMENT INITIATIVES TO PROMOTE SAFE, TIMELY, EFFECTIVE, EFFICIENT, EQUITABLE, AND PATIENT-CENTERED CARE

The design of quality improvement initiatives must be empirically based and dependent on sources of knowledge that include research evidence; clinical experience; reasoning; authority; quality improvement data; and the patient's situation, values, and experience (Brown, 2005).

These are the tools that can help the DNP-prepared nurse decide whether the clinical guidelines and scientific evidence are consistent with the context, values, and desires of the patient (Glanville, Schirm, & Wineman, 2000).

For the past century, most outcome measurement has focused on the outcomes of medical care, particularly negative outcomes. However, during the past several years, there has been a greater focus on positive indicators of nursing care delivery (Melnyk & Fineout-Overholt, 2005). The development of nurse-sensitive patient outcomes (NSPOs) was an outgrowth of public demand for greater accountability by healthcare providers.

Some examples of nurse-sensitive indicators of quality include health-promoting behaviors (Mitchell, Ferketich, & Jennings, 1998), compliance/adherence (Ingersoll, McIntosh, & Williams, 2000), quality of life (Ingersoll et al., 2000), support systems available to assist with caregiver burden (Craft-Rosenburg, Krajicek, & Shin, 2002), trust in care provider (Ingersoll et al., 2000), and length of stay (Hodge, Asch, Olson, Kravitz, & Sauve, 2002). **Table 22-7**

TABLE 22-7	Selected Evidence-Based Outcome Indicators for Advanced Practice Nursing

Outcomes	Examples and Indicators
Patient satisfaction	Ambulatory care: Survey
Risk	Morbidity and mortality: Summary
	Patient falls: Reports
	Medication errors: Medication administration records (MARs); comprehensiveness of exams
Knowledge	Blood pressure medication: Blood pressure control
Condition-specific	Postoperative pain: Pain management scale
	Diabetes management: Blood glucose levels
Infection control	Surgical procedures: Hand washing; nosocomial infection rates
Compliance	Fluid restriction: Daily weights
	Prenatal and postpartum visits

presents additional examples of evidence-based outcome indicators.

The success of evidence-based practice depends on asking the right questions at the right time, critically analyzing results of other studies for fit in a given situation, observing for differences in responses, and evaluating. In this regard, quality improvement evaluation is important in advanced practice to ascertain the impact of interventions and their effect on cost-effective care. DNP and APN interventions are appropriately evaluated on the basis of physiological, psychosocial, functional, behavioral, and knowledge-focused effectiveness (Glanville et al., 2000). The evaluation process involves the selection of appropriate measurement instruments. Glanville et al. (2000) made the point that instruments that measure effectiveness in care processes are not the same as those that measure outcomes. For example, a tool that measures risk for patient infections is not the same tool as one that actually tracks infection rates in a group of postsurgical patients. Similarly, in process management, the focus is on which components produce or contribute to practice variations that may ultimately affect, but are not the same as, outcomes (Ingersoll, 2005).

Some basic provisions for an effective outcomes model are to keep the outcomes as short as possible; to use outcomes, not activities or processes; and to use singular, not compound, outcomes (Duignan, 2006). Components of an effective outcomes management model include the following:

> 1) identification of the problem, 2) scanning the existing evidence and standards of care, 3) identification of benchmark targets, 4) determination and selection of outcomes measuring and monitoring tools, 5) development of specific guidelines to drive care delivery processes, 6) assessment of existing processes, 7) measurement and monitoring of processes and outcomes of care, 8) reporting findings to key stakeholders and decision makers, and 9) refining care delivery processes and data collection techniques based on findings. (Ingersoll, 2005, pp. 314–315)

A significant time commitment is required for designing systems for promoting safe, timely, patient-centered care. However, the benefits are efficiency and effectiveness. Since the Institute of Medicine (IOM) studies, patient safety has been a primary focus of quality improvement initiatives. Safety issues are of concern in every care setting—primary, secondary, and tertiary. A review of the literature from 2000 to 2011 in the Medline and CINAHL databases produced 217 (Medline/PubMed) and 78 (CINAHL) nondissertation nursing studies that involved quality improvement projects with safety as a focus. Only 4 studies included the word *evidence* in the title. Topics included studies on drug errors, environment, technology, acute care, pediatrics, critical care, culture, intravenous infusions, long-term care and home health, rural health, legislation and oversight, policy, diabetes, anesthesia, health education, chemotherapy, childhood vaccines, blood and HIV, neuroscience issues, food and drug issues, nurse injury, radiation, emergency services, and behavioral health. In addition to safety issues, a number of studies dealt with issues of timely (24 studies in CINAHL), effective (13,000 studies in CINAHL), and equitable care (467 studies in CINAHL), which are also important dimensions of quality that need to be addressed, especially as they affect safety and quality outcomes. Patient-centered care was addressed in 6,100 CINAHL studies. Direct care providers, including DNP-prepared nurses, must take a lead role in continuing the effort to improve care delivery systems that benefit patients, families, and providers of care.

USING PRACTICE GUIDELINES TO IMPROVE PRACTICE AND THE PRACTICE ENVIRONMENT

As Goolsby, Meyers, Johnson, Klardie, and McNaughton (2004) have noted, "clinical practice guidelines are protocol-driven, step-wise recommendations for diagnosing, and treating specific conditions, or patient populations"

(p. 178). Clinical decision making is grounded in the use of clinical research, expert opinion, and clinical practice guidelines. Further, clinical practice guidelines "minimize differences in practice patterns and the risk of misdiagnosis or treatment failures" (Goolsby, Meyers, et al., 2004, p. 178). Unfortunately, practice guidelines are not always used for a variety of reasons. Time, communication, involvement, resources, patient expectations, and perceived priority are all facilitators of or barriers to the implementation of evidence-based practice guidelines (DiCenso, Cullum, & Ciliska, 1998; Gagan & Hewitt-Taylor, 2004; Lopez-Bushnell, 2002; McCaughan, Thompson, Cullum, Sheldon, & Thompson, 2002; Rutledge & Bookbinder, 2002).

One way to eliminate some of the barriers is through the use of "linkage agents." As described by Cooke et al. (2004), APNs, particularly DNP-prepared nurses, are in an excellent position to propose scientifically based recommendations to reduce cost and improve quality, documentation, and outcomes. In developing an institutional change model to promote evidence-based practice with cancer patients, the linking agents from the nursing research department at one hospital functioned as rotating consultants 3 to 4 hours per month. The linking agent consultants rotated to clinical units for 1 hour of monthly case presentation and analysis to assist clinical nurses in translating research into practice. The theoretical framework used was a quality of life model with four domains: psychological, social, physical, and spiritual (Padilla, Ferrell, Grant, & Rhiner, 1990). Each month, one or more topics related to the four domains relevant to a case study were discussed. A brief 5-minute lecture was presented on EBP principles at the beginning of the session. The program started as a research outreach program and evolved into an EBP program that linked a case study format with critical thinking and practical application. This approach could be modified and used in a variety of clinical practice settings.

EVALUATION OF PRACTICE

He who every morning plans the transaction of the day and follows out that plan, carries a thread that will guide him through the maze of the most busy life. But where no plan is laid, where the disposal of time is surrendered merely to the chance of incidence, chaos will soon reign.

—Victor Hugo

Evaluating practice and changes in practice is essential to the successful implementation of any quality improvement or evidence-based practice initiative. Evaluation is an ongoing process that must start early in a project and be continual. Planning for evaluation is as important as the change itself and must be a systematic process. Classification schemes allow for an organized approach to evaluating outcomes. Outcomes may be classified according to population served (e.g., pediatric, adult, geriatric), time (long term, medium term, or short term), or type (care related, patient related, or performance related) (Schmidt & Brown, 2009).

USING BENCHMARKS TO EVALUATE CLINICAL OUTCOMES AND TRENDS

One method of evaluating practice is to evaluate practice patterns against national benchmarks to determine variances in clinical outcomes and population trends. Benchmarking is "the continual process of measuring services and practices against the toughest competitors in the industry" (Hebda & Czar, 2009). Organizations that regularly collect data on outcomes in health care are state boards of health and the Centers for Medicare and Medicaid Services (CMS). The Joint Commission and the Magnet Recognition Program (American Nurses Credentialing Center, 2005) also have performance measurement standards that are based on quality indicators. In addition to these organizations, many hospitals and healthcare facilities have memberships in organizations that benchmark indicators of

TABLE 22-8	Websites for Healthcare Outcome Information

Organization	Website
AcademyHealth	http://www.academyhealth.org
Agency for Healthcare Research and Quality	http://www.ahrq.gov/research/findings/evidence-based-reports/index.html
Centers for Medicare and Medicaid Services	http://www.cms.gov
Institute for Healthcare Improvement	http://www.ihi.org
International Society for Pharmacoeconomics and Outcomes Research	http://www.ispor.org
The Joint Commission	http://www.jointcommission.org
National Cancer Institute	http://appliedresearch.cancer.gov
National Committee for Quality Assurance	http://www.ncqa.org
National Quality Forum	http://www.qualityforum.org/Home.aspx
University of Iowa College of Nursing	http://www.nursing.uiowa.edu/cncce/nursing-outcomes-classification-overview

Source: Modified from Rich, K. A. (2009). Evaluating outcomes of innovations. In N. A. Schmidt & J. M. Brown (Eds.), *Evidence-based practice for nurses* (p. 388). Sudbury, MA: Jones and Bartlett.

quality in specialty services (Schmidt & Brown, 2009).

Nursing services are an important aspect of outcome evaluation and reporting at any healthcare institution because nurses make up such a large part of the healthcare workforce. Effectiveness of nursing care is determined by nurse-sensitive indicators. Nursing administrators are responsible for maintaining evaluation systems and reporting nurse-sensitive outcomes. As leaders in clinical care and outcome evaluation, DNP-prepared nurses must be in the forefront of designing outcome evaluation plans for advanced practice.

DNP-prepared nurses in advanced practice roles are also included in medical outcome working groups within their scope of practice. The American Medical Association Physician Consortium for Performance Improvement (AMA-PCPI) has performance measures

available for 31 topics or conditions (Gallagher, 2009). The general approach to measurement includes six steps: "1) identifying the opportunities for improvement, 2) involving representation from medical specialties and other care disciplines, 3) linking measures to an evidence base, 4) supporting clinical judgment and patient preferences, 5) testing measures, and 6) promoting a single set of measures for widespread use and multiple purpose" (Gallagher, 2009, p. 185). **Table 22-8** contains a brief listing of websites for healthcare outcomes and data.

DATABASE DESIGN TO GENERATE MEANINGFUL EVIDENCE FOR NURSING PRACTICE

A systematic process for patient care and practice data is essential to guide practice. This requires the development of standardized databases to guide outcomes research for practice. Clinical databases from computerized medical records and disease registries are the result of documentation of care or research protocols. Outcome data are also available from birth logs, death records, discharge summaries, and clinical pathways. Most important, the outcome must be measurable, and the data must relate to the care processes or interventions (Arthur, Marfell, & Ulrich, 2009).

Another useful resource for evidence-based outcomes is the National Guideline Clearinghouse (NGC), an initiative of the AHRQ, the American Medical Association, and America's Health Insurance Plans. Users can subscribe to the NGC weekly email update service. The site provides information about new and updated guidelines from the Centers for Disease Control and Prevention (CDC), the National Institute for Clinical Excellence, the Program for

Evidence-Based Care, and others. Conference information is also available, as well as food and drug advisory information.

The *Cochrane Collaboration Review* is another source that provides reprints online of the newest intervention reviews. The *Review* lists authors and their affiliations; an abstract, including background, objectives, search strategies, selection criteria, data collection, and analysis; authors' conclusions; and a plain-language summary. The library contains sections for clinicians, researchers, patients, and policy makers. The Cochrane Library, a collection of medical and healthcare databases, is available online through Wiley InterScience. Podcasts are also available.

These and other evidence-based resources are effective tools to aid in the efficient delivery of evidence-based care. **Table 22-9** provides a brief description of other available databases.

TABLE 22-9   Evidence Databases

Source	Content
American College of Physicians (ACP) Journal Club	Articles reporting original studies and systematic reviews.
AHRQ	Produces guidelines and technology assessments on selected topics from 12 evidence-based practice centers.
AIDSLINE	Indexes the published literature on HIV and AIDS. The index includes journal articles; monographs; meeting abstracts; and papers, newsletters, and government reports (Fain, 2009).
Bandolier	Reviews literature; offers subjects by medical specialty.
CANCERLIT	Includes cancer literature from journal articles, government reports, technical reports, meeting abstracts and papers, and monographs.
CDC Sexually Transmitted Disease Treatment Guidelines	Includes Web-browsable source with crosslinks.

| **TABLE 22-9** | Evidence Databases *(continued)* |

Source	Content
Cochrane Database of Systematic Reviews	"Reviews individual clinical trials and summarizes systematic reviews from over 100 medical journals" (Fain, 2009, p. 277).
DynaMed	Point-of-care resource to support clinical decision making.
EPPI Centre	Evidence for Policy and Practice Information and Co-ordinating Centre, Institute of Education, University of London.
Essential Evidence Plus (formerly InfoPOEMs)	Includes reviews and commentary of recently published articles by the *Journal of Family Practice*.
Evidence-Based Practice at the University of Iowa	Includes an evidence-based practice toolkit, information about recent evidence-based practice projects, and an evidence-based practice model and resources.
HealthLinks: Evidence-Based Practice	Includes metasearch engines and links to peer-reviewed journals, a DNP toolkit, and other publications.
HSTAT	Health Services Technology Assessment Text, full-text guidelines.
The Joanna Briggs Institute	International institute that provides resources for evidence-based practice for healthcare professionals in nursing, medicine, midwifery, and allied health.
Johns Hopkins Evidence-Based Practice Center	Includes systematic reviews of evidence.
MD Consult	Includes full-text access to journal articles, textbooks, practice guidelines, patient education handouts, and drug awareness information. MD Consult is a good, quick source for background information on a topic.
MEDLINE	A compilation of information from Index Medicus, Index to Dental Literature, and the International Nursing Index. It includes published research in allied health, biological sciences, information sciences, physical sciences, and the humanities.
MedPage Today	Includes daily research updates, news by specialty, policy news, continuing medical education (CME), and surveys. Includes an excellent tool, MedPage Tools Guide to Biostatistics, that can be used as a reference guide when reading research articles.
National Guideline Clearinghouse	Provides nonintegrated evidence-based practice clinical guidelines and recommendations on selected topics from a number of organizations.

(continues)

TABLE 22-9 Evidence Databases *(continued)*

Source	Content
Prescriber's Letter	Includes evidence-based information on new drug developments, with links to articles and continuing education offerings.
PubMed	Provides source for queries and evidence-based filters for MEDLINE.
ScHarr	School of Health and Related Research. Comprehensive up-to-date evidence on the Web.
University of Illinois http://researchguides.uic.edu/cat.php?cid=5873	Resources, links, video presentations, and learning modules.
University of Minnesota https://www.lib.umn.edu/apps/instruction/ebp	Links and EBP tutorial with case scenarios.

Source: Data from Fain, J. A. (2009). Understanding evidence-based practice. In *Reading, understanding and applying nursing research* (3rd ed., pp. 276–278). Philadelphia, PA: F. A. Davis.

The use of these resources is valuable when combined with the best empirical knowledge and judgment. The true measure of their effectiveness is in the evaluation of the outcomes of management and care decisions and delivery processes.

As nursing takes on larger, more autonomous roles in the delivery of health care through advanced practice, the need for accountability will continue to increase. DNP-prepared nurses, with their knowledge of clinical practice, research, and informatics, can best represent advanced practice nursing by participating in and guiding the development of databases that are relevant to the care that DNP-prepared nurses and APNs provide. Becoming involved in professional organizations that have quality initiatives is an excellent way for DNPs to become knowledgeable in research that contributes to quality care and the profession.

The American Nurses Association (ANA) and specialty organizations such as the Oncology Nursing Society, the Advanced Practice Registered Nurses' Research Network, and the Midwest Nursing Centers Consortium Research Network, a practice-based research network funded by the AHRQ, provide avenues for collaboration and dissemination of information on quality and outcomes (Burns & Grove, 2009).

INFORMATION TECHNOLOGY, DATABASES, AND EVIDENCE FOR PRACTICE

Computers have changed the face of clinical care, making them a necessary tool for research and evidence-based practice. They provide efficiency in the inputting of statistical data and the retrieval of the most current information on relevant clinical trial outcomes, supportive research, and accepted practice protocols. It is essential to pay attention to the kinds of data that are retrieved and how they are used to make clinical decisions and evaluate practice.

COLLECTING APPROPRIATE AND ACCURATE DATA

Data and observations from practice can be augmented and strengthened through evidence from clinical trials. Several electronic databases provide access to clinical trial data and other peer-reviewed research and outcome data. However, clinical trial data and data from other aggregate sources do not always address the outcomes that can be uniquely attributed to APN or DNP-prepared nurse practice. For APNs and DNP-prepared nurses to assess and demonstrate their effectiveness, data are needed that reflect what they do. Although the primary goal of outcome data and analysis is to improve care, DNP-prepared nurses in direct practice may be asked to justify their roles in terms of factors such as cost, time, patient outcomes, and revenue generation, among other indicators (Burns, 2009).

Most institutions rely on aggregated data to determine nursing outcomes. Unfortunately, most aggregated data do not show the APN's or DNP-prepared nurse's specific contribution to the outcomes (Burns, 2009). For this reason, it is important that measures be selected that truly reflect the APN/DNP role. This means developing role-sensitive indicators and collecting data that are specific to those indicators in a systematic way. Indicators such as satisfaction with APN and DNP-prepared nurse care related to a particular program or procedure that the APN or DNP-prepared nurse initiates, controls, or coordinates are better than trying to extrapolate the APN's or DNP-prepared nurse's role in a multidisciplinary effort. Time savings or clinical outcomes related to a change in practice coordinated by the APN or DNP-prepared nurse may also be role sensitive.

A well-designed assessment plan uses a model that considers organizational factors, employee behavior, patient characteristics, patient experience, and outcomes (Minnick & Roberts, 1991, Figure 4-1, as cited in Minnick, 2009). Instruments for measuring outcomes are also a necessary component in the assessment process. A systematic search of the databases mentioned in Table 22-9, such as AHRQ, PubMed, and CancerLit may be helpful as a starting place for appropriate measurement tools.

ANALYZING DATA FROM CLINICAL PRACTICE

Data from practice are rich and can be analyzed in a number of ways, depending on the nature of the research question. Computer-based statistical tools such as absolute risk (AR) and absolute risk reduction (ARR) calculations, relative risk (RR) and relative risk reduction (RRR) calculations, number needed to treat (NNT), survival curves, hazard ratios, and sensitivity and specificity are helpful measures for assessing risk of disease in studies of different cohort groups and in aiding clinical decision making. In an excellent article in the *Journal of the American Academy of Nurse Practitioners*, Goolsby, Klardie, Johnson, McNaughton, and Meyers (2004) analyzed the implementation of clinical practice guidelines (CPGs) and their outcomes in a hypothetical patient situation. The analysis includes a review of commonly used statistical concepts, including some of those just mentioned, with examples of their application in interpreting and reporting research. Johnston (2005) also provides a detailed section on statistical measures and their meaning in a chapter entitled "Critically Appraising Quantitative Evidence."

DESIGNING EVIDENCE-BASED INTERVENTIONS

Selecting and defining the problem is one of the most critical steps in the design of any evidence-based intervention. The problem statement provides the direction for the study design and is usually stated at the beginning. Essential to good design is adequate background information that includes a rationale for pursuing an intervention, evidence from research that has already been done on the topic, and the goals to be achieved (Fain, 2009). Depending on the problem to be addressed, evidence-based interventions may be generated from quantitative research, qualitative research, outcome studies, patient concerns and choices, or clinical judgment.

Models serve as good frameworks for design. Several models that were originally designed for research utilization were the historical precursors to evidence-based practice. Three well-known models for research utilization and evidence-based practice are the conduct and utilization of research in nursing (CURN) model (Horsely, Crane, & Bingle, 1978), the Kitson model (Kitson et al., 1998), the Stetler/Marram model (Stetler, 1994; Stetler & Marram, 1976), and the Iowa model of research utilization (Titler et al., 1994). As evidence-based practice has evolved, these models have been adapted, and other models have been developed. Some later models include the Advancing Research and Clinical Practice Through Close Collaboration (ARCC) model (Melnyk & Fineout-Overholt, 2002), the Rosswurm and Larrabee model (1999), the Iowa model of evidence-based practice to promote quality care (Titler, 2002), and the Johns Hopkins model (Newhouse et al., 2008). Each of these models has been successful in disseminating research or in facilitating change toward evidence-based practice. **Figure 22-4** shows a schematic of the Iowa model.

It is beyond the scope of this chapter to detail the specifics of each model. However, although there are nuances and structural differences, all the models support some form of practice change through the systematic review of research and other evidence, such as clinical practice guidelines, to create a culture of research conduct and research utilization. Certainly, the first step in the design of any practice intervention is to define the clinical practice questions. Once that is accomplished, critical questions include the following: What patients will be affected? What treatment or intervention or practice change is involved? What old practice would need to be discontinued? What outcomes are expected? (Collins et al., 2008).

The next step is to review the evidence, basing the analysis on the hierarchy of evidence (see Table 22-1) and a search of all relevant databases (e.g., Cochrane, CINAHL, National Guideline Clearinghouse). Once the evidence has been verified, assessing applicability to the population and environment is crucial. Questions to be considered may include the following: Will implementing this practice increase patient safety? Are there ethical or legal considerations? Will other departments or providers be affected? How will the change affect practitioner time? How will patients react to the change? The next step is to develop a plan for the change. Who are the key stakeholders? How will they be apprised and included? Who has final sign-off authority? Is a pilot study indicated before full-scale implementation? Finally, determine the methods of education and communication. How much time, money, and personnel resources will be needed?

When implementing the plan, the following questions should be considered: Who is responsible for coordinating the effort? What contingency plans are in place in the event that a change must be made? Who is managing issues that may arise? Evaluate the implementation on an ongoing basis. How will feedback be generated? Who will conduct the evaluation? What is the method of analysis? What are the measurement tools? How will results of the evaluation be presented? (Collins et al., 2008). Some specific strategies to promote guideline implementation are outlined by Carey, Buchan, and Sanson-Fisher (2009). **Table 22-10** summarizes their recommendations.

FIGURE 22-4 The Iowa model of evidence-based practice to promote quality care.

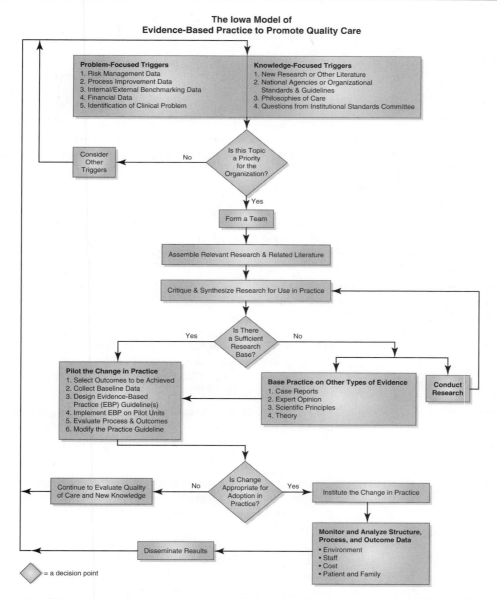

The Iowa Model of Evidence-Based Practice to Promote Quality Care

Source: Used/Reprinted with permission from the University of Iowa Hospitals and Clinics and Marita G. Titler, PhD, RN, FAAN. Copyright 1998. For permission to use or reproduce the model, please contact the University of Iowa Hospitals and Clinics at (319)384-9098

TABLE 22-10	Strategies to Promote Guideline Implementation: Theoretical Constructs and Examples of Application

Strategy	Relevant Constructs	Key Illustrative Examples
Phase 1		
Concrete and specific recommendations	Knowledge, executability, decidability	Concrete and specific recommendations were more likely to be adopted by general practitioners (GPs) than were vague, nonspecific recommendations. Observational study. (Grol et al., 1998)
Identify priorities	Goal setting, action planning	Of 228 primary care patients with cardiovascular disease risk factors who made an action plan to identify behavioral change goals, 53% also reported making behavioral change related to their action plan. Descriptive study. (Handley et al., 2006)
Set targets for implementation	Goal setting	
Present a rationale	Beliefs, attitudes, perceived relative advantage	Recommendations compatible with current values were more likely to be adopted by GPs than were those perceived as controversial or incompatible with values. Observational study. (Grol et al., 1998)
Highlight clinical norms	Normative beliefs, attitudes, modeling/verbal persuasion	An intervention to improve myocardial infarction care that involved using local medical opinion leaders to influence peers through small-group discussions, informal consultation, and revisions of clinical protocols was compared with performance feedback alone. Hospitals in both groups improved from baseline to follow-up on indicators of quality; however, the improvement was greatest for those allocated to the peer intervention. Randomized controlled trial. (Soumerai et al., 1998)
Orient to the need of the end user	Complexity	Among the guideline characteristics most commonly endorsed to promote use by GPs was "clarity, simplicity and availability of a short format." Descriptive study of 391 GPs. (Watkins et al., 1999)
Phase 2		
Skills training	Skills, knowledge, self-efficacy	Continuing medical education (CME) improves knowledge, skills, attitudes, and patient outcomes. CME that is interactive, uses multimedia, live media, and involves multiple exposures is more effective than other types. Systematic review. (Marinopoulos et al., 2007)
Social influences	Normative beliefs, attitudes, modeling, verbal persuasion	The use of local opinion leaders in hospital settings can be effective in promoting evidence-based practice. Systematic review of 12 studies. (Doumitt, Gattelliari, Grimshaw, & O'Brien, 2007)

| | **TABLE 22-10** | Strategies to Promote Guideline Implementation: Theoretical Constructs and Examples of Application *(continued)* |

Strategy	Relevant Constructs	Key Illustrative Examples
Environmental influences	Cues to action, environmental triggers	Guideline adherence improved due to the implementation of a computerized clinical decision aid that gave clinicians real-time recommendations for venous thromboembolism prophylaxis. Time series study. (Durieux, Nizard, Ravaud, Mounier, & Lepage, 2000)
Patient-mediated	Knowledge, skills, and attitudes of patients	Patient request for a new drug and patient acceptability were cited as contributing to decisions to prescribe a new drug in approximately 20% of cases. Descriptive study. (Prosser, Almond, & Walley, 2003)
Feedback	Positive/negative reinforcement; goal setting; skill development	Audit and feedback are effective strategies for improving care, particularly when baseline adherence to the recommended practice is low. Systematic review of 118 studies. (Jamtvedt, Young, Kristofferson, O'Brien, & Oxman, 2006)
Incentives	Positive/negative reinforcement	Five of six studies examining physician-level incentives, and seven of nine studies examining provider group–level incentives demonstrated partial or positive effects on quality indicators. Systematic review. (Peterson, Woodward, Urech, Daw, & Sookanan, 2006)
Phase 3		
Pilot testing with iterative refinement of implementation strategies	Perceived advantages; beliefs; trialability	Breakthrough collaborative model intervention that involved a series of iterative plan-do-study-act cycles was found to be effective in improving care for chronic heart failure. Quasi-experimental, controlled study. (Asch et al., 2005)

Source: Carey, M., Buchan, H., & Sanson-Fisher, R. (2009). The cycle of change: Implementing the best-evidence clinical practice. *International Journal for Quality in Health Care, 21*(1), 37–43. Reproduced with permission.

PREDICTING AND ANALYZING OUTCOMES

Often in clinical practice, the occurrence of one event in time may be the basis for predicting a future event. In such instances, a predictive relationship is established. In this case, the practitioner or researcher is looking for a correlation between the two events that may predict the outcome of a future intervention or occurrence that could be designed to affect or influence the independent variable. Although correlational prediction is not the same as cause and effect, it is stronger than a purely descriptive study (Melnyk & Cole, 2005). This type of study would be appropriate if, for example, the DNP-prepared nurse was interested in how a person's initial attitude toward insulin affected compliance with the regimen 3, 6, or 12 months after the therapy began.

Correlation statistics would be used to measure the relationship between the two variables. The results of the correlation could later be used to design interventions, such as educational strategies or follow-up programs, that would help those with negative attitudes toward therapy learn, adapt, and achieve more positive outcomes. Correlational statistics are also used to measure the strength of relationship between two variables. A direct correlation is seen in correlation coefficients between the values of 0 (no correlation) and 1 (large positive correlation) and means that when there is a large change in the value of one predictor, there is a large change in the value of the other predictor; likewise, a small change in one predictor is accompanied by a small change in the other predictor. A relationship that has a correlation coefficient of 0.5 is stronger than 0, but less than 1.0. Conversely, in a negative correlation—between 0 (no correlation) and –1 (large negative correlation)—large changes in the value of one predictor would be accompanied by small changes in the other, or small changes in one would be accompanied by large changes in the other. Therefore, a negative correlation coefficient of –0.6 shows a stronger negative relationship between two variables than a coefficient of 0, but not as strong as a coefficient of –1.0 (Lanthier, 2002).

An example of this kind of analysis is shown in a correlation study on salary and income levels. **Table 22-11** shows salary levels and corresponding years of education. **Figure 22-5** shows an example of a correlation scatter plot, with years of education on the y axis and income on the x axis. Each point on the plot shows one person's answers to the questions regarding years of education and income. In a positive correlation such as this, the line is always in the upward direction. In another example, **Table 22-12** and **Figure 22-6** show a negative

TABLE 22-11   Salary and Years of Education

Participant	Income	Years of Education
1	125,000	19
2	100,000	20
3	40,000	16
4	35,000	16
5	41,000	18
6	29,000	12
7	35,000	14
8	24,000	12
9	50,000	16
10	60,000	17

Source: Lanthier, E. (2002). Correlation samples. http://www.nvcc.edu/home/elanthier/methods/correlation-samples.htm. Copyright 2002 by Elizabeth Lanthier, PhD. Reproduced with permission.

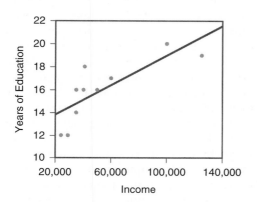

FIGURE 22-5 Regression scatter plot, salary, and education in years.

Source: Lanthier, E. (2002). Correlation samples. http://www.nvcc.edu/home/elanthier/methods /correlationsamples.htm. Copyright 2002 by Elizabeth Lanthier, PhD. Reproduced with permission.

TABLE 22-12 Grade Point Average and TV Use

Participant	GPA	TV Use (hr/wk)
1	3.1	14
2	2.4	10
3	2.0	20
4	3.8	7
5	2.2	25
6	3.4	9
7	2.9	15
8	3.2	13
9	3.7	4
10	3.5	21

Source: Lanthier, E. (2002). Correlation samples. http://www.nvcc.edu/home/elanthier/methods /correlation-samples.htm. Copyright 2002 by Elizabeth Lanthier, PhD. Reproduced with permission.

FIGURE 22-6 Regression scatter plot, hours of television use, and grade point average.

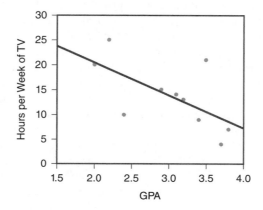

Source: Lanthier, E. (2002). Correlation samples. http://www.nvcc.edu/home/elanthier/methods /correlationsamples.htm. Copyright 2002 by Elizabeth Lanthier, PhD. Reproduced with permission.

relationship between grade point average (GPA) and number of hours spent watching television. The scatter plot (Figure 22-6) shows the direction of the line when the correlation is negative. In these cases, the researcher is measuring conditions that already exist and looking for relationships—either positive or negative.

Examining Patterns of Behavior and Outcomes

Although much of the research and evidence for practice is focused on cause and effect, patterns of behavior, dispositions, and attitudes are also outcomes that require examination. Behavioral theories can be classified as intrapersonal (individual), interpersonal (relational), and community based. The stages of change model (Prochaska & DiClemente, 1986), the health belief model (Rosenstock, 1966), and the theory of reasoned action (Fishbein & Ajzen, 1980) are useful in examining behaviors and their relationship to outcomes.

One way of examining data is through the use of aggregated data derived from large data sets. Organizations such as AHRQ, the CDC, the National Institute for Child Health and Development, and the National Institutes of Health (NIH) have large national data sets from various sources, such as quality of life surveys, hospital discharge data, and infection control data. The data sets can be accessed or purchased to allow researchers to develop clinical, behavioral, or interventional outcome questions that can be statistically analyzed. The advantage of this kind of analysis is that the data sets are large enough to provide an adequate sample and effect size from which to generalize intervention effects. AHRQ also maintains a database of comparative effectiveness reviews that synthesizes information from the most current studies on numerous diseases through the Evidence-Based Practice Centers (AHRQ, 2009).

In addition to aggregated evidence, clinical trial data, and comparative effectiveness reviews, some innovative healthcare systems are bringing " 'practice-based evidence' to the bedside or work setting in aggregate form so that providers have the most up-to-date information available on outcomes before evidence based interventions are begun" (Lambert & Burlingame, 2009, p. 1). As an example, this kind of decision support has been trialed in the Mental Health Services Centers for the state of Utah. The state partnered with an outcomes measurement vendor (OQ, LLC) to provide aggregated evidence from clinical trials and laboratory research that resulted in a 5-minute self-report outcome measurement for patients in any setting—outpatient, inpatient, or residential. Adult patients use a handheld personal digital assistant (PDA), computer kiosk, or paper survey to report information to clinicians based on the domains of symptomatic distress, interpersonal relations, and functional ability. Adolescents and parents/guardians provide information on age-normed questionnaires. The scoring is derived from empirically tested software that alerts the provider that a patient is at risk for a less than optimal outcome from treatment and gives the care provider options for consideration using a clinical decision support tree. According to the designers, the advantage of this kind of tracking is that the system provides immediate evidence-based support for direct patient care. Furthermore, it provides a method for storing data for future review, evaluation, and benchmarking (Lambert & Burlingame, 2009). Use and expansion of this kind of system to document and support clinical practice and scholarship would be an easy transition for nurses who are familiar with the use of PDAs "to support the application of current standards, and knowledge for clinical decision making" (Stroud, Erkel, & Smith, 2005).

Identifying Gaps in Evidence for Practice

In a systematic analysis of reviews published by the Joanna Briggs Institute between 1998 and 2002, high-quality evidence to support nursing interventions was not evident (Averis & Pearson, 2003). Further, the report identified considerable gaps in the evidence base available for nurses in relation to 22 discrete areas of practice that were examined in the analysis. However, the impetus to improve patient safety generated by the IOM reports *To Err Is Human* (Kohn, Corrigan, & Donaldson, 2000), *Crossing the Quality Chasm* (Institute of Medicine [IOM], 2001), and *Health Professions Education: A Bridge to Quality* (IOM, 2003) and the availability of support for EBP through educational restructuring and systems support are increasing.

Nevertheless, gaps in the evidence remain. Research by nurses and family physicians suggests that a translational model to fill the gaps is necessary (Armson et al., 2007; Gumei, Tiedje, & Oweis, 2007). One such model, developed in Canada, uses a small, self-formed group-discussion format within local communities. The impetus for this model was the need to stay competent in view of the vast amount of medical information currently available. In these groups, a facilitator guides physicians' discussion using sample patient cases and prepared modules on selected clinical topics. The groups have been ongoing for 15 years and have attracted international interest (Armson et al., 2007; Kelly, Cunningham, McCalister, Cassidy, & MacVicar, 2007). Nurses engage in similar forums in hospital grand rounds, within their professional specialty organizations, and at regional and national conferences. However, collaborative engagement needs to be broader and more systematic. DNP-prepared nurses are in an excellent position to initiate this kind of practice-based dialogue in community-based practice settings.

The AMA, the AACN, the NONPF, and other professional nursing organizations in each specialty all have agendas for advancing research and evidence for practice in their respective areas. As examples, the American Academy of Nurse Practitioners, Nurse Practitioner Associates for Continuing Education, and the Practicing Clinicians Exchange provide excellent forums for translating current research into practice and for networking with peers about research and clinical outcome information.

The Joint Commission, the National Database of Nursing Quality Indicators, and individual hospital report cards may be used as sources of research or outcome analysis to identify gaps in care delivery or in patient or staff education in particular institutions or practice groups. Examples include adverse events, smoking cessation, rates of adherence to best practice, blood glucose control, patient satisfaction rates, time spent with patients, tests ordered, and number of consultations (care related); knowledge, functional status, and access to care (patient related); and collaboration, technical quality, exam comprehensiveness, and adherence to guidelines (performance related) (Kleinpell, 2009). Within these and other categories, the gaps may be identified through the development of a specific plan based on target areas of APN practice. Planning questions should include the following: What exactly can be measured? How can it be measured? What will be done with the information? When should it be done? (Kleinpell, 2007). **Figure 22-7** shows a sample time line for outcome assessment.

As advanced practice nursing evolves into the DNP role, it will be imperative that direct care providers, senior-level nurse executives, and doctorally prepared nurse educators take lead roles in quality improvement to positively affect patient safety (O'Grady, 2008). Identifying, testing, and disseminating information about nurse-sensitive quality indicators is essential to close the gap in quality care delivery. All advanced practice nurses prepared at the clinical doctorate level must be involved in this effort.

FIGURE 22-7 Timeline for occurrence assessment for APN practice.

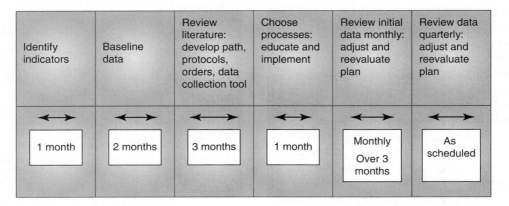

Identify indicators	Baseline data	Review literature: develop path, protocols, orders, data collection tool	Choose processes: educate and implement	Review initial data monthly: adjust and reevaluate plan	Review data quarterly: adjust and reevaluate plan
1 month	2 months	3 months	1 month	Monthly Over 3 months	As scheduled

Source: Adapted from Kleinpell, R. M. (2007, May). APN's invisible champions. *Nursing Management, 38*(5), 18–22.

PARTICIPATION IN COLLABORATIVE RESEARCH

It is a credit to the profession of nursing and its leaders that there are several evidence-based practice centers in the United States: the ANA National Center for Nursing Quality, Sigma Theta Tau International, the National Institute of Nursing Research at the NIH, and centers at many of the major university schools of nursing. However, as O'Grady (2008) noted, turf battles have limited collaboration. On the macrolevel, "APN organizations along with governmental and private research enterprise must come together to develop a research plan that identifies the most critical research questions" (O'Grady, 2008, p. 12). On the micro- and macrolevels, APNs individually and as a group must "demonstrate specific clinical performance and patient outcomes" (p. 12). This means "clearly distinguishing APNs in the context of interdisciplinary practice" (p. 12). Individual studies can demonstrate gaps in care in smaller samples, but the time has come for a more comprehensive and collaborative agenda

for research that focuses on such issues as roles, functions, outcomes, access improvements for vulnerable populations, interdisciplinary collaboration impacts, cost-effectiveness, safety, and other indicators. To discover gaps in care that are of concern to APNs and DNP-prepared nurses, nurses must have representatives from their ranks on research decision-making bodies. The AHRQ is positioned to take the lead in outcomes research, whereas the NIH focuses on biomedical aspects of disease management (O'Grady, 2008). To have their voices heard and their studies funded and disseminated, DNP-prepared nurses must use the power of their professional organizations to garner positions on national and international research collaboratives.

Participating in collaborative research is an excellent way for advanced practice nurses to resolve clinical dilemmas and highlight their expertise through well-constructed questions that interest scientists and engage professional peers within and outside nursing. The dynamic nature of scientific evidence and the speed with which it is now possible to generate new knowledge through the use of technology demand that all care providers combine their expertise to interpret, plan, and evaluate the outcomes of interventions based on these new discoveries. Collaboration "implies collective action toward a common goal in a spirit of trust and harmony" (D'Amour, Ferrada-Videla, San Martin-Rodriquez, & Beaulieu, 2005, p. 116). Even within nursing, specialization demands collaboration between peers and patients to resolve complex clinical dilemmas if patients are to be treated holistically instead of as a collection of organ systems. In fact, as Nolan (2005) noted, patients must be included as "shapers of knowledge and action" (p. 503).

Nursing now has a body of knowledge, separate and unique from that of medicine, that provides the basis for unique contributions to science and to the care of individuals. At the same time, "nursing scholarship remains contextual and contingently situated" (Fairman, 2008, p. 10). Nurses have shown in practice that they are creative and capable of managing changing circumstances and dynamic cultural milieus, thus ensuring that APNs with both research and clinical skills are in a prime position to function as practice consultants in collaborative knowledge-generating research (AACN, 2006). This role is illustrated in the following example.

A DNP-prepared nurse was a voluntary member of an advisory board of a suburban primary healthcare network that provided care to uninsured patients. The members of the board were very interested in ascertaining information about the effectiveness of the organization and its efforts to provide cost-effective, timely primary care. Questions of particular interest were, "Are emergency department visits decreased by the offering of this service? If they are, how much cost is actually saved?" The DNP-prepared nurse collaborated with the organization's administrator and developed an initial research question and a preliminary plan

for presentation to a grant funding agency. The DNP-prepared nurse researched the literature and took the preliminary plan to her institution's research group; with the help of a colleague from the college's health administration program, the DNP designed a study that was submitted to a grant funding agency specializing in grants to medical centers and community health agencies. The agency did not fund the grant that year. However, the following year, the original proposal was reframed as a cohort study, "Emergency Room Usage Among Uninsured Patients with Access to a Primary Care Provider" (Tymkow, Shen, & MacMullen, 2006) and resubmitted as a subproject of a much larger NIH grant that was funded. A primary aim of the larger National Center on Minority Health and Health Disparities grant was to build capacity for research in healthcare disparities through mentoring by senior-level researchers (Samson, 2006). The DNP-prepared nurse, who was a mentee, became the primary investigator, working with two co-investigators on this project.

In another example of collaborative research, Oman, Duran, and Fink (2008) described a collaborative EBP project to institute evidence-based policy and procedure development at the University of Colorado Hospital using the hospital's evidence-based multidisciplinary practice model. The model established the evidence base through valid and current research and through other forms of evidence or benchmark data, including cost-effectiveness analysis; pathophysiology; retrospective or concurrent chart review; quality improvement and risk data; international, national, and local standards; infection control data; patient preferences; and clinical expertise. The more sources that are added to the research core, the stronger the evidence. However, all sources are contributory to the evidence.

The Evidence-Based Practice Council used the levels of evidence of Stetler (1994) to guide the process of gathering evidence. As described by Oman et al. (2008), because there was nothing addressing policy and procedure in the literature, the members identified steps and created an algorithm to describe the process. Once developed, the algorithm was piloted on the units using six nurse champions, mentored by a researcher. The champions and researcher reviewed an orthostatic vital sign policy that was scheduled for update. After obtaining 12 research-based articles, 8 clinical articles, 1 national guideline, and anecdotal recommendations, the group was divided into subgroups, and each person was assigned two reports to review using a standardized critique form. Each nurse was responsible for reading the articles, completing the critique form (with levels of evidence), and presenting the findings at a journal club. The policy being reviewed was checked for references and levels of evidence by the research scientist. A comparison of agreement between the policy author and reviewers was then determined, and the percentage of agreement between reviewer and author tabulated. Only clinically based policies were reviewed. This process is a good example of how collaboration between practice and education could be merged in any number of areas.

Whether collaboration involves clinical research or quality improvement, DNP-prepared nurses in clinical and leadership roles are key stakeholders in the process. As identified in the IOM report *Crossing the Quality Chasm* (IOM, 2001), communication and collaboration are requisites to the achievement of quality systems and patient outcomes. These skills are also a necessary part of a culture of collaboration that begins in educational programs and continues in the professional work setting. Collaborative efforts may include small, unit-based or practice-based efforts or large, system-wide initiatives. These efforts have been driven by consumer demand for excellence, accountability, and transparency in quality care, patient safety, and patient satisfaction (Freshman, Rubino, & Chassiakos, 2010). In any collaborative initiative, three levels of expertise are required: system leadership, including the authority to implement change; clinical technical expertise (guidance and know-how); and day-to-day leadership (details of the system) (Baker, Reising, Johnson, Stewart, & Baker, 1997, cited in Freshman et al., 2010).

DISSEMINATING FINDINGS FROM EVIDENCE-BASED PRACTICE

A primary reason for disseminating research is to use the findings to improve practice and health outcomes. Communicating the results of research and evidence-based practice trials is the culminating step of the research and research utilization processes. It is one of *the* most important steps in research and the application of research in practice because it is the communication of research findings that provides the basis for meaningful critique, development of new questions, and testing of research evidence in practice (Lyder & Fain, 2009).

The methods used to communicate evidence from practice trials are similar to those used for communicating research findings: journal publications, podium or poster presentations, Internet webinar sessions, media communications, journal clubs, and community presentations. However, the forums for dissemination may be broader because the audience of interest may be more diverse, including those with practice, research, and community development interests. In addition, the choice of method for communicating information depends on a number of important factors. For example, a journal publication may be personally advantageous to the author, but the time from submission to actual publication and dissemination may delay utilization of important evidence-based treatments in practice. Oral reports at national conferences may facilitate timelier dissemination. Webinars may be the fastest way to disseminate information but may not reach all the desired audiences. Journal clubs are useful forums for discussions of research findings in academic settings. Reports of community-based studies to advisory boards or media venues may also become the basis for further research and political support that help nonprofit and other community organizations. Nevertheless, because theory, research, and practice must be constantly intertwined, the circular and reciprocal relationship among these elements must be apparent regardless of where the research is presented (McEwen & Wills, 2007).

PREPARING A JOURNAL PUBLICATION

Preparing a journal article for publication is time consuming and at times tedious, but the rewards of feeling that you have made a contribution and seeing your work in print are worth the effort. Once the topic for an article has been established, the next step is selecting the journal. Peer-reviewed journals have the most rigorous review criteria. Therefore, publication in one of these journals is considered to be more credible. The actual content will be determined by the editorial guidelines of the journal, which may be found in the "Information for Authors" section of the journal. In most cases, the guidelines may also be obtained from the journal's website. Generally, the submission requirements cover technical details such as page length, margins, font style and size, reference format, use of graphics and figures, and method of submission. It is very important to follow the submission requirements because many journals will not review articles that are not submitted in the correct format.

Once submitted, articles in peer-reviewed journals are blind (anonymously) reviewed by several reviewers. It is not uncommon for the review process to last several weeks or months; articles may be rejected, accepted with revisions, or accepted. It is common to have articles returned for revision. The key to success is to be persistent, correct those things that can be corrected, give an explanation for those that cannot, and return the submission in the agreed-upon time frame.

PREPARING A RESEARCH PRESENTATION

Regardless of where or how evidence is reported, the essential element is that it combines the knowledge and values of the study patients or population with practitioner expertise and the best in available and current research evidence. Reporting evidence also requires knowledge of the audience and their needs. Specifically, the presenter must ask: What is the specific content to be addressed? How will the audience use the information? What is the knowledge level of those who are to receive the information? What is the time allowed for the presentation? What audiovisual resources are available for the presentation? Once these questions have been answered, specific learning objectives should be developed in order to guide and organize the presentation.

Table 22-13 shows an outline for presentation of research study findings. Important points of each aspect of the study can be

TABLE 22-13	Outline for Research Presentation

I. Introduction

II. Purpose of the study

III. Theoretical framework

IV. Hypothesis

V. Design

    A. What kind of study

    B. Intervention

    C. Sample

        1. Population

        2. Inclusion/Exclusion criteria

    D. Instruments

VI. Analysis

    A. Method

    B. Types of statistical tests used

VII. Findings

VIII. Discussion

IX. Implications

    A. Research

    B. Clinical practice

TABLE 22-14	Resources and Websites for Developing Multimedia and PowerPoint Presentations
PosterPresentations.com (Scientific Template)	http://www.posterpresentations.com
University of South Florida	http://etc.usf.edu/presentations/index.html
University of Texas Medical Branch	http://ar.utmb.edu
Virginia Commonwealth University	http://www.eric.vcu.edu/home/scholarship/presentation.html
Vanderbilt University	http://web.vanderbilt.edu/2010/08/bruff-tech-classroom
WebAim	http://www.webaim.org/techniques/powerpoint/alternatives.php

displayed as a PowerPoint presentation to aid in maintaining the presentation within the designated time frame and keep the audience focused on the important elements of the presentation. **Table 22-14** lists some useful websites concerning PowerPoint presentations.

PREPARING A POSTER PRESENTATION

Disseminating information from scholarship—original research, practice innovations, clinical projects—through poster presentations has become an accepted medium for the exchange of ideas in a more personal and less formal environment than the podium presentation. It is both efficient and effective. Presenters and participants have the freedom to engage in a dialogue that allows for education, clarification, and networking. Posters also allow for the formatting of data in creative ways. As Berg (2005) noted, "imagery can be substituted for words and this is a powerful way to convey information" (p. 245). Like any presentation, posters require preparation. The following steps are essential.

Plan Ahead

A good poster presentation takes considerable time. The planning stage is a most important step. In this stage, considerable thought should be given to the message you are trying to convey. What is the purpose? The format for a research presentation will be different from that of a practice innovation. Is the conference only for nurses, only for advanced practice nurses, or for a multidisciplinary audience? How much background information or detail do you need to include? Is the audience generally familiar with the topic or not? If they are, do not include familiar details, but if they are not, do not make the information so specific that those who are not familiar with the topic will be put off. Avoid using abbreviations that only a select audience will understand. These and other considerations specific to the venue should be thought about during the planning stage (Berg, 2005; Hardicre, Devitt, & Coad, 2007).

Decide on Layout and Format

Most people read top to bottom, and left to right. This is the usual sequence for poster layout. Generally, the layout for a research poster presentation is as follows: title, abstract, introduction, methods, results, discussion, and acknowledgments. If the presentation is a practice innovation, the layout will be different. The innovation is usually in the center, with explanatory text at the periphery or below the diagram or explanation of the protocol or change (Hardicre et al., 2007). References are also included, as in the research poster. "The poster should be easy to read from a distance of up to 6 feet. Section heads should be at least 40 pt. and supporting text 32 pt." (Halligan, 2005, p. 49). Titles should be short, with letters 2 to 3 inches high (Berg, 2005).

Determine the Content

If the purpose of the poster is to display a research project, it will not be the same as one that is designed to describe a clinical innovation. The content of the research poster should follow the guidelines established by the conference guidelines. If the study is funded by an outside or government agency, some grant-funded studies require specific wording of the acknowledgment; this should be determined during the poster planning. If an abstract is required, it should include the main purpose of the study, be clearly worded, and be succinct. A key component is to keep it simple because posters "show," they do not "tell" (Miracle, 2008).

Clinical project content will vary according to the specific topic and scope. The title for either a research study or clinical innovation should be creative, but, most important, it should accurately reflect the content of the project. The title banner should also include authors and affiliations in order of authorship and/or contribution to the effort. In many instances, the organization's logo will be included as well (Hardicre et al., 2007).

Prepare a Brief Presentation

"The poster is a story board of information" (Jackson & Sheldon, 1998, as cited in Hardicre et al., 2007, p. 398). However, it also gives the presenters an opportunity to present themselves. As with any kind of communication, you want to convey confidence and knowledge. Preparing a short presentation script or handouts for participants allows you to organize your thoughts and prepare for possible questions. The handouts are always welcomed by participants, who are inundated with information during a conference. Be sure to include your name and contact number or attach a business card so that participants may contact you with questions. This is a very effective networking tool (Miracle, 2008).

MEDIA COMMUNICATIONS

Communicating with large audiences is often facilitated through professional media communications. This kind of communication is essential when there is a major event or change, such as a policy to be initiated. It is usually best to engage the resources of a professional organization to make the preliminary contact and to aid in constructing the message.

JOURNAL CLUB PRESENTATIONS

Another way to facilitate the communication of evidence-based research is through journal club presentations. Journal clubs are not new, especially in academic and many professional settings. However, using them to facilitate evidence-based practice is a more recent development, especially as a forum for clinical guideline development (Kirchoff & Beck, 1995, as cited in McQueen, Miller, Nivison, & Husband, 2006). In a small survey study of the use of journal clubs to determine changes in practice, McQueen et al. (2006) found that journal clubs were effective in "1) focusing staff on clinical evidence in discussions, 2) increasing confidence as they became more aware of evidence, and, 3) bridging the evidence-practice gap" (p. 315). Additionally, with the aid of the Internet, evidence-based articles or studies can be posted in advance and facilitated online, thus increasing the possibility of wider participation. In one pilot study of this format, nurses in New Zealand branded the journal club's website and the articles for discussion. An article is posted for one month and removed on the Friday before the following month's posting (Trim, 2008). **Table 22-15** presents an outline of a journal club.

TABLE 22-15   Online Journal Club

Outline of the Journal Club

1. A specific clinical question is chosen.

2. All evidence-based literature related to the question is derived from online databases.

3. A reference list of all literature for review is generated.

4. High-level-evidence randomized controlled trials and systematic reviews are critiqued and given more weight than quasi-experimental case studies and opinions.

5. Participants critically appraise the relevant literature before attending the journal club.

6. Journal club discussions center on the critical appraisal of evidence found for clinical interventions.

7. Implications for practice and further research are discussed, with key findings recorded in minutes.

8. A resource folder that includes a reference list of resource critiques, guidelines for practice, treatment resources, standardized assessments, disease management strategies, and gaps in evidence is created.

9. A system for ongoing evaluation of outcomes and changes in practice is developed and communicated.

Source: Adapted from McQueen, J., Miller, C., Nivison, C., & Husband, V. (2006). An investigation into the use of a journal club for evidence-based practice. *International Journal of Therapy and Rehabilitation, 13*(7), p. 313. Modified with permission.

Whether live or Internet-based, journal clubs provide a mechanism for promoting professional debate, increasing confidence, and, most important, improving practice and quality care (Sheratt, 2005, as cited in McQueen et al., 2006). With their educational background and advanced skills, DNP-prepared nurses are in an excellent position to implement this kind of strategy in a collaborative, interdisciplinary format.

SUMMARY

Scholarship and evidence-based practice are not the same, but each has elements that support the other. Scholarship involves research and application, as does evidence-based practice. Whereas scholarship may be a joint or singular effort, evidence-based practice requires teamwork and collaboration. The outcome of scholarship is a scholarly product, a new way of thinking, or a change in awareness about a subject or phenomenon—an end in itself. Evidence-based practice is based on the scholarship of research and evidence gathering and synthesis. It is a means for improving care for patients or effecting a change in a system that results in better care for patients, providers, and communities. It is a transformation of knowledge to new levels of understanding and integration. Changing to a model of evidence-based practice does not just happen; it requires the integration of a number of skills, such as the use of good research and the synthesis of best information and other "evidences," including patient choice and professional expertise at its core. The DNP-prepared nurse, with the advantage of expertise in practice built on a strong base of education and knowledge, is—and will continue to be—in the forefront of this movement to transform care.

DISCUSSION QUESTIONS

1. How will the Iowa model of evidence-based practice help to promote quality care in the clinical practice setting?

2. Which role will the advanced practice nurse play in intradisciplinary and interdisciplinary collaborative research teams?

3. As an advanced practice nurse leading a research team, which strategies would you employ to encourage your team members to critically appraise research articles?

REFERENCES

Academy of Breastfeeding Medicine. (2004). *Breastfeeding the near term infant (35–37 weeks gestation)*. New Rochelle, NY: Academy of Breastfeeding Medicine.

Adib-Hajbaghery, M. (2007). Factors facilitating and inhibiting evidence-based practice in Iran. *Journal of Advanced Nursing, 58*(6), 566–575.

Agency for Healthcare Research and Quality. (2002). *Systems to rate the strength of scientific evidence, summary* (Technical Report No. 47). Retrieved from http://archive.ahrq.gov/clinic/epcsums/strengthsum.htm

Agency for Healthcare Research and Quality. (2009). *Evidence-based practice centers*. Retrieved from http://www.ahrq.gov/research/findings/evidence-based-reports/overview/index.html

AGREE Collaboration. (2001). AGREE instrument. Retrieved from http://www.agreetrust.org/?o=1085

Allen, M. (1996). *Celebrating nursing history: What to keep*. Retrieved from http://nahrs.mlanet.org/home/weeding

American Association of Colleges of Nursing. (1999). *Position statement on defining scholarship for the discipline of nursing*. Retrieved from http://www.aacn.nche.edu/Publications/positions/scholar.htm

American Association of Colleges of Nursing. (2006). *The essentials of doctoral education for advanced nursing practice*. Retrieved from http://www.aacn.nche.edu/DNP/pdf/Essentials.pdf

American Association of Colleges of Nursing. (2010). New AACN data show growth in doctoral nursing programs. Retrieved from http://www.aacn.nche.edu/news/articles/2010/enrollchanges

American Nurses Credentialing Center. (2005). Magnet recognition program overview. Retrieved from http://www.medscape.com/partners/ancc/public/ancc

Andrews, T. (2008). Under pressure for a diagnosis: A case study review of pheochromocytoma genetics. *Clinical Scholars Review: The Journal of Doctoral Nursing Practice, 1*(2), 96–100.

Annells, M. (1996). Grounded theory method: Philosophical perspectives, paradigms of inquiry, and postmodernism. *Qualitative Health Research 6*(3), 379–393.

Armson, H., Kinzie, S., Hawes, D., Roder, S., Wakefield, J., & Elmslie, T. (2007). Translating learning into practice. *Canadian Family Physician, 53*(9), 1477–1485.

Arthur, R., Marfell, J., & Ulrich, S. (2009). Outcomes measurement in nurse-midwifery practice. In R. M. Kleinpell (Ed.), *Outcome assessment in advanced practice nursing* (2nd ed., pp. 229–255). New York, NY: Springer.

Asch, S. M., Baker, D. W., Keesey, J., Broder, M., Schonlau, M., Rosen, M., . . . Keeler, E. B. (2005). Does the collaborative model improve care for chronic heart failure? *Medical Care, 43*(7), 667–675.

Averis, A., & Pearson, A. (2003). Filling the gaps: Identifying nursing research priorities through the analysis of completed systematic reviews. *JBI Reports, 1*(3), 49–126.

Baker, C. M., Reising, D. L., Johnson, D. R., Stewart, R. L., & Baker, S. D. (1997). Organizational effectiveness: Toward an integrated model for schools of nursing. *Journal of Professional Nursing, 13*(4), 246–255.

Barnes, D. M. (1996). An analysis of the grounded theory method and the concept of culture. *Qualitative Health Research, 6*(3), 429–441.

Batalden, P. B., Nelson, E. C., & Roberts, J. S. (1994). Linking outcome measurements to continual improvement: The serial "V" way of thinking about improving clinical care. *Journal of Quality Improvement, 20*(4), 167–180.

Batalden, P. B., & Stoltz, P. K. (1993). A framework for the continual improvement of healthcare: Building and applying professional and improvement knowledge to test changes in daily work. *Joint Commission Journal of Quality Improvement, 19*(10), 424–447.

Berg, J. A. (2005). Creating a professional poster presentation: Focus on nurse practitioners. *Journal of the American Academy of Nurse Practitioners, 17*(7), 245–248.

Bickerton, J., Procter, S., Johnson, B., & Medina, A. (2011). Socio-phenomenology and conversation analysis: Interpreting video lifeworld healthcare interactions. *Nursing Philosophy, 12*(4), 271–281.

Bond, A. E., Draeger, C. R., Mandleco, B., & Donnelly, M. (2003). Needs of family members of patients with severe traumatic brain injury. *Critical Care Nurse, 23*(4), 63–71.

Boyer, E. L. (1990). *Scholarship reconsidered: Priorities of the professoriate*. The Carnegie Foundation for the Advancement of Teaching. San Francisco, CA: Jossey-Bass.

Boyer, E. L. (1997). *Scholarship reconsidered: Priorities of the professoriate* (Rev. ed.). The Carnegie Foundation for the Advancement of Teaching. San Francisco, CA: Jossey-Bass.

Brown, S. J. (2005). Direct clinical practice. In A. B. Hamric, J. A. Spross, & C. M. Hanson (Eds.),

Advanced practice nursing: An integrative approach (3rd ed., pp. 143–185). Philadelphia, PA: W. B. Saunders.

Burns, N., & Grove, S. K. (2005). *The practice of nursing research: Conduct, critique, and utilization* (5th ed.). St. Louis, MO: Elsevier Saunders.

Burns, N., & Grove, S. K. (2009). *The practice of nursing research, appraisal, synthesis, and generation of evidence* (6th ed.). St. Louis, MO: Elsevier Saunders.

Burns, S. (2009). Selecting advanced practice nurse outcome measures. In R. M. Kleinpell (Ed.), *Outcomes assessment in advanced practice nursing* (2nd ed.). New York, NY: Springer.

Carey, M., Buchan, H., & Sanson-Fisher, R. (2009). The cycle of change: Implementing the best-evidence clinical practice. *International Journal for Quality in Health Care, 21*(1), 37–43. Retrieved from http://www.medscape.com/viewarticle/587370

Carnegie Foundation for the Advancement of Teaching. (1996). *Ernest L. Boyer* (Ninety-first Annual Report of the Carnegie Foundation for the Advancement of Teaching). Princeton, NJ: Author.

Celik, H., Lagro-Janssen, T. A., Widdershoven, G. G., & Abma, T. A. (2011). Bringing gender sensitivity into healthcare practice: A systematic review. *Patient Education and Counseling, 84*(2), 143–149.

Chism, L. A. (2009). The relationship of nursing students' spiritual care perspective to their expressions of spiritual empathy. *Journal of Nursing Education, 48*(1), 597–605. doi:10 .3928/01484834-20090716-05

Cochrane Collaboration. (2004). *Cochrane reviewers' handbook*. London, England: Cochrane Group.

Coe, R. (2002, September). *It's the effect size, stupid: What effect size is and why it is so important*. Paper presented at the annual conference of the British Educational Research Association, University of Exeter, England.

Collins, P. M., Golembeski, S. M., Selgas, M., Sparger, K., Burke, N., & Vaughn, B. B. (2008, January 25). Clinical excellence through evidence-based practice: A model to guide practice changes. *Topics in Advanced Practice E-Journal*. Retrieved from http://www.medscape.com/viewarticle/567682

Conger, M. M., & Plager, K. A. (2008). Advanced nursing practice in rural areas: Connectedness versus disconnectedness. *Online Journal of Rural Nursing and Healthcare, 8*(1), 24–38.

Cooke, L., Smith-Idell, C., Dean, G., Gemmill, R., Steingass, S., Sun, V., . . . Borneman, T. (2004). "Research to practice": A practical program to enhance the use of evidence-based practice at the unit level. *Oncology Nursing Forum, 31*(4), 825–832.

Craft-Rosenburg, M., Krajicek, M. J., & Shin, D. (2002). Report of the American Academy of Nursing Child-Family Expert Panel: Identification of quality and outcome indicators for maternal child nursing. *Nursing Outlook, 50*(2), 57–60.

Crotty, M. (1996). *Phenomenology and nursing research*. Melbourne, Australia: Churchill Livingstone.

D'Amour, D., Ferrada-Videla, M., San Martin-Rodriquez, L., & Beaulieu, M. D. (2005). The conceptual basis for interprofessional collaboration: Core concepts and theoretical frameworks. *Journal of Interprofessional Care, 19*(Suppl. 1), 116–131.

Decker, S., & Iphofen, R. (2005). Developing the profession of radiography: Making uses of oral history. *Radiography, 11*(4), 262–271.

Deming, E. W. (1986). *Out of crisis*. Cambridge, MA: MIT Press.

DePalma, J. A., & McGuire, D. B. (2005). Research. In A. B. Hamric, J. A. Spross, & C. Mittenson (Eds.), *Advanced nursing practice: An integrative approach* (3rd ed., pp. 217–249). Philadelphia, PA: Elsevier Saunders.

Diaz-Granados, N., Pitzul, K. B., Dorado, L. M., Wang, F., McDermott, S., Rondon, M. B., . . . Stewart, D. E. (2011). Monitoring gender equity in health using gender-sensitive indicators: A cross-national study. *Journal of Women's Health, 20*(1), 145–153.

DiCenso, A., Cullum, N., & Ciliska, D. (1998). Implementing evidence-based nursing: Some misconceptions. *Evidence-Based Nursing, 1*(2), 38–39.

Dohrn, J. (2008). Scaling up HIV treatment for pregnant women: Components of a midwifery model of care as identified by midwives in Eastern Cape, South Africa. *Clinical Scholars Review: The Journal of Doctoral Nursing Practice, 1*(1), 50–54.

Doran, D. M., & Sidani, S. (2007). Outcomes-focused knowledge translation: A framework for knowledge translation and patient outcomes improvement. *Worldviews on Evidence-Based Nursing, 4*(1), 3–13.

Dorn, K. (2004). Caring-healing inquiry for holistic nursing practice: Model for research and evidence based practice. *Topics in Advanced Practice Nursing E-Journal, 4*(4). Retrieved from http://www.medscape.com/viewarticle/496363

Doster, J. A., Purdum, M. D., Martin, L. A., Goven, A. J., & Moorefield, R. (2009). Gender differences, anger expression, and cardiovascular risk. *Journal of Nervous and Mental Diseases, 197*(7), 552–554.

Doumitt, G., Gattelliari, M., Grimshaw, J., & O'Brien, M. A. (2007). Local opinion leaders: Effects on professional practice and healthcare outcomes. *Cochrane Database of Systematic Reviews, 4,* CD000125. doi:10.1002/14651858.CD000125.pub3

Doyle-Lindrud, S. (2008). Gestational breast cancer. *Clinical Scholars Review: The Journal of Doctoral Nursing Practice, 1*(1), 23–31.

Dreher, M. (1999). Clinical scholarship: Nursing practice as an intellectual endeavor. In Sigma Theta Tau International Clinical Scholarship Task Force, *Clinical scholarship resource paper* (pp. 26–33). Retrieved from http://www.nursingsociety.org/aboutus/PositionPapers/Documents/clinical_scholarship_paper.pdf

Duignan, P. (2006). *Outcomes model standards for systematic outcome analysis.* Retrieved from http://www.parkerduignan.com/oiiwa/toolkit/standards1.html

Dunlop, W. L., & Beauchamp, M. R. (2011). En-gendering choice: Preferences for exercising in gender-integrated and gender-segregated groups and consideration of overweight status. *International Journal of Behavioral Medicine, 18,* 216–220. doi:10.1007/s12529-010-9125-6

Durieux, P., Nizard, R., Ravaud, P., Mounier, N., & Lepage, E. (2000). A clinical decision support system for prevention of venous thromboembolism: Effect on physician behavior. *Journal of the American Medical Association, 283*(21), 2816–2821.

Edwards, S. D. (2001). *Philosophy of nursing: An introduction.* New York, NY: Palgrave.

Fain, J. A. (2009). *Reading, understanding, and applying nursing research* (3rd ed.). Philadelphia, PA: F. A. Davis.

Fairman, J. (2008). Context and contingency in the history of post World War II scholarship in the United States. *Journal of Nursing Scholarship, 40*(1), 4–11.

Fawcett, J., & Garrity, J. (2009). *Evaluating research for evidence-based nursing practice.* Philadelphia, PA: F. A. Davis.

Fawcett, J., Watson, J., Neuman, B., Hinton Walker, P., & Fitzpatrick, J. (2001). On nursing theories and evidence. *Journal of Nursing Scholarship, 33*(2), 115–119.

Fishbein, I., & Ajzen, M. (1980). *Understanding attitudes and predicting social behavior.* Englewood Cliffs, NJ: Prentice Hall.

Fitzpatrick, M. L., & Munhall, P. L. (2001). Historical research: The method. In P. L. Munhall (Ed.), *Nursing research: A qualitative perspective* (3rd ed.). Sudbury, MA: Jones and Bartlett.

French, P. (1999). The development of evidence-based nursing. *Journal of Advanced Nursing, 29*(1), 72–78.

Freshman, B., Rubino, L., & Chassiakos, Y. R. (2010). *Collaboration across the disciplines in health care.* Sudbury, MA: Jones and Bartlett.

Gagan, M., & Hewitt-Taylor, J. (2004). The issues involved in implementing evidence based practice. *British Journal of Nursing, 13*(20), 1216–1220.

Gallagher, R. M. (2009). Participation of the advanced practice nurse in managed care and quality initiatives. In L. A. Joel (Ed.), *Advanced practice nursing: Essentials of role development* (2nd ed., p. 185). Philadelphia, PA: F. A. Davis.

Giddens, A. (1982). *Profiles and critiques in social theory.* London, England: Macmillan.

Gifford, W., Davies, B., Edwards, N., Griffin, P., & Lybanon, V. (2007). Managerial leadership for nurses' use of research evidence: An integrative review of the literature. *World Views on Evidence Based Practice, 4*(3), 126–145.

Giorgi, A. (2000). Concerning the application of phenomenology to caring research. *Scandinavian Journal of Caring Science, 14*(1), 11–15.

Glanville, I., Schirm, V., & Wineman, N. M. (2000). Using evidence-based practice for managing clinical outcomes in advanced practice nursing. *Journal of Nursing Care Quality, 15*(1), 1–11.

Glaser, B. G., & Strauss, A. (1967). *The discovery of grounded theory.* Chicago, IL: Aldine.

Goolsby, M. J., Klardie, K. A., Johnson, J., McNaughton, M. A., & Meyers, W. (2004). Integrating the principles of evidence-based practice into clinical practice. *Journal of the American Academy of Nurse Practitioners, 16*(3), 98–105.

Goolsby, M. J., Meyers, W. C., Johnson, J. A., Klardie, K., & McNaughton, M. A. (2004). Integrating the principles of evidence-based practice: Prognosis and the metabolic syndrome. *Journal of the American Academy of Nurse Practitioners, 16*(5), 178–186.

Graling, P. R. (2011). Designing an applied model of perioperative patient safety. *Clinical Scholars Review, 4*(2), 104–114.

Griffin-Sobel, J. P. (2003). Evaluating an instrument for research. *Gastroenterology Nursing, 26*(3), 135–136.

Grol, R., Dalhuijsen, J., Thomas, S., Veld, C., Rutten, G., & Mokkink, H. (1998). Attributes of clinical guidelines that influence use of guidelines in general practice: Observational study. *British Medical Journal, 317*(7162), 858–861.

Gumei, M. K., Tiedje, L. B., & Oweis, A. (2007). Vaginal or cesarean birth: Toward evidence based practice.

American Journal of Maternal Child Nursing, 32(6), 388.

Hallett, C. (1995). Understanding the phenomenological approach to research. *Nurse Researcher, 3*(2), 55–56.

Halligan, P. (2005). Poster perfect. *World of Irish Nursing and Midwifery, 13*(8), 49.

Hammersley, M. (1989). *The dilemma of qualitative method.* London, England: Routledge.

Handley, M., MacGregor, K., Schillinger, D., Sharifi, C., Wong, S., & Bodenheimer, T. (2006). Using action plans to help primary care patients adopt healthy behaviors: A descriptive study. *Journal of the American Board of Family Medicine, 19*(3), 224–231.

Hardicre, J., Devitt, P., & Coad, J. (2007). Ten steps to successful poster presentation. *British Journal of Nursing, 16*(7), 398–401.

Hawkins, R. C., & Clement, P. F (1984). Binge eating: Measurement problems and a conceptual model. In R. E. Hawkins, W. J. Fremouw, & P. F. Clement (Eds.), *The binge-purge syndrome: Diagnosis, treatment, and research* (pp. 229–251). New York, NY: Springer.

Hebda, T., & Czar, P. (2009). *Handbook of informatics for nurses and healthcare professionals* (4th ed.). Upper Saddle River, NJ: Pearson/Prentice Hall.

Hodge, M. B., Asch, S. M., Olson, V. A., Kravitz, R. L., & Sauve, M. J. (2002). Developing indicators of nursing quality to evaluate nurse staffing ratios. *Journal of Nursing Administration, 32*(6), 338–345.

Holleman, G., Eliens, A., van Vliet, M., & van Acterburg, T. (2006). Promotion of evidence based practice by professional nursing associations: Literature review. *Journal of Advanced Nursing, 53*(6), 702–709.

Horsely, J. A., Crane, J., & Bingle, J. D. (1978). Research utilization as an organizational process. *Journal of Nursing Administration, 8*(7), 4–6.

Imberg, W. C. (2008). *The meaning of U.S. childbirth for Mexican immigrant women* (Doctoral dissertation). Available from ProQuest Dissertations and Theses database. (UMI No. 3318193)

Ingersoll, G. (2005). Generating evidence through outcomes management. In B. M. Melnyk & E. Fineout-Overholt (Eds.), *Evidence-based practice in nursing and healthcare: A guide to best practice.* Philadelphia, PA: Lippincott Williams & Wilkins.

Ingersoll, G. L., McIntosh, E., & Williams, M. (2000). Nurse sensitive outcomes of advanced practice. *Journal of Advanced Nursing, 32*(5), 1272–1281.

Institute of Medicine. (2001). *Crossing the quality chasm: A new health system for the 21st century.* Washington, DC: National Academies Press.

Institute of Medicine. (2003). *Health professions education: A bridge to quality.* Washington, DC: National Academies Press.

International Development Research Centre. (2009). *Confounding variables.* Retrieved from http://www.idrc.ca/en/ev-1-201-1-DO_TOPIC.html

Ironside, P. M. (2006). Reforming doctoral curricula in nursing: Creating multiparadigmatic, multipedagogical researchers. *Journal of Nursing Education, 45*(2), 51–52.

Israni, R. K. (2007). Guide to biostatistics. *MedPage Today.* Retrieved from http://www.medpagetoday.com/lib/content/Medpage-Guide-to-Biostatistics.pdf

Jackson, K. I., & Sheldon, J. M. (1998). Poster presentation: How to tell a story. *Pediatric Nurse, 10*(9), 36–37.

Jamtvedt, G., Young, J. M., Kristofferson, D. T., O'Brien, M. A., & Oxman, A. D. (2006). Audit and feedback: Effects on professional practice and healthcare outcomes. *Cochrane Database of Systematic Reviews, 2,* CD000259.

Johnston, L. (2005). Critically appraising quantitative evidence. In B. M. Melnyk & E. Fineout-Overholt (Eds.), *Evidence-based practice in nursing and healthcare: A guide to best practice.* Philadelphia, PA: Lippincott Williams & Wilkins.

The Joint Commission (2009). Universal protocol. Retrieved from http://www.jointcommission.org/standards_information/up.aspx

Kelly, D. R., Cunningham, D. E., McCalister, P., Cassidy, J., & MacVicar, R. (2007). Applying evidence in practice through small group learning: A qualitative exploration of success. *Quality in Primary Care, 15*(2), 93–99.

Kirchoff, K., & Beck, S. (1995). Using the journal club as a component of the research utilization process. *Heart and Lung: The Journal of Acute and Critical Care, 24*(3), 246–250.

Kitson, A., Harvey, G., & McCormack, B. (1998). Enabling the implementation of evidence-based practice: A conceptual framework. *Quality in Healthcare, 7*(3), 149–158.

Kleinpell, R. M. (2007). APNs invisible champions? *Nursing Management, 38*(5), 18–22.

Kleinpell, R. M. (2009). Measuring outcomes in advanced nursing practice. In R. M. Kleinpell (Ed.), *Outcome assessment in advanced nursing practice* (2nd ed., pp. 1–63). New York, NY: Springer.

Kohn, L. T., Corrigan, J. M., & Donaldson, M. S. (2000). *To err is human: Building a safer health system.* A report of the Committee on Quality of Health Care in America, Institute of Medicine. Washington, DC: National Academies Press.

Kovarsky, D. (2008). Representing voices from the life-world in evidence-based practice. *International Journal of Language and Communication Disorders, 43*(S1), 47–57.

Lambert, M. J., & Burlingame, G. M. (2009). Measuring outcomes in the state of Utah: Practice based evidence. *Behavioral Healthcare, 27,* 16–20.

Lanthier, E. (2002). Correlation samples. Retrieved from http://www.nvcc.edu/home/elanthier/methods/correlation-samples.htm

Leedy, P. D., & Ormrod, J. E. (2010). *Practical research: Planning and design.* Boston, MA: Pearson.

Library of Congress. (n.d.). *American memory collection.* Retrieved from http://memory.loc.gov/ammem/index.html

Libster, M. M., & McNeil, B. A. (2009). *Enlightened charity.* Farmville, NC: Golden Apple Publications.

Long, C. O. (2009). Adapted from Weighing in on the evidence. In N. A. Schmidt & J. M. Brown (Eds.), *Evidence-based practice for nurses.* Sudbury, MA: Jones and Bartlett.

Lopez-Bushnell, K. (2002). Get research-ready. *Nursing Management, 33*(11), 41–44.

Lowell, J. R. (n.d.). Knowledge. Retrieved from http://quotationsbook.com/quote/22196

Luttik, M. L., Jaarsma, T., Lesman, I., Sanderman, R., & Hagedoorn, M. (2009). Quality of life in partners of people with congestive heart failure: Gender and involvement in care. *Journal of Advanced Nursing, 65*(7), 1442–1451.

Lyder, C., & Fain, J. A. (2009). Interpreting and reporting research findings. In J. A. Fain (Ed.), *Reading, understanding, and applying research* (3rd ed., pp. 233–250). Philadelphia, PA: F. A. Davis.

Maggs-Rapport, F. (2001). "Best research practice": In pursuit of methodological rigour. *Journal of Advanced Nursing, 35*(3), 373–383.

Mak, Y. (2003). Use of hermeneutic research in understanding the meaning of desire for euthanasia. *Palliative Medicine, 17,* 395–402.

Marineau, M. L. (2005). *Exploring the lived experience of individuals with acute infections transitioning in the home with support by an advanced practice nurse using telehealth* (Unpublished doctoral dissertation). University of Hawaii at Manoa. (UMI Order No. AA13198369)

Marinopoulos, S. S., Dorman, T., Ratanawongsa, N., Wilson, L. M., Ashar, B. H., Magaziner, J. L., . . . Bass, E. B. (2007). Effectiveness of continuing medical education. *Evidence Reports in Technology Assessment, 14,* 1–69.

Masharani, V., Goldfine, I. D., & Youngren, J. F. (2009). Influence of gender on the relationship between insulin sensitivity, adiposity, and plasma lipids in lean nondiabetic subjects. *Metabolism, 58*(11), 1602–1608. Retrieved from http://www.ncbi.nlm.nih.gov/pubmed/19604524

McCaughan, D., Thompson, C., Cullum, N., Sheldon, T. A., & Thompson, D. R. (2002). Acute care nurses' perceptions of barriers to using research information in clinical decision-making. *Journal of Advanced Nursing, 39*(1), 46–60.

McCloskey, D. J. (2008). Nurses' perceptions of research utilization in a corporate health care system. *Journal of Nursing Scholarship, 40*(1), 39–45.

McCollum, M., Hanson, L. S., Lu. L., & Sullivan, P. W. (2005). Gender differences in diabetes mellitus and effects on self-care activity. *Gender Medicine, 2*(4), 246–254.

McEwen, M., & Wills, E. M. (2007). *Theoretical basis for nursing* (2nd ed.). Philadelphia, PA: Lippincott Williams & Wilkins.

McQueen, J., Miller, C., Nivison, C., & Husband, V. (2006). An investigation into the use of a journal club for evidence-based practice. *International Journal of Therapy and Rehabilitation, 13*(7), 311–316.

McSherry, R. (2002). *Evidence informed nursing: A guide for clinical nurses.* London, England: Routledge.

Melnyk, B., & Cole, R. (2005). Generating evidence through quantitative research. In B. Melnyk & E. Fineout-Overholt (Eds.), *Evidence-based practice in nursing and healthcare* (pp. 239–281). Philadelphia, PA: Lippincott Williams & Wilkins.

Melnyk, B., & Fineout-Overholt, E. (2002). Putting research into practice. Rochester ARCC. *Reflections on Nursing Leadership, 28*(2), 22–25.

Melnyk, B., & Fineout-Overholt, E. (2005). *Evidence-based practice in nursing and healthcare.* Philadelphia, PA: Lippincott Williams & Wilkins.

Minnick, A. (2009). General design and implementation challenges in outcomes assessment. In R. M. Kleinpell (Ed.), *Outcomes assessment in advanced practice nursing* (2nd ed., pp. 107–119). New York, NY: Springer.

Miracle, V. (2008). Effective poster presentations. *Dimensions of Critical Care Nursing, 27*(3), 122–124.

Mitchell, P. H., Ferketich, S., & Jennings, B. M. (1998). Quality health outcomes model. *Image: Journal of Nursing Scholarship*, 30(1), 43–36.

Monico, E. P., Moore, C. L., & Calise, A. (2005). The impact of evidence-based medicine and evolving technology on the standard of care in emergency medicine. *The Internet Journal of Law, Healthcare and Ethics*, 3(2).

Munhall, P. (1994). *In women's experience*. New York, NY: National League for Nursing.

Munhall, P. (2007). A phenomenological method. In P. L. Munhall (Ed.), *Nursing research: A qualitative perspective* (4th ed.). Sudbury, MA: Jones and Bartlett.

National Organization of Nurse Practitioner Faculties. (2005). *Nurse practitioner faculty practice: An expectation of professionalism*. Retrieved from http://c.ymcdn.com/sites/www.nonpf.org/resource/resmgr/imported/FPStatement2005Final.pdf

Newhouse, R. P., Dearholt, S. L., Poe, S. S., Pugh, L., & White, K. M. (2008). *Johns Hopkins nursing evidence-based practice model and guidelines: Instructor's guide*. Indianapolis, IN: Sigma Theta Tau International.

Nolan, M. (2005). Reconciling tensions between research, evidence-based practice and user participation: Time for nursing to take the lead. *International Journal of Nursing Studies*, 42(5), 503–505.

O'Grady, E. T. (2008). Advanced practice registered nurses: The impact on patient safety and quality. In *Patient safety and quality: An evidence-based handbook for nurses*. Retrieved from http://www.ahrq.gov/qual/nurseshdbk/

Oman, K. S., Duran, C., & Fink, R. (2008). Evidence-based policy and procedures: An algorithm for success. *Journal of Nursing Administration*, 38(1), 47–51.

Padilla, G. V., Ferrell, B., Grant, M. M., & Rhiner, M. (1990). Defining the content domain of quality of life for cancer patients with pain. *Cancer Nursing*, 13(2), 108–115.

Patton, M. Q. (1990). *Qualitative evaluation and research methods* (2nd ed.). Newbury Park, CA: Sage.

Pesut, B., & Johnson, J. (2007). Reinstating the "Queen": Understanding philosophical inquiry in nursing. *Journal of Advanced Nursing*, 61(1), 115–121.

Peterson, L. A., Woodward, L. D., Urech, T., Daw, C., & Sookanan, S. (2006). Does pay-for-performance improve the quality of health care? *Annals of Internal Medicine*, 145(4), 265–272.

Polit, D. F., & Hungler, B. P. (1997). *Essentials of nursing research: Methods, appraisal, and utilization* (4th ed.). Philadelphia, PA: Lippincott-Raven.

Porter, S. (1996). Qualitative research. In D. F. S. Cormack (Ed.), *The research process in nursing* (3rd ed., pp. 113–122). Oxford, England: Blackwell Science, as cited in Maggs-Rapport, F. (2001). "Best research practice": In pursuit of methodological rigour. *Journal of Advanced Nursing*, 35(3), 373–383.

Pravikoff, D. S., Tanner, A. B., & Pierce, S. T. (2005). Readiness of U.S. nurses for evidence-based practice. *American Journal of Nursing*, 105(9), 40–51.

Prochaska, J. O., & DiClemente, C. C. (1986). Toward a comprehensive model of change. In W. R. Miller & N. Heather (Eds.), *Treating addictive behaviors: Processes of change*. New York, NY: Plenum Press.

Prosser, H., Almond, S., & Walley, T. (2003). Influences on GP's decision to prescribe new drugs: The importance of who says what. *Family Practice*, 20(1), 61–68.

Raines, C. F. (2010, March). *The Doctor of Nursing Practice: A report on progress*. Presentation at the annual meeting of the American Association of Colleges of Nursing. Retrieved from http://www.aacn.nche.edu/leading-initiatives/dnp/DNPForum3-10.pdf

Reavy, K., & Tavernier, S. (2008). Nurses reclaiming ownership of their practice: Implementation of an evidence-based model and process. *Journal of Continuing Education in Nursing*, 39(4), 166–172.

Reed, P., & Shear, N. C. (2004). *Perspectives on nursing theory* (4th ed.). Philadelphia, PA: Lippincott Williams & Wilkins.

Reeves, M. J., Fonarow, G. G., Zhao, X., Smith, E. E., Schwamm, L. H., & Get With the Guidelines Stroke-Steering Committee and Investigators. (2009). Quality of care in women with ischemic stroke in the GWTG program. *Stroke*, 40(4), 1127–1133. doi:10:1161./Stroke AHA.108.543/57

Rich, K. A. (2009). Evaluating outcomes of innovations. In N. A. Schmidt & J. M. Brown, (Eds.), *Evidence-based practice for nurses* (p. 388). Sudbury, MA: Jones and Bartlett.

Rosenstock, I. M. (1966). Why people use health services. *Milbank Fund Quarterly*, 44, 94–127.

Rosswurm, M. A., & Larrabee, J. (1999). A model for change to evidence based practice. *Image: Journal of Nursing Scholarship*, 31(4), 317–322.

Russell, C., & Gregory, D. (2003). Evaluation of qualitative research studies. *Evidence-Based Nursing*, 6(2), 36–40.

Rutledge, D. N., & Bookbinder, M. (2002). Processes and outcomes of evidence-based practice. *Seminars in Oncology Nursing*, 18(1), 3–10.

Rycroft-Malone, J., Kitson, A., Harvey, G., McCormack, B., Seers, K., Titchen, A., & Estabrooks, C. (2002). Ingredients for change: Revisiting a conceptual framework. *Quality and Safety in Health Care, 11*(2), 174–180.

Rycroft-Malone, J., Seers, K., Titchen, A., Harvey, G., Kitson, A., & McCormack, B. (2004). What counts as evidence in evidence-based practice? *Journal of Advanced Nursing, 47*(1), 81–90.

Sackett, D. L., Richardson, W. S., Rosenberg, W. T., & Haynes, R. B. (1997). *Evidence-based medicine: How to practice and teach evidence-based medicine.* New York, NY: Churchill Livingstone.

Samson, L. (2006). *Building capacity for health disparities research.* Grant 1P20MD001816-01 from the National Center on Minority Health and Health Disparities, National Institutes of Health, Bethesda, MD.

Santucci, S. (2011). A system change: Expansion of primary and secondary prevention services in a marginalized community. *Clinical Scholars Review, 4*(2), 98–103.

Schmidt, N., & Brown, J. M. (2009). *Evidence-based practice for nurses: Appraisal and application of research.* Sudbury, MA: Jones and Bartlett.

Schulman, L. S. (1993). Teaching as community property: Putting an end to pedagogical solitude. *Change, 25*(6), 6–7.

Scott-Findley, S., & Pollack, C. (2004). Evidence, research and knowledge: A call for conceptual clarity. *Worldviews on Evidence Based Nursing, 1*(2), 92–97.

Sheratt, C. (2005). The journal club: A method for occupational therapists to bridge the theory-practice gap. *British Journal of Occupational Therapy, 68*(7), 301–306.

Sigma Theta Tau International Clinical Scholarship Task Force. (1999). *Clinical scholarship resource paper.* Retrieved from http://www.nursingsociety.org/aboutus/PositionPapers/Documents/clinical_scholarship_paper.pdf

Simmons-Mackie, N. N., & Damico, J. S. (2001). Intervention outcomes: Clinical applications of qualitative methods. *Topics in Language Disorders, 22*(1), 21–36, as cited in Kovarsky, D. (2008). Representing voices from the life-world in evidence-based practice. *International Journal of Language and Communication Disorders, 43*(S1), 47–57, p. 51).

Singleton, J., & Levin, R. (2008). Strategies for learning evidence-based practice: Critically appraising clinical practice guidelines. *Journal of Nursing Education, 47*(8), 380–383.

Slutsky, J. (2005). Using evidence-based practice guidelines: Tools for improving practice. In B. M. Melnyk & E. Fineout-Overholt (Eds.), *Evidence-based practice in nursing and healthcare: A guide to best practice* (pp. 221–227). Philadelphia, PA: Lippincott Williams & Wilkins.

Soumerai, S. B., McLauglin, T. J., Gurwitz, J. H., Guadagnoli, E., Hauptman, P. J., Borbas, C., . . . Gobel, F. (1998). Effect of local medicine opinion leaders on quality of care for acute myocardial infarction. *Journal of the American Medical Association, 279*(17), 1358–1363.

Spitzer, R. L., Devlin, M., Walsh, B. T., Hasin, D., Wing, R., Marcus, M., . . . Nonas, C. (1992). Binge eating disorder: A multi-site field trial of the diagnostic criteria. *International Journal of Eating Disorders, 11*(3), 191–203.

Stetler, C. B. (1994). Refinement of the Stetler/Marram model for application of research findings to practice. *Nursing Outlook, 42*(1), 15–25.

Stetler, C. B., & Marram, G. (1976). Evaluating research findings for applicability in practice. *Nursing Outlook, 24*(9), 559–563.

Stoekel, P. (2010). Leadership and management role of the Doctor of Nursing Practice in the care of older persons in the USA. *Journal of Clinical Nursing, 19*(Suppl. 1), 145–146.

Strauss, A., & Corbin, J. (1994). *Basics of qualitative research: Grounded theory procedures and techniques.* Newbury Park, CA: Sage.

Strauss, A., & Corbin, J. (1998). *Basics of qualitative research: Techniques and procedures for developing grounded theory.* Thousand Oaks, CA: Sage.

Stroud, S. D., Erkel, E. A., & Smith, C. A. (2005). The use of personal digital assistants by nurse practitioner students and faculty. *Journal of the American Academy of Nurse Practitioners, 17*(2), 67–75.

Stull, A., & Lanz, C. (2005). An innovative model for nursing scholarship. *Journal of Nursing Education, 44*(11), 493–497.

Tanyi, R. A., McKenzie, M., & Chapek, C. (2009). How family practice physicians, nurse practitioners, and physicians assistants incorporate spiritual care in practice. *Journal of the American Academy of Nurse Practitioners, 21*, 690–697.

Timmerman, G. M. (1999). Using a women's health perspective to guide decisions made in quantitative research. *Journal of Advanced Nursing, 30*(3), 640–645.

Titler, M. G. (2002). Use of research in practice. In G. LoBiondo & J. Haber (Eds.), *Nursing research methods: Critical appraisal and utilization* (5th ed.) St. Louis, MO: Mosby.

Titler, M. G., Klieber, C., Steelman, V., Goode, C., Rakel, B., Barry-Walker, J., . . . Buckwalter, K. (1994). Infusing research into practice to promote quality care. *Nursing Research, 43*(5), 307–313.

Trim, S. (2008). Journal club offers new opportunities. *Kai Tiaki Nursing New Zealand, 14*(11), 23.

Tropello, P. G. D. (2000). *Origins of the nurse practitioner movement: An oral history* (Doctoral dissertation). Rutgers, State University of New Jersey–New Brunswick, and University of Medicine and Dentistry of New Jersey. (UMI Order No. AAI9970979)

Tymkow, C., Shen, J. J., & MacMullen, N. (2006). Project 2: Emergency room usage among uninsured patients with access to a primary care provider. In L. Samson (Ed.), *Building capacity for health disparities research*. Grant 1P20MD001816-01 from the National Center on Minority Health and Health Disparities, National Institutes of Health, Bethesda, MD.

van Manen, M. (1990). *Researching lived experiences: Human science for an action sensitive pedagogy*. Albany: State University of New York Press.

Wall, B. M., Edwards, N. E., & Porter, M. L. (2007). Textual analysis of retired nurses' oral histories. *Nursing Inquiry, 14*(4), 279–288.

Watkins, C., Harvey, I., Langley, C., Gray, S., & Faulkner, A. (1999). General practitioners' use of guidelines in the consultation and their attitudes to them. *British Journal of General Practice, 49*(438), 11–15.

Webber, P. B. (2008). The doctor of nursing practice degree and research: Are we making an epistemological mistake? *Journal of Nursing Education, 47*(10), 466–472.

Zuzelo, P. R. (2007). Evidence-based nursing and qualitative research: A partnership imperative for real-world practice. In P. L. Munhall (Ed.), *Nursing research: A qualitative perspective* (4th ed., pp. 533-553). Sudbury, MA: Jones and Bartlett.

PART 5

The Role of Race, Culture, Ethics, and Advocacy in Advanced Nursing Practice

© A-R-T/Shutterstock

The fifth section of this text covers other core concepts as recommended by the American Association of Colleges of Nursing for advanced practice nursing knowledge—namely, diversity and ethics. Diversity in this context incorporates two complementary issues: diversity of the population cared for by nurses and diversity of the nursing workforce itself. As the U.S. population moves toward a more diverse and pluralistic society, the nursing profession is challenged to develop greater cultural competence.

Given the multicultural, multiethnic, and multilingual society now found in the United States, Dayer-Berenson (Chapter 23) provides working definitions for transcultural nursing, cultural competence, and diversity as it relates to patient care. The chapter provides a review of theoretical models that have shaped the thinking of the nursing profession as related to cultural diversity and cultural competence.

Chapter 24 considers diversity as a global phenomenon and its influence on the nursing profession. The author compares and contrasts healthcare delivery systems of the United States and the United Kingdom, Australia, Canada, and South Africa, considering the impact of racial and ethnic disparities in health care.

In Chapter 25, Shi and Singh provide a comprehensive overview of the major characteristics of select U.S. population groups whose members face challenges and barriers in accessing healthcare services. These groups include racial/ethnic minorities, children and women, persons living in rural areas, persons who are homeless, those who are mentally ill, and individuals with HIV/AIDS. The health needs of these population groups are summarized, and the services available to them are described. The gaps that currently exist between these population groups and the rest of the population indicate that the nation must make significant efforts to address the unique healthcare disparities of U.S. subpopulations.

In Chapter 26, Pozgar introduces basic ethics concepts and definitions. Scattered throughout this chapter are examples of ethical situations the reader can use to apply ethical principles to nursing practice.

Chapter 27 comprises a discussion by Grace on the individual and environmental factors that interfere with ethical nursing actions. Issues regarding informed consent, proxy decision making, and advanced directives are analyzed. The author also addresses contemporary issues regarding the role of social media as it pertains to privacy and confidentiality in healthcare settings.

CHAPTER 23

Birth of Transcultural Nursing to Current Theories and Conceptual Models for Cultural Diversity

Linda Dayer-Berenson

CHAPTER OBJECTIVES

1. Provide working definitions for transcultural nursing, cultural competence, and diversity.

2. Identify various areas of diversity that the nurse should assess for and be aware of in order to provide culturally appropriate care.

3. Describe three nursing theories that promote the delivery of competent nursing care to culturally diverse patients.

4. Select a theoretical model of cultural competency that is complementary to the reader's nursing philosophy of patient care.

INTRODUCTION

Whether a nursing student in the clinical setting, a seasoned nurse, or nurse practitioner, you observe diversity within your patient population on a daily basis. Our patients come from many different races and ethnic groups, which means they often do not look, feel, or respond like we do. These differences result in a cultural mismatch. Helping you to develop a plan for proceeding in the face of a cultural mismatch is the guiding force behind this chapter. The Office of Minority Health in 2000 published recommendations for 14 national standards for culturally and linguistically appropriate services in health care to provide the knowledge necessary for nurses to work respectfully and effectively with patients and each other in a culturally diverse work environment. These standards are called CLAS for short and were revised in 2012.

How have we come to this point where the federal government has provided mandates, guidelines, and recommendations? It would appear that all members of the healthcare team need to do a better job. The CLAS standards were developed with input from national leaders (including the American Nurses Association [ANA]) and are based on an analysis of current standards in use that are deemed essential and appropriate.

The members of the expert panel on cultural competence of the American Academy of Nursing (AAN) have developed recommendations (**Box 23-1**) to ensure that measurable outcomes be achieved to reduce or eliminate health disparities commonly found among racial, ethnic, uninsured, underserved, and/or underrepresented populations residing throughout the United States.

Achieving cultural competence suggests possession of the ability to respond effectively to the cultural needs of our patients. This view would be too narrow, however. We must recognize that diversity exists among patients but also within the members of the healthcare team (nurses, physicians, and other allied health professionals). As we continue to struggle with a nursing shortage, one ongoing solution has been for large numbers of immigrant nurses to enter and work within the American healthcare system. Not only will the immigrant nurses have the challenge of adapting to our healthcare delivery system but often their ethnocultural background may be different from that of the dominant culture and of the patients to whom they are to deliver nursing care. Since the 1960s, the Philippines has been the number one source of foreign-trained nurses in the United States;

BOX 23-1 | Twelve Recommendations of the Expert Panel on Cultural Competence of the American Academy of Nursing

---

1. The AAN, through its publications, mission statements, and yearly conferences, must make an explicit commitment to quality, culturally competent care that is equitable and accessible by targeting four groups: healthcare customers, healthcare providers, healthcare systems, and communities.

2. The AAN will collaborate with other organizations and communities in developing guidelines.

3. The AAN shall develop mechanisms to synthesize existing theoretical and research knowledge concerning nursing care of ethnic/minorities and other vulnerable populations.

4. The AAN, through its expert panels and commissions, must create an interdisciplinary knowledge base that reflects healthcare practices within various cultural groups, along with human communication strategies that transcend interdisciplinary boundaries to provide a foundation for education, research, and action.

5. The AAN, through its expert panels and commissions, must identify, describe, and examine methods, theories, and frameworks appropriate for utilization in the development of knowledge related to health care of minority, stigmatized, and vulnerable populations.

6. The AAN shall seek resources to develop and sponsor studies to describe and identify principles used by organization magnets that provide an environment that enhances knowledge development related to cross-cultural, ethnic minority/stigmatized populations, and attract

| BOX 23-1 | Twelve Recommendations of the Expert Panel on Cultural Competence of the American Academy of Nursing *(continued)* |

and retain minority and other vulnerable students, faculty, and clinicians.

7. The AAN, through its various structures, must identify healthcare system delivery models that are the most effective in the delivery of culturally competent care to vulnerable populations and develop mechanisms to promote the necessary changes in the United States healthcare delivery system toward the identified models.

8. The AAN must collaborate with other organizations in establishing ways to teach and guide faculty and nursing students to provide culturally competent nursing care practices to clients in diverse clinical settings in local, regional, national, and international settings.

9. The AAN must collaborate with racial/ethnic nursing organizations to develop models of recruitment, education, and retention of nurses from racial/ethnic minority groups.

10. The AAN will collaborate with other organizations in promoting the development of a document to support the regulation of content reflecting diversity in nursing curricula. In addressing regulations, specific attention needs to be given to the National Council Licensure Examinations, continuing education, and undergraduate curricula.

11. The AAN must take the lead in promulgating support of research funding for investigation with emphasis on interventions aimed at eliminating health disparities in culturally and racially diverse groups and other vulnerable populations in an effort to improve health outcomes. The AAN must take a more proactive stance to encourage policy makers to create policies that address the elimination of health disparities and ultimately improve health outcomes.

12. The AAN must encourage funding agencies' requests to solicit proposals focusing on culturally competent interventions designed to eliminate health disparities.

Source: Giger, J., Davidhizar, R. E., Purnell, L., Harden, J. T., Phillips, J., & Strickland, O. (2007). American Academy of Nursing Expert Panel Report: Developing cultural competence to eliminate health disparities in ethnic minorities and other vulnerable populations. *Journal of Transcultural Nursing, 18*(2), 95–102.

this trend is continuing in the twenty-first century (Marquand, 2006). Cultural differences not only will affect the nursing care that is provided but also may negatively affect the ability of the immigrant nurse to assimilate effectively as an essential member of the healthcare team. The growing diversity that has been seen and that continues to widen in the U.S. population has not been seen within the population of healthcare professionals. This lack of parallel growth in diversity among healthcare professionals affects healthcare delivery and suggests that many patients are receiving culturally discordant care. Culturally discordant care arises from unaddressed cultural differences between healthcare providers and patients. Research has shown that significant disparities exist in health status, treatment, and medical outcomes between groups of patients who differ on the basis of gender, race, or ethnicity. A provider's unconscious bias about a particular race, ethnicity, or culture, or his or her lack of effective cross-cultural communication skills, may contribute to discordant medical care and health disparities. This suggests that all healthcare providers should know how to interact effectively with and provide care for patients whose ethnic or cultural background differs from their own.

The population growth in the United States between 2000 and 2012 was almost entirely minority driven with more than one in three U.S. residents being a member of a minority group (U.S. Census Bureau, 2012). According to the most recent census, our country continues toward diversity, as demonstrated by significant increases in the numbers and proportion of populations such as Hispanics, Asians, and Pacific Islanders (U.S. Census Bureau, 2012). Data from the 2010 census released in 2011 reveal that the Caucasian population (White or European American) of the United States is 223.5 million (72.4% of total population) and that there are 38.0 million Blacks (12.6% of total population), 14.6 million Asians (4.8%), and 50.5 million Latinos (16.4% of total population) (U.S. Census Bureau, 2010).

BICULTURAL/MULTICULTURAL

Another important consideration is that in contemporary U.S. society many individuals are bicultural (McGrath, 1998). Membership in more than one culture, being bicultural, is not the same as being biracial or multiracial. Bicultural people identify with core elements of their culture of origin as well as those of the dominant culture. They self-identify with more than one cultural group, and the bicultural person sees both sides and can function in both worlds. The degree of biculturalism and acculturation that has occurred can influence intergenerational differences in health beliefs and behaviors for certain U.S. ethnic groups (English & Le, 1999). Bicultural individuals

successfully integrate into and participate in important aspects of the values and belief systems of both cultures.

In today's increasingly diverse and mobile world, growing numbers of individuals have internalized more than one culture and can be described as bicultural or multicultural. In fact, 12.5% of U.S. residents are immigrants and have presumably internalized more than one culture (Battalova & Terrazas, 2010). We must also consider that U.S.-born ethnic and cultural minorities (descendants of immigrants) identify with their ethnic culture and the mainstream culture of the United States. It is a process for the bicultural or multicultural person to navigate between these different cultural identities.

Biculturalism can be associated with feelings of pride, uniqueness, and a rich sense of community and history, while also bringing to mind identity confusion, dual expectations, and value clashes (Benet-Martínez & Haritatos, 2005).

ACCULTURATION

Acculturating immigrants and ethnic minorities have to deal with two central issues. The first issue is the extent to which they are motivated or permitted to retain their identification with their culture of origin (their ethnic culture), and the second is the extent to which they are motivated or are permitted to identify with the dominant mainstream American culture. The dominant mainstream American culture is usually defined as having a Northern European cultural tradition while utilizing the English language. As the immigrant wrestles and negotiates with this, he or she can end up in one of four identified acculturation positions. According to Berry (1990), the four distinct acculturation positions are assimilation (identification mostly with the dominant culture), integration (high identification with both cultures), separation (identification largely with the ethnic culture), or marginalization (low identification with both cultures).

Acculturation is not a linear process—one does not move forward in a direct line from one position to the next. This is why individuals can simultaneously hold two or even more cultural orientations. People who are bicultural can move easily between their two cultural identities by engaging in cultural frame switching (Hong, Morris, Chiu, & Benet-Martínez, 2000). Cultural frame switching occurs in response to cultural cues. The important point is the individual response. There will be individual variation in the way the bicultural identity is negotiated and organized. Some bicultural individuals will find both cultural identities are compatible, integrated, and easy to negotiate. Others may struggle if they find the two cultures are oppositional or difficult to integrate or negotiate. Various terms for the acculturation process of biculturals have been developed by different theorists. Some examples of these terms are "fusion" (Chuang, 1999), "blendedness" (Padilla, 1994), and "alternating biculturalism" (Phinney & Devich-Navarro, 1997).

OTHER AREAS OF DIVERSITY

Although racial diversity is becoming more known, it is not the only potential area of diversity encountered by healthcare providers. Diversity can be categorized as dimensions of human diversity, dimensions of cultural diversity, or systems diversity dimensions. Examples of human diversity are race, gender, physical ability, marital status, family status, ethnicity, and age. A person's dimensions of cultural diversity are characterized by that person's beliefs, attitudes, values, personal characteristics, lifestyle, communication, and religion. There are also systems diversity dimensions, such as teamwork, empowerment, education, and strategic alliances (Guillory, 2001).

Healthcare providers increasingly have to care for and communicate with patients of varying backgrounds, preferences, and cultures. Diversity may even have an impact on treatment response. Some researchers suggest that there may be subtle differences in the way that members of different racial and ethnic groups respond to treatment, particularly with regard to some pharmaceutical interventions, suggesting that variations in some forms of treatment may be justified on the basis of patient race or ethnicity. Diversity may also influence rejection of treatment recommendations by patients. As an example, it was cited in the Institute of Medicine report (IOM, 2003) that a number of studies concluded that Black Americans are slightly more likely to reject medical recommendations for some treatments, but these differences in refusal rates are generally small (Black Americans are only 3% to 6% more likely to reject recommended treatments, according to these studies). The IOM report recommends that more research is needed to fully understand the reasons for the refusal of treatment, as this may lead to the development of different strategies to help patients make informed treatment decisions. The IOM report hypothesizes that stereotypes, bias, and clinical uncertainty may influence clinicians' diagnostic and treatment decisions; education may be one of the most important tools as part of an overall strategy to eliminate healthcare disparities. Clearly, there is much to consider, and we have much more that we need to learn.

OVERVIEW OF CONCEPTUAL MODELS FOR CULTURAL DIVERSITY

For more than five decades, nurses have recognized cultural diversity as an important variable and have attempted to provide culturally specific and appropriate care to a population that is continuing to become even more racially and ethnically diverse. This desire to provide appropriate care was based on the knowledge that people belonging to different cultures have different kinds of demands and needs in terms of health and illness. People having different cultural values should be respected, and the health care offered and provided should be inclusive of the patient's cultural values whenever possible. Transcultural nursing models provide nurses with the foundation to become knowledgeable about the various cultures seen in their practice settings. Nurse scholars continue to develop and refine a vast number of cultural theories, models, and assessment guides that are used internationally. Dr. Madeline Leininger has provided the basic foundation for cultural competency in nursing practice. Today, arguably the most well-known and commonly used nursing cultural competency models are by Leininger (1991), Purnell (Purnell, 2013; Purnell & Paulanka, 1998), and Giger and Davidhizar (Giger, 2013; Giger et al., 2007). After the passing of Ruth Davidhizar, Joyce Giger published the sixth edition of the textbook *Transcultural Nursing: Assessment and Intervention* in 2013 (Giger, 2013). Each of these theories and models will be discussed in greater detail in this chapter because it is essential for the nurse to utilize the knowledge gained from these models to deliver culturally appropriate care. In today's diverse world, our nursing care must be grounded in the knowledge and science of transcultural nursing. Through these theories, nursing has made an important contribution to the provision of all health care by all types of practitioners.

Because of our global relationships and the leadership in the area of healthcare delivery in the United States, many people from other countries come to the United States for medical care. As a result, U.S. nurses are often called upon to assess clinically, in a short period of time, individuals who, in many cases, are very different culturally, racially, and ethnically from themselves. An area of formal study and practice developed in response to this fact; the knowledge and understanding of different cultures is called transcultural nursing (Leininger, 1995). Transcultural nursing is a learned branch of nursing that focuses on the comparative study and analysis of cultures as they apply to nursing and health/illness practices, beliefs, and values. Transcultural nursing was developed in the mid-1960s by Madeline Leininger, a nurse anthropologist. In the 1960s, the field received financial

support for nurses who wished to obtain doctoral degrees and become nurse anthropologists. These nursing pioneers were convinced that an understanding of cultural diversity relative to health and illness was an essential component of nursing knowledge. The essential foundation of transcultural nursing is that cultures exhibit both diversity and universality.

The first course in transcultural nursing was offered by Dr. Leininger in 1966 at the University of Colorado (one year after she earned her PhD in anthropology from the University of Seattle). Dr. Leininger stated that transcultural nursing developed in response to nurses having increased exposure to diverse groups of patients. This increase was because of the changing demographics in the United States as well as the leadership of the United States in healthcare delivery, resulting in many people from other countries coming to the United States for medical care. Dr. Leininger and other transcultural nursing scholars refer to care as a universal phenomenon that transcends cultural boundaries. Because we provide direct patient care, it is critical for nurses to understand how to work effectively within a diverse cultural atmosphere.

Transcultural nursing, as defined by Leininger (1984), is a humanistic and scientific area of formal study and practice in nursing that is focused on the comparative study of cultures. Focusing on differences and similarities in care, health, and illness patterns based on cultural values, beliefs, and practices of different cultures in the world, transcultural nursing uses knowledge to provide culturally specific and universal nursing care to people. The goal of transcultural nursing is to provide care that is congruent with cultural values, beliefs, and practices—culturally specific care (Leininger, 1984). Today, transcultural nursing concepts are found in the curricula for nursing programs in the United States and Canada. This theory has provided the basic foundation for transcultural nursing practice.

The Transcultural Nursing Society was founded in 1974. It publishes a monthly journal (*Journal of Transcultural Nursing*) and provides a certification process for transcultural nursing for nurses in the United States and Canada.

Although the importance of the work done by Dr. Leininger cannot be denied, there have been some problems identified in her transcultural nursing framework by nurse scholars. The major flaw, according to Tripp-Reimer and Fox (1990), is that it was based on the anthropological theory of functionalism. Dr. Leininger did, after all, receive her doctorate in anthropology. Functionalism in anthropology stresses understanding culture by emphasizing specific customs, folkways, and patterns such as diet preferences, religious practices, communication styles, and health beliefs and practices (Tripp-Reimer & Fox, 1990). Critics (Brink, 1990; Browning & Woods, 1993; Sprott, 1993; Tripp-Reimer & Fox, 1990) believe that this "narrow view" of people results in stereotyping. This is by no means a small concern. The fear of stereotyping is often cited as the major criticism of the cultural competency movement. It is important that this process of identifying the characteristics that may be associated with certain cultural groups be done with an extremely open mind and for the nurse to realize that, just like in anything, exceptions can be found. It is important that we do not proceed with blinders on as the nurse must continually assess for affirmation or for exceptions.

Although the concern about stereotyping is an important one, there are other nurse scholars who argue that a reliance on generalizations about race, ethnicity, and culture are necessary to expand a nurse's knowledge about a particular patient population (Giger, 2013; McGoldrick, 1993; Valente, 1989). Looking at the situation from both sides, it is clear that it is important for the nurse to be cautious and to use these generalizations as a flexible guide that permits individualization of patient care at all times. We must strive to avoid stereotyping and oversimplification of the impact of culture

(Betancourt, 2003), and the nurse must attempt to possess cultural humility, openness, and inquisitiveness toward each individual patient (Tervalon & Murray-Garcia, 1998).

In the twenty-first century, with the emergence of evidence-based medicine (EBM), a new challenge of integration with cultural competence has risen. There is some concern in the literature that cultural competence and evidence-based medicine can be contradictory goals. This is because the overriding goal of EBM is to provide quality health care through standardization of care, not individualized care. The overriding goal of cultural competence is the delivery of individualized health care that acknowledges and understands cultural diversity, with respect for individual health beliefs, values, and behaviors. Combining these approaches can result in optimal patient-centered care. Future research needs to focus on determining the best way to integrate EBM and cultural competence to ensure demonstrably improved patient outcomes. Nurses need to assess for a patient's explanatory model of the patient's health status (how the person understands the illness) to avoid stereotyping and oversimplification of the impact of culture.

All of nursing's largest professional organizations—the ANA in 1991, the National League for Nursing in 1993, and the American Association of Colleges of Nursing in 1998—have cited the need for nurses to practice cultural competence.

The ANA established the American Academy of Nursing in 1973. Its purpose is to advance health policy and practice, and it is often referred to as the think tank of nursing. The AAN has a number of expert panels, including the Expert Panel on Cultural Competence. From 1991 to 1992, the Expert Panel on Cultural Competence proposed 10 recommendations in an attempt to address health disparities. This panel developed its most recent position paper in 2007 to help serve as a catalyst for substantive nursing action to promote outcomes that reduce or eliminate health disparities commonly found among racial, ethnic, uninsured, underserved, and underrepresented populations residing throughout the United States (Giger et al., 2007). Membership on any of the expert panels within the AAN are by invitation only to fellows of the AAN. Fellowship in the AAN is considered one of the highest honors a nurse can achieve. The members consist of major nursing theorists and scholars.

The Expert Panel on Cultural Competence developed a comprehensive list of 12 recommendations (Box 23-1) that can serve as a starting point for all health professionals who seek to address the problem of health disparities in the United States through cultural competency with the hope that measurable outcomes be achieved to reduce or eliminate health disparities commonly found among the minority and vulnerable populations in the United States (Giger et al., 2007).

Based on the work of the Expert Panel on Cultural Competence, a set of universally applicable standards of practice for culturally competent care were developed that nurses can use when providing care. The 12 standards were developed based on the social justice framework, which is the belief that each and every person is entitled to fair and equal rights and participation in healthcare opportunities (Douglas et al., 2009). The standards (**Box 23-2**)

BOX 23-2   Standards of Practice for Culturally Competent Nursing Care

Standard	Description
1. Social Justice	Professional nurses shall promote social justice for all. The applied principles of social justice guide nurses' decisions related to the patient, family, community, and other healthcare professionals. Nurses will develop leadership skills to advocate for socially just policies.
2. Critical Reflection	Nurses shall engage in critical reflection of their own values, beliefs, and cultural heritage in order to have an awareness of how these qualities and issues can impact culturally congruent nursing care.
3. Transcultural Nursing Knowledge	Nurses shall gain an understanding of the perspectives, traditions, values, practices, and family systems of the culturally diverse individuals, families, communities, and populations they care for, as well as a knowledge of the complex variables that affect the achievement of health and well-being.
4. Cross-Cultural Practice	Nurses shall utilize cross-cultural knowledge and culturally sensitive skills in implementing culturally congruent nursing care.
5. Healthcare Systems and Organizations	Healthcare organizations should provide the structure and resources necessary to evaluate and meet the cultural and language needs of their diverse clients.

BOX 23-2   Standards of Practice for Culturally Competent Nursing Care *(continued)*

Standard	Description
6. Patient Advocacy and Empowerment	Nurses shall recognize the effect of healthcare policies, delivery systems, and resources on their patient populations and shall empower and advocate for their patients as indicated. Nurses shall advocate for the inclusion of their patient's cultural beliefs and practices in all dimensions of their health care.
7. Multicultural Workforce	Nurses shall be activists in the global effort to ensure a more multicultural workforce in healthcare settings.
8. Education and Training	Nurses shall be educationally prepared to promote and provide culturally congruent health care. Knowledge and skills necessary for ensuring that nursing care is culturally congruent shall be included in global healthcare agendas that mandate formal education and clinical training, and ongoing, continuing education for all practicing nurses will be required.
9. Cross-Cultural Communication	Nurses shall use effective, culturally competent communication with clients that takes into consideration the client's verbal and nonverbal language, cultural values and context, and unique healthcare needs and perceptions.
10. Cross-Cultural Leadership	Nurses shall have the ability to influence individuals, groups, and systems to achieve outcomes of culturally competent care for diverse populations.
11. Policy Development	Nurses shall have the knowledge and skills to work with public and private organizations, professional associations, and communities to establish policies and standards for comprehensive implementation and evaluation of culturally competent care.
12. Evidence-Based Practice and Research	Nurses shall base their practice on interventions that have been systematically tested and shown to be the most effective for the culturally diverse populations that they serve. In areas where there is a lack of evidence of efficacy, nurse researchers shall investigate and test interventions that may be the most effective in reducing the racial and ethnic inequalities in health outcomes.

Source: Data from Douglas, M. K., Pierce, J. U., Rosenkoetter, M., Callister, L. C., Hattar-Pollara, M., Lauderdale, J., . . . Pacquiao, D. (2009). Standards of practice for culturally competent nursing care: A request for comments. *Journal of Transcultural Nursing, 20*(3), 257–269.

were collaboratively developed by Douglas et al. (2009), with participation from members of the Expert Panel on Cultural Competence, among others.

Nurses are ideally suited to strive toward cultural competence. When nurses consider the race, ethnicity, culture, and cultural heritage of their patients, they become more sensitive to each patient's individual needs. This is by no means an easy feat, as evidenced by the vast number of cultures and subcultures that exist on our planet (estimated to be more than 2,500 by Leininger), but a highly complex issue that requires a lifelong commitment (McGee, 2001).

It is important to learn from our mistakes, as each cultural gaffe provides the opportunity to learn, improve, and grow professionally. We must also realize that the practice of nursing should never be done by using a "cookbook approach." There is as much variation within certain races, cultures, or ethnic groups as there is across cultural groups. The informed nurse is being asked to consider the significance of culture to ensure that patients are then approached and cared for from a more informed perspective—this is the crux of transcultural nursing care delivery.

NONNURSING MODELS FOR CULTURAL ASSESSMENT

There are both nonnursing and nursing models for cultural assessment from which to choose. Arguably, the two most well-known nonnursing models are the Outline of Cultural Materials by Murdock (1971) and Brownlee's (1978) *Community, Culture, and Care: A Cross-Cultural Guide for Health Workers*. The Murdock tool was designed for use by anthropologists and as such does not utilize the nursing process. The Brownlee tool is considered difficult by some and also is not a nursing tool. This lack of nursing focus has been a driving point behind the development of nursing-specific cultural assessment models.

SELECTED NURSING MODELS FOR CULTURAL ASSESSMENT

Culture Care, Diversity, and Universality: A Theory of Nursing

The first nursing cultural assessment model was developed by Dr. Madeline Leininger. She developed her theory—Culture Care, Diversity, and Universality—from both anthropology and nursing principles. She first published her theory in *Nursing Science Quarterly* in 1985. In 1988, the theory was further described in the same journal, and in 1991, she published her textbook, *Culture Care Diversity and Universality: A Theory of Nursing*. The theory states that nurses must take into account the cultural beliefs, caring behaviors, and values of individuals, families, and groups to provide effective, satisfying, and culturally congruent nursing care (Leininger, 1991). The central purpose of the theory is to discover and explain diverse and universal culturally based care factors influencing the health, well-being, illness, or death of individuals or groups. The goal is to identify ways to provide culturally congruent nursing care to people of diverse or similar cultures (Leininger, 2002). The foundation of the theory is that cultures exhibit both diversity and universality. Leininger (1985) defined diversity as perceiving, knowing, and practicing care in different ways and defined universality as commonalities of care.

To fully understand any nursing theory or nursing care model, one must understand the operational definitions for key terms. Traditionally, nursing has four metaparadigms: the concepts of person, environment, health, and nursing. Leininger believes that the paradigm of nursing is too limited in its definition, so that construct was replaced by caring. Caring, according to Leininger, has a better ability to explain nursing. She feels that the concept of person is too limiting and culture-bound to explain nursing, because the concept of person does not exist in every culture. The term *person* is often used globally to refer to families, groups, and communities. Leininger also views the paradigm of health as belonging to many other healthcare disciplines and as such it is not unique to nursing. The fourth paradigm is environment, which Leininger has replaced with environmental context. Environmental context includes events with meanings and interpretations given to them in particular physical, ecological, sociopolitical, and/or cultural settings (Leininger, 1995).

Leininger (1985) defines culture as a group's values, beliefs, norms, and life practices that are learned, shared, and handed down. Culture guides thinking, decision making, and our actions in specific ways. Culture is the framework people use to solve human problems. In that sense, culture is universal yet also diverse. Cultural values are usually long-term and are very stable. Caring is defined by Leininger (1985) as assisting, supporting, or enabling behaviors that ease or improve a patient's condition. Leininger (1985) states that the essence of nursing is caring; caring is unique to nursing. It is essential to life, survival, and human development. It is through caring that people can deal with life's events. *Caring* is the verb counterpart to the noun *care* and is a feeling of compassion, interest, and concern for people. Caring has different meanings in different cultures. Individual cultural definitions of caring can be discovered by examining the cultural group's view of the world, social structure, and language (Leininger, 1985). *Culture care* refers to the values and beliefs that assist, support, or enable another person or group to maintain well-being, improve personal condition, or face death or disability. Culture care, according to Leininger (1985), is universal, but the actions, expressions, patterns, lifestyles, and meanings of care may be different. A nurse cannot provide appropriate cultural care without having a knowledge and understanding of cultural diversity. Worldview is defined as the outlook a group or person has, based on the view of the world or universe. Worldview consists of both a social structure and environmental context. The social structure provides organization to a culture, and it can come from religion, education, or economics. The environmental context is any event or situation that gives meaning to human expressions. Folk health, or well-being systems, are care practices that have a special meaning within the culture. These practices are used to heal or assist people in their homes or within the community at large. Folk or well-being systems have the potential to supplement traditional healthcare delivery systems. Person is defined as a human being that is capable of being concerned about others. A key construct of all nursing theory is environment. Leininger did not specifically define environment in her theory other than providing an operational definition for environmental context. Health is viewed as a state of well-being. Most importantly, though, health is culturally defined, valued, and practiced. Health is viewed as a universal concept across all cultures but is defined differently by each to reflect its specific values and beliefs. Nursing is defined as a learned humanistic art and science that focuses on personalized behaviors, functions, and processes to promote and maintain health or recovery from illness. According to Leininger (1985), nursing uses three modes of action to deliver care: culture care preservation or maintenance, culture care accommodation or negotiation, and culture care restructuring or repatterning.

Leininger's Sunrise Model (1991) illustrates the major components and interrelationships of the culture care, diversity, and universality. Nurses can use the Sunrise Model when caring for patients to ensure that nursing actions are culture specific. It requires that the nurse understand the values, beliefs, and practices of the patient's culture. The Sunrise Model symbolizes the rising of the sun (the sun represents care). The model depicts a full sun with four foci. Within the circle in the upper portion of the model are components of the social structure and worldview factors that influence care and health.

When applying Leininger's model, it is important for the nurse to consider whether there is a cultural mismatch present. A cultural mismatch is what occurs when people violate each other's cultural expectations. The healthcare provider needs to develop awareness into his or her personal style of interaction, because he or she may have a personal style of interaction that does not match the patient's. An example of a cultural mismatch would be the healthcare provider, attempting to keep to a tight schedule, interrupting the prayer session of a devoutly Muslim patient (Leininger, 1995). This interruption would definitely result in a cultural mismatch, but it could also result in causing cultural pain to the Muslim patient, which is a much more serious situation. Leininger (1997) states cultural pain occurs when hurtful, offensive, or inappropriate words are spoken to an individual or group. These spoken words are experienced by the receiver as being insulting, discomforting, or stressful. Cultural pain occurs because of a lack of awareness, sensitivity, and understanding by the offender of differences in the cultural values, beliefs, and meanings of the offended persons. When these types of events occur during a patient–provider encounter, they can result in significant consequences. It is essential that if a cultural mismatch or the infliction of cultural pain does occur, it be recognized, or we risk the development of consequences, one of which would be the inability to establish a therapeutic alliance with the patient. If a cultural mismatch or mistake is made, it is best for the healthcare provider to attempt to recover quickly from the mistake and to avoid becoming defensive. If the provider suspects that the mismatch has been serious enough to have caused cultural pain (as evidenced by seeing a sudden negative change in attitude), the health professional must act on this feeling and ask whether he or she did or said anything offensive. Cultural pain occurs if the clinician inadvertently ignores an important cultural obligation or violates a cultural taboo. Making this type of adjustment requires

cultural flexibility—this is only possible in those healthcare providers who have taken the time to develop self-awareness and who have examined their own cultural background and biases.

Leininger (2002) identified eight unique features of her model. The eight features include (1) the fact that it is one of the oldest nursing theories (1950s), (2) its focus is on the interrelationships of culture on health and illness, (3) its focus on comparative cultures, (4) it is holistic and multidimensional, (5) it was designed to discover global diversities (both differences and similarities), (6) it has its own associated research method (ethnonursing), (7) it consists of both abstract and practical modes for delivering culturally congruent care, and (8) it has a focus on ethnohistory for use in diverse environmental contexts (Leininger, 2002).

Leininger (2002) advocates the concurrent use of her theory and the Sunrise Model in order to discover factors that may influence the patient's response, such as cultural stresses and pain, and to reduce the incidence of anger and noncompliance.

The importance of Leininger's theory with the Sunrise Model is substantial and invaluable as the theory has served as the prototype for the development of other culturally specific nursing models and tools.

Giger and Davidhizar's Transcultural Assessment Model

Giger and Davidhizar's model provides a framework for assessment that focuses on the six cultural phenomena that they believe shape care: communication, space, social organization, time, environmental control, and biologic variations (Giger, 2013). They also systematically explore the variations that exist in caregivers' responses and recipients' perspectives relative to the cultural diversity that is present in the United States. The model serves as a resource for healthcare professionals when they are called upon to provide culturally discordant care. The authors advocate that the model can and should be used in a variety of clinical settings (primary, secondary, and tertiary) (Giger, 2013).

The model was first developed in 1988 to help undergraduate nursing students assess and provide care for patients who were culturally diverse. Giger and Davidhizar state that although all cultures are not the same, they share the same basic organizational factors (Giger, 2013). In its present form, the model provides a framework to systematically assess the role of culture on health and illness and has been used extensively in a variety of settings and by diverse disciplines. In 1993, Spector combined this model with the Cultural Heritage Model, which appears in Potter and Perry's *Fundamentals of Nursing*. Spector (1993) used the model's six phenomena, but placed them in a different hierarchical arrangement and then used this hierarchy as a guide for cultural assessment of people from a variety of racial and cultural groups. The model has been utilized in other healthcare disciplines such as medical imaging, dentistry, education, and administration. The model has also been the theoretical framework for dissertations and other research studies.

Giger (2013) provides the following definition of culture:

> Culture is a patterned behavioral response that develops over time as a result of imprinting the mind through social and religious structures and intellectual and artistic manifestations. Culture is also the result of acquired mechanisms that may have innate influences but are primarily affected by internal and external environmental stimuli. Culture is shaped by values, beliefs, norms and practices that are shared by members of the same ethnic group. Culture guides our thinking, doing and being and becomes patterned expressions of who we are. These patterned expressions are passed down from one generation to the next. . . . [Cultural values are] unique expressions of a particular culture that have been accepted as appropriate over time. (p. 2)*

The model postulates that every individual is culturally unique and requires culturally competent care. Culturally competent care is defined by Giger (2013) as

> a dynamic, fluid, continuous process whereby an individual, system, or healthcare agency finds meaningful and useful care delivery strategies based on knowledge of the cultural heritage, beliefs, attitudes, and behaviors of those to whom they render care. Cultural competence connotes a higher, more sophisticated level of refinement of cognitive skills and psychomotor skills, attitudes, and personal beliefs. To develop cultural competency, it is essential for the healthcare professional to use knowledge gained from conceptual and theoretical models of culturally appropriate care. Attainment of cultural competence can assist the astute nurse in devising meaningful interventions to promote optimal health among individuals regardless of race, ethnicity, gender identity, sexual identity, or cultural heritage. (p. 8)†

Patients should be assessed according to the six cultural phenomena. It is important to emphasize that the model does not presuppose that every person within an ethnic or cultural group will act or behave in a similar manner. In fact, Giger (2013) informs us that a culturally appropriate model must recognize differences in groups while also avoiding stereotypical approaches to client care. In addition, the six cultural phenomena described are not mutually exclusive but are related and often interacting. Whereas the phenomena vary with application across cultural groups, the six concepts of the model are evident in every cultural group. The six cultural phenomena will be discussed individually.

The Phenomena

Communication The first phenomenon is communication. Communication embraces the entire world of human interaction and behavior, and it is how we relate or connect to others. Communication is the way by which culture is

---

transmitted and preserved. It is a continuous and complex process as it can be transmitted through written or oral language and nonverbal behaviors, such as gestures, facial expressions, body language, and the use of space. Although the factors that influence communication are universal, they vary among culture-specific groups in terms of language spoken, voice quality, pronunciation, use of silence, and use of nonverbal communication (Giger, 2013). Effective communication is essential for effective healthcare delivery because it motivates both the patient and the nurse to work together to manage the patient's health because the patient is better informed and empowered to participate more fully. Motivating our patients to take action on behalf of their own health is one of the tenets of Healthy People 2020.

Communication can present a barrier between the nurse and the patient, as well as the patient's family, especially when the nurse and the patient are from different cultural backgrounds. This feeling of alienation or powerlessness can occur if the language spoken is the same or if it is different. Impaired communication can result in a poor outcome. There are many different types of communication differences that the nurse may experience. Even when the language is shared between patient and nurse, misunderstandings can occur because of cultural orientation. Even though people may speak the same language, word meanings may differ between the sender and the receiver. This is because vocabulary words have both a connotative and denotative meaning. A denotative meaning is the meaning that is used by most people who share that common language, but the connotative meaning comes from the person's personal experience. Differences in the meaning of words can cause numerous conflicts among various cultural groups. Overcoming language differences is probably the most difficult hurdle when attempting to provide cross-cultural health care. Clear and effective communication is essential. Nurses often become frustrated and find it difficult when faced with a language difference between patient and nurse. All parts of the nursing process are affected negatively when we are unable to speak with our patients. When verbal communication is not possible, then we must rely instead on interpretation of the patient's nonverbal language. When patients are unable to communicate with us, they may withdraw or become hostile or uncooperative.

Both verbal and nonverbal communication are learned within one's culture. Communication and culture are intertwined. Our culture determines how our feelings are expressed and what is and is not appropriate. It is believed that cultural patterns of communication are firmly a part of us as early as age 5. Communication is essential to human interaction—it discloses information or provides a message. Through communication, we become aware of how another is feeling. Often, communication issues cause the most significant problems when working with people from a different culture. One of the most common barriers to communication is overcoming ethnocentrism (viewing one's culture as superior to another), particularly when assessing patients. An example of how to ensure that a patient's communication needs for patient education are met would be to provide oral instructions if the patient feels less comfortable with written materials. In contrast, when educating the Asian population, it is helpful to know that the majority of Asians prefer written materials over oral instructions.

Language differences need to be overcome with the use of competent interpreters. When a nurse cares for a patient who does not speak the dominant language, an interpreter is a must. In 1998, the National Council on Interpreting in Health Care was founded with the goal of promoting culturally competent healthcare interpretation. The Office of Minority Health recommends against the use of a patient's friends or family members as interpreters. One reason for this is that the patient may not be comfortable disclosing certain symptoms or behaviors to friends or family.

Differences between patient and provider influence communication and clinical decision making. There is strong evidence that provider–patient communication is directly linked to patient satisfaction. When these differences are not acknowledged or explored, they result in poor patient satisfaction, poor adherence, and, most alarmingly, a poor outcome (Betancourt, Green, Carrillo, & Ananeh-Firempong, 2003). Failure to recognize the uniqueness of all of our patients can result in stereotyping and biased and discriminatory treatment.

Space   The second of the six phenomena is space. *Space* refers to the distance between people when they interact. Personal space is the area that surrounds the body. All communication occurs within the context of space. Rules concerning personal distance vary from culture to culture; therefore, views of appropriate spatial distance vary among persons of different cultures. Discomfort occurs when individuals feel their personal space has been violated (Giger, 2013). Personal space is perceived through our biological senses, and the degree of comfort one feels in proximity to others, in body movement and perception of personal, intimate, and public space, is culturally based (Giger, 2013). European North Americans are aware of zones associated with personal space: the intimate zone, personal distance, social distance, and public distance. Other cultures may not be aware of these distinctions. Humans are similar to felines in that we wish to establish territoriality, and we become uncomfortable when our territory is encroached upon. How large our territorial space is depends on individual and cultural preferences. Encroachment into one's intimate zone by another can cause many different types of reactions. One possible outcome is embarrassment and modesty. Modesty may pose a significant barrier that may be difficult to overcome when it is time to examine the patient.

Giger and Davidhizar identified four aspects of behavior patterns related to space that must be assessed to promote a healthy interaction: (1) proximity to others, (2) attachment with objects in the environment, (3) body posture, and (4) movement in the setting (Giger, 2013).

These four concepts are particularly important during periods when family members are experiencing emotional chaos, such as during the grieving process. Although the desired degree of physical proximity between the client and provider is based on the degree of intimacy and the trust that has been mutually established, as a general rule, Hispanics and Asians tend to stand closer to each other than do Euro-Americans.

Social Organization   The third phenomenon is social organization. Cultural behavior, or how one acts in certain situations, is socially acquired, not genetically inherited. Patterns of cultural behavior are learned through a process called enculturation (also referred to as socialization), which involves acquiring knowledge and internalizing values (Giger, 2013). Most people achieve competence in their own culture through enculturation/socialization. Social organization refers to the manner in which a cultural group organizes itself around the family group. Family structure and organization, religious values and beliefs, and role assignments all relate to ethnicity and culture. Where we grow up and choose to live in adulthood plays an essential role in our socialization process. There is a strong need among many cultural groups to maintain social congruency. This need can negatively affect health care. Access to healthcare providers does not necessarily translate into positive lifestyle behaviors or risk-reduction activities as prescribed by the dominant society. People from some cultures may verbally agree with a treatment plan out of respect for the provider but then defer to folk remedies or alternative health practices upon discharge. Social organization consists of the family unit and the social organizations in which one may have membership. Social organizations are structured in a variety of groups, including family, religious, ethnic, racial, and special interest groupings. Membership in groups, except for ethnic or racial groups, is voluntary. Social barriers also exist and can influence access to health care, as was pointed out in the IOM (2003) report. These social barriers include unemployment, socioeconomic status, and lack of health insurance.

Time The fourth phenomenon of the Giger and Davidhizar model is time (Giger, 2013). Time has two meanings. The first is duration (interval of time), and the second is specified instances or points in time (Giger, 2013). As a result of these two distinct meanings, time is very culture-bound, as it is perceived, measured, and valued differently across cultures (Giger, 2013). In essence, time is conceptualized in reference to our chronologic age, in relation to events, and as an external entity that is outside of our control (Giger, 2013).

Although it may not be readily apparent on the surface, time is an important aspect of interpersonal communication. The concept of time not only is based on clock hours and social influences (e.g., meals and holidays) but is culturally perceived. Clock time is frequently more highly valued by the majority of Western cultures, in which appointments tend to be kept at the prescribed time. In a culture in which places and persons are more important than social time, activities start when a previous social event has been completed, and to be dominated by adherence to clock time is often considered rude. Persons in different cultures may have a time orientation that focuses on either the past, present, or future. This can tremendously influence preventive health care because a patient must have at least a small degree of future time orientation to be motivated by a future-situated reward (improved health down the road or a longer life). People who are future oriented are more likely to embrace preventive health measures as they are concerned about the onset of illness in the future. People who are present oriented are often late for medical appointments or may skip them entirely. Recognizing the patient's time orientation has value for the nurse. Considering the time orientation can provide a bridge to increase compliance with a medication regimen or with recommended health screenings.

Environmental Control The fifth phenomenon is the environment and locus of control, individuals' perception of whether they can control events and plan and direct factors in the environment that may affect them. Many Americans believe they have internal control over nature, which influences the decision to seek health care. If the patient comes from a culture in which there is less belief in internal control and more in external control, there may be a fatalistic view in which seeking health care is viewed as useless.

Human attempts to control nature and the environment are as old as recorded history. At its most basic level, locus of control is a significant variable in how people react within the American healthcare system. In general, the willingness to accept responsibility for one's health is considered an internal locus of control. Persons who have an external locus of control believe the healthcare delivery system exists to provide essential care, and they can become especially frustrated with the complexities of health care in the United States and the myriad of options available.

The environment also encompasses a person's health and illness beliefs and whether the person expands health delivery from that provided only by Western medicine with that provided by complementary or alternative practitioners. Understanding the patient's perspective on alternative therapies is essential when developing an optimal plan of care.

Biologic Variations The last of the six phenomena is biologic variations (Giger, 2013). Biologic differences, especially genetic variations, exist between individuals in different ethnic groups. Although there is as much difference within cultural and ethnic groups as there is across and among cultural and racial groups, knowledge of general baseline data relative to the specific cultural group is an excellent starting point to provide culturally appropriate care. This is also an important area when it comes to racial differences in how pharmaceuticals are metabolized and utilized (ethnopharmacology).

Ethnopharmacologic research has revealed that ethnicity significantly affects drug response. Genetic or cultural factors, or both, may influence a given drug's pharmacokinetics (its absorption, metabolism, distribution, and elimination) and pharmacodynamics (its mechanism of action and effects at the target site), as well as patient adherence and education. In addition, the tremendous variation within each of the broader racial and ethnic categories defined by the U.S. Census Bureau (categories often used by researchers) must be considered. For example, some researchers use the terms *race*, *ethnicity*, and *culture* synonymously, even though each term has a distinct and unique definition. Improper labeling can result in inaccuracies with data collection, and the nurse should consider that when critically evaluating ethnopharmacologic research findings. In addition, most clinical drug trials are conducted on adult White males, with the results then generalized to all patients who might be prescribed and administered the drugs. Despite the growing evidence that ethnicity influences drug response, many nurses and healthcare providers still remain largely unaware of this. Research has shown that genetic variations in certain enzymes may cause differing drug responses (although the precise mechanisms are unknown); also, certain ethnic groups have more of these variations than others do. Individual factors, such as diet and alcohol and tobacco usage, can also influence gene expression, and therefore drug metabolism (Muñoz & Hilgenberg, 2005).

Nurses need to become knowledgeable about drugs that are likely to elicit varied responses in people with different ethnic backgrounds, as well as the potential for adverse effects. The existing ethnopharmacologic research focuses primarily on psychotropic and antihypertensive agents (Muñoz & Hilgenberg, 2005). The nurse should utilize caution and consider the possibility of biologic variations when administering

antihypertensives and psychotropic drugs to culturally diverse patients. Some patients will have a therapeutic response at a dose lower than typically recommended for a particular agent. The nurse must carefully monitor the patient to help prevent unnecessary increases in dosage, which will increase the likelihood of adverse events.

The nurse must also be on guard in the event a therapeutic substitution is required. Sometimes substitution is done to contain costs or because a drug is not on an institution's formulary. Drugs may vary in how they are metabolized, and substitution may be more clinically risky for patients from non-White racial and ethnic groups. Although individual differences exist and should be considered, the nurse would be wise to be extra vigilant when drug substitutions occur in their non-White patients.

Healthcare providers must understand the biologic differences and susceptibility that exist in persons from different cultures. For example, Black Americans have a higher prevalence of cardiovascular disease, cancer, and diabetes than do others. Cultural differences can also contribute to either noncompliance or poor compliance with therapy. Unfortunately, in many cases, lack of knowledge limits the ability of healthcare professionals to differentiate environmental, familial, and genetic predisposition to disease states. Although research is being conducted on biologic differences relating to ethnic groups, it lags behind the knowledge available regarding other cultural phenomena. An important example of this is that the development of pain measurement instruments remains culturally centered even though significant differences exist in how members of different cultural groups perceive and respond to pain management.

There are several ways that people from one cultural group differ biologically from members of other cultural groups. These differences are called biologic variants. They can include stature or size, skin color, genetic differences, disease susceptibility, and nutritional variants. Asians traditionally are smaller in stature than are members of other racial or ethnic groups. Skin color differences among races also affect hair and nail texture. Genetic differences can result in enzyme deficiencies such as a lack of lactase, which causes lactose intolerance. Certain ethnic groups, such as Hispanics and Black Americans, have higher morbidity rates than do other groups because of differences in disease susceptibility. Even the diets that are followed by our patients can be culture-bound, such as a Jewish patient's kosher diet or balancing hot and cold foods, as is common in many Hispanic homes.

Another area that is under intense study is biocultural differences. This area of study is also known as biocultural ecology, and it focuses on human adaptation and homeostasis (Giger, 2013). Biocultural ecology may help to lessen the fragmentation that has occurred in the past where culture, biology, ecology, and the environment have been looked at separately or in isolation.

Clinical Application of the Model

It is essential for all healthcare professionals to be aware that not all patients with the same medical diagnosis are likely to have the same experience. Following this model permits the patient to be an equal partner with the nurse. A cultural assessment can be obtained by utilizing the questions posed by Giger and Davidhizar, which will provide a better understanding of patient behaviors that might, if not understood within the context of ethnic values, be regarded as puzzling or even negative (Giger, 2013). This approach is not meant to be stereotypical. By carefully listening and observing and questioning appropriately, the nurse should be able to discover the health traditions or beliefs of an individual patient.

The recognition of the importance of providing culturally appropriate clinical approaches has developed in response to the easily discernible fact that the United States is rapidly becoming a multicultural, heterogeneous, pluralistic society. As the demographics of the population of the United States continue to expand, and especially when the demographics of the healthcare professional and the patient do not match, it is essential that the healthcare professional embark on a journey to develop sensitivity and cultural competence in order to provide safe and effective care. This can be achieved by performing cultural assessment according to the guidelines established by any transcultural nursing model.

See **Box 23-3** for examples of cultural gaffes that can occur within each aspect of Giger and Davidhizar's Transcultural Assessment Model.

Purnell Model for Cultural Competence

One of the unique components of the Purnell Model for Cultural Competence (Purnell & Paulanka, 1998) is—as a holographic theory—its applicability: it can be used by all disciplines and healthcare team members. Nurses who are members of interdisciplinary teams may wish to use this model for this reason. Not only can this model be used by all team members but also it is unique in that it includes the recognition of biocultural ecology and workforce issues and the impact of these on the culturally diverse patient. Often, team members can be from various cultures, and this model can be helpful when they try to forge a greater understanding of what is similar and different among the various cultures that make up the healthcare team. Purnell (2013) identifies many benefits to the use of his model. The model provides a framework for all healthcare providers to utilize when learning about the inherent concepts and characteristics of new cultures.

The Purnell Model for Cultural Competence consists of circles. The outermost circle represents the global society, the second represents

BOX 23-3	Six Phenomena of the Giger and Davidhizar Model and Examples of Cultural Gaffes

Phenomenon	Event	Response
Time	Visiting hours are not being respected.	Explain institution's time expectations.
Space	Poor eye contact on the part of your patient.	Make sure you are aware of the customs regarding contact, such as eye contact and touch, for many different cultural groups (optimally, all that you will come in contact with in practice). Poor eye contact is a sign of respect in some cultures (Vietnamese Americans, American Indian, Appalachians); excessive eye contact may be perceived as rude by Chinese Americans.
Communication	Family member is using a lot of hand gesturing when communicating.	Gestures do not have universal meaning; what is acceptable to one group may be taboo to another.
Social Organization	Prayer sessions in a hospital room by patient and family members.	Be aware of the expected rituals and how religious services are conducted for many different groups.
Biologic Variations	Family members repeatedly bring home-prepared meals for the patient with foods that are in violation of the prescribed diet plan.	Look for foods that are not in violation of the prescribed diet and encourage the family to only bring in foods from the approved list.
Environmental Control	Family members wish to bring in a folk medicine healer as a member of the healthcare team.	Advocate for the patient for inclusion of the complementary provider as a member of the team.

Source: This article was published in *Transcultural nursing: Assessment and intervention* (6th ed), Giger, J. N., p. 7, Copyright 2013 Elsevier.

community, and the third represents the family. The innermost circle represents the person. The interior circle is divided into 12 pie-shaped wedges. Each wedge depicts one of the 12 cultural domains. The dark center of the circle represents all unknown phenomena. There is a jagged line at the bottom that represents the concept of cultural consciousness, which is nonlinear (Purnell, 2013).

The model provides a link between historical perspectives and their impact on one's cultural worldview. It also provides a link for the central relationships of culture so that congruence can occur and to facilitate the delivery of consciously competent care.

Consciously competent care is an important concept because when we are conscious of the care we provide, we ensure that it is culturally competent and we can replicate that care delivery for this patient and for other patients in the future. The model also provides a framework that allows the nurse to reflect on and consider each patient's unique human characteristics such as motivation, intentionality, and meaning when planning for and providing patient care. The model provides a structure for analyzing cultural data, and it permits the nurse to view the individual, family, or group within its own unique and ethnocultural environment. The model encourages the nurse to consider communication strategies to overcome identified barriers. Effective communication depends on not only verbal language skills, including the dominant language, dialects, and the contextual use of the language, but also other important factors such as the paralanguage variations of voice volume, tone, intonations, reflections, as well as the openness of the patient (willingness to share thoughts and feelings). Another important component is nonverbal communication. The varied and numerous components of nonverbal communication must also be considered. For example, the nurse must know whether to engage in the use of eye contact or to avoid it, depending on the cultural norms of the patient. This consideration must also be given to the type of facial expressions to utilize, as not all facial expressions will be acceptable to all patients. Whether or when to touch a patient is also culturally dependent, as is our use of body language and interpretation of the patient's body language. Even how close we are to our patients communicates information about us. Nurses must become aware of the spatial-distancing practices and acceptable greetings associated with the various cultural groups that come under their care. The nurse's worldview in terms of whether the nurse or the patient utilizes a past, present, or future orientation must be considered and planned for. Does the patient place a focus on clock time (as is the case with the Western Biomedical Model) or on social time? Consideration must even be given to how we address our patients. Miscalculating the degree of formality in the use of names can result in breaking trust or blocking the establishment of a therapeutic alliance between nurse and patient. Communication styles may vary between insiders (family and close friends) and outsiders (strangers and unknown healthcare providers). Purnell (2013) reminds us that in regard to verbal and nonverbal communication, there is indeed much to consider.

The Purnell (2013) model has an organizing framework of 12 universal domains:

- Overview, inhabited localities, and topography
- Communication
- Family roles and organization
- Workforce issues
- Biocultural ecology
- High-risk health behaviors
- Nutrition
- Pregnancy and childbearing practices
- Death rituals
- Spirituality
- Healthcare practices
- Healthcare practitioners

An important consideration for the nurse to keep in mind is the higher level of regard or esteem that nurses are given in the United States compared to what is given to nurses in other parts of the world. This higher regard may be due to the amount of educational preparation required and the nurse's need to pass a licensing examination to become a nurse in the United States. In some ethnic or cultural groups, however, folk healers or other nonlicensed healthcare providers (e.g., shamans, medicine men, lay midwives) are held in higher regard than are nurses who are educationally prepared and who practice within the Western Biomedical Model. When providing care to patients from a culture where this may be an issue, the nurse should spend time establishing a good interpersonal relationship in order to bridge the cultural gap and to improve the patient's outcome and the overall healthcare experience of the patient.

SUMMARY

By now, it should be clear that it is impossible to practice high-quality nursing with our culturally diverse patient population unless we gain knowledge in transcultural health care and cultural competency models. See **Table 23-1**

TABLE 23-1	Cultural Factors

Family structure and characteristics

Education levels

Family assets

Family in the community

Communication style

Health beliefs and practice

Help-seeking style

View of professional and family roles

View of early intervention

Knowledge of health and education system

Time orientation

Socioeconomic status

TABLE 23-2	Process for Attaining Cultural Competence

Develop awareness of own cultural biases

Understand facets of culture

Acknowledge and honor range of diversity in families' values and beliefs

Develop cultural sensitivity

Develop collaborative partnerships with families

Develop methods of cross-cultural communication

Learn to collaborate with interpreters

Minimize cultural bias in assessments

Identify and address barriers to assessment and intervention

for more information on cultural factors and **Table 23-2** for a process to follow to develop cultural competence. It is not enough to just gain this knowledge, however. In order to deliver high-quality culturally diverse nursing care, nurses need to utilize this unique nursing knowledge; nurses must not only know but also attempt to do. Utilizing any of the described nursing models allows the nurse to gain knowledge and to deliver culturally appropriate care. The use of transcultural models is beneficial for nurses to become knowledgeable about and for evaluating society in terms of culture, to find the cultural data in a more systematic and standardized way, and to improve the field of transcultural nursing. Having a greater knowledge of the cultures served by the nurse will play an important role in improving the quality of health care. It is well known that the meaning of health and illness is different for various cultural groups. Nurses who utilize transcultural theories are in an ideal position to demonstrate how the provision of culturally competent care will shape health care in the future. These and other models provide a starting point for assessment of patients who are culturally diverse. The nurse just needs to select the one that fits him or her best. The key is to remember that patients' cultural behaviors are relevant to health assessment and should be considered when planning care. Nurses can be guided in this process by selecting and following one of the available nursing models. A description of three of these models was provided in this chapter—Leininger's Culture Care, Diversity, and Universality Theory and the Sunrise Model; Giger and Davidhizar's Transcultural Assessment Model; and Purnell's Model for Cultural Competence—to help you select the model that is best for you. You are now ready to begin to develop your transcultural nursing practice.

PERTINENT RESEARCH STUDIES OF SELECTED MEDICAL DISORDERS AND CULTURAL COMPETENCY

Tuberculosis

Many studies have found that worldwide patients who stopped treatment for tuberculosis (TB) did so because they felt better, their symptoms abated, or they thought that they were cured. In addition, patient beliefs about TB may differ from the medical model, such as believing that the disease has a mystical, superstitious, or religious origin. Compliance can also be a factor, especially if a patient was a refugee, as the patient may perceive the healthcare worker as a government representative or as an oppressor. Various rumors have also spread among different cultures that TB is caused by smoking, pollution, or even hard labor.

Vietnamese Patients

Hoa, N. P., Thorson, A. E. K., Long, N. H., & Diwan, V. K. (2003). Knowledge of tuberculosis and associated health-seeking behaviour among rural Vietnamese adults with a cough for at least three weeks. *Scandinavian Journal of Public Health*, 31(Suppl. 62), 59–65.

Houston, H. R., Herada, N., & Makinodan, T. (2002). Development of a culturally sensitive educational intervention program to reduce the high incidence of tuberculosis among foreign-born Vietnamese. *Ethnicity and Health*, 7(4), 255–265.

Johannson, E., Long, N. H., Diwan, V. K., & Winkvist, A. (1999). Attitudes to compliance with tuberculosis treatment among women and men in Vietnam. *International Journal Tuberculosis and Lung Disease*, 3(10), 862–868.

Asian Indian Patients

Asghar, R. J., Pratt, R. H., Kammerer, J. S., Navin, T. R. (2008). Tuberculosis in South Asians living in the United States, 1993–2004. *Archives of Internal Medicine*, 168(9), 936–942.

Singh, V., Jaiswal, A., Porter, J. D., Ogden, J. A., Sarin, R., Sharma, P. P., . . . Jain, R. C. (2002). TB control, poverty and vulnerability in Delhi, India. *Tropical Medicine & International Health*, 7(8), 693–700.

Gambian Patients

Harper, M., Ahmadu, F. A., Ogden, J. A., McAdam, K. P., & Lienhardt, C. (2003). Identifying the determinants of tuberculosis control in resource poor countries: Insights from a qualitative study in The Gambia. *Transactions of the Royal Society of Tropical Medicine and Hygiene*, 97(5), 506–510.

Diabetes Patients

According to the Centers for Disease Control and Prevention (CDC), there are 900,000 new cases of diabetes mellitus (DM) annually, which translates to more than 2,600 new cases each and every day. The worst-case scenario results when a strong genetic predisposition is combined with poor lifestyle choices. When this occurs repeatedly, it results in escalating rates of type 2 diabetes. It is believed that this is one of the primary reasons why minority populations are experiencing such a high type 2 diabetes incidence. This is a worldwide problem because the burden of diabetes is growing even more rapidly in other countries than it is growing in the United States. This will result in a huge economic burden in some countries that are not in a financial position to handle it. Type 2 diabetes is becoming epidemic in areas with higher proportions of at-risk ethnic groups.

In these areas, a child as young as 12 years old is more likely to have type 2 diabetes than type 1 diabetes (sometimes still referred to as juvenile diabetes).

Recognition that poor diabetes outcomes may be related to inadequate cultural competency could result in a reduction or elimination of poor outcomes in these high-risk ethnic groups. These poor outcomes can be eliminated or reduced by enhanced awareness and improved skills in cross-cultural encounters. This understanding needs to extend to the complications that can be associated with DM in minorities as well. The following contributing factors have been identified to explain the high incidence of long-term complications of diabetes in ethnic minorities: high prevalence rate of DM, earlier age of onset that results in a longer duration of diabetes, poor glycemic control, delayed diagnosis, limited access to health care, less intense or comprehensive healthcare encounters, and a genetic susceptibility to complications (IOM, 2001).

Type 2 diabetes affects different populations in different ways. The prevalence is significantly higher in minority groups in comparison to the White population. This important disparity is beginning to be shared with the public through public service announcements. The American Diabetes Association has used the public service campaign of "Diabetes Favors Minorities." These facts were included in that public service announcement: diabetes strikes 1 out of 3 Native Americans, 1 out of 7 Hispanics, and 1 out of 14 Blacks.

The Translating Research Into Action for Diabetes (TRIAD) study was published in *Medical Care* in December 2006 by Duru et al. TRIAD's overall goal is to understand and influence the quality of care (both processes and outcomes of care) for patients with diabetes in managed care settings. TRIAD is a 10-year project funded by the Centers for Disease Control and Prevention and the National Institute of Diabetes and Digestive and Kidney Diseases. It is a six-center prospective study of managed care and diabetes quality of care, costs, and outcomes in the United States.

The goal of this study was to determine whether the utilization of clinical care strategies in managed care (diabetes registry, physician feedback, and physician reminders) is associated with attenuation of known racial/ethnic disparities in diabetic care. The study found that, for the most part, high-intensity implementation of a diabetes registry, physician feedback, and physician reminders—three clinical care strategies similar to those strategies that are used in many healthcare settings—are not associated with an attenuation of known disparities of diabetes care in managed care. The authors also reported that disparities in care do exist, particularly among the Black American population.

DISCUSSION QUESTIONS

1. Differentiate the terms *culture*, *cultural assessment*, and *cultural competency*.

2. List the six cultural phenomena of the Giger and Davidhizar model.

3. Purnell identifies the 12 domains of culture in his model. What are the similarities and differences between those 12 domains and the 6 cultural phenomena that are in the Giger and Davidhizar model?

4. Provide two nursing implications for a nurse administering antihypertensives or psychotropics to a non-White patient (ethnopharmacology principles).

5. What was the theoretical framework used to develop the 12 standards of culturally competent nursing care practice that were published in the *Journal of Transcultural Nursing* in 2009?

6. Describe the process of how to attain cultural competency.

7. Which nursing theorist gave birth to the transcultural nursing movement?

8. Identify and describe three potential areas of diversity.

9. Describe the potential consequences of culturally discordant care.

10. What can the nurse do to decease the likelihood of committing a cultural gaffe?

REFERENCES

Battalova, J., & Terrazas, A. (2010). Frequently requested statistics on immigrants and immigration in the United States. Retrieved from http://www.migrationinformation.org/feature/display.cfm?ID=818

Benet-Martínez, V., & Haritatos, J. (2005). Bicultural identity integration (BII): Components and psychosocial antecedents. *Journal of Personality, 73*(4), 1015–1049. Retrieved from University of California Postprints website: http://escholarship.org/uc/item/4vh6z3s2

Berry, J. W. (1990). Psychology of acculturation. In N. R. Goldberger & J. B. Veroff (Eds.), *The culture and psychology reader* (pp. 457–488). New York, NY: New York University Press. Reprinted from Nebraska symposium on motivation: Berman, J. J. (Ed.). (1989). *Cross-cultural perspectives.* Lincoln: University of Nebraska Press.

Betancourt, J. R. (2003). Cross-cultural medical education: Conceptual approaches and frameworks for evaluation. *Academic Medicine, 78*(6), 560–569.

Betancourt, J. R., Green, A. R., Carrillo, J. E., & Ananeh-Firempong, O. (2003). Defining cultural competence: A practical framework for addressing racial/ethnic disparities in health and health care. *Public Health Reports, 118*(4), 293–302.

Brink, P. J. (1990). *Transcultural nursing: A book of readings.* Prospect Heights, IL: Waveland Press.

Browning, M. A., & Woods, J. H. (1993). Cross-cultural family nurse partnerships. In S. I. Feetham, S. B. Meister, & J. M. Bell (Eds.), *The nursing of families: Theories, research, education, and practice.* Newbury Park, CA: Sage.

Brownlee, A. T. (1978). *Community, culture, and care: A cross-cultural guide for health workers.* St. Louis, MO: Mosby.

Chuang, Y. (1999). *Fusion: The primary model of bicultural competence and bicultural identity development in a Taiwanese-American family lineage.* Unpublished doctoral dissertation.

Douglas, M. K., Pierce, J. U., Rosenkoetter, M., Callister, L. C., Hattar-Pollara, M., Lauderdale, J., . . . Pacquiao, D. (2009). Standards of practice for culturally competent nursing care: A request for comments. *Journal of Transcultural Nursing, 20*(3), 257–269.

Duru, O. K., Mangione, C. M., Steers, N. W., Herman, W. H., Karter, A. J., Kountz, D., . . . Brown, A. F. (2006). The association between clinical care strategies and the attenuation of racial/ethnic disparities in diabetes care: The Translating Research Into Action for Diabetes (TRIAD) study. *Medical Care, 44*(12), 1121–1128.

English, J. G., & Le, A. (1999). Assessing needs and planning, implementing, and evaluating health promotion and disease prevention programs among Asian American population groups. In R. M. Huff & M. V. Klein (Eds.), *Promoting health in multicultural populations: A handbook for practitioners* (pp. 357–374). Thousand Oaks, CA: Sage.

Giger, J. N. (2013). *Transcultural nursing: Assessment and intervention* (6th ed.). Philadelphia, PA: Elsevier.

Giger, J., Davidhizar, R. E., Purnell, L., Harden, J. T., Phillips, J., & Strickland, O. (2007). American Academy of Nursing Expert Panel report: Developing cultural competence to eliminate health disparities in ethnic minorities and other vulnerable populations. *Journal of Transcultural Nursing, 18*(2), 95–102.

Guillory, W. (2001). *Business of diversity: The case for action.* Salt Lake City, UT: Innovations International.

HealthyPeople.gov. (2014). Healthy People 2020. Retrieved from http://www.healthypeople.gov/2020/default.aspx

Hong, Y. Y., Morris, M. W., Chiu, C. Y., & Benet-Martínez, V. (2000). Multicultural minds: A dynamic constructivist approach to culture and cognition. *American Psychologist, 55*(7), 709–720.

Institute of Medicine. (2001). *Exploring the biological contributions to human health: Does sex matter?* Washington, DC: National Academies Press.

Institute of Medicine. (2003). *Patient safety: Achieving a new standard of care.* Washington, DC: National Academies Press.

Leininger, M. M. (1984). Transcultural nursing: An overview. *Nursing Outlook, 32*(2), 72–73.

Leininger, M. M. (1985). Transcultural care, diversity, and universality: A theory of nursing. *Nursing & Health Care, 6*(4), 208–212.

Leininger, M. M. (1991). *Culture care diversity and universality: A theory of nursing.* New York, NY: National League for Nursing Press.

Leininger, M. M. (1995). *Transcultural nursing: Concepts, theories, research and practices* (2nd ed.). New York, NY: McGraw-Hill.

Leininger, M. M. (1997). Understanding cultural pain for improved health care. *Journal of Transcultural Nursing, 9*(1), 32–35.

Leininger, M. (2002). Culture care theory: A major contribution to advance transcultural nursing knowledge and practices. *Journal of Transcultural Nursing, 13*(3), 189–192.

Leininger, M., & McFarland, M. (2002). *Transcultural nursing: Concepts, theories, research, and practice* (3rd ed.). New York, NY: McGraw Hill.

Marquand, B. (2006). Philippine nurses in the US—yesterday and today. MinorityNurse.com. Retrieved from http://www.minoritynurse.com/article/philippine-nurses-us%E2%80%94yesterday-and-today

McGee, C. (2001). When the Golden Rule does not apply: Starting nurses on the journey toward cultural competence. *Journal for Nurses in Staff Development, 17*(3), 105–112.

McGoldrick, M. (1993). *Ethnicity, cultural diversity and normality.* New York, NY: Guilford Press.

McGrath, B. B. (1998). Illness as a problem of meaning: Moving culture from the classroom to the clinic. *Advances in Nursing Science, 21*(2), 17–29.

Muñoz, C., & Hilgenberg, C. (2005). Ethnopharmacology: Understanding how ethnicity can affect drug response is essential to providing culturally competent care. *American Journal of Nursing, 105*(8), 40–48.

Murdock, G. P. (1971). Ethnographic atlas. *Ethnology World Cultures, 19*(1), 24–136.

Office of Minority Health. (2000). *Assuring cultural competence in health care: Recommendations for national standards and an outcomes-focused research agenda.* Washington, DC: U.S. Department of Health and Human Services.

Padilla, A. M. (1994). Bicultural development: A theoretical and empirical examination. In R. Malgady & O. Rodriguez (Eds.), *Theoretical and conceptual issues in Hispanic mental health* (pp. 20–51). Melbourne, FL: Krieger.

Parsons, T. (1951). *The social system.* Glencoe, IL: Free Press.

Phinney, J. S., & Devich-Navarro, M. (1997). Variations in bicultural identification among African American and Mexican American adolescents. *Journal of Research on Adolescence, 7*(1), 3–32.

Purnell, L. D. (Ed.). (2013). *Transcultural health care: A culturally competent approach* (4th ed.). Philadelphia, PA: F. A. Davis.

Purnell, L., & Paulanka, B. (1998). *Transcultural health care: A culturally competent approach.* Philadelphia, PA: F. A. Davis.

Spector, R. (1993). Culture, ethnicity and nursing. In P. Potter & A. Perry (Eds.), *Fundamentals of nursing: Concepts, process and practice.* St. Louis, MO: Mosby.

Sprott, J. E. (1993). The Black box in family assessment: Cultural diversity. In S. L. Feetham, S. B. Meister, J. M. Bell, & C. L. Gilliss (Eds.), *The nursing of families: Theory, research, education, & practice.* Thousand Oaks, CA: Sage.

Tervalon, M., & Murray-Garcia, J. (1998). Cultural humility versus cultural competence: A critical distinction in defining physician training outcomes in multicultural education. *Journal of Health Care for the Poor and Underserved, 9*(2), 117–125.

Tripp-Reimer, T., & Fox, S. (1990). *Beyond the concept of culture.* St. Louis, MO: Mosby.

U.S. Census Bureau. (2010). American fact finder. Retrieved from http://factfinder2.census.gov/faces/nav/jsf/pages/index.xhtml

U.S. Census Bureau. (2012). Census data. Retrieved from http://www.census.gov

Valente, S. M. (1989). Overcoming cultural barriers. *California Nurse, 85*(8), 4–5.

CHAPTER 24

Global Diversity

Linda Dayer-Berenson

© A-R-T/Shutterstock

CHAPTER OBJECTIVES

1. Define diversity.
2. Recognize that diversity is a global phenomenon.
3. Describe the impact of diversity on healthcare disparities.

INTRODUCTION

The movement toward cultural competency is in no small part a response to the growing diversity occurring in the United States. The population of the United States is extremely diverse and becoming even more so with each passing year. Depending on what Congress decides to do about immigration—curtail it, expand it, and so forth—the United States is facing a future population just 40 years away that could vary by more than 135 million residents. Our population is going to be growing in any case, largely because of immigrants who have arrived in the past few generations, but that growth could be limited to about 72 million persons (a 24.6% increase) if illegal immigration is significantly curtailed (Martin & Fogel, 2006). Alternatively, if current proposals of immigration reform, such as giving legal status to those currently here illegally, and the creation of a new guest worker program are adopted, we will likely be facing the prospect of a population in 2050 of half a billion people. That would be about 200 million more persons than live here today (a 67% increase) (Martin & Fogel, 2006). What is known from the 2010 census data is that the U.S. population grew by 9.7% since the year 2000. There was growth seen in the Latino population, but overall immigration to the United States has slowed, reversing a trend of steady growth over the past 30 years (U.S. Census Bureau, 2010a).

What is the cultural makeup of our current and projected population? For the first time, racial and ethnic minorities make up more than half the children born in the United States. At the same time the Hispanic/Latino population boom appears to have peaked due to the overall decline in immigration (Census 2012 estimates). Minorities increased 1.9% to 114.1 million (36.9%) of the total U.S. population. The recent slowdown in the growth of the Hispanic/Latino and Asian populations has resulted in a change to the projection on when the true tipping point in diversity will arrive—the time when non-Hispanic Whites become the minority. Initial review of the 2010 census data (U.S. Census Bureau, 2010a) suggested that this tipping point may occur as early as 2040, but now experts believe this date needs to be pushed back several more years. In 2011, non-White babies outnumbered non-Hispanic White babies for the first time (Livingston & Cohn, 2012).

Hispanic/Latinos and Asians remain the fastest growing minority groups. Hispanic/Latinos make up approximately 16.7 % of the U.S. population, and Asians account for 4.8% of the total U.S. population. Blacks, who compose about 12.3% of the population, have maintained a population increase rate of about 1% annually, while the proportion of Whites in the United States has increased very little in recent years (U.S. Census Bureau, 2010a).

In 1970, about 83% of the 203 million U.S. residents were non-Hispanic Whites and only 6% were either Hispanic/Latino or Asian. In 2010, the United States had 310 million residents, of which 66% were non-Hispanic White, 13% were Black, 16% were Hispanic/Latino, 4% were Asian, and 2% were identified as "other" (U.S. Census Bureau, 2010a).

Recent immigration patterns and policies show both continuity and change. Continuity is reflected in the arrival to the United States of an average of 104,000 foreigners per day. This group includes 3,100 persons who have received immigrant visas that allow them to settle and become naturalized citizens after 5 years, and 99,200 others who are made up of tourists and those with either business or student visas. On average, approximately 2,000 people enter the United States without authorization per day. More than half of these come from Mexico. The other half initially enter the country legally but then violate the terms of their visa by either going to work illegally or by failing to depart the country when their visa expires (Passel & Taylor, 2010). From 2005 to 2009, the number of people entering the United States illegally declined by nearly 67%, according to the Pew Hispanic Center, from 850,000 yearly average in the early 2000s to 300,000 (Passel & Taylor, 2010).

Immigration, legal and otherwise, affects not only the United States but also the country from which the immigrants come. Previously, Mexico was the primary source of immigration into the United States—both legal and illegal. Mexico accounted for approximately 18% of legal immigration admissions between 1993 and 2002. Net migration from Mexico to the United States, both legal and illegal, now stands at zero—or less. In other words, the number of migrants coming here from Mexico is equal to, or less than, the number of migrants leaving or being deported from the United States and returning to Mexico (Passel & Taylor, 2010).

Racial and ethnic minorities, especially those with low incomes and limited English proficiency, experience multiple barriers to health care, encounter lower access to and availability of health care, and experience less favorable health outcomes, according to the groundbreaking Institute of Medicine report (IOM, 2003) *Patient Safety: Achieving a New Standard of Care*. There is also evidence that stereotypes associated with sex, age, diagnosis, sexual orientation, socioeconomic status, obesity, and race/ethnicity influence providers' beliefs about and expectations of patients.

CULTURAL DIVERSITY DEFINED

The very nature of nursing encompasses the need to be aware of cultural diversity. The culture of the United States is made up of cultures from throughout the world. This complexity of cultural diversity within the healthcare system requires dedication and an ongoing commitment by the nurse to master—it cannot be achieved overnight, and in reality should be a career-long endeavor (Lowe & Archibald, 2009). The continuing and ongoing changes of the cultural makeup of patients within the U.S. healthcare delivery system result in a daily challenge for the nurse not only to recognize the diverse needs of each and every patient but also to incorporate patient needs into the quality nursing care that must be provided. The prevalence of cultural diversity requires the nurse to strive for cultural competence so he or she may meet society's expectations regarding nursing care delivery. The cultural makeup of the nursing workforce indicates that nursing does not have sufficient numbers of minority nurses. The minority nursing workforce totals only 16.8% of the total registered nurse (RN) workforce. The RN minority workforce is made up of 5.4% Black American, 3.6% Hispanic/Latino, 5.8% Asian/ Native Hawaiian, and 0.3% American Indian and Alaska Native. The remaining 1.7% identified as multiracial (National Sample Survey of Registered Nurses [NSSRN], 2008).

Healthcare disparities persist for the millions of Americans who are members of minority groups because they are not attaining patient outcomes that reflect the progress in medical technology and medical research. Just how different are minority patient outcomes? Members of ethnic minority groups (even those who are well educated and well insured and who possess adequate financial means) have shorter lifespans and die faster from every type of disease or illness—with the exception of suicide (Lowe & Archibald, 2009). To combat this phenomenon, it is therefore essential that every nurse is prepared to meet the unique healthcare needs for each and every culturally diverse patient who enters his or her care. The nurse must not lose site of the risk of falling prey to stereotyping. All patients must be individually assessed to see which (if any) cultural beliefs they possess that differ from the nurse's beliefs (Lowe & Archibald, 2009). The nurse must also avoid being ethnocentric. The avoidance of ethnocentrism means that you view yourself as being different rather than the "others" as being different, and you value each culture for its unique contributions to society and to the world at large.

CULTURAL FACTORS THAT AFFECT THE CLINICAL RELATIONSHIP

An awareness of a person's cultural frame of reference is essential. Cultural frame of reference is defined as those elements that cause a cultural group to interpret the world in a particular manner. This can also be described as the filter through which perceptions of, encounters with, and understandings of the outside world are ordered and made meaningful. Culture can be assessed according to four specific areas: cultural identity of the individual, cultural explanations of the individual, cultural factors regarding social environment, and lifestyle and cultural factors affecting relationships with others.

Unaddressed cultural differences between the nurse and the patient can result in difficulties with diagnosis, nonadherence, and mutual frustration when the patient or the nurse does not meet the implicit, culturally determined expectations of the other. There can, in some circumstances, be a benefit when there are cultural differences between nurse and patient. For example, some patients may report symptoms and more readily accept treatment from an empathetic nurse who is not of the same culture as the patient, because they may believe that confidentiality will be maintained and the stigma will be lessened (Rubio-Stipec, Hsiao-Rei Hicks, & Tsuang, 2000).

Nurses should be aware that in their assessments no one is culture-free. The encounter between the patient and the nurse is an interaction between two explanatory models of illness. This is true even when both are from the same cultural background because intracultural differences in how sickness and the healthcare system are viewed can be as great as any existing intercultural differences. To avoid any misunderstandings, the nurse must be aware of his or her own belief system and take care not to stereotype or make assumptions about the patient.

The physician's model, which is the Western Biomedical Model, is disease oriented, with the goal of determining the biologic or pathologic cause and executing a cure for that disease process. Nurses, by virtue of working in the healthcare system and following medical orders, often share this disease-oriented view. Many nurse practitioner programs educate using this model for diagnosis and treatment as well. Not only is the biomedical model in contrast to the illness model of the patient but also it is flawed because medicine is commonly viewed as a reductionist science. Medicine is considered to be objective and neutral, dealing only in the truth or facts. In reality, medicine is grounded in social and cultural behaviors. Therefore, the nurse, to be truly culturally sensitive, must be aware of assumptions about medical systems and recognize that other systems may be considered equally valid for patients. The patient's explanatory model will be illness oriented. This model is culturally determined and provides the meaning of the sickness for individuals: how they decide that they are ill, what they believe is the reason for the illness, how they cope, and when or if they decide they are no longer ill.

Although the patient's explanatory model is culturally determined, it may differ in the same individual with different illnesses or different stages of illness. Therefore, the nurse must determine the model for each illness episode for each patient. For instance, a patient may have a relatively biomedical approach to a sickness episode until the stress of end-of-life issues results in a reversion to original values and traditions.

It is also important to consider whether the explanatory framework is a physical or psychosocial one. Utilizing a physical explanatory framework (illness is a result of a disruption of a bodily or physiologic process) instead of a psychosocial explanatory framework (illness is a response to thoughts or emotions that are a result of social factors) results in a very different view of the illness itself. This can be problematic when the nurse's and patient's explanatory frameworks are different.

An attempt should be made to determine how culture-bound the patient may be for each illness, and again periodically throughout a prolonged illness. The nurse should ask for an explanation, as a part of the history of present illness, as to what the patient believes caused the illness, the expected course, and expectations of treatment. Determining the patient's explanatory model should be a routine part of taking a patient's history (Kleinman, 1988). See **Table 24-1** for questions the nurse can ask to determine the patient's explanatory model for illness.

If necessary, ask for clarifications of the patient's illness along the way. If you feel the explanation is unusual or unfamiliar, consider that it may have a cultural explanation rather than being indicative of or a result of a psychiatric disorder (e.g., the African patient who feels he may have a spell cast on him). It is also important not to automatically use culture as the sole explanation—striking a balance is the key. Culture can be a red herring, which means it can be overattributed as the cause or

TABLE 24-1	Questions the Nurse Can Ask to Determine a Patient's Explanatory Model of Illness

1. What do you call this illness? Does it have a name?
2. What do you think caused it?
3. Why did it happen at this time?
4. How does the illness affect you?
5. What does it do to you?
6. How bad is it?
7. How long do you think it will last?
8. Do you think treatment will work for it?
9. What kind of treatment do you think you should have?
10. Have you tried any other treatments already?

Source: Hanson, M., Russel, L., Robb, A., & Tabak, D. (1996). *Cross-cultural interviewing: A guide for teaching and evaluation*. Toronto, Ontario: University of Toronto.

reason for symptoms to be present. This can result in mistakes in diagnosis and treatment (Stein, 1985).

The questions associated with the patient's explanatory model of illness address the major issues of concern to the nurse and nurse practitioner: etiology, pathophysiologic alteration, usual or expected course, and treatment. Neither the medical nor the patient's model is sufficient alone. Both approaches are needed for the provision of culturally sensitive, patient-centered care. Once the nurse has a working knowledge of the patient's model, the nurse can determine whether treatments (such as herbal or alternative therapies) are previously or concurrently being used by the patient and whether they are beneficial, harmful, or neutral. If a treatment is determined to be beneficial or neutral, it is recommended to incorporate the patient's intervention into the plan of care. If an intervention is deemed harmful, it requires that the nurse develop a culturally competent

teaching plan and that the nurse ensures the patient is fully informed of the danger, or potential risk for danger, the intervention poses. The nurse's view of illness can be shared with the patient, and then a negotiation must take place to achieve a shared understanding of the illness so that a treatment plan can be put in place.

THE IMPORTANCE OF STRIVING FOR UNDERSTANDING

The progression toward cultural understanding, and ultimately to competency, is vital to be an effective nurse in the multicultural twenty-first century. The impact of global health work can only be as strong as its cultural relevance. As much as we would like to jump in and begin the encounter, there are many cultural nuances and ethnic differences that are not readily apparent. Success of the nursing interaction rests on the nurse's ability to work with patients within their cultural context. The successful nurse today must be able to function in cross-cultural patient encounters. Developing this ability begins with first having the willingness to learn as much as possible, maintaining cultural humility, and taking the time for self-reflection to evaluate your progress along the way.

The degree of family involvement in patient illness is also culturally driven. Many patients come from cultures in which the family and community involvement in the individual's illness episode is much more than occurs in other cultures, such as those from countries in Europe and North America. This has implications for how the nurse approaches important issues such as consent, patient confidentiality, and controversy over how to proceed with treatment and ethical dilemmas (e.g., do not resuscitate orders, transplantation, organ donation, assisted suicide). Obtaining information regarding the family structure is a good starting point: Who is the head of the family? Is this the same person who will be making the medical decisions? Is this the same person as the patient? Another important consideration is what community resources are available and, if the patient utilizes those services, whether confidentiality will be maintained (this may be more of an issue in small geographic areas or if limited resources or agencies are available). Other relevant questions include the patient's and medical decision maker's educational backgrounds, as well as the patient's health literacy level. It is important that these factors be assessed prior to planning any educational interventions.

LANGUAGE BARRIERS

The nurse needs to assess the patient's fluency in English if the patient is communicating without an interpreter and he or she speaks English as a second language. Do not automatically assume that a patient with a heavy accent is not fluent or that just because it appears a patient is fluent that he or she comprehends the conversation. The easiest and quickest way to assess comprehension is to ask the patient to repeat back an explanation or instruction.

Do not rely on nonverbal cues for comprehension, as many patients will nod or indicate agreement out of respect or embarrassment, even when they do not understand. Even the apparent proper use of language in seemingly fluent individuals can result in misunderstandings. In addition, violations in the rules of grammar may make a person seem vague and indecisive. The nurse should consciously avoid the use of idioms when speaking with patients and especially when providing patient education. The use of idiomatic expressions may baffle a person not well versed in English (e.g., quitting "cold turkey" when discussing smoking cessation).

Proper Use of Interpreters

Because it is essential that the nurse and patient be fully able to communicate effectively with each other, if it is determined that an interpreter is needed, request one. It is essential that all medical and cultural issues be fully explored, which cannot occur if there is a language barrier not bridged by the use of a qualified professional interpreter. If an interpreter is used, he or she becomes a critical component of the encounter. It is highly recommended to use only professional interpreters who are culturally competent in the patient's culture. This is so important that it is recommended that if the medical situation is not urgent, and it is safe to do so, it is preferable to postpone the interview until the services of a cultural or professional interpreter can be obtained. This is often very time consuming and frustrating, but it will be well worth the effort because of the quality of information that will be obtained. Often, because of time constraints or other variables, this may not be possible, and poor choices can be made.

The use of or reliance on family members to serve as translators should be avoided unless absolutely necessary. This is very important to emphasize because there can be serious negative consequences if family members are used as translators/interpreters. The family member or the patient may editorialize extensively, and the nurse would have no way of knowing this was occurring. Editing questions and responses greatly reduces the amount and accuracy of the information transmitted from and to the patient. Role strain can be another serious consequence resulting from this practice. Both editorializing and role strain can occur if a child is asked to translate sensitive issues regarding the child's parents (e.g., a male child translating for his mother who is having a gynecological issue such as extensive vaginal bleeding).

Access to a professional interpreter does not mean adequate communication is guaranteed. There are some skills associated with the effective use of interpreters that the nurse should be aware of. Ascertain the interpreter's qualifications. If a trained professional interpreter is available, this person probably needs no instructions or reminders about confidentiality or the process of triadic interviewing. A professional interpreter is capable of culturally interpreting the patient's meaning, which saves time. If there is no professional interpreter available and you must use a nonprofessional who speaks the same language, such as a hospital employee, you will need to spend time explaining the process in much more detail and emphasizing the interpreter's responsibility to maintain confidentiality and not to editorialize. Brief the interpreter by informing him or her about the situation and the need for interpreter services. Let the interpreter know how you wish to proceed. Just because the interpreter may work in the hospital does not mean this person is familiar with or comfortable dealing with a patient encounter, especially if it is an acute or urgent situation. Let the interpreter know that you expect and need him or her to translate exactly what is said by both parties. Assure the interpreter that you will use brief sentences to allow the interview to proceed more quickly and to increase accuracy. Let the interpreter know that you will be looking at and speaking to the patient and that you

will be seated in a triad during the interview process. Be alert for signs that all of the information is not being translated accurately (e.g., a long conversation in the patient's language, followed by a short translation to you, or vice versa).

CULTURAL HUMILITY

A nurse who possesses cultural humility recognizes the limitations of his or her cultural perspective and works toward overcoming this perspective in order to provide better nursing care to all patients. It is an acknowledgment that you are aware of the inherent barriers that exist from your own culture—that indeed your own perspective is limited. Having this focus makes it much easier for nurses to be reflective and proactive about any prejudices or assumptions they have so that these are less likely to have an impact on a cross-cultural nursing interaction. This is not the whole description, however. The nurse must also not assume that all members of a certain culture conform to a certain stereotype and must acknowledge that each patient is a unique individual and deserves to be treated as such.

The nurse who has cultural humility is less likely to act in an authoritarian way or assume a power position over the patient. Cultural humility is seen as an important step in redressing the power imbalance between provider and patient, because the nurse who recognizes that his or her own perspective is full of assumptions is more likely to maintain an open mind, be respectful of all people, and not act as if his or her way is the only or best way to proceed. Cultural humility should always be practiced, even if nurse believe they have worked and developed true cultural competency. This is necessary because even though nurses may have extensive knowledge of a culture, they are not "living" that culture, which means there will still be differences between nurses' perspectives and those of the actual members of the learned culture.

IMPACT OF DIVERSITY

The data presented here provide you with an overview of demographics from the 2010 U.S. census and from other government agencies (U.S. Census Bureau, 2010a). There is no doubt that the population of the United States is extremely diverse and becoming even more so with each passing year.

According to the U.S. Census Bureau estimates from 2011, the minority population now accounts for 36.9% of the total U.S. population. This means one in three U.S. residents is a minority (U.S. Census Bureau, 2010a). The nation's Black population is 12.8% of the total U.S. population, a 12.3% increase from the 2000 census data (U.S. Census Bureau, 2010a).

According to the 2012 estimate from the U.S. Census Bureau (2010a), the current population of the United States is 314,454,829. Of that number, 72.4% are considered White (non-Hispanic). Hispanic/Latinos make up 16.3% (a 43% increase from the 2000 census data) of the population, African Americans 12.8% (an increase of 12.3% from the 2000 census data), Asians 4.8% (an increase of 43.3%), American Indian and Alaska Native 0.9% (an increase of 18.4%), Native Hawaiian/Pacific Islander 0.2% (an increase of 35.4%), and 2.9% of our population was identified as belonging to two or more races (an increase of 32%) (U.S. Census Bureau, 2010a). Our country continues toward even more diversity, as demonstrated by significant increases in the numbers and proportion of minority populations.

Another key consideration in attempting to understand diversity is that in contemporary U.S. society, many individuals, probably the majority, are or consider themselves to be bicultural. Membership in more than one culture is not the same as being biracial or multiracial (McGrath, 1998). A person may self-identify with more than one cultural group, and that bicultural person sees both sides and can function in both worlds (McGrath, 1998).

There is a correlation among race, economic status, and poor health (**Boxes 24-1** and **24-2**): 12% of nonelderly (age 65 years or younger) Whites (non-Hispanics) are considered poor, as they fall below the federal poverty level, and 8% self-rated their health as fair or poor; 29% of nonelderly Hispanic/Latinos are considered poor and 13% have fair or poor health; 33% of nonelderly Black Americans are considered poor and 15% have fair or poor health; 17% of nonelderly Asians are considered poor and 9% have fair or poor health; 34% of nonelderly American Indians are considered poor and 17% have fair or poor health; and 21% of the nonelderly members of two or more races are considered poor and 13% have fair or poor health (U.S. Census Bureau, 2006). The federal poverty level was set by the government as income below $19,971 for a family of four.

Diversity also affects health insurance coverage (**Box 24-3** and **Box 24-4**). The racial group with the highest percentage of people lacking health insurance is the nonelderly American Indian/Alaska Native population at 32.9%.

| BOX 24-1 | Nonelderly Population by Race/Ethnicity as of 2005 |

White	African American	Hispanic	Asian	American Indian/ Alaska Native	Two or More Races
166.6 million	32.6 million	40.8 million	11.8 million	1.5 million	4.2 million

Source: U.S. Census Bureau. (2006). Income, poverty and health insurance coverage in the United States: 2005; current population reports. Retrieved from http://www.census.gov/prod/2006pubs/p60-231.pdf

BOX 24-2

Poverty Status of the Nonelderly Population by Race/Ethnicity as of 2005

White	African American	Hispanic	Asian	American Indian/Alaska Native	Two or More Races
74% Nonpoor	46% Nonpoor	42% Nonpoor	68% Nonpoor	43% Nonpoor	59% Nonpoor
(200% + FPL)	(200% + FPL)	(200% + FPL)	(200% + FPL)	(200% + FPL)	(200% + FPL)

Note: FPL = federal poverty level.

Source: U.S. Census Bureau. (2006). Income, poverty and health insurance coverage in the United States: 2005; current population reports. Retrieved from http://www.census.gov/prod/2006pubs/p60-231.pdf

BOX 24-3

Uninsured (Health Insurance) Percentage of the Nonelderly by Race/Ethnicity as of 2007

White	African American	Hispanic	Asian	American Indian/ Alaska Native	Two or More Races
14.3%	19.2%	32.1%	16.8%	32.9%	19.5%

Source: Institute of Medicine. (2009). *America's uninsured crisis: Consequences for health and health care*. Washington, DC: National Academies Press.

BOX 24-4

Percentage of Adults (Ages 18–64) Without a Usual Source of Health Care by Race/Ethnicity as of 2005

White	African American	Hispanic/ Latino	Asian	American Indian/ Alaska Native	Two or More Races
15%	18%	31%	19%	21%	18%

Source: U.S. Census Bureau. (2006). Income, poverty and health insurance coverage in the United States: 2005; current population reports. Retrieved from http://www.census.gov/prod/2006pubs/p60-231.pdf

Whites, at 14.3%, have the lowest percentage of people lacking health insurance coverage (Institute of Medicine, 2009). Lack of health insurance coverage is a significant barrier, and clearly this burden is felt more severely by minority patients. The Institute of Medicine (2004, p. 11) states in its report, *Insuring America's Health*, "health insurance contributes essentially to obtaining the kind and quality of health care that can express the equality and dignity of every person." Clearly, the lack of health insurance is an important barrier to the elimination of healthcare disparities.

Historically, our cultural diversity has identified, separated, bound, and evolved us. The implication is that some cultural features are not only different from others but also better. This is supported by the fact that all people have repeatedly chosen to abandon some feature of their own culture in order to replace it with something from another culture, because the replacement feature is deemed more effective. Some examples of this are the switch from Roman numerals (even in countries whose own cultures derived from Rome) to Arabic numerals and the fact that produce indigenous to one area of a country is now being produced and exported from a different country (most rice is now grown in Africa but originated in Asia). One should view cultural diversity both internationally and historically as a dynamic competition in which what serves humankind survives, and what does not disappears (Sowell, 1991). The will to survive is a common link as exemplified by the explorers that moved around the globe to explore "new" worlds and lands. Just as the colonists in America learned survival skills from Native Americans, the first Europeans who entered Australia with its rough terrain learned from the Australian aborigines. The goal was survival, and meeting that objective often required change and adaptation. A given culture may not be superior in all settings and at all times, but certain cultural features of that specific culture may be superior for certain purposes and at certain times.

Certain countries and civilizations have experienced different levels of cultural leadership over time (Sowell, 1991). There have been rises and falls of nations and empires throughout history: the Roman Empire, the Golden Age of Spain, the technology explosion in Japan, and the West of today. Certain cultural groups have been associated with certain skills or talents and occupations. Italians are known for wine production, Germans for beer making, and Jews in the apparel industry (Sowell, 1991). Geography has a role to play through not only the provision of or lack of natural resources but also the allowance or limits on opportunity for cultural interaction among different groups. The more isolated the geography, the more isolated the culture associated with that area. Access to water (either the sea at a port on the coastline or a river near or in a city) is another very important geographical determinant associated with sustaining life. Positive geographical features permit humans to interact with each other and with others, sharing their culture. Culture can exist in isolation as well. Culture dictates how we do all of the things that have to be done to live life where we are living it. Culture exists to serve the practical requirements of life: to structure society, to perpetuate life, to pass on hard-earned knowledge and skills, and to spare the next generation the trial and error of learning how to live life.

How much culture a person chooses to retain is a personal decision. Every culture makes changes over time—how much of the old to retain and how much of the new to embrace—and as such culture is dynamic.

CULTURALLY DISCORDANT CARE

Although this growing diversity has been seen and continues to widen within the American population, the same cannot be said for our country's population of healthcare professionals. This lack of a parallel growth in the diversity of healthcare professionals affects healthcare delivery and suggests that many patients are receiving culturally discordant medical care. Culturally discordant care arises from unaddressed cultural differences between healthcare providers and their patients. Research has shown that significant disparities in health status, treatment, and medical outcomes between groups of patients who differ on the basis of gender, race, or ethnicity exist. A provider's unconscious bias about a particular race, ethnicity, or culture or lack of effective cross-cultural communication skills may contribute to discordant medical care and health disparities. Racial discordance in medical encounters is prevalent and often inevitable as a result of the lack of diversity in the healthcare workforce in the United States. A relatively small percentage of minority patients are likely to have access to health professionals who are from the same race or ethnic group (only 23% of Black Americans, 26% of Hispanic/Latinos, and 39% of Asian Americans). This is a significantly lower percentage than the 82% of White patients who have a physician from the same racial or ethnic group (Collins et al., 2002). Although research supports the desire for patients to have a provider from their racial/ethnic group, the lack of workforce diversity makes this very difficult, if not impossible, for everyone except White patients. To compensate for the lack of diversity, all healthcare providers should know how to interact effectively with and provide care for patients whose ethnic or cultural background differs from their own to lessen the impact of culturally discordant care on health disparities.

HEALTH DISPARITIES

It is also important to recognize that perception can influence our understanding of health disparities. Two studies conducted by the Kaiser Family Foundation (2004) are revelatory when physician and patient perceptions are compared to each other (**Box 24-5**). There was no significant difference found between physicians and the public in the perception of how often they thought our healthcare system treats people unfairly based on whether a patient had insurance (72% doctors and 70% patients).

BOX 24-5   Physician Versus Public Perceptions of Disparities in Health Care

---

Question: Generally speaking, how often do you think our healthcare system treats people unfairly based on:

Percentage Stating Very/Somewhat Often

What their race or ethnic background is?

     29% physicians

     47% patients

Whether they are male or female?

     15% physicians

     27% patients

How well they speak English?

     43% physicians

     58% patients

Healthcare disparities refers to differences in access to or availability of facilities and services (National Library of Medicine, 2012). *Health status disparities* refers to the variation in rates of disease occurrence and disabilities among socioeconomic or geographically defined population groups and differences in the incidence, prevalence, mortality, and burden of diseases and other adverse health conditions that exist among specific population groups (National Library of Medicine, 2012). Despite scientific medical advances, the poor and non-White ethnic minorities are ranked lower in health status on numerous measures. The literature reveals that the reasons for the lower health status rankings are potentially many: genetic differences, gender differences, stereotyping, perceived discrimination, mistrust of the medical community, ineffective or poor communication, economic differences, clinical uncertainty by provider, biologic treatment variations, and lack of access. This problem is so significant that in 2010 the National Institutes of Health (NIH) transitioned the National Center on Minority Health and Health Disparities to the National Institute on Minority Health and Health Disparities, because an institute can have a more defined research agenda within the NIH than a center can.

IMPACT OF DIVERSITY ON DIAGNOSIS AND TREATMENT

At no time in the history of the United States has the health status of minority populations—Black Americans, Native Americans, Hispanic/Latinos, and some Asian subgroups—equaled or even approximated that of White Americans (Geiger, 2003). Despite the medical and scientific advances that occurred in the twentieth century, the excess morbidity and decreased life expectancy for people of color have persisted. In 1995, the overall Black American mortality rate was 60% higher than that of Whites—precisely what it had been in 1950. Black Americans today continue to die disproportionately from chronic disease (Geronimus, Bound, & Colen, 2011). Despite steady improvement in the overall health of Americans, racial and ethnic minorities, with few exceptions, experience higher rates of morbidity and mortality than do nonminorities. **Table 24-2** lists barriers to cross-cultural communication that can affect the advanced practice nurse's or the nurse's ability to properly diagnose and treat patients. **Table 24-3** provides strategies to improve cross-cultural communication that the nurse can utilize.

TABLE 24-2	Barriers to Cross-Cultural Communication That Can Impact Diagnosis and Treatment

1. Belief that cross-cultural communication entails learning the details of every existing cultural belief system.
2. Belief that such skills are impractical in that learning them is too time consuming.
3. Belief that the Western Biomedical Model is the only valid model of health care.
4. Physician/nurse lack of experience.

Source: Hanson, M., Russel, L., Robb, A., & Tabak, D. (1996). *Cross-cultural interviewing: A guide for teaching and evaluation.* Toronto, Ontario: University of Toronto.

TABLE 24-3	Strategies to Improve Cross-Cultural Communication

1. Do not rush through the encounter; take time to establish a human connection.

2. Use plain language whenever possible (avoid medical jargon and never assume the patient understands any medical terminology).

3. Use pictures (show them or draw them) to better illustrate the content.

4. Provide just enough information; do not overload the patient with too much information.

5. Use the "teach back" technique (in a nonthreatening way, have the patient repeat back what was discussed during the encounter).

6. Encourage questions through the provision of a comfortable and open environment.

Source: Data from Mandell, B. F. (2012). Talking to patients: Barriers to overcome. *Cleveland Clinic Journal of Medicine, 79*(2), 90; Misra-Hebert, A. D., & Isaccson, J. H. (2012). Overcoming health care disparities via better cross-cultural communication and health literacy. *Cleveland Clinic Journal of Medicine, 79*(2), 127–133; and Weiss, B. D. (2007). *Health literacy and patient safety: Help patients understand* (2nd ed.). Chicago, IL: American Medical Association Foundation and American Medical Association. Retrieved from http://psnet.ahrq.gov/resource.aspx?resourceID=5839

BARRIERS TO HEALTH CARE

In order for people to receive adequate health care, a number of potential barriers need to be addressed, including the "11 A's": availability, accessibility, affordability, appropriateness, accountability, adaptability, acceptability, awareness, attitudes, approachability, and alternative practices and additional services availability. Other barriers include fragmentation of care and cultural insensitivity of healthcare providers. Quality care is not possible if the provider lacks sensitivity to the patient's culture (Giger, 2013; Purnell, 2013; Saha, Komaromy, Koepsell, & Bindman, 1999). Effective patient care can be enhanced through awareness of one's own culture and how it may differ from other individuals' sociocultural experiences (Purnell, 2013). A healthcare provider who lacks awareness of cultural issues is culturally blind, and this type of provider requires the patient to accept the Western Biomedical Model of health, which may be in conflict with the patient's own views and beliefs. This type of narrow view, which is cultural blindness or cultural dogmatism, can lead to disaster, a tragic example of which is detailed in the book *The Spirit Catches You and You Fall Down*, by Fadiman (1997). The healthcare provider can overcome barriers and learn a lot by watching for varying interpretations of language, nonverbal interactions, and patient and provider responsibility.

Another barrier is the lack of understanding of the impact of cultural epidemiology. Cultural epidemiology is often not emphasized in health professions training, even though the epidemiology of diseases and individual interpretation varies among populations. This means that a commitment to continuing education must be a focus of the nurse, and the nurse must seek out learning opportunities to learn more about various cultures. It is important to remember that with the vast number of ethnic and cultural groups in the United States, it is impossible for anyone to gain knowledge of all of the groups. A more reasonable approach may be to use the culture general approach.

With the culture general approach, healthcare professionals develop the knowledge, skills, and approaches that may be effectively used with any group or individual who comes from a different cultural background (Taylor, 2005). This skill set includes acknowledgment of differences, advocacy for marginalized clients, and intolerance of inequity, bias, and stereotyping.

ETHNOPHARMACOLOGY

Ethnopharmacology is also an important consideration when attempting to provide culturally appropriate care. Ethnopharmacology (or ethnic pharmacology) is a field of study that investigates variant responses to drugs in ethnic and racial groups. Ethnopharmacologic research has revealed that ethnicity significantly affects response to some drugs. Genetic or cultural factors, or both, may influence a given drug's pharmacokinetics (absorption, metabolism, distribution, and elimination) and pharmacodynamics (mechanism of action and effects at the target site), as well as whether a patient will be adherent to the drug therapy and the necessary patient education that would be required for maximum benefit. As the nurse attempts to consider the impact of ethnopharmacology on a patient encounter, it leads to an important consideration—in a world of mixed heritages, how does a nurse or physician even determine a patient's race? Promoting certain drugs for race-specific markets could lead to stereotyping and discrimination. The issue is further complicated because some feel that racial categories are a societal construct and not a scientific one. In an attempt to overcome these factors, new drug research focuses on designing drugs to target certain genes, eliminating the need to weigh race or ethnicity.

REASONS FOR HEALTH DISPARITIES

The many reasons for health disparities are complex and require further investigation. This research initiative is being spearheaded by the National Institutes of Health. What has been discovered so far indicates that socioeconomic differences, differences in health-related risk factors, environmental factors, discrimination, and barriers such as access all play a role. An important concept for the nurse to understand is that the differences in health that certain populations experience are due to factors that are beyond the individual patient's control. Not only is it not the patient's fault but also the patient is often powerless to change the situation, because the root causes of health disparities are systemic, institutionalized, and have accumulated after many decades or even centuries. The relationships among the root causes of health disparities are multidirectional and cyclical, exacerbating one another and calling for intervention at every level. As nurses, we have a role to play in lessening the impact of health disparities through the delivery of culturally competent care. Keep in mind that Hispanics, Asian Americans, American Indians, Alaska Natives, and Black Americans are all less likely than are Whites to have health insurance, have more difficulty getting health care, and have fewer choices in where to receive that care. Hispanic and Black American patients are more likely to receive care in hospital emergency rooms and are less likely than Whites to have a primary care provider.

Perhaps most disturbing is that when adjustments have been made to correct access issues, disparity still persists. Even when equivalent access to care exists, racial and ethnic minorities experience a lower quality of health services and are less likely to receive even routine medical procedures than are White Americans. An example of this is that Black Americans and Hispanics are less likely than Whites to receive appropriate cardiac medication (thrombolytic therapy, aspirin, and beta-blockers) or to undergo coronary artery bypass surgery (Mickelson, Blum, & Geraci, 1997).

In summary, racial and ethnic minorities are less likely than Whites to possess health insurance, are more likely to be beneficiaries of publicly funded health insurance, and, even when insured, may face additional barriers to care because of other socioeconomic factors, such as high copayments, geographic factors such as the scarcity of healthcare providers in some minority communities, and insufficient transportation. Access-related factors pose a most significant barrier to equitable care, and access must be addressed systemically in order to have any chance of eliminating healthcare disparities.

GLOBAL HEALTHCARE DISPARITIES

Public health experts have identified a significant deficit of resources to deal with the diseases that have a global impact. This deficit is referred to as the 10/90 gap. This means only 10% of the world's health research budget is spent on diseases that affect 90% of the world's population (Resnik, 2004). The existence of global health disparities is such an apparent and pressing issue that the United Nations has set global mandates entitled the United Nations Millennium Development Goals (United Nations Development Programme, 2008). Poverty is an important component of global health disparities. The World Health Organization (WHO) estimates that diseases associated with poverty, such as tuberculosis, malaria, and HIV/AIDS, account for 45% of the disease burden in the poorest countries of the world (WHO, 2004). This does not need to be the case because many of these diseases are preventable or can be treated with medications that are already available. Vitamin A deficiency, a cause of blindness, can be eradicated through vitamin A supplementation. If there are solutions and treatments available, why does this global problem persist? It appears that lack of access is the culprit. Lack of access is an intractable political and economic problem. According to the World Health Organization (2004), an estimated 30% of the world population lacks regular access to existing drugs, with this figure rising to over 50% in the poorest parts of Africa and Asia.

Some of these patients are coming to the United States for treatment, which means nurses and other healthcare providers are being called on to care for patients from a widening and expanding range of cultural backgrounds. This explosion in diversity has resulted in an evolution in conceptualizing how nurses should function in global healthcare settings. The evolution has been from an initial awareness of or sensitivity to cultural differences, to striving for competence or being able to interact effectively with people from a different culture than one's own, to cultural humility. Cultural humility does not have an end point or the objective of mastery (which some experts claim is a lofty standard that few, if any, nurses will attain). Cultural humility places the emphasis on the evolution of the nurse in a continual, active process of self-reflection and self-critique (which is an activity that any nurse can participate in) and is seen as a way of engaging in the world and developing a therapeutic relationship with those who are culturally different from ourselves.

As members of the global healthcare community, all nurses must engage in an ongoing dialogue with themselves about the differences culture exerts on health outcomes, their own attitudes toward cultural differences, and their ability to objectively understand descriptions of cultural behaviors that are taken as explanatory. It is important that the descriptions they develop do not stereotype or constrain the different cultural groups that they work with and care for.

Nurses and nursing programs in the United States are expanding their focus to other healthcare systems. Nursing schools are offering cultural immersion experiences in various parts of the world, and more and more nurses and nursing faculty are having global nursing experiences. There will be more opportunities for collaboration, and learning more about our fellow nurses utilizing cultural humility may permit us to find common ground and a true appreciation for the diversity of our global partners.

GLOBAL DIVERSITY: THE ROLE OF NURSING

One would be mistaken to assume that health disparities are a problem confined to the United States. Differential treatment of minorities is not a uniquely American phenomenon. Nursing practice is a critical place to build diverse relationships for the purpose of globally providing optimal health for all. The National League for Nursing (NLN, 2011) has identified the role of nursing in global diversity as a critical priority. Our world is more open to migration than ever before. Despite our advancing technology and communication tools, there are still significant global healthcare needs and a worldwide shortage of nurses who are prepared to care for a racially and ethnically diverse patient population. The NLN is calling for nursing educational institutions to prepare an ethnically and racially diverse workforce, including faculty to mentor future nurses, and researchers to help to find solutions to the issues posed by our global diversity. What is known now is that the building of diverse relationships is key during times of a global nursing shortage. Nurses are challenged to view their patients from a variety of perspectives because of diverse global populations. Bridging the nurse–patient cultural gap can be a challenge. We must become aware of our differences to meet this challenge. Nurses are likely to feel helpless or powerless in effecting change when working with patients from another culture. Learning more about our differences may be helpful.

Disparities in health care continue to be a troubling issue for nursing, and despite attention being given to the issue, it is still a worldwide problem. Research and evidence-based nursing care are crucial to improving health care for all patients. Evidence-based nursing practice directed at how to effectively manage and treat diseases related to ethnic and racial minorities is imperative in overcoming current disparities in health care. In addition, more studies that listen to the voices of minority clients related to effective health interventions are needed to improve the quality of health care rendered to minority populations.

Cultural, ethnic, racial, language, and religious diversity exist in most nations in the world. One of the challenges to diverse democratic nation-states is to provide opportunities for different groups to maintain aspects of their community cultures while at the same time building a nation in which these groups are structurally included and to which they feel allegiance. A delicate balance of diversity and unity should be an essential goal of democratic nation-states and of teaching and learning in a democratic society. The challenge of balancing diversity and unity is intensifying as democratic nation-states such as the United States, Canada, Australia, the United Kingdom, and Japan become more diversified and as racial and ethnic groups within these nations try to attain cultural, political, and economic rights.

These nations share the democratic ideal of inclusion of diverse groups into the mainstream society, but they are also characterized by widespread inequality through racial, ethnic, and class stratification. The discrepancy between this democratic ideal and reality can result in protest. During the 1960s and 1970s in the United States, the civil rights movement resulted in major change. A similar civil rights movement continues to spread throughout the world.

Because of technology, we are no longer just citizens of our country of origin, but we are global citizens, and as such we need the knowledge, skills, and attitudes to function in this cultural community and to maintain our diversity and unity. We are becoming a multicultural global community.

Culture of Poverty

Poverty is a global phenomenon. The cycle of poverty perpetuates itself from generation to generation. Often, the motivation for immigration is the search for a better life or as a way out of poverty—to break the cycle. A child born into poverty is likely to have poor intellectual and physical development. Often, the child lives in substandard housing in either a densely populated or remotely located rural area where water or other resources are scarce, resulting in poor nutrition and health. All of these poverty-related conditions result in high morbidity, substance abuse, and increased incidence of accidents and injury caused by violence.

United States

According to the U.S. Census Bureau (2012) and international census data (2010), the United States is the third most populous country on Earth with a population of 312.8 million people. Despite this, the U.S. population composes only 4.5% of the total world's population. As a basis of comparison, China, with 1,339,724,852 inhabitants, makes up 58% of the world's total population. This relationship is not likely to change significantly in the future, because the world's population is continuing to grow at a rate of 1.1% annually.

The size of a country's total population tells only a small part of its demographic story. A country's population growth rate and its age–sex composition indicate the challenges it faces in providing health care for its children and elderly, providing education to its youth, providing employment opportunities for its young adults, and supporting its elderly population. According to 2010 census data, 21.2% of the U.S. population is younger than the age of 16 and 13% are 65 years old and older. Our country is benefitting from an increase in longevity for some populations, with 1.8% of our population now composed of people older than age 84 years. Females are now the slight majority, encompassing 50.8% of the U.S. population.

For the past 50 years, the United States (along with other more developed countries and moderately developed countries [MDCs], such as all of North America, Europe, Japan,

Australia, and New Zealand) has differed from other less developed countries in fertility, mortality, and overall growth. The United States and all MDCs have typically had lower fertility, mortality, and population growth rates. This is now less true than in the past and in the area of relative population growth is particularly alarming. From 1990 to 2000, the U.S. population increased by 13% (compared with only 2.5% for other MDCs combined). According to the most recent census data, the U.S. population continues to grow but at a slower rate than in the previous decade (1990–2000), with a 9.8% increase (U.S. Census Bureau, 2010b). Access to these population numbers is essential for planning public policy to address many global issues. The distribution of the world's children and elderly older than age 80 indicates where the needs for children and elderly healthcare services are greatest in the world, and it is also used to predict where the needs for schooling and elderly support will be greatest in the coming years.

The country's age structure, its support ratios, and its national wealth indicate the extent to which it will be likely to address all of these age-related needs. Alarmingly, 60% of the world's children younger than 5 years of age live in just 10 countries, of which the United States is one. Although people 24 years old or younger make up almost half of the world's population (with 1.2 billion between the ages of 10 and 19), their percentage of the population in some major developing countries is already at its peak, according to the Population Division of the United Nations Department of Economic and Social Affairs (2010a) in its *World Population Prospects: The 2010 Revision*. For example, in Mexico, reductions in fertility are already having a major impact. Mexico's population "pyramid" has been steadily shrinking at the bottom, with the birth-to-14-years age group down from 38.6% of the total national count in 1990 to 34.1% in 2000, and 29.3% in 2010 (Population Division, 2010b). The country's median age has consequently risen from 19 to 26 in two decades.

The 2012 U.S. Census Bureau predicts that by 2025, the U.S. population will grow by 13%. This statistic in itself is alarming enough, but when immigration numbers are factored in, the increase swells to 22%. Industrial nations as a group, including the United States, will be forced to support a growing elderly population with a smaller number of working adults. Despite this decrease in work support, the impact is expected to be less in the United States than elsewhere worldwide because fertility and immigration tend to replenish our younger populations.

As of May 31, 2012, the population of the world was 7,016,939,519 and 313,647,805 in the United States. See **Figure 24-1** for the top 10 countries of the world ranked by population as of 2008.

United Kingdom

As of July 1, 2010, the population of the United Kingdom was ranked at 22 with a population of 62,262,000. The life expectancy at birth was 80.1 years of age (World Bank, 2009). See **Figure 24-2** for population pyramids for all countries described in this chapter from the year 2008 and estimated for the year 2025.

The transition of uniting the former countries into what today is the United Kingdom was a gradual process. Even after being recognized as one nation, there still remained hostility and cultural barriers. There had to be a new set of rules and guiding principles put into play in order to keep all satisfied. These guiding principles, such as the division of property, capitalism, and parliamentary democracy, along with technological advancements, are now present not only in the United Kingdom but also around the world. See **Figure 24-3** for demographic information related to the United Kingdom.

Despite a high caloric diet and minimal exercise, the average life span in the United Kingdom is 80.1 years of age. Healthcare dollars are almost entirely derived from taxes. The National Health Service has been criticized for long waiting periods and obsolete equipment and praised for its high number of qualified physicians.

There have been published reports, since as early as 1981, that describe racism within the National Health Service in the United Kingdom. Language other than English and social class have been associated with impaired continuity of care (Hemingway, Saunders, & Parsons, 1997). Another study found that non-White patients are referred for coronary revascularization less often than are White patients with similar severity of disease (Hemingway et al., 2001). According to Nazroo (2003), mortality data are not kept by ethnic group in the United Kingdom. When evaluating data on immigrant mortality rates and morbidity, heterogeneity of experience across minority groups was found. For most outcomes, Bangladeshi and Pakistani people report the poorest health, followed by Caribbean people and then Indian people,

FIGURE 24-1 Top 10 countries of the world by population.

Rank	Country or Area	Population
1	China	1,355,692,576
2	India	1,236,344,631
3	United States	318,892,103
4	Indonesia	253,609,643
5	Brazil	202,656,788
6	Pakistan	196,174,380
7	Nigeria	177,155,754
8	Bangladesh	166,280,712
9	Russia	142,470,272
10	Japan	127,103,388

Source: U.S. Census Bureau. (2008). International data base. Retrieved from http://www .census.gov/population/international/data /countryrank/rank.php

with Chinese and White people having the best health (Nazroo, 2003). Obviously, diversity is having an impact on health outcomes in the United Kingdom as well.

Australia

The cultural competency movement is a global one, and it is making itself known in Australia. Australia is an extremely diverse nation.

FIGURE 24-2

Population pyramids showing statistics from 2008 and projections for 2025. (A) United Kingdom. (B) Australia. (C) Canada. (D) South Africa.

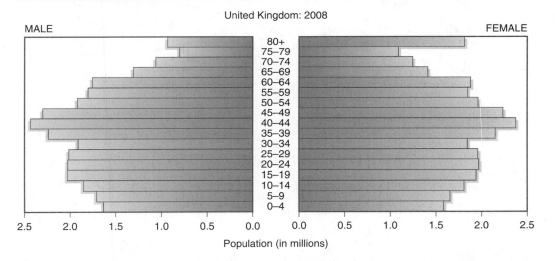

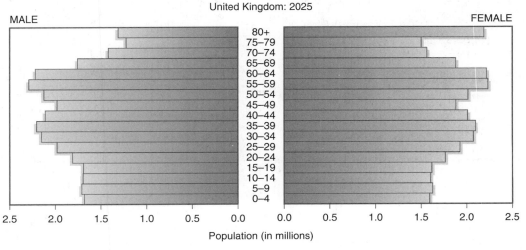

Source: Data from World Bank.

(continues)

FIGURE 24-2
Population pyramids showing statistics from 2008 and projections for 2025. (A) United Kingdom. (B) Australia. (C) Canada. (D) South Africa. *(continued)*

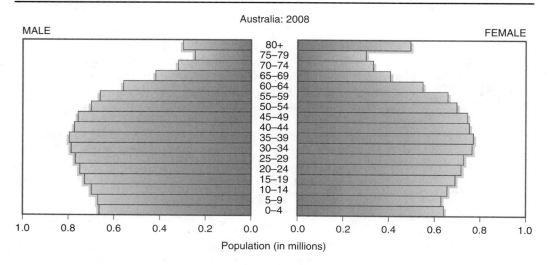

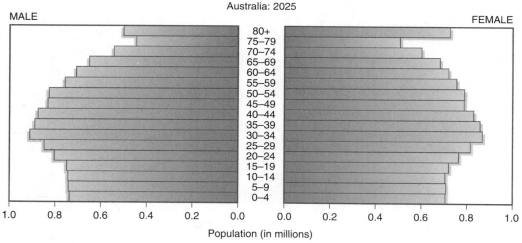

Source: Data from World Bank.

FIGURE 24-2

Population pyramids showing statistics from 2008 and projections for 2025. (A) United Kingdom. (B) Australia. (C) Canada. (D) South Africa.

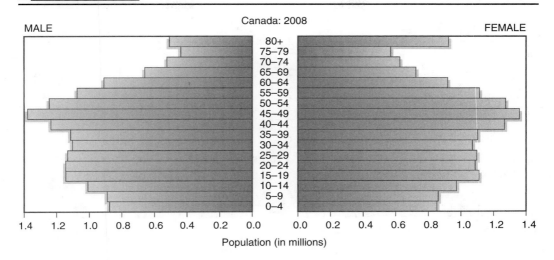

Canada: 2008

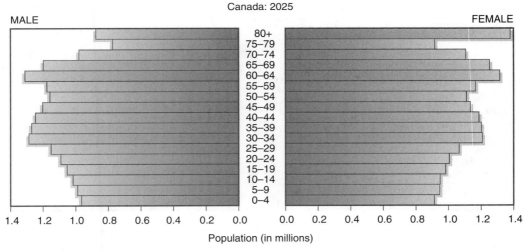

Canada: 2025

Source: Data from World Bank.

(continues)

FIGURE 24-2 Population pyramids showing statistics from 2008 and projections for 2025. (A) United Kingdom. (B) Australia. (C) Canada. (D) South Africa. *(continued)*

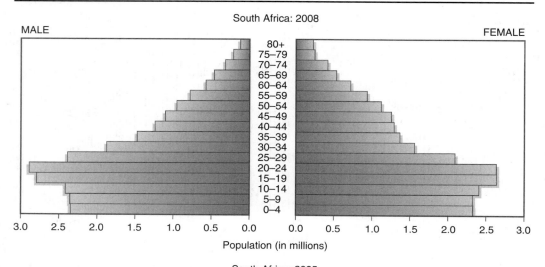

South Africa: 2008

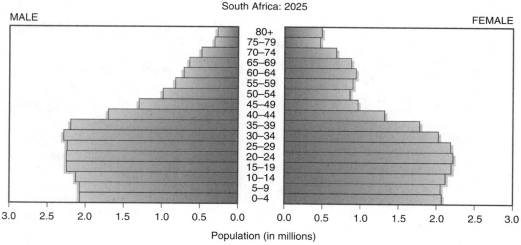

South Africa: 2025

Source: Data from World Bank.

The population of Australia as of June 2012 was 22,922,915 (Australian Bureau of Statistics, 2012). Australia's population comprises people with more than 200 different ancestries. Over 200 languages are spoken and over 100 religions are observed. Almost one-quarter of the population (22%) were born overseas and approximately 15% speak a language other than English at home (Australian Bureau of Statistics, 2012). In addition to this is the diversity within Australia's

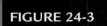

FIGURE 24-3 Breakdown of the demographics of the United Kingdom.

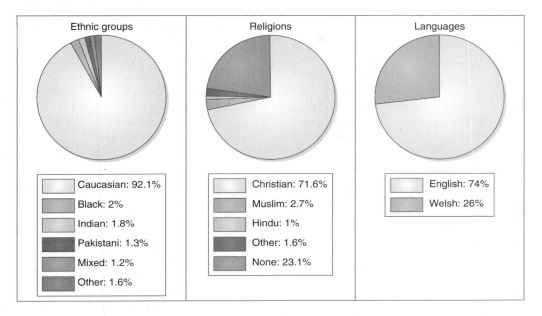

Ethnic groups

- Caucasian: 92.1%
- Black: 2%
- Indian: 1.8%
- Pakistani: 1.3%
- Mixed: 1.2%
- Other: 1.6%

Religions

- Christian: 71.6%
- Muslim: 2.7%
- Hindu: 1%
- Other: 1.6%
- None: 23.1%

Languages

- English: 74%
- Welsh: 26%

Source: United Kingdom demographics profile (2012). *CIA World Factbook.*

indigenous population who, at the last census, made up 2.4% of Australia's population (Australian Bureau of Statistics, 2012). Australia, like the United States, provides medical care according to the Western Biomedical Model. As has been discussed previously, for many client groups, this approach does not fit with their belief systems. When there is a mismatch between belief systems, health outcomes are likely to be poorer. The tendency of the health system (or more specifically medicine) to represent itself as a "culture of no culture" thus results in a culture-blind and ethnocentric approach. This effectively creates an exclusionary system that must be avoided.

An additional issue is the lack of health insurance among many Australians. According to the Australian Bureau of Statistics (2012), slightly more than half of the population aged

15 years and older had private health insurance (53%) in 2007–2008. Of those persons with private health insurance, 77% had both hospital and ancillary coverage, 15% had hospital coverage only, and 7% had ancillary coverage only. The level and type of coverage differed across age groups, with the highest overall coverage in the 45- to 54-year and 55- to 64-year age groups (59% and 62%, respectively) and the lowest in the 25- to 34-year and 75 years and older age groups (both 45% with some form of private health insurance coverage). There is some flicker of improvement, however, for the Aboriginal Australian population. Healthcare expenditures for Aboriginal people were 3.5% of the total health expenditures for the years 2008–2009, which was an increase of 0.4% from the previous 2 years. The Aboriginal people make up about

2.5% of Australians. Healthcare expenditures are higher for this population ($1.39 per capita) compared to expenditures for the non-Aboriginal Australian population ($1 spent per capita) (Australian Bureau of Statistics, 2012).

There is a growing body of work being produced to respond to Australasian contexts, some of it addressing the relationship between cultural respect and working with Aboriginal peoples. The health care of Aboriginal people in Australia has been criticized repeatedly during the past 20 years. It is well documented that the health status of Aboriginal and Torres Strait Islander people is substantially poorer than that of nonindigenous Australians. Disadvantages across a range of socioeconomic factors negatively affects the health of Aboriginal and Torres Strait Islander people.

Both morbidity and mortality rates are higher, and indigenous people are more likely to experience disability and reduced quality of life because of ill health. Life expectancy of indigenous Australians is estimated to be approximately 20 years lower than for other Australians (Australian Bureau of Statistics & Australian Institute of Health and Welfare, 2003). Discrimination and stereotyping impacting the allocation of healthcare resources has also been described recently and historically (Awofeso, 2011; Lowe, Kerridge, & Mitchell, 1995). Encouragingly, Awofeso (2011) advocates for improved cultural competency skills as an effective strategy to improve healthcare outcomes for the indigenous populations of Australia

Canada

In Canada, the population in general, and thus the service area for health care, is becoming more diverse. As of May 2011, the total population of Canada was 33,476,688 (Statistics Canada, 2011b). This is almost twice as many Canadians as there were in 1961. The average life span in Canada is 81.23 years. It has been estimated that one in eight Canadians is a member of a visible minority in a proportion

that grew by 25% between 1996 and 2001, while overall population growth was just 4%. The population of First Nations peoples increased 22.2%, and there are now 1 million First Nations people in Canada. According to 2006 Canadian census data, 3.75% of the population is Canadian Aboriginal, which includes First Nations, Metis, and Inuit (Statistics Canada, 2011a). Thus, the diversity of the country has grown rapidly and will continue to do so in the coming 50 years.

Canada has also been experiencing a tremendous growth in immigration, specifically of internationally trained professionals. These "new Canadians" are changing the culture of Canada. Canada has recognized the need for its nurses to become culturally competent, and the Registered Nurses' Association of Ontario has established nursing best practice guidelines on this important issue (Registered Nurses' Association of Ontario, 2007). The recommendation of this best practice guideline is that as Canada becomes more diverse, so must its healthcare system. Men and women from all cultures need to be recruited and welcomed into a profession that is committed to the care of others so they can learn from these diverse groups to create an environment that capitalizes on diversity and furthers the profession and the broader healthcare system (Registered Nurses' Association of Ontario, 2007).

Although Canada has a long-standing multicultural identity and a tradition of acceptance of diversity, reinforced, for example, by the federal government's 1971 Multiculturalism Policy, government intentions have not been sufficient to achieve equity and integration. Racism and cultural oppression have been realities for many minority groups living in Canada, especially the First Nations peoples, resulting in poverty, poor health, loss of identity, and marginalization.

Numerous problems with the differential treatment of the Inuit people of Canada have also been described. These problems have resulted in a call for cultural competency in

Canada to better meet the healthcare needs of the Inuit population.

South Africa

South Africa is characterized as a multicultural society and has great diversity in geography, language, and culture. The total population in South Africa in 2011 was 50.59 million (Statistics South Africa, 2011). The family structure in many families tends to be extended rather than nuclear and may also be multigenerational. There tends to be a fatalistic approach to disability that can result in passivity when seeking out treatment or rehabilitation. Traditional healers may form an integral part of a family's approach to health and illness. Technology and Western medical practices may be viewed as an intrusion on accepted and respected traditional activities and rituals. The community view within South Africa is that the group takes precedence over the individual, and time is only a two-dimensional phenomenon. The concept of time is one of having a long past, a present, and no future.

During the time of apartheid in South Africa, profound inequality existed in the availability and content of medical and public health services, which resulted in serious consequences for the majority non-White population (Nightingale et al., 1990). Despite the fall of apartheid, there is evidence that discrimination in treatment persists (Geiger, 2003). This painful part of South Africa's history has resulted in a push toward cultural competency within the country. The Truth and Reconciliation Commission of South Africa was established by former South African President Nelson Mandela; the commission's work has allowed the people of South Africa to openly discuss the pain and suffering caused by the intentional and enforced racial and cultural divisions within their country. The commission's activities have been credited with opening the doors to deeper cultural knowledge and positive change—key elements in the journey toward cultural competence.

RECOMMENDATIONS

It is necessary to increase recognition among all healthcare providers that racial bias persists and can be overt or covert. These biases continue to influence treatment decisions of minority patients. Quality assurance programs should be expanded to track patterns of patient care by race and ethnicity. The elephant in the room must be acknowledged, and nursing students need to be made aware that this bias is out there and that they need to advocate for their patients when treatment decisions are not evidence-based. Curriculum should be expanded, not just as has been done with cultural competency concepts but also including the importance of the nurse developing self-awareness and understanding the culture of medicine and how it may affect the patient experience.

For example, nurse practitioners are taught to present a case according to the medical model. This approach has traditionally included the patient's race in the clinical presentation. It has been argued that labeling a patient by race is necessary to clarify biologic risk for particular diseases, critical for differential diagnosis formation, that it provided information about socioeconomic status by proxy, and that the practice should be continued (South-Paul, 2001). Others feel that the placement of the patient's race should be moved from its traditional position in the initial patient description and placed with the other psychosocial patient data (Anderson, Moscou, Fulchon, & Neuspiel, 2001). On the surface, the placement of the patient's race in the clinical presentation may appear trivial, but small changes may ultimately result in effective change within the culture of medicine (Geiger, 2003).

SUMMARY

Diversity is a global phenomenon. As people who later become patients and as healthcare professionals immigrate into the United States, this global diversity will contribute to even greater diversity within the United States.

DISCUSSION QUESTIONS ──────────

1. Identify your own primary and secondary characteristics of culture.

2. How have these characteristics influenced you and your worldview?

3. Determine the racial and ethnic characteristics of the community where you practice or will practice nursing.

4. Define *race* and *ethnicity*. Differentiate the two terms.

5. Compare and contrast the healthcare delivery systems of the United States and the United Kingdom, Australia, Canada, and South Africa.

REFERENCES ──────────

Anderson, M. R., Moscou, S., Fulchon, C., & Neuspiel, D. R. (2001). The role of race in the clinical presentation. *Family Medicine, 33*(6), 430–434.

Australian Bureau of Statistics. (2012). Retrieved from http://www.abs.gov.au/

Australian Bureau of Statistics & Australian Institute of Health and Welfare. (2003). *The burden of disease and injury in Australia 2003.* Retrieved from http://www.aihw.gov.au/WorkArea/DownloadAsset .aspx?id=6442459747

Awofeso, N. (2011). Racism: A major impediment to optimal indigenous health and health care in Australia. *Australian Indigenous Health Bulletin, 11*(3). Retrieved from http://healthbulletin.org.au /articles/racism-a-major-impediment-to-optimal -indigenous-health-and-health-care-in-australia

Collins, K. S., Hughes, D. L., Doty, M. M., Ives, B. L., Edwards, J. N., & Tenney, K. (2002). *Diverse communities, common concerns: Assessing health care quality for minority Americans.* New York, NY: Commonwealth Fund.

Fadiman, A. (1997). *The spirit catches you and you fall down.* New York, NY: Farrar, Straus, and Giroux.

Geiger, H. J. (2003). Racial and ethnic disparities in diagnosis and treatment: A review of the evidence and a consideration of causes. In B. D. Smedley, A. Y. Stith, & A. R. Nelson (Eds.), *Unequal treatment: Confronting racial and ethnic disparities in health care* (pp. 417–454). Washington, DC: National Academies Press.

Geronimus, A. T., Bound, J., & Colen, C. G. (2011). Excess black mortality in the United States and in selected black and white high-poverty areas, 1980–2000. *American Journal of Public Health, 101*(4), 720–729.

Giger, J. N. (2013). *Transcultural nursing: Assessment and intervention* (6th ed.). Philadelphia, PA: Elsevier.

Hanson, M., Russell, L., Robb, A., & Tabak, D. (1996). *Cross-cultural interviewing: A guide for teaching and evaluation.* Toronto, Ontario: University of Toronto.

Hemingway, H., Crook, A. M., Feder, G., Banerjee, S., Dawson, J. R., Magee, P., ... Timmis, A. D. (2001). Underuse of coronary revascularization procedures in patients considered appropriate candidates for revascularization. *New England Journal of Medicine, 344*(9), 645–654.

Hemingway, H., Saunders, D., & Parsons, L. (1997). Social class, spoken language and pattern of care as determinants of continuity of care in maternity services in East London. *Journal of Public Health Medicine, 19*(2), 156–161.

Institute of Medicine. (2003). *Patient safety: Achieving a new standard of care.* Washington, DC: National Academies Press.

Institute of Medicine. (2004). *Insuring America's health: Principles and recommendations.* Washington, DC: National Academies Press.

Institute of Medicine. (2009). *America's uninsured crisis: Consequences for health and health care.* Washington, DC: National Academies Press.

Kaiser Family Foundation. (2004). National survey on consumers' experiences with patient safety and quality information. Retrieved from http: //kaiserfamilyfoundation.files.wordpress .com/2013/01/national-survey-on-consumers -experiences-with-patient-safety-and-quality -information-survey-toplines.pdf

Kleinman, A. (1988). *Rethinking psychiatry: From cultural category to personal experience.* New York, NY: Free Press.

Livingston, G., & Cohn, D. (2012). Pew Research: Social and demographic trends: U.S. birth-rate falls to a record low; decline is greatest among immigrants. Retrieved from http://www .pewsocialtrends.org/2012/11/29/u-s-birth-rate -falls-to-a-record-low-decline-is-greatest-among -immigrants

Lowe, J., & Archibald, C. (2009). Cultural diversity: The intention of nursing. *Nursing Forum, 44*(1), 11–18.

Lowe, M., Kerridge, I. H., & Mitchell, K. R. (1995). "These sorts of people don't do very well": Race and allocation of health care resources. *Journal of Medical Ethics, 21*(6), 356–360.

Mandell, B. F. (2012). Talking to patients: Barriers to overcome. *Cleveland Clinic Journal of Medicine, 79*(2), 90.

Martin, J., & Fogel, S. (2006). *Projecting the US population to 2050: Four immigration scenarios* (Federation for American Immigration Reform report). Retrieved from http://www.fairus.org/site/DocServer/pop_projections.pdf?docID5901

McGrath, B. B. (1998). Illness as a problem of meaning: Moving culture from the classroom to the clinic. *Advances in Nursing Science, 21*(2), 17–29.

Mickelson, J. K., Blum, C. M., & Geraci, J. M. (1997). Acute myocardial infarction: Clinical characteristics, outcome in metropolitan veterans. *Journal of the American College of Cardiology, 29*(5), 915–925. Retrieved from http://content.onlinejacc.org/article.aspx?articleid=1121666

Misra-Hebert, A. D., & Isaccson, J. H. (2012). Overcoming health care disparities via better cross-cultural communication and health literacy. *Cleveland Clinic Journal of Medicine, 79*(2), 127–133.

National Center on Minority Health and Health Disparities. (2002). *Strategic research plan and budget to reduce and ultimately eliminate health disparities: Volume II.* Retrieved from http://www.nimhd.nih.gov/documents/VolumeII.pdf

National League for Nursing. (2011). Global/diversity initiatives. Retrieved from http://www.nln.org/aboutnln/globaldiversity/index.htm

National Library of Medicine. (2012). Health disparities. Retrieved from http://www.nlm.nih.gov/hsrinfo/disparities.html

National Sample Survey of Registered Nurses. (2008). *The registered nurse population.* Retrieved from http://bhpr.hrsa.gov/healthworkforce/rnsurveys/rnsurveyfinal.pdf

Nazroo, J. Y. (2003). The structuring of ethnic inequalities in health: Economic position, racial discrimination, and racism. *American Journal of Public Health, 93*(2), 277–284.

Nightingale, E. O., Hannibal, K., Geiger, H. J., Hartmann, L., Lawrence, R., & Spurlock, J. (1990). Apartheid medicine: Health and human rights in South Africa. *Journal of the American Medical Association, 264*(16), 2097–2102.

Passel, J., Livingston, G., & Cohn, D. (2012). Explaining why minority births now outnumber white births. Retrieved from http://www.pewsocialtrends.org/2012/05/17/explaining-why-minority-births-now-outnumber-white-births/#more-12006

Passel, J., & Taylor, P. (2010). Unauthorized immigrants and their U.S.-born children. Retrieved from http://www.pewhispanic.org/2010/08/11/unauthorized-immigrants-and-their-us-born-children

Population Division of the United Nations Department of Economic and Social Affairs. (2010a). World population prospects: The 2010 revision. Retrieved from http://esa.un.org/wpp/

Population Division of the United Nations Department of Economic and Social Affairs. (2010b). World population prospects: The 2010 revision: Frequently asked questions. Retrieved from http://esa.un.org/wpp/other-information/faq.htm

Purnell, L. D. (Ed.). (2013). *Transcultural health care: A culturally competent approach* (4th ed.). Philadelphia, PA: F. A. Davis.

Registered Nurses' Association of Ontario. (2007). *Embracing cultural diversity in health care: Developing cultural competence.* Toronto, Canada: Author.

Resnik, D. B. (2004). The distribution of biomedical research resources and international justice. *Developing World Bioethics, 4*(1), 42–57.

Rubio-Stipec, M., Hsiao-Rei Hicks, M., & Tsuang, M. T. (2000). Cultural factors influencing the selection, use, and interpretation of psychiatric measures. In *Handbook of psychiatric measures* (pp. 33–41). Washington, DC: American Psychiatric Association.

Saha, S., Komaromy, M., Koepsell, T. D., & Bindman, A. B. (1999). Patient–physician racial concordance and the perceived quality and use of health care. *Archives of Internal Medicine, 159*(9), 997–1004.

South-Paul, J. E. (2001). Racism in the examining room: Myths, realities, and consequences. *Family Medicine, 33*(6), 473–475.

Sowell, T. (1991). A worldview of cultural diversity. *Society, 29*(1), 37–44.

Statistics Canada. (2011a). Canadian Census release topics, 2006. Retrieved from http://www12.statcan.ca/census-recensement/2006/rt-td/index-eng.cfm

Statistics Canada. (2011b). 2011 census. Retrieved from http://www12.statcan.gc.ca/census-recensement/index-eng.cfm

Statistics South Africa. (2011). *Mid-year population estimates 2011*. Retrieved from http://www.statssa.gov.za/publications/P0302/P03022011.pdf

Stein, H. F. (1985). The culture of the patient as a red herring in clinical decision making: A case study. *Medical Anthropology Quarterly, 17*(1), 2–5.

Taylor, R. (2005). Addressing barriers to cultural competence. *Journal for Nurses in Staff Development, 21*(4), 135–142.

United Nations Development Programme. (2008). *UNDP annual report: Capacity development: Empowering people and institutions*. Retrieved from http://www.undp.org/content/undp/en/home/librarypage/corporate/undp_in_action_2008.html

U.S. Census Bureau. (2006). Income, poverty and health insurance coverage in the United States: 2005; current population reports. Retrieved from http://www.census.gov/prod/2006pubs/p60-231.pdf

U.S. Census Bureau. (2008). International data base. Retrieved from http://www.census.gov/population/international/data/idb/sysmessage.php

U.S. Census Bureau. (2010a). 2010 Census data. Retrieved from http://www.census.gov/2010census/data

U.S. Census Bureau. (2010b). U.S. population clock. Retrieved from http://www.census.gov/population/www/popclockus.html

U.S. Census Bureau. (2012). Census and international census data. Retrieved from http://www.census.gov/population/international/data/idb/informationGateway.php

Weiss, B. D. (2007). *Health literacy and patient safety: Help patients understand* (2nd ed.). Chicago, IL: American Medical Association Foundation and American Medical Association. Retrieved from http://psnet.ahrq.gov/resource.aspx?resourceID=5839

World Bank. (2009). Life expectancy at birth, total (years). Retrieved from http://data.worldbank.org/indicator/SP.DYN.LE00.IN

World Health Organization. (2004). *Diseases of poverty and the 10/90 gap*. Retrieved from http://www.who.int/intellectualproperty/submissions/InternationalPolicyNetwork.pdf

CHAPTER 25

Health Services for Special Populations

Leiyu Shi and Douglas A. Singh

CHAPTER OBJECTIVES

1. Identify population groups facing greater challenges and barriers in accessing healthcare services.

2. Understand the racial and ethnic disparities in health status.

3. Explore the health concerns of America's children and the health services available to them.

4. Discuss the challenges faced in rural health and learn about measures taken to improve access to care.

5. Analyze the characteristics and health concerns of the homeless population.

6. Develop an understanding of the US mental health system.

7. Comprehend the AIDS epidemic in America, the population groups affected by it, and the services available to HIV/AIDS patients.

INTRODUCTION

Certain population groups in the United States face greater challenges than does the general population in accessing timely and needed health care services (Shortell et al. 1996). They are at greater risk of poor physical, psychological, and/or social health (Aday 1993). Various terms are used to describe these populations, such as "underserved populations," "medically underserved," "medically disadvantaged," "underprivileged," and "American under-classes." The causes of their vulnerability are largely attributable to unequal social, economic, health, and geographic conditions. These population groups consist of racial and ethnic minorities, uninsured children, women, those living in rural areas, those who are homeless, those who are mentally ill, those who are chronically ill and disabled, and those with human immunodeficiency virus (HIV)/ acquired immune deficiency syndrome (AIDS). These population groups are more vulnerable than is the general population and experience greater barriers in access to care, financing of care, and racial or cultural acceptance. After presenting a conceptual framework to study vulnerable populations, this chapter defines these population groups, describes their health needs, and summarizes the major challenges they face. The potential impact of the Affordable Care Act (ACA) on vulnerable populations will also be discussed.

FRAMEWORK TO STUDY VULNERABLE POPULATIONS

The vulnerability framework (see **Exhibit 25-1**) is an integrated approach to studying vulnerability (Shi and Stevens 2010). From a health perspective, *vulnerability* refers to the likelihood of experiencing poor health or illness. Poor health can be manifested physically, psychologically, and/or socially. Because poor health along one dimension is likely to be compounded by poor health along others, the health needs are greater for those with problems along multiple dimensions than for those with problems along a single dimension.

According to the framework, vulnerability is determined by a convergence of (1) predisposing, (2) enabling, and (3) need characteristics at both individual and ecological (contextual)

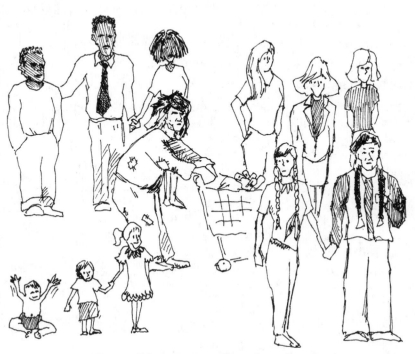

They all have something in common.

EXHIBIT 25-1   The Vulnerability Framework

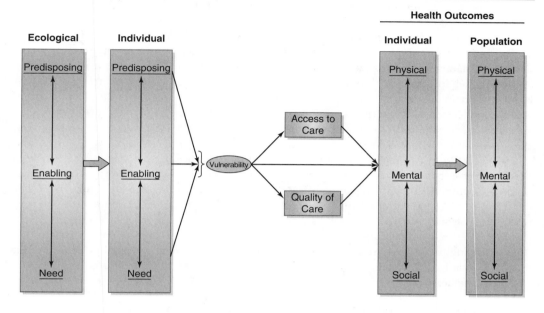

levels (see **Exhibit 25-2**). Not only do these predisposing, enabling, and need characteristics converge and determine individuals' access to health care but also they ultimately influence individuals' risk of contracting illness or, for those already sick, recovering from illness. Individuals with multiple risks (i.e., a combination of two or more vulnerability traits) typically experience worse access to care, care of lesser quality, and inferior health status than do those with fewer vulnerability traits.

Understanding vulnerability as a combination or convergence of disparate factors is preferred over studying individual factors

EXHIBIT 25-2   Predisposing, Enabling, and Need Characteristics of Vulnerability

Predisposing Characteristics

- Racial/ethnic characteristics
- Gender and age (women and children)
- Geographic location (rural health)

Enabling Characteristics

- Insurance status (uninsured)
- Homelessness

Need Characteristics

- Mental health
- Chronic illness/disability
- HIV/AIDS

separately because vulnerability, when defined as a convergence of risks, best captures reality. This approach not only reflects the co-occurrence of risk factors but underscores the belief that it is difficult to address disparities in one risk factor without addressing others.

This vulnerability model has a number of distinctive characteristics. First, it is a comprehensive model, including both individual and ecological attributes of risk. Second, this is a general model, focusing on the attributes of vulnerability for the total population rather than focusing on vulnerable traits of subpopulations. Although we recognize individual differences in exposure to risks, we also think there are common, crosscutting traits affecting all vulnerable populations. Third, a major distinction of our model is the emphasis on the convergence of vulnerability. The effects of experiencing multiple vulnerable traits may lead to cumulative vulnerability that is additive or even multiplicative.

RACIAL/ETHNIC MINORITIES

The 2010 census questionnaire lists 15 racial categories, as well as places to write in specific races not listed on the form (US Census Bureau 2009). These are White, Black, American Indian or Alaska Native, Asian Indian, Chinese, Filipino, Japanese, Korean, Vietnamese, Other Asian, Native Hawaii, Guamanian or Chamorro, Samoan, Other Pacific Islander, or some other race. Respondents can choose more than one race.

The US Census Bureau estimated that, in 2010, more than 36% of the US population was made up of minorities: Black or African Americans (12.3%), Hispanics or Latinos (16.3%), Asians (4.7%), Native Hawaiians and Other Pacific Islanders (0.2%), and American Indian and Alaska Natives (0.7%). In addition, 1.9% identified as two or more races (US Census Bureau 2010a).

Significant differences exist across the various racial/ethnic groups on health-related lifestyles and health status. For example, in 2010, the percentage of live births weighing less than 2,500 grams (low birth weight) was greatest among Blacks, followed by Asians or Pacific Islanders, American Indians or Native Americans, Whites, and Hispanics (**Figure 25-1**). Asians and Pacific Islanders were most likely to begin prenatal care during their first trimester, followed by Whites, Hispanics, Blacks, and American Indians or Alaska Natives (**Table 25-1**). Mothers of Asian and Pacific Islander origin are least likely to smoke cigarettes during pregnancy, followed by Hispanics, Blacks, Whites, and American Indians or Alaska Natives, who have a smoking rate more than double that of any other group (19.6%) (**Figure 25-2**). The White adult population is more likely to consume alcohol than other races (**Figure 25-3**). Among women 40 years of age and older, utilization of mammography is the highest among Whites and lowest among Hispanics (**Figure 25-4**).

Black Americans

Black Americans are more likely to be economically disadvantaged than Whites are. They also fall behind in health status, despite progress made during the past few decades. Blacks have shorter life expectancies than do Whites (**Figure 25-5**); higher age-adjusted death rates for a majority of leading causes of death (**Table 25-2**); higher age-adjusted maternal mortality rates (**Figure 25-6**); and higher infant, neonatal, and postneonatal mortality rates (**Table 25-3**). On self-reported measures of health status, Blacks are more likely to report fair or poor health status than Whites (**Figure 25-7**). In terms of behavioral risks, Black males are slightly more likely to smoke cigarettes than are White males (23.2% versus 21.4%), but White females are more likely to smoke than Black females are (17.7% versus 15.2%) (**Figure 25-8**), although smoking among Black females has increased. Conversely, Blacks have lower levels of serum cholesterol than do Whites (**Table 25-4**).

FIGURE 25-1 Percentage of US live births weighing less than 2,500 grams by mother's detailed race.

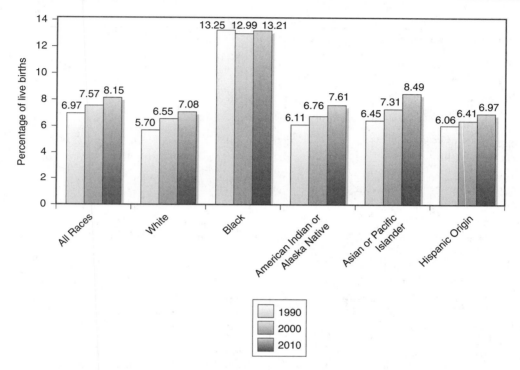

Source: Data from National Center for Health Statistics. 2013. *Health, United States, 2012.* Hyattsville, MD: Department of Health and Human Services, p. 56.

TABLE 25-1 Characteristics of US Mothers by Race/Ethnicity

Item	1970	1980	1990	2000	2010
Prenatal care began during 1st trimester					
All mothers	68.0	76.3	75.8	83.2	83.2
White	72.3	79.2	79.2	85.0	84.7
Black	44.2	62.4	60.6	74.3	76.0
American Indian or Alaska Native	38.2	55.8	57.9	69.3	69.5
Asian or Pacific Islander	—	73.7	75.1	84.0	84.8
Hispanic origin	—	60.2	60.2	74.4	77.3

(continues)

| TABLE 25-1 | Characteristics of US Mothers by Race/Ethnicity *(continued)* | | | | |

Item	1970	1980	1990	2000	2010
Education of mother 16 years or more					
All mothers	8.6	14.0	17.5	24.7	26.6*
White	9.6	15.5	19.3	26.3	27.9*
Black	2.8	6.2	7.2	11.7	13.4*
American Indian or Alaska Native	2.7	3.5	4.4	7.8	8.5*
Asian or Pacific Islander	—	30.8	31.0	42.8	47.1*
Hispanic origin	—	4.2	5.1	7.6	8.7*
Low birth weight (less than 2,500 grams)					
All mothers	7.93	6.84	6.97	7.57	8.15
White	6.85	5.72	5.70	6.55	7.08
Black	13.90	12.69	13.25	12.99	13.21
American Indian or Alaska Native	7.97	6.44	6.11	6.76	7.61
Asian or Pacific Islander	—	6.68	6.45	7.31	8.49
Hispanic origin (selected states)	—	6.12	6.06	6.41	6.97

Note: Numbers are percentages.

* Data from 2003.

Source: Data from National Center for Health Statistics. 2013. *Health, United States, 2012.* Hyattsville, MD: Department of Health and Human Services, p. 144; National Center for Health Statistics. 2010. *Health, United States, 2009.* Hyattsville, MD: Department of Health and Human Services, pp. 159, 163.

Hispanic Americans

The Hispanic segment of the US population is growing at a significantly higher rate than other population segments are. Between 2000 and 2010, the Hispanic segment increased by 43%, compared to the 10% increase in the total population (US Census Bureau 2011a, 2011b). In 2008, the Hispanic population numbered nearly 47 million, and it is projected to reach 57 million by the year 2015. Hispanic Americans are also one of the youngest groups. In 2009, the median age among Hispanic Americans was 27.4, compared to 41.2 years for non-Hispanic Whites; 11.3% were younger than age 5, compared to 5.5% of non-Hispanic Whites (US Census Bureau 2012). In 2011, 25.3% of Hispanic persons lived below the federal poverty level (FPL), compared to 9.8% of non-Hispanic White persons (US Census Bureau 2010b).

Many Hispanic Americans experience significant barriers in accessing medical care. This represents a greater problem for those from Central America (79% foreign born) and South America (75% foreign born) than those from Spain (17% foreign born) or Mexico (28% foreign born). Place of birth is also related to Hispanic people's inability to speak English, which is another factor associated with reduced access to medical services (Solis et al. 1990). Because of low education

FIGURE 25-2 Percentage of US mothers who smoked cigarettes during pregnancy according to mother's race.

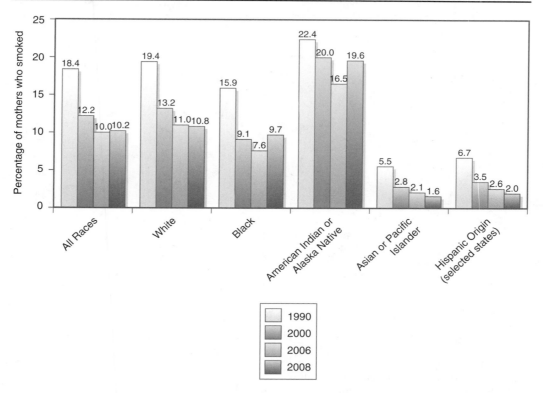

Source: Data from National Center for Health Statistics. 2012. *Health, United States, 2011.* Hyattsville, MD: Department of Health and Human Services, p. 84.

levels, Hispanic Americans have higher unemployment rates than do non-Hispanic Whites (11.5% versus 7.9% in 2011; US Bureau of Labor Statistics [BLS] 2012) and are more likely to be employed in semiskilled, non-professional occupations (US Census Bureau 2011a). Consequently, Hispanic Americans are more likely to be uninsured or underinsured than are non-Hispanic Whites. In 2007, 30.7% of Hispanic persons were uninsured compared to 12.8% of non-Hispanic Whites and 18.5% of non-Hispanic Blacks or African Americans (National Center for Health Statistics [NCHS]

2013). Among Hispanics, 33% of Mexican Americans were uninsured, followed by 28.1% of Cubans, 15.8% of Puerto Ricans, and 31.8% of other Hispanics (NCHS 2013).

Homicide was the seventh leading cause of death for Hispanic males in 2006. They have the highest ranking, along with Blacks, for this cause of death (NCHS 2013).

Hispanic Americans are less likely to take advantage of preventive care than are non-Hispanic Whites and certain other races. Hispanic women 40 years of age or older were least likely to use mammography (64.2% versus

| FIGURE 25-3 | Alcohol consumption by persons 18 years of age and older. |

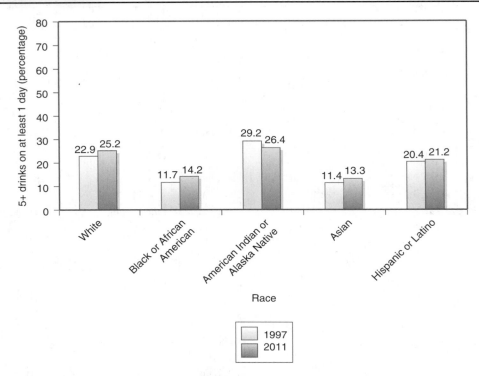

Race

1997
2011

Source: Data from National Center for Health Statistics. 2013. *Health, United States, 2012.* Hyattsville, MD: Department of Health and Human Services, p. 202.

67.8% for non-Hispanic Whites and 67.4% for non-Hispanic Blacks; see Figure 25-4). In 2010, fewer Hispanic mothers began their prenatal care during the first trimester than did mothers of other ethnic groups (77.3% for Hispanic mothers versus 84.7% for White mothers and 84.8% for Asian and Pacific Islander mothers; see Table 25-1). Among Hispanics 2 years of age and older in 2011, 57.2% had at least one dental visit during a year compared to 69% for non-Hispanic Whites (NCHS 2013).

People of Hispanic origin also experience greater behavioral risks than Whites and certain other racial/ethnic groups do. For example, among individuals 18 years of age or older

in 2011, a higher proportion of Hispanics drank five or more alcoholic drinks per day than did people of other ethnic origins (21.2% for Hispanics versus 14.2% for Blacks and 13.3% for Asians; see Figure 25-3). However, fewer Hispanics smoked compared to people from other ethnic groups. In 2011, 16.4% of Hispanic males 18 years of age and older identified themselves as "current smokers" compared to 27.9% of non-Hispanic White males and 18.6% of non-Hispanic Black males (NCHS 2013). Among female adults, 9.1% of Hispanics smoked in 2011 compared to 19.4% of non-Hispanic Whites and 17.3% of non-Hispanic Blacks (NCHS 2013).

| FIGURE 25-4 | Use of mammography by women 40 years of age and older, 2008. |

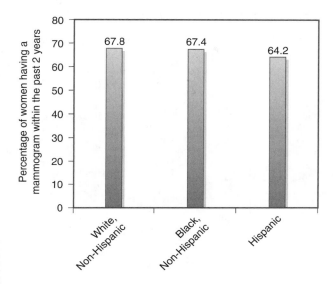

Source: Data from National Center for Health Statistics. 2013. *Health, United States, 2012.* Hyattsville, MD: Department of Health and Human Services, p. 256.

Asian Americans

Minority health epidemiology has typically focused on Blacks, Hispanics, and American Indians or Alaska Natives because Asian Americans (AAs) have relatively small numbers. In 2009, Asians accounted for only 4.5% of the US population and numbered 14 million (US Census Bureau 2012). To include the diversity of AAs, the National Center for Health Statistics (NCHS) has expanded the race codes into nine categories: White, Black, Native American, Chinese, Japanese, Hawaiian, Filipino, Other Asian/Pacific Islanders, and other races. But even the category of "Other Asian/Pacific Islander" is extremely heterogeneous, encompassing 21 subgroups with different health profiles.

AAs constitute one of the fastest growing population segments in the United States. The percentage of change in the Asian population

was 32% between 2000 and 2009, compared to 9% for the population as a whole (US Census Bureau 2012). The US Census Bureau (2010b) projects that the AA population will reach 16.5 million by 2015.

In education, income, and health, Asian Americans and Pacific Islanders (AA/PI) are very diverse. In 2010, 88.9% of AA/PIs 25 years of age or older had at least graduated from high school, compared with 87.6% of non-Hispanic Whites; in addition, the percentage of AA/PIs with a bachelor's degree or higher was 52.4% compared to 30.3% for non-Hispanic Whites (US Census Bureau 2012). Educational attainment varies greatly among the subgroups. For example, between 2007 and 2009, 94% of adults of Japanese descent had graduated from high school, whereas among Vietnamese it was 72% and only 61% among Hmong adults (US Census

FIGURE 25-5   US life expectancy at birth, 1970–2006.

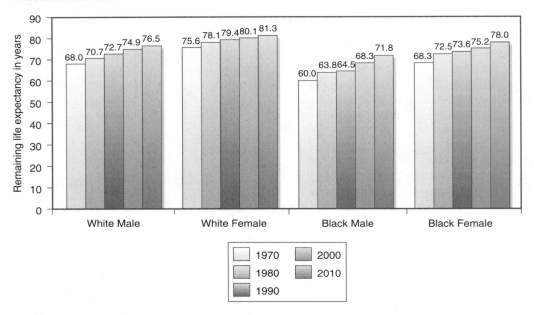

Source: Data from National Center for Health Statistics. 2013. *Health, United States, 2012.* Hyattsville, MD: Department of Health and Human Services, p. 76.

TABLE 25-2   Age-Adjusted Death Rates for Selected Causes of Death (1970–2010)

Race and Cause of Death	1970	1980	1990	2000	2010
All persons	**Deaths per 100,000 Standard Population**				
All causes	1,222.6	1,039.1	938.7	869.0	747.0
Diseases of the heart	492.7	412.1	321.8	257.6	179.1
Ischemic heart disease	—	345.2	249.6	186.8	113.6
Cerebrovascular diseases	147.7	96.2	65.3	60.9	39.1
Malignant neoplasms	198.6	207.9	216.0	199.6	172.8
Chronic lower respiratory diseases	21.3	28.3	37.2	44.2	42.2
Influenza and pneumonia	41.7	31.4	36.8	23.7	15.1
Chronic liver disease and cirrhosis	17.8	15.1	11.1	9.5	9.4

| TABLE 25-2 | Age-Adjusted Death Rates for Selected Causes of Death (1970–2010) |

Race and Cause of Death	1970	1980	1990	2000	2010
Diabetes mellitus	24.3	18.1	20.7	25.0	20.8
Human immunodeficiency virus (HIV) disease	—	—	10.2	5.2	2.6
Unintentional injuries	60.1	46.4	36.3	34.9	38.0
Motor vehicle–related injuries	27.6	22.3	18.5	15.4	11.3
Suicide	13.1	12.2	12.5	10.4	12.1
Homicide	8.8	10.4	9.4	5.9	5.3
White					
All causes	1,193.3	1,012.7	909.8	849.8	741.8
Diseases of the heart	492.2	409.4	317.0	253.4	176.9
Ischemic heart disease	—	347.6	249.7	185.6	113.5
Cerebrovascular diseases	143.5	93.2	62.8	58.8	37.7
Malignant neoplasms	196.7	204.2	211.6	197.2	172.4
Chronic lower respiratory diseases	21.8	29.3	38.3	46.0	44.6
Influenza and pneumonia	39.8	30.9	36.4	23.5	14.9
Chronic liver disease and cirrhosis	16.6	13.9	10.5	9.6	9.9
Diabetes mellitus	22.9	16.7	18.8	22.8	19.0
Human immunodeficiency virus (HIV) disease	—	—	8.3	2.8	1.4
Unintentional injuries	57.8	45.3	35.5	35.1	40.3
Motor vehicle–related injuries	27.1	22.6	18.5	15.6	11.7
Suicide	13.8	13.0	13.4	11.3	13.6
Homicide	4.7	6.7	5.5	3.6	3.3
Black					
All causes	1,518.1	1,314.8	1,250.3	1,121.4	898.2
Diseases of the heart	512.0	455.3	391.5	324.8	224.9
Ischemic heart disease	—	334.5	267.0	218.3	131.2
Cerebrovascular diseases	197.1	129.1	91.6	81.9	53.0
Malignant neoplasms	225.3	256.4	279.5	248.5	203.8
Chronic lower respiratory diseases	16.2	19.2	28.1	31.6	29.0
Influenza and pneumonia	57.2	34.4	39.4	25.6	16.8
Chronic liver disease and cirrhosis	28.1	25.0	16.5	9.4	6.7

(continues)

| | TABLE 25-2 | Age-Adjusted Death Rates for Selected Causes of Death (1970–2010) *(continued)* |

Race and Cause of Death	1970	1980	1990	2000	2010
Diabetes mellitus	38.8	32.7	40.5	49.5	38.7
Human immunodeficiency virus (HIV) disease	—	—	26.7	23.3	11.6
Unintentional injuries	78.3	57.6	43.8	37.7	31.3
Motor vehicle–related injuries	31.1	20.2	18.8	15.7	10.9
Suicide	6.2	6.5	7.1	5.5	5.2
Homicide	44.0	39.0	36.3	20.5	17.7

Source: Data from National Center for Health Statistics. 2013. *Health, United States, 2012.* Hyattsville, MD: Department of Health and Human Services, Table 20, pp. 80–83.

| | FIGURE 25-6 | Age-adjusted maternal mortality rates. |

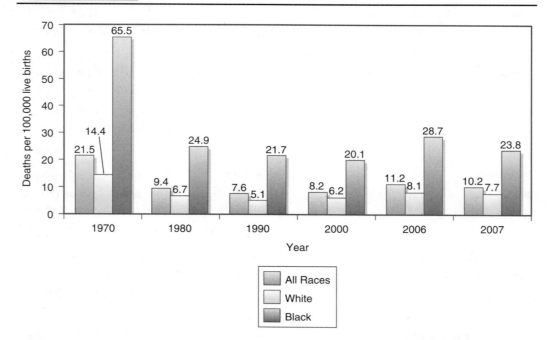

Source: Data from National Center for Health Statistics (NCHS). 2011. *Health, United States, 2010.* Hyattsville, MD: Department of Health and Human Services, p. 231.

TABLE 25-3	Infant, Neonatal, and Postneonatal Mortality Rates by Mother's Race (per 1,000 live births)											
Race of Mother	Infant Deaths				Neonatal Deaths				Postneonatal Deaths			
	1983	1990	2000	2008	1983	1990	2000	2008	1983	1990	2000	2008
All mothers	10.9	8.9	6.9	6.6	7.1	5.7	4.6	4.3	3.8	3.2	2.3	2.3
White	9.3	7.3	5.7	5.6	6.1	4.6	3.8	3.6	3.2	2.7	1.9	2.0
Black	19.2	16.9	13.5	12.4	12.5	11.1	9.1	8.1	6.7	5.9	4.3	4.3
American Indian or Alaska Native	15.2	13.1	8.3	8.4	7.5	6.1	4.4	4.2	7.7	7.0	3.9	4.2
Asian or Pacific Islander	8.3	6.6	4.9	4.5	5.2	3.9	3.4	3.1	3.1	2.7	1.4	1.4
Hispanic origin(selected states)	9.5	7.5	5.6	5.6	6.2	4.8	3.8	3.9	3.3	2.9	1.8	1.8

Source: Data from National Center for Health Statistics. 2013. *Health, United States, 2012.* Hyattsville, MD: Department of Health and Human Services, p. 66.

Bureau 2010a). In 2007, the median income for Asian males (aged 15 years and older) was $37,193, compared to $35,141 for non-Hispanic White males (US Census Bureau 2010a). In addition, in 2010, a smaller percentage of Asians (12.1%) lived below the FPL, compared to Blacks (27.4%), and Hispanics (26.6%; US Census Bureau 2011c). One study found that Chinese, Asian Indian, Filipino, and other AA/PI children were more likely to be without contact with a health professional compared to non-Hispanic White children. Citizenship/nativity status, maternal education attainment, and poverty status were all significant independent risk factors for health care access and utilization (Yu et al. 2004). In addition, cultural practices and attitudes may prevent AA/PI women from receiving adequate preventive care, such as Pap smears and breast cancer screening. Overall, the AA/PI population reported lower Pap smear test utilization, with a median rate of 74.4% over the course of 3 years, compared to Blacks (85%),

American Indians (83.5%) and Hispanics (83.1%; Centers for Disease Control and Prevention [CDC] 2010c).

The heterogeneity of the AA/PI population is reflected in the various indicators of health status. For instance, people of Vietnamese descent are more than twice as likely to assess their own health status as fair or poor, compared to people of Korean, Chinese, Filipino, Asian Indian, and Japanese descent (NCHS 2013). The incidence of overweight and obesity varies greatly, from 47.1% among Filipinos to 24.4% among Vietnamese. Although, in the US population, overall smoking rates are the lowest among AA/PIs, 22% of Koreans are current smokers, a rate higher than that of Black (21%) and Hispanic adults (15%). Compared with Whites, Asian Indians are more than twice as likely to have diabetes (NCHS 2013). Unawareness of this heterogeneity sometimes contributes to the myth of a minority population that is both healthy and economically successful.

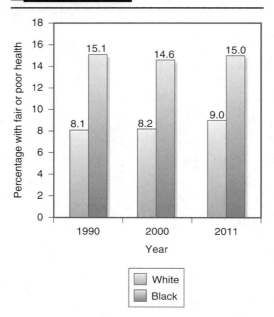

FIGURE 25-7 Respondent-assessed health status.

Source: Data from National Center for Health Statistics (NCHS). 1996. *Health, United States, 1995.* Hyattsville, MD: Department of Health and Human Services, p. 172; National Center for Health Statistics. 2013. *Health, United States, 2012.* Hyattsville, MD: Department of Health and Human Services, p. 168.

American Indians and Alaska Natives

More than three-quarters of the American Indian and Alaska Native (AIAN) population resides in rural and urban areas outside of reservations or off-reservation trust lands (US Census Bureau 2011d). According to the Census Bureau, the AIAN population is growing at a rate of 26.7% per year (US Census Bureau 2011d). Concomitantly, demand for expanded health care has been on the rise for several decades and is becoming more acute. The incidence and prevalence of certain diseases and conditions, such as diabetes, hypertension, infant mortality and

morbidity, chemical dependency, and AIDS- and HIV-related morbidity, are all high enough to be matters of prime concern. Compared to the general US population, Native Americans also have much higher death rates from alcoholism, tuberculosis, diabetes, injuries, suicide, and homicide (Indian Health Service [IHS] 2010a).

It is also no secret that Native Americans continue to occupy the bottom of the socioeconomic strata. AIANs are approximately twice as likely to be poor and unemployed (US Census Bureau 2011d). The health status of American Indians appears to be improving. For example, the mortality rate among Native American expectant mothers dropped from 28.5 per 100,000 live births in 1972–1974 to 11.1 per 100,000 live births by 2002–2004; infant mortality declined from 25 per 1,000 births to 6.9 per 1,000 births (IHS 2009). Still, Native Americans experience significant health disparities compared to the general US population. The life expectancy of Native Americans is 4.6 years fewer than the US population as a whole (IHS 2010a). Native Americans die at higher rates than other Americans from alcohol (519% higher), tuberculosis (500% higher), diabetes (195% higher), unintentional injuries (149% higher), homicide (92% higher), and suicide (72% higher; IHS 2010a).

The provision of health services to American Indians by the federal government was first negotiated in 1832, as partial compensation for land cessions. Subsequent laws have expanded the scope of services and allowed American Indians greater autonomy in planning, developing, and administering their own health care programs. These laws explicitly permit the practice of traditional as well as Western medicine.

Indian Health Care Improvement Act

The Indian Health Care Improvement Act of 1976, and later amendments in 1980, outlined a 7-year effort to help bring American Indian health to a level of parity with the general population. Although health parity still remains unachieved, the act has at least been successful

FIGURE 25-8

Current cigarette smoking by persons 18 years of age and older, age adjusted, 2011.

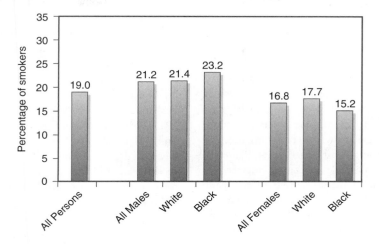

Source: Data from National Center for Health Statistics (NCHS). 2013. *Health, United States, 2012.* Hyattsville, MD: Department of Health and Human Services, p. 182.

TABLE 25-4

Selected Health Risks Among Persons 20 Years and Older, 2007–2010

Sex and Race*	Percentage of Persons 20 Years of Age and Older with Hypertension	Mean Serum Cholesterol Level (mg/dl) of Persons 20 Years of Age and Older	Percentage of Overweight Persons 20 Years of Age and Older
Both sexes	30.6	196	68.5
White			
Male	31.1	193	73.6
Female	28.1	199	60.3
Black			
Male	40.5	191	70.0
Female	44.3	192	80.0

* 20–74 years, age adjusted.

Source: Data from National Center for Health Statistics. 2013. *Health, United States, 2012.* Hyattsville, MD: Department of Health and Human Services, pp. 207, 211, 221.

in minimizing prejudice, building trust, and putting responsibility back into the hands of American Indians.

Indian Health Service

The goal of the Indian Health Service is to ensure that comprehensive and culturally acceptable health services are available to AIANs (IHS 2013). The IHS serves the members and descendants of more than 560 federally recognized AIAN tribes (IHS 2010b). However, the health care needs of a rapidly expanding American Indian population have grown faster than medical care resources, and most American Indian communities continue to be medically underserved.

IHS is divided into 12 area offices, each responsible for program operations in a particular geographic area. Each area office is composed of branches dealing with various administrative and health-related services. Delivery of health services is the responsibility of 161 tribally managed service units operating at the local level (IHS 2010b). The IHS mandate has been made particularly difficult because the locations of Indian reservation communities are among the least geographically accessible (Burks 1992).

Besides rendering primary and preventive care, special initiatives focus on areas such as injury control, alcoholism, diabetes, mental health, maternal and child health, Indian youth and children, elder care, and HIV/AIDS (IHS 1999a). Additional areas of focus include domestic violence and child abuse, oral health, and sanitation (IHS 1999b). However, despite limitations in the IHS's scope of service, many American Indians do not avail themselves of the system's services.

THE UNINSURED

Although uninsurance among adults has increased, lack of health insurance coverage among children declined from 13.2% in 2009 to 6.5% in 2011 (CDC 2011a), mainly because of the success of the CHIP program.

Ethnic minorities are more likely than Whites to lack health insurance. The US Census Bureau (2011e) estimated that, in 2011, 30.1%

of Hispanic residents were uninsured, compared with 17.8% of Blacks, 16.2% of AAs, and 14.9% of Whites. Most of the uninsured population is composed of young workers (O'Neill and O'Neill 2009). Lack of coverage is also more prevalent in the South and the West of the United States and among individuals who lack a college degree. Generally, the uninsured are in poorer health than the general population (CDC 2010a). Studies have also shown that the uninsured use fewer health services than the insured (CDC 2010a). In 2011, 53% of uninsured people reported having no regular source of health care (Kaiser 2012a). Decreased utilization of lower cost preventive services can ultimately result in an increased need for more expensive emergency health care. Even when the uninsured can access health care, they often have serious problems paying medical bills. In 2011, 30% of uninsured people postponed seeking medical care because of cost compared to 12% of those with public insurance and 7% of privately insured people (Kaiser 2012b).

The plight of the uninsured affects those who have insurance. Medical expenditures for uncompensated care to the uninsured were estimated to be $57 billion in 2008 (Kaiser 2012b). Much of this cost was absorbed by Medicaid, federal grants to nonprofit hospitals, and charitable organizations.

Without the Affordable Care Act (ACA), the number of uninsured would be 56 million (Congressional Budget Office 2012). Yet, it is estimated that between 29.8 million and 31 million will remain uninsured after the ACA goes into effect (Nardin et al. 2013). Hence, the problem of the uninsured will continue to haunt the US health care system.

CHILDREN

In 2011, 38.2% of children under the age of 18 were covered under Medicaid and 53.7% under private insurance (NCHS 2013). Vaccinations of children for selected diseases differ by race, poverty status, and area of residence (**Table 25-5**). White children have greater vaccination rates for diphtheria-tetanus-pertussis (DTP), polio,

TABLE 25-5 Vaccinations of Children 19–35 Months of Age for Selected Diseases According to Race, Poverty Status, and Residence in a Metropolitan Statistical Area (MSA), 2011 (%)

Vaccination	Total	Race White	Race Black	Poverty Status Below Poverty	Poverty Status At or Above Poverty	Inside MSA Central City	Inside MSA Remaining Areas
DTP[1]	85	85	81	81	87	86	84
Polio[2]	94	94	94	94	94	94	93
Measles containing (MMR)[3]	92	91	91	91	92	92	91
HIB[4]	80	81	75	82	76	81	80
Combined series[5]	69	69	64	64	72	70	68

[1] Diphtheria-tetanus-pertussis, four doses or more.

[2] Three doses or more.

[3] Respondents were asked about measles-containing or MMR (measles-mumps-rubella) vaccines.

[4] Haemophilus B, three doses or more.

[5] The combined series consists of four doses of DTP vaccine, three doses of polio vaccine, and one dose of measles-containing vaccine (4 : 3 : 1 : 3 : 3 : 1).

Source: Data from National Center for Health Statistics (NCHS). 2013. *Health, United States, 2012.* Hyattsville, MD: Department of Health and Human Services, p. 247.

measles, *Haemophilus influenzae* serotype b (Hib), and combined series than do Blacks. Children who come from families with incomes below the FPL, or who live in central city areas, have lower vaccination rates than other children do.

When children have inadequate access to health care, their ability to learn is compromised. Some children stay home and miss school for long periods when they do not receive needed medical care. Some sick children go to school because of unavailability of child care or inability of working parents to get leave. Once in school, children may also expose other children to contagious illnesses (Wenzel 1996).

In 2013, the United Nations (UN) published *The State of the World's Children*, which focuses on how the health of children with disabilities is affected by social and environmental barriers. This report suggests that greater social inclusiveness will lead to profound and positive impacts on children's health, well-being, and development (UN 2013).

Children's health has certain unique aspects in the delivery of health care. Among these are children's developmental vulnerability, dependency, and differential patterns of morbidity and mortality. *Developmental vulnerability* refers to the rapid and cumulative physical and emotional changes that characterize childhood and the potential impact that illness, injury, or disruptive family and social circumstances can have on a child's life-course trajectory. *Dependency* refers to children's special circumstances that require adults—parents, school officials, caregivers, and sometimes neighbors—to recognize and respond to their health needs, seek health care services on their behalf, authorize treatment, and comply with recommended treatment regimens. These dependency relationships can be complex, change over time, and affect utilization of health services by children.

Children increasingly are affected by a broad and complex array of conditions, collectively referred to as "new morbidities." *New morbidities* include drug and alcohol abuse, family and neighborhood violence, emotional disorders, and learning problems from which older generations do not suffer. These dysfunctions originate in complex family or socioeconomic conditions rather than exclusively biological causes. Hence, they cannot be adequately addressed by traditional medical services alone. Instead, these conditions require comprehensive services that include multidisciplinary assessment, treatment, and rehabilitation, as well as community-based prevention strategies.

Although serious chronic medical conditions that lead to disability are less prevalent among children, by conservative estimates, at least 3 million children 18 years of age and under are disabled, and 1 million children in the United States have a severe chronic illness. Medical problems in children are usually related to birth or congenital conditions rather than degenerative conditions that affect adults. These differences call for an approach to the delivery of health care that is uniquely designed to address the needs of children.

Oral health among children is particularly affected by socioeconomic and demographic factors. Among Hispanic children only 46.7% are reported to have teeth in excellent or very good condition by their parents/guardians, compared to 76.4% for White children (Health Resources and Service Administration [HRSA] Maternal and Child Health Bureau 2005). There is a clear relationship between family income and child oral health. At less than 100% FPL, less than half of children have teeth in excellent or very good condition, compared to 82.8% of children at 400% FPL or greater (HRSA Maternal and Child Health Bureau 2005). In addition to tooth loss, poor oral health in children can result in missed school (Gift et al. 1992), increased emergency department visits (Sheller et al. 1997), and decreased productivity and quality of life in the long term (General Accounting Office 2000).

Children and the US Health Care System

The various programs that serve children have distinct eligibility, administrative, and funding criteria that can present barriers to access. The patchwork of disconnected programs also makes it difficult to obtain health care in an integrated and coordinated fashion. These programs can be categorized into three broad sectors: the personal medical and preventive services sector, the population-based community health services sector, and the health-related support services sector.

Personal medical and preventive health services include primary and specialty medical services, which are delivered in private and public medical offices, health centers, and hospitals. Personal medical services are principally funded by private health insurance, Medicaid, and out-of-pocket payments.

The population-based community health services include community-wide health promotion and disease prevention services. Examples are immunization delivery and monitoring programs, lead screening and abatement programs, and child abuse and neglect prevention. Other health services include special child abuse treatment programs and rehabilitative services for children with complex congenital conditions or other chronic and debilitating diseases. Community-based programs also provide assurance and coordination functions, such as case management and referral programs, for children with chronic diseases and early interventions and monitoring for infants at risk for developmental disabilities. Funding for this sector comes from federal programs, such as Medicaid's Early Periodic Screening, Diagnosis, and Treatment (EPSDT) program; Title V (Maternal and Child Health) of the Social Security Act; and other categorical programs.

The health-related support services sector includes such services as nutrition education, early intervention, rehabilitation, and family support programs. An example of a rehabilitation service is education and psychotherapy for children with HIV. Family support services include parent education and skill building in families with infants at risk for developmental delay because of physiological or social conditions, such as low birth weight or very low income. Funding for these services comes from diverse agencies, such as the Department of Agriculture, which funds the Supplemental Food Program for Women, Infants, and Children (WIC), and the Department of Education, which funds the Individuals with Disabilities Education Act (IDEA).

WOMEN

Women are playing an increasingly important role in the delivery of health care. Not only do women remain the leading providers of care in the nursing profession but also they are well represented in various other health professions, including allopathic and osteopathic medicine, dentistry, podiatry, and optometry (**Figure 25-9**).

Women in the United States can expect to live about 4.8 years longer than men (NCHS 2013), but they suffer greater morbidity and poorer health outcomes. Morbidity is greater among women than among men, even after childbearing-related conditions are factored out. For instance, nearly 38% of women report having chronic conditions that require ongoing medical treatment compared to 30% of men (Salganicoff et al. 2005). Women also have a higher prevalence of certain health problems than men over the course of their lifetimes (Sechzer et al. 1996). Heart disease and stroke account for a higher percentage of deaths among women than men at all stages of life. In contrast to 24% of men, 42% of women

FIGURE 25-9 Percentage of female students of total enrollment in schools for selected health occupations, 2006–2007.

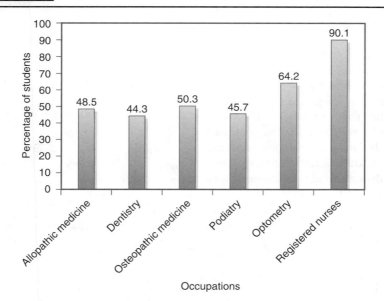

Source: Data from National Center for Health Statistics (NCHS). 2010. *Health, United States, 2009.* Hyattsville, MD: Department of Health and Human Services, p. 383.

who have heart attacks die within a year (Misra 2001). Research has also demonstrated that women are more likely than men to experience functional limitations due to health (35% and 26%, respectively; NCHS 2013).

According to the 2012 Health in the United States Report, 88% of women had at least one visit to a health care provider in the previous year compared to 80% of men (NCHS 2013). Compared to men, women have only a slightly higher mean number of specialty care visits and emergency department visits. However, women have higher annual charges than men for all types of care, including primary, specialty, emergency, and diagnostic services, which indicates that women receive more intensive services (Bertakis et al. 2000). Women are more likely to delay seeking care than men (13% compared to 9.6%, respectively; HRSA Maternal and Child Health Bureau 2011). In addition, women (9.3%) are more likely than men (7.8%) to forgo needed care (HRSA Maternal and Child Health Bureau 2011).

The differences between men and women are equally pronounced for mental illness. For example, anxiety disorders and major depression affect two to three times as many women as men (McLean et al. 2011). Clinical depression is a major mental health problem for both men and women; however, 4.0% of women, compared to 2.7% of men, had depression during 2006–2008 (CDC 2010b). An estimated 12% of women in the United States, compared with 7% of men, will suffer from major depression during their lifetime (Misra 2001). Certain other mental disorders also affect more women at different stages of life.

Eating disorders are among the illnesses predominantly affecting women and have been the subject of relatively little rigorous study to date. Up to 3% of women are affected by eating disorders (e.g., anorexia nervosa and bulimia), although between 29% and 38% report dieting at any given time (Misra 2001). At least 90% of all eating disorder cases occur in young women, and eating disorders account for the highest mortality rates among all mental disorders (Misra 2001).

Some disorders once thought to primarily affect men are now affecting women in increasing numbers. For example, death rates related to alcohol abuse are 50–100% higher among women than among men (Misra 2001). Compared to older men, older women are at substantially greater risk of Alzheimer's disease, a disease responsible for 60–70% of all cases of dementia and one of the leading causes of nursing home placement for older adults (Herzog and Copeland 1985).

In addition to the differences experienced in health care utilization and health outcomes between women and men there are large disparities by race and ethnicity, income, and education among women. New HIV cases are greatest among minorities. In 2009, per 100,000 women, 47.8 Black, 13.3 Native American or Pacific Islander, and 11.9 Hispanic were newly diagnosed with HIV compared to only 2.4 White women (HRSA Maternal and Child Health Bureau 2011). The prevalence of diabetes among women also varies: 14% of American Indian or Alaska Natives and 11.9% of Native Hawaiian or Other Pacific Islanders have diabetes compared to only 6.4% of White women (HRSA Maternal and Child Health Bureau 2011).

Office on Women's Health

The Public Health Service's Office on Women's Health (OWH) is dedicated to the achievement of a series of specific goals that span the spectrum of disease and disability. These goals range across the life cycle and address cultural and ethnic differences among women. The OWH promotes, coordinates, and implements a comprehensive women's health agenda on research, service delivery, and education across various government agencies.

The OWH was responsible for implementing the National Action Plan on Breast Cancer (NAPBC), a major public–private partnership, dedicated to improving the diagnosis, treatment, and prevention of breast cancer through research, service delivery, and education. The OWH also worked to implement measures to prevent physical and sexual abuse against women, as delineated in the Violence Against Women Act of 1994. The OWH is also active in projects promoting breastfeeding, women's health education and research, girl and adolescent health, and heart health.

Within the Substance Abuse and Mental Health Services Administration (SAMHSA), the Advisory Committee for Women's Services has targeted six areas for special attention: physical and sexual abuse of women; women as caregivers; women with mental and addictive disorders; women with HIV infection or AIDS, sexually transmitted diseases, and/or tuberculosis; older women; and women detained in the criminal justice system. The Women's Health Initiative, supported by the National Institutes of Health (NIH), was the largest clinical trial conducted in US history, involving more than 161,000 women (NIH 2002). It focused on diseases that are the major causes of death and disability among women—heart disease, cancer, and osteoporosis. In 2002, the Women's Health Initiative published a groundbreaking study, finding detrimental effects of postmenopausal hormone therapy on women's development of invasive breast cancer, coronary heart disease, stroke, and pulmonary embolism (NIH 2002).

Women and the US Health Care System

Women face a distinct disadvantage in employer-based health insurance coverage because they are more likely than men to work part time, receive lower wages, and have interruptions in their work histories. Hence, women are more likely to be covered as dependents under their husbands' plans and are at a higher risk of being uninsured. Women also place greater reliance on Medicaid for their health care coverage. In 2011, 15.6% of women were uninsured compared to 18.8% of men, while 19.3% of women compared to 16.3% of men were covered by Medicaid (NCHS 2013).

Women are more likely than men to use contraceptives (**Figure 25-10**), but contraceptives have been among the most poorly covered reproductive health care services in the United States. As of September 2013, 28 states required private health insurance plans to cover prescription contraceptives if they covered other prescription drugs (Guttmacher Institute 2013).

The ACA requires private insurance to cover, with no cost sharing, a wide variety of preventive services and additional services for women, including FDA-approved prescription contraceptives, domestic violence screening, breastfeeding supports, and human papillomavirus (HPV) testing. Although such services are not required under Medicaid, several states have started to cover all preventive services important for women with or without cost sharing (Kaiser Family Foundation 2013a).

RURAL HEALTH

For rural citizens, access to health care may be affected by poverty, long distances, rural topography, weather conditions, lack of transportation, and being uninsured. Consequently, residents of rural areas are less likely to utilize health services and have poorer health outcomes than those in more urban areas. A greater percentage of persons residing in a rural area report being in fair or poor health compared to those in urban areas (CDC 2012a, 2012b). In addition, rural residents are more likely to report health problems, such as headaches and back and neck pain, than urban residents (17.2% compared to 14.7%, respectively; CDC 2012a, 2012b).

Among residents whose family incomes are below 100% FPL, those in rural areas are more likely than urban residents to forgo or delay care due to cost (27.1% compared to 21.4%, respectively; CDC 2012a, 2012b). Across race and ethnicity, rural residents have lower levels of insurance coverage. Among Hispanic rural

FIGURE 25-10 Percentage of women using contraception is 62.2.

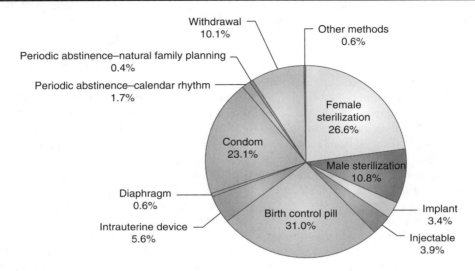

Percentage of women using contraception is 62.2.

Source: Data from National Center for Health Statistics (NCHS). 2013. *Health, United States, 2012.* Hyattsville, MD: Department of Health and Human Services, pp. 60–62.

residents, 48.3% do not have health insurance, compared to 42.5% of urban Hispanics. Among Whites, 22.5% of rural residents were uninsured compared to 14.2% of urban residents (CDC 2012a, 2012b). The uninsured often do not have a usual source of care (Larson and Fleishman 2003).

Geographic maldistribution that creates a shortage of health care professionals in rural settings results in barriers in access to care. As of January 2013, there were about 5,900 designated primary care health professional shortage areas (HPSAs), 4,600 dental HPSAs, and 3,800 mental health HPSAs (HRSA 2013b). About 21% of the US population resides in areas where primary care health professionals are in short supply (HRSA National Health Service Corps 2013). More than 33 million Americans live in a nonmetropolitan federally designated health

professional shortage area (HRSA National Health Service Corps 2013). The scarcity of health care providers encompasses a broad spectrum of professionals, including pediatricians, obstetricians, internists, dentists, nurses, and allied health professionals (Patton and Puskin 1990). Rural hospitals are often under financial strain, which results in smaller hospitals that provide fewer services than urban hospitals.

Various measures have been taken to improve access in rural America, including the promotion of the National Health Service Corps (NHSC), the designation of Health Professional Shortage Areas (HPSAs) and Medically Underserved Areas (MUAs), the development of Community and Migrant Health Centers (C/MHCs), and the enactment of the Rural Health Clinics Act. In addition, the Office of Rural Health Policy, within the Health

Resources and Services Administration of the US Department of Health and Human Services (DHHS), was established in 1987 to promote better health care in rural America (HRSA Office of Rural Health Policy 2007).

The National Health Service Corps

The NHSC was created in 1970, under the Emergency Health Personnel Act, to recruit and retain physicians to provide needed services in physician shortage areas. A 1972 amendment created a scholarship program targeting HPSAs. The scholarship and loan repayment program apply to doctors, dentists, nurse practitioners, midwives, and mental health professionals who serve a minimum of 2 years in underserved areas. Since 1972, more than 40,000 health professionals have been placed in medically underserved communities in hospitals and clinics (HRSA National Health Service Corps 2013). Currently, nearly 10,000 health professionals are providing services under NHSC (HRSA National Health Service Corps 2013).

Health Professional Shortage Areas

The Health Professions Educational Assistance Act of 1976 provided the designation criteria for Health Manpower Shortage Areas, later renamed Health Professional Shortage Areas (Greene 1976). The act provided that three different types of HPSAs could be designated: geographic areas, population groups, and medical facilities. A geographic area must meet the following three criteria for designation as a primary care HPSA: (1) The geographic area involved must be rational for the delivery of health services. (2) One of the following conditions must prevail in the area: (a) the area has a population to full-time equivalent primary care physician (PCP) ratio of at least 3,500:1, or (b) the area has a population to full-time equivalent PCP ratio of less than 3,500:1 but greater than 3,000:1 and has unusually high needs for primary care services or insufficient capacity of existing primary care providers. (3) Primary

care professionals in contiguous areas are over-utilized, excessively distant, or inaccessible to the population of the area under consideration (HRSA Bureau of Health Professions 2007).

A population group can be designated as an HPSA for primary care if it can be demonstrated that access barriers prevent members of the group from using local providers. Medium- and maximum-security federal and state correctional institutions and public or nonprofit private residential facilities can be designated as facility-based HPSAs. HPSAs are classified on a scale of 1 to 4, with 1 or 2 signifying areas of greatest need.

Medically Underserved Areas

The primary purpose of the MUA designation in the HMO Act of 1973 was to target the community health center and rural health clinic programs. The statute required that several factors be considered in designating MUAs, such as available health resources in relation to area size and population, health indices, and care and demographic factors affecting the need for care. To meet this mandate, the Index of Medical Underservice was developed, comprising four variables: (1) percentage of population below poverty income levels, (2) percentage of population 65 years of age and older, (3) infant mortality rates, and (4) primary care practitioners per 1,000 population. The index yields a single numerical value on a scale from zero to 100; any area with a value less than 62 (the median of all counties) is designated an MUA.

MIGRANT WORKERS

Migrant workers are farmworkers who travel long distances from their primary residence or lack a primary residence entirely, either due to seasonal crop changes or work availability. While their exact number is difficult to assess due to citizenship issues and the transient nature of the population, it is widely accepted that there are at least 3 million migrant workers in the United States (Larson and Plascencia

1993; Migrant Health Promotion 2014; Rust 1990). The migrant population is largely composed of racial and ethnic minorities. As of 2009, 72% of migrant workers were born in Mexico or Central America (US Department of Labor 2011).

The average annual income of a family in which at least one member is a migrant worker was between $17,500 and $19,999 in 2009. Furthermore, only 57% of workers were currently receiving any public assistance (US Department of Labor 2011). As of 2000, approximately 85% of migrant workers were uninsured and only 20% of all workers reported utilizing any health service within the prior 2 years (Rosenbaum and Shin 2005). Furthermore, only 42% of female migrant workers sought prenatal care during their first trimester compared with the national average of 72% (Rosenbaum and Shin 2005). In addition to the occupational health risks that this population is exposed to, the lack of access to and utilization of health services translates to poor health outcomes.

The rate of obesity among migrant workers has risen to 81% of males and 76% of females (Villarejo et al. 2000). This rate is not found among migrant workers within their first year in the United States; therefore, dietary changes in later years likely account for the rates of obesity (Ikeda 1990). In addition to higher rates of chronic conditions, migrant populations are also at greater risk for infectious disease. In part due to their living conditions, migrant workers are at greater risk of tuberculosis, with studies finding rates between 17% (McCurdy et al. 1997) and 44% (Villarino et al. 1994). The rate of HIV/AIDS is also considerably higher than in the general population, with observed rates between 5% and 13% (Organista and Organista 1997).

To address the growing health needs of this population, services have been provided to migrant workers and their families through state programs and federally through HRSA's Migrant Health Program.

Community and Migrant Health Centers (C/MHCs)

Community and migrant health centers provide services to low-income populations on a sliding-fee scale, thereby addressing both geographic and financial barriers to access. Although community health centers must be located in areas designated as MUAs, migrant centers must be located in "high-impact" areas, defined as areas that serve at least 4,000 migrant and/or seasonal farm workers for at least 2 months per year. For more than 4 decades, C/MHCs have provided primary care and preventive health services to populations in designated MUAs. Because of a shortage of physicians, C/MHCs heavily rely on nonphysician providers (NPPs). In 2012, C/MHCs served approximately 900,000 migrants and seasonal farm workers.

The Rural Health Clinics Act

The Rural Health Clinics Act was developed to respond to the concern that isolated rural communities could not generate sufficient revenue to support the services of a physician. In many cases, the only source of primary care or emergency services was NPPs, who were ineligible at that time for Medicare or Medicaid reimbursement. The act permitted physician assistants (PAs), nurse practitioners (NPs), and certified nurse midwives (CNMs) associated with rural clinics to practice without the direct supervision of a physician; enabled rural health clinics (but not NPPs directly) to be reimbursed by Medicare and Medicaid for their services; and tied the level of Medicaid payment to the level established by Medicare. To be designated as a rural health clinic, a public or private sector physician practice, clinic, or hospital must meet several criteria, including location in an MUA, geographic HPSA, or a population-based HPSA. More than 3,000 rural health clinics provide primary care services to over 7 million people in 47 states (National Association of Rural Health Clinics [NARHC] 2007).

THE HOMELESS

Although an exact number is unknown, an estimated 3.5 million people (1.35 million of them children) are likely to experience homelessness in a given year (National Law Center on Homelessness and Poverty 2004). Nationally, approximately 1 in 200 people became homeless in 2011 (US Department of Housing and Urban Development [HUD] 2012). Although most homeless persons live in major urban areas, a surprising 27.7% live in suburban and rural areas (HUD 2012).

The adult homeless population is comprised of 63% men and 37% women, 22.8% are children younger than age 18 years, 35.8% are families with children, and 14% are veterans (HUD 2012). Homeless women in particular face major difficulties: economic and housing needs and special gender-related issues that include pregnancy, child care responsibilities, family violence, fragmented family support, job discrimination, and wage discrepancies. The economic standing of women is often more unstable than that of men, and women are more likely to live in poverty than men are. In 2010, 17 million women were living in poverty, of which 7.5 million were in extreme poverty (National Women's Law Center 2011). The low wages and extreme poverty faced by women increases their risk for becoming homeless. In addition, domestic violence has been found to be a contributing factor to family homelessness, with 18% of families citing this as the main cause (United States Conference of Mayors 2011). Among all homeless women, one in four states that her homelessness was a direct result of violence committed against her (Jasinski 2005). Homeless women, regardless of parenting status, should be linked with social services, family support, self-help, and housing resources. Mentally ill women caring for children need additional consideration, with an emphasis on parenting skills and special services for children. Thus, homelessness is a multifaceted problem related to personal, social, and economic factors.

The economic picture of homeless persons is dismal, as would be expected, and suggests that they are severely lacking in the financial and educational resources necessary to access health care. A majority of mothers living in poverty that have ever been homeless did not complete high school (60%; Institute for Children, Poverty, & Homelessness 2011). In addition, it is estimated that approximately 38% of the homeless population is unsheltered (National Alliance to End Homelessness 2012). Receipt of public benefits among the homeless is low. For example, among more than 9,000 clients served by Maryland's Health Care for the Homeless, 75% were uninsured (Health Care for the Homeless 2012). These numbers remain low because of federal restrictions that prohibit federal help to those without a physical street address.

The shortage of adequate low-income housing is the major precipitating factor for homelessness. Unemployment, personal or family life crises, rent increases that are out of proportion to inflation, and reduction in public benefits can also directly result in the loss of a home. Illness, on the other hand, tends to result in the loss of a home in a more indirect way. Other indirect causes of homelessness include deinstitutionalization from public mental hospitals, substance abuse programs, and overcrowded prisons and jails.

Community-based residential alternatives for mentally ill individuals vary from independent apartments to group homes staffed by paid caregivers. Independent living may involve either separate apartments or single-room occupancy units in large hotels, whereas group homes are staffed during at least a portion of the day and traditionally provide some on-site mental health services (Schutt and Goldfinger 1996).

The homeless, adults and children, have a high prevalence of untreated acute and chronic medical, mental health, and substance abuse problems. The reasons are debatable. Some argue that people may become homeless because of a physical or mental illness. Others argue that homelessness itself may lead to the development of physical and mental disability because homelessness produces risk factors, which include excessive use of alcohol, illegal drugs, and cigarettes; sleeping in an upright position, which results in venous stasis and its consequences; extensive walking in poorly fitting shoes; and grossly inadequate nutrition. While the reasons may not be agreed upon, the outcomes are easily seen. Homeless adults typically have eight to nine medical conditions or illnesses (Breakey et al. 1989). Homeless children have a nearly doubled risk of mortality than housed children (Kerker et al. 2011).

Homeless persons are also at a greater risk of assault and victimization regardless of whether they live in a shelter or outdoors. They are also subject to exposure to extreme heat, cold, and other weather conditions. The homeless are also exposed to illness because of overcrowding in shelters and overexposure to weather.

Barriers to Health Care

The homeless face barriers to ambulatory services but incur high rates of hospitalization. A high use of inpatient services in this manner amounts to the substitution of inpatient care for outpatient services. Both individual factors (competing needs, substance dependence, and mental illness) and system factors (availability, cost, convenience, and appropriateness of care) account for the barriers to adequate ambulatory services.

Other barriers include accessible transportation to medical care providers and competing needs for basic food, shelter, and income than obtaining health services or following through with a prescribed treatment plan. Homeless individuals who experience psychological distress and disabling mental illness may be in the greatest need of health services and yet may be the least able to obtain them. This inability to obtain health care may be attributable to such individual traits of mental illness as paranoia,

disorientation, unconventional health beliefs, lack of social support, lack of organizational skills to gain access to needed services, or fear of authority figures and institutions resulting from previous institutionalization. The social conditions of street life also affect compliance with medical care because of a lack of proper sanitation and a stable place to store medications. They also lack resources to obtain proper food for a medically indicated diet necessary for conditions like diabetes or hypertension.

Federal efforts to provide medical services to the homeless population are primarily through the Health Care for the Homeless (HCH) program. Community health centers supported by the 1985 Robert Wood Johnson Foundation/Pew Memorial Trust HCH program (subsequently covered by the 1987 McKinney Homeless Assistance Act) have addressed many of the access and quality-of-care issues faced by the homeless. In 2012, community health centers served approximately 1.1 million homeless patients (HRSA Bureau of Primary Health Care 2012b). A walk-in appointment system reduces access barriers at these medical facilities. Medical care, routine laboratory tests, substance abuse counseling, and some medications are provided free of charge to eliminate financial barriers.

The Mental Health Services for the Homeless Block Grant program sets aside funds for states to implement services for homeless persons with mental illness. These services include outreach services; community mental health services; rehabilitation; referrals to inpatient treatment, primary care, and substance abuse services; case management services; and supportive services in residential settings.

Services for homeless veterans are provided through the Department of Veterans Affairs (VA). The Homeless Chronically Mentally Ill Veterans Program provides outreach, case management services, and psychiatric residential treatment for homeless mentally ill veterans in community-based facilities in 45 US cities. The Domiciliary

Care for Homeless Veterans Program addresses the health needs of veterans who have psychiatric illnesses or alcohol or drug abuse problems, operating 1,800 beds at 31 sites across the country (US Department of Veterans Affairs 2014).

The Salvation Army also provides a variety of social, rehabilitation, and support services for homeless persons. Its centers include adult rehabilitation and food programs and permanent and transitional housing.

MENTAL HEALTH

Mental disorders are common psychiatric illnesses affecting adults and present a serious public health problem in the United States. Mental disorders are among the leading causes of disability in the United States (World Health Organization [WHO] 2012). Mental illness is a risk factor for death from suicide, cardiovascular disease, and cancer. Suicide is currently the 11th leading cause of death in the United States and the 4th leading cause of death among persons aged 18–65 (CDC 2010e). Non-Hispanic White men 85 years of age and older have one of the highest rates of suicide, with approximately 52 suicide deaths per 100,000 (CDC 2010e). AIANs are at higher risk for suicides as well, with approximately 11 suicide deaths per 100,000 (CDC 2010e).

Mental health disorders can be either psychological or biological in nature. Many mental health diseases, including mental retardation (MR), developmental disabilities (DD), and schizophrenia, are now known to be biological in origin. Other behaviors, including those related to personality disorders and neurotic behaviors, are still subject to interpretation and professional judgment.

National studies have concluded that the most common mental disorders include phobias; substance abuse, including alcohol and drug dependence; and affective disorders, including depression. Schizophrenia is considerably less common, with estimates ranging from 0.7% (McGrath et al. 2008) to 1.1% of the population (Regier et al. 1993).

About one in four adults suffers from a diagnosable mental disorder every year (Kessler et al. 2005). In 2009, 45.1 million adults (18 years of age or older) had a mental illness, including 11 million with severe mental illness (SMI; Substance Abuse and Mental Health Services Administration [SAMHSA] 2012a, 2012b). Among adults with any diagnosable mental disorder, 62.1% did not seek mental health treatment (SAMHSA 2012a, 2012b). Prevalence of SMI was higher among Medicaid recipients, women, and individuals in the 18–25 age group (SAMHSA 2012a, 2012b).

The mental health of children has drawn increasing concern in recent years. Approximately one in five children has a mental disorder, a similar rate to that of adults; approximately 4 million children or adolescents have a serious mental illness (US Department of Health and Human Services 2001). Only half of those diagnosed receive mental health services (US Public Health Service 2000). If left untreated, mental health in children can lead to more severe and/or co-occurring mental illness (Kessler et al. 2005).

Most mental health services are provided in the general medical sector—a concept first described by Regier and colleagues (1988) as the de facto mental health service system—rather than through formal mental health specialist services. The de facto system combines specialty mental health services with general counseling services, such as those provided in primary care settings, nursing homes, and community health centers by ministers, counselors, self-help groups, families, and friends. Specifically, mental health services are provided through public and private resources in both inpatient and outpatient facilities. These facilities include state and county mental hospitals, private psychiatric hospitals, nonfederal general hospital psychiatric services, VA psychiatric services, residential treatment centers, and freestanding psychiatric outpatient clinics (**Table 25-6**). Total expenditures for mental disorders have increased from $31 billion in 1986 to $113 billion in 2005

TABLE 25-6	Mental Health Organizations (Numbers in Thousands), 2008

Service and Organization	Number of MH Organizations
All organizations	3,130
State psychiatric hospitals	241
Private psychiatric hospitals	256
Nonfederal general hospital psychiatric services	1,292
Residential treatment centers for emotionally disturbed children	538
All other	673

Source: Data from National Center for Health Statistics. 2012. *Health, United States, 2011.* Hyattsville, MD: Department of Health and Human Services, p. 358.

(SAMHSA 2012a). Despite the cost of mental health care for individuals with any mental illness, only 37.9% received mental health services and only 48.5% of individuals covered under Medicaid/CHIP received care (SAMHSA 2012a, 2012b). The nation's *mental health system* is composed of two subsystems: one primarily for individuals with insurance coverage or private funds and the other for those without private coverage.

Barriers to Mental Health Care

Two main barriers to access for mental health care are commonly experienced across the United States: prohibitive costs of services and shortage of available mental health professionals. In 2009, among adults who delayed or did not seek needed mental health care, 50.1% stated that it was the result of the prohibitive cost of treatment (SAMHSA 2012a, 2012b). In addition to the inability to cover the high cost of care, many individuals currently reside in a Mental Health Care Health Professional Shortage Area. A Mental Health HPSA is defined as an area in which the population to mental health profession ratio equals 6,000 people to 1 mental health professional and 20,000 people to 1 psychiatrist (HRSA Bureau of Health

Professions 2013). As of 2013, there were more than 3,700 shortage areas across the United States (Kaiser Family Foundation 2013c). This shortage translates to the available services being able to meet only 54% of need, leaving a large number of patients without needed care (Kaiser Family Foundation 2013c).

The Uninsured and Mental Health

Patients without insurance coverage or personal financial resources are treated in state and county mental health hospitals and in community mental health clinics. Care is also provided in short-term, acute care hospitals and emergency departments. Local governments are the providers of last resort, with the ultimate responsibility to provide somatic and mental health services for all citizens regardless of ability to pay.

The Insured and Mental Health

For patients who have insurance coverage or personal ability to pay, availability of both inpatient and ambulatory mental health care has expanded tremendously. Inpatient mental health services for patients with insurance are usually provided through private psychiatric hospitals. These hospitals can be operated on either a nonprofit or a for-profit basis. There has been substantial growth in national chains of for-profit mental health hospitals. Patients with insurance coverage are also more likely to receive care through the offices of private psychiatrists, clinical psychologists, and licensed social workers. Mental health services are also provided by the VA and by the military health care system; however, access to these services is limited by eligibility.

Managed Care and Mental Health

Managed care has expanded its services into mental health delivery. State and local governments are also contracting with MCOs to manage a full health care benefit package that includes mental health and substance abuse services for their Medicaid enrollees.

Many health maintenance organizations (HMOs) contract with specialized companies that provide managed behavioral health care, an arrangement called a carve out. This is mainly because HMOs lack the in-house capacity to provide treatment. Using case managers and reviewers, most of whom are psychiatric nurses, social workers, and psychologists, these specialized companies oversee and authorize the use of mental health and substance abuse services. The case reviewers, using clinical protocols to guide them, assign patients to the least expensive appropriate treatment, emphasizing outpatient alternatives over inpatient care.

Working with computerized databases, a reviewer studies a patient's particular problem and then authorizes an appointment with an appropriate provider in the company's selective network. On average, psychiatrists constitute about 4.5% of any given provider network, psychologists constitute 17%, counselors constitute 24%, and psychiatric social workers constitute another 45% (SAMHSA 2012a).

Mental Health Professionals

A variety of professionals provide mental health services (**Table 25-7**), including but not limited

TABLE 25-7 Full-Time-Equivalent Patient Care Staff in Mental Health Organizations, 2000

Staff Discipline	Number	Percentage
All patient care staff	426,558	74.9
Professional patient care staff	243,993	42.9
Psychiatrists	20,233	3.6
Other physicians	2,962	0.5
Psychologists	19,003	3.3
Social workers	70,208	12.3
Registered nurses	70,295	12.4
Other mental health professionals	53,271	9.4
Physical health professionals and assistants	8,023	1.4
Other mental health workers	182,566	32.1

Source: Modified from Section V, Chapter 22, Table 19.7, *Mental Health, United States, 2004.* Ronald W. Manderscheid, Joyce T. Berry, eds. Rockville, MD: US Department of Health and Human Services, Substance Abuse and Mental Health Services Administration, Center for Mental Health Services.

to psychiatrists, psychologists, social workers, nurses, counselors, and therapists.

Psychiatrists are physicians who specialize in the diagnosis and treatment of mental disorders. Psychiatrists receive postgraduate specialty training in mental health after completing medical school. Psychiatric residencies cover medical, as well as behavioral, diagnosis, and treatments. A relatively small proportion of the total mental health workforce consists of psychiatrists, but they exercise disproportionate influence in the system by virtue of their authority to prescribe drugs and admit patients to hospitals.

Psychologists usually hold a doctoral degree, although some hold master's degrees. They are trained in interpreting and changing the behavior of people. Psychologists cannot prescribe drugs; however, they provide a wide range of services to patients with neurotic and behavioral problems. Psychologists use such techniques as psychotherapy and counseling, which psychiatrists typically do not engage in. Psychoanalysis is a subspecialty in mental health that involves the use of intensive treatment by both psychiatrists and psychologists.

Social workers receive training in various aspects of mental health services, particularly counseling. Social workers are trained at the master's degree level. They also compete with psychologists for patients.

Nurses are involved in mental health through the subspecialty of psychiatric nursing. Specialty training for nurses had its origins in the latter part of the 1800s. Nurses provide a wide range of mental health services.

Many other health care professionals contribute to the array of available services, including marriage and family counselors, recreational therapists, and vocational counselors. Numerous people work in related areas, such as adult day care (ADC), alcohol and drug abuse counseling, and as psychiatric aides in institutional settings.

THE CHRONICALLY ILL

Chronic diseases are now the leading cause of death in the United States—heart disease, cancer, and stroke account for more than 50% of deaths each year. Seven out of 10 deaths each year are from chronic diseases (Kung et al. 2008). Heart disease is the number one cause of death in the United States, at 179.1 per 100,000 persons (NCHS 2013). The prevalence of heart disease from 2010 to 2011 was 11.6%, which is equal to 36.1 million Americans (NCHS 2013). In 2010, more than one in four adults had more than one chronic illness, roughly 80 million Americans (Ward and Schiller 2013).

This large prevalence of disease results in adverse consequences such as limitations on daily living activities. Among normal weight adults with one or more chronic illnesses it is estimated that, as a result of the number of sick or unhealthy days they experience each month, the resulting cost due to loss of productivity is more than $15 billion per year (Witters and Agrawal 2011). For overweight or obese adults with one or more chronic illnesses, this loss more than doubled to $32 billion annually. Overall, the total loss due to overweight, obesity, or other chronic illnesses is estimated at more than $153 billion each year.

The loss in human potential and work days notwithstanding, chronic disease is expensive. Chronic disease places a huge economic demand on the nation. In 2010, the estimated annual direct medical expenditures for the most common chronic diseases were more than $107 billion (Agency for Healthcare Research and Quality [AHRQ] 2010). In 2008, expenditures on obesity were estimated to total $147 billion (Finkelstein et al. 2009). The estimated cost to treat diabetes in 2007 totaled more than $116 billion (American Diabetes Association 2008). In addition, costs related to heart disease totaled more than $475 billion in 2009 (Lloyd-Jones et al. 2009).

Much of the burden of chronic diseases is the result of four modifiable risk behaviors:

physical activity, nutrition, smoking, and alcohol (CDC 2010c). Only 21% of the US population met the 2008 Physical Activity Guidelines for Americans standards for aerobic and muscle strengthening (NCHS 2013). There has also been a decline in participation in physical education classes among high school students, from 42% in 1991 to 31% in 2011. The nation also suffers from poor nutrition. Less than 25% of adults and children eat the required five or more servings of fruit and vegetables, although the majority consumes more than the recommended amount of saturated fat (CDC 2012b).

Disability

As of 2010, approximately 56.7 million people in the United States had a disability, of which more than 38 million were severely disabled (Brault 2012). The prevalence of disability increases with age, with 70.5% of adults aged 80 and older having a disability (Brault 2012). The chronic conditions most responsible for disabilities are arthritis, heart disease, back problems, asthma, and diabetes (Kraus et al. 1996). Persons with disabilities tend to receive coverage from public insurance (30% by Medicare and 10% by Medicaid) compared to those who have no disabilities and are more likely to have private health insurance (US Census Bureau 2011f).

Disability can be categorized as mental, physical, or social; tests of disability tend to be more sensitive to some categories than others. Physical disability usually addresses a person's mobility and other basic activities performed in daily life, mental disability involves both the cognitive and emotional states, and social disability is considered the most severe disability because management of social roles requires both physical and mental well-being (Ostir et al. 1999).

Two commonly used measures of disability are activities of daily living (ADLs) and instrumental activities of daily living (IADLs). Another tool for assessing disability is the Survey of Income and Program Participation (SIPP), which measures disability by asking participants about functional limitations (difficulty in performing activities such as seeing, hearing, walking, having one's speech understood, etc.), but ADL and IADL scales are more widely used.

Despite the availability of community-based and institutional long-term care services for people with functional limitations, many people are not getting the help they need with the basic tasks of personal care. It is estimated that approximately one in five individuals with an ADL limitation do not receive needed assistance (Newcomer et al. 2005). Furthermore, racial minorities are more likely to experience unmet personal assistance needs (Newcomer et al. 2005).

HIV/AIDS

Figure 25-11 illustrates trends in AIDS reporting. The number of AIDS cases reported increased between 1987 and 1993, decreased between 1994 and 1999, increased between 2000 and 2004, and decreased again since 2005 (US Census Bureau 2010c).

Deaths from AIDS declined 11% between 2007 and 2008 (CDC 2010d). Declines in reported AIDS cases are ascribed to new treatments; decreasing death rates may reflect the fact that benefits from new treatments are being fully realized. Consequently, the number of people living with AIDS has continued to increase. In 2010, 487,692 people were living with AIDS; in 2001, the figure was 341,332 (CDC 2011b).

For Blacks, Hispanics, and minority women, AIDS/HIV is still a major public health concern. In 2010, males and Blacks continued to have significantly higher rates of HIV/AIDS than females and Whites did (**Table 25-8**). Also, only among Black males is HIV a leading cause of death (CDC 2012c). In 2011, rates of AIDS cases per 100,000 people were 51.3 in the Black population, 16.2 in the Hispanic population,

FIGURE 25-11 US AIDS cases reported, 1987–2008.

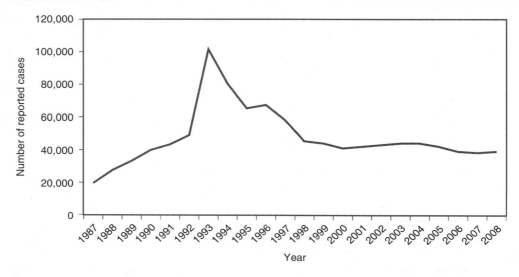

Source: Reprinted from US Census Bureau, *Statistical Abstracts of the United States, 2001*, p. 119; *Statistical Abstracts of the United States, 2007*, p. 120; *Statistical Abstracts of the United States, 2008*, p. 121; *Statistical Abstracts of the United States, 2009*, p. 120; *Statistical Abstracts of the United States, 2010*, p. 122; and *Statistical Abstracts of the United States, 2012*, p. 125. Available at: http://www.census.gov/prod/www /statistical_abstract.html

and 4.9 in the White population (CDC 2012d). Blacks accounted for a rate of annual diagnoses eight times greater than the rate for Whites in 2009 (CDC 2013d). Racial differences in HIV/AIDS infection probably reflect social, economic, behavioral, and other factors associated with HIV transmission risks.

HIV Infection in Rural Communities

Spread of HIV in the rural United States has grown. In 2006, CDC reported 2,696 new cases of AIDS and estimated 26,154 adults and adolescents to be living with AIDS in the rural United States (CDC 2008).

Rural persons with HIV and AIDS are more likely to be young, non-White, and female and to have acquired their infection through heterosexual contact. Additionally, a growing number of these HIV-infected persons live in the rural South, a region historically characterized by a disproportionate number of poor and minority persons, strong religious beliefs and sanctions, and decreased access to comprehensive health services (CDC 1995). Trends in new cases of HIV and AIDS in rural areas indicate that poor and non-White residents are disproportionately affected (Aday 1993; Lam and Liu 1994).

HIV in Children

In the absence of specific therapy to interrupt transmission of HIV, an infected woman has a 20% chance of having a child born with HIV (Cooper et al. 2000). Building on previous

TABLE 25-8	US AIDS Cases Reported Through 2010			
	All Years		**2010**	
Characteristic	Number	Percentage	Number	Percentage
Total	1,129,127	100.0	33,942	100.0
Sex				
Male (13 years and older)	810,676	71.8	24,507	73.3
Female (13 years and older)	198,544	17.6	8,242	26.6
Children younger than 13 years	9,209	0.8	23	0.1
Race/Ethnic Group				
White	429,804	38.1	8,875	26.1
Black	473,229	41.9	16,188	47.7
Hispanic	197,449	17.5	6,636	19.6
Asian	8,759	0.8	479	1.4
Native Hawaiian or other Pacific Islander	870	0.1	44	0.1
American Indian/Alaska Native	3,721	0.3	170	0.5

Source: Data from National Center for Health Statistics. 2013. *Health, United States, 2012.* Hyattsville, MD: Department of Health and Human Services, p. 140.

success with zidovudine monotherapy in the 1990s, clinical studies established the efficacy of antiretroviral therapy on reducing the mother-to-child transmission rate when administered prenatally (Cooper et al. 2000). Use of antiretroviral therapy resulted in a decrease of the rate of mother-to-child transmission to only 2% (Cooper et al. 2000). Guidelines on the use of antiretroviral drugs in pregnant HIV/AIDS-infected women have since been established (NIH 2012; WHO 2004). The importance of preventing perinatal transmission is underscored by the fact that 75% of all AIDS cases among US children are caused by mother-to-child transmission in pregnancy, labor, delivery, or breastfeeding (CDC 2012e). Children who are born with AIDS suffer from failure to thrive, the inability to grow and develop as healthy children. Without intervention, this failure to thrive may lead to developmental delays that can have negative lifetime consequences for the child and his or her family.

HIV in Women

Women are a rapidly growing proportion of the population with HIV/AIDS. In 2010, women made up more than one-half of HIV/AIDS cases worldwide (UNAIDS 2010). For Black US women 15 to 44 years of age and Hispanic women aged 25 to 44, HIV/AIDS was among the top 10 leading causes of death in 2010 (CDC 2013b). For women, heterosexual exposure to HIV, followed by injection drug use (IDU), is the greatest cause for exposure (US Census Bureau 2012). Aside from the inherent risks in IDU, drug use overall contributes to a higher risk of contracting HIV if heterosexual sex with an IDU user occurs or when sex is traded for drugs or money (CDC 2013c). Black and Hispanic minority women are at particular risk. Despite representing less than one-fourth of the total US female population, Black and Hispanic women represent more than three-fourths (79%) of all AIDS cases in women (CDC 2012c).

HIV/AIDS-Related Issues

Need for Research

HIV-related research seeks to develop a vaccine to prevent HIV-negative people from acquiring HIV. Researchers are also seeking to develop a therapeutic vaccine to prevent HIV-positive people from developing symptoms of AIDS.

People with HIV/AIDS represent a broad spectrum of social classes, races, ethnicities, sexual orientations, and genders. Behavioral intervention research, therefore, should focus particularly on populations that are most vulnerable to HIV infection and are in urgent need of preventive interventions. These populations include gay youth and young adults, especially Black and Hispanic; disenfranchised and impoverished women; heterosexual men, again, Black and Hispanic in particular; inner-city youth; and out-of-treatment substance abusers and their sexual partners. Research should be aimed not only at the individual but also at the impact of broader interventions (e.g., among drug users or those involved in sexual networks or communitywide groups) that change behavioral norms and, consequently, affect individual behavior (Merson 1996).

Public Health Concerns

AIDS underscores the synergy between poverty and intravenous drug use. Further, control of the HIV epidemic among the poor is hampered by their preoccupation with other problems related to survival, such as homelessness, crime, and lack of access to adequate health care.

Additionally, a relationship exists between the current tuberculosis epidemic and HIV. Indeed, tuberculosis, an *opportunistic infection*, is the worldwide leading cause of death among HIV-infected people. Tuberculosis in HIV-infected persons is also a particular public health concern because HIV persons are at greater risk of developing multidrug-resistant tuberculosis. Multidrug-resistant tuberculosis is understandably difficult to treat and can be fatal (CDC 1999a, 1999b).

Reducing the spread of AIDS requires the understanding and acceptance of a variety of sexual issues, ranging from the likelihood that even heterosexual men may engage in anonymous homosexual intercourse to the difficulty that adolescents may have controlling their sexual urges. Prejudice against gays and lesbians is manifested as *homophobia*, a fear and/or hatred of these individuals. Homophobia explains the initial slow policy-related response to the HIV epidemic.

Unfortunately, testing for HIV may not limit its spread because many people who learn their HIV status do not change the behaviors that contribute to its spread. HIV has no cure, and current treatments do not affect the transmissibility of HIV.

Criminal law has also been used to contain the spread of HIV and to protect public health. For example, several laws nationwide require that those convicted of sex offenses be tested for HIV. Most of these laws, however, are disproportionately enforced against prostitutes. These laws suggest that those who test HIV-positive may receive greater prison sentences; however, it is questionable whether this type of punishment actually reduces the spread of HIV.

Health promotion efforts, including those used to reduce the transmission of HIV, are often hamstrung by psychosocial and other factors. For example, humans generally have difficulty changing their behaviors. Further, much human behavior is associated with functional needs (e.g., unsafe sex might fulfill a need for intimacy). The social learning theory explains that behavior change, first, requires knowledge, followed by a change of attitude or perspective.

Discrimination

HIV-positive people may experience discrimination in access to health care. The policies of various government agencies intended to help have also had a discriminatory impact on people with HIV/AIDS. For example, the Social Security Administration has not historically considered many of the HIV-related symptoms of women and IV drug users in adjudicating disability claims. Although the Department of Defense provides adequate medical care to individuals who acquire HIV in the military, recruits who test HIV-positive cannot join the military.

Provider Training

Knowledge about HIV and personal contact with people who have HIV has improved the attitudes of health care providers toward individuals with HIV and contributed to their willingness to care for people with HIV. Training should encompass not only medical and treatment-related information but also a range of competencies related to interpersonal skills.

In the area of psychosocial skills, the following characteristics are essential for an effectively trained provider: good communication skills (ability to establish rapport, ask questions, and listen), positive attitudes (respect, empowerment, trust), and an approach that incorporates principles of holistic care. In the area of cultural competence, essential elements include understanding of and respect for the person's specific culture; understanding that racial and ethnic minorities have important and multiple subdivisions or functional units; acknowledging the issues of gender and sexual orientation within the context of cultural competence; and respecting the customs, including modes of communication, of the person's culture. In the area of

substance abuse, the following key elements are essential for primary care providers: understanding the complex medical picture presented by a person who suffers both from HIV and addiction; understanding the complicated psychosocial, ethical, and legal issues related to care of addicted persons; and being aware of the personal attitudes about addiction that may impair the providers' ability to give care objectively and nonjudgmentally (e.g., in the administration of pain medication; Gross and Larkin 1996).

Cost of HIV/AIDS

Medical care for an HIV/AIDS patient is extremely expensive. Pharmaceutical companies claim that the high prices they charge for AIDS drugs are related to their extensive investment in research and development of drugs. Medicaid covers more than 220,000 people with HIV (Kaiser Family Foundation 2013b). In fiscal year (FY) 2012, combined federal and state Medicaid spending on HIV totaled $9.6 billion, making it the largest source of public financing for HIV/AIDS care in the United States. Of this, the federal share was $5.3 billion in FY 2012, or 55% of federal HIV care spending (Kaiser Family Foundation 2013b). Lack of insurance and underinsurance represent formidable financial barriers to HIV/AIDS care.

The US government also invests substantial amounts of money in research and development through research supported at NIH and CDC. Government programs spend money in several areas for HIV (**Figure 25-12**). Seventy-three percent of the cost is for antiretroviral medications, 13% for inpatient care, 9% for outpatient care, and 5% for other HIV-related medications and laboratory costs. For patients who initiate highly active antiretroviral therapy (HAART) when the CD4 cell count is 200/L, projected life expectancy is 22.5 years, discounted lifetime cost is $354,100 and undiscounted cost is $567,000 (Schackman et al. 2006). Indirect costs include lost productivity, largely because

FIGURE 25-12	US federal spending for HIV/AIDS by category, FY 2001 budget request.

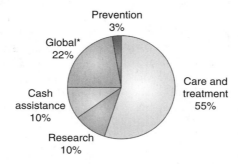

Prevention
3%

Global*
22%

Cash
assistance
10%

Research
10%

Care and
treatment
55%

*Categories may include funding across multiple
agencies/programs; global category includes
international HIV research at NIH.

Source: Adapted from Kaiser Family Foundation. *US Federal Funding for HIV/AIDS: The President's FY 2011 Budget Request.* HIV/AIDS Policy Fact Sheet, February 2010.

of worker morbidity and mortality. However, other factors affect cost projections associated with the HIV epidemic, including the level of employment of HIV-positive people; regional differences in the cost of care, which is often associated with the lack of subacute care in many parts of the country; and the rate at which HIV spreads.

Containment of escalating medical costs, including the coordination of medical care, is the objective of two HIV-specific efforts: the Medicaid waiver program and the Ryan White Comprehensive AIDS Resources Emergency (CARE) Act. Through the *Medicaid waiver program*, states may design packages of services to specific populations, such as elderly adults, persons with disabilities, and those who test positive for HIV. At this time, it is unknown whether the program is cost effective.

The passage of the Ryan White CARE Act in 1990 provided federal funds to develop treatment and care options for persons with HIV/AIDS (Summer 1991). Title II of this legislation is administered by states and has been used to establish HIV clinics and related services in areas lacking the resources needed to offer this specialty care. Some public health systems have used Ryan White money to provide HIV/AIDS services in rural communities in which poor or medically underserved persons lack access to adequate care. Federal spending for Ryan White was estimated to total $2.4 billion in 2012 (HRSA 2013a).

AIDS and the US Health Care System

The course of AIDS is characterized by a gradual decline in a patient's physical, cognitive, and emotional function and well-being. Such a comprehensive decline requires a continuum of care, including emergency care, primary care, housing and supervised living, mental health and social support, nonmedical services, and hospice care. The continuum can encompass elements like outreach and case finding, preventive services, outpatient and inpatient care, and coordination of private and public insurance benefits.

As HIV disease progresses, many persons become disabled and rely on public entitlement or private disability programs for income and health care benefits. These programs include Social Security Disability Income and Supplemental Security Income, administered by the Social Security Administration. Medicare and Medicaid become primary payers for health care because of the onset of disability and depletion of personal funds. Many HIV/AIDS patients are expected to gain health insurance under the ACA, which prohibits denial of health insurance because of preexisting medical conditions.

SUMMARY

This chapter examines the major characteristics of certain US population groups that face challenges and barriers in accessing health care services. These population groups are racial/ethnic minorities, children and women, those living in rural areas, those who are homeless, migrants, those who are mentally ill, and those with HIV/AIDS. The health needs of these population groups are summarized, and services available to them are described. The gaps that currently exist between these population groups and the rest of the population indicate that the nation must make significant efforts to address the unique health concerns of US subpopulations.

DISCUSSION QUESTIONS

1. How can the framework of vulnerability be used to study vulnerable populations in the United States?
2. What are the racial/ethnic minority categories in the United States?
3. Compared with White Americans, which health challenges do minorities face?
4. Who are the AA/PIs?
5. What is the Indian Health Service?
6. What are the health concerns of children?
7. Which childhood characteristics have important implications for health system design?
8. Which health services are currently available for children?
9. What are the health concerns of women?
10. What are the roles of the Office on Women's Health?
11. What are the challenges faced in rural health?
12. Which measures are being taken to improve access to care in rural areas?
13. What are the characteristics and health concerns of the homeless population?
14. How is mental health provided in the United States?
15. Who are the major mental health professionals?
16. How does AIDS affect different population groups in the United States?
17. Which services and policies are currently being used to combat AIDS in the United States?

REFERENCES

Aday, L.A. 1993. *At risk in America: The health and health care needs of vulnerable populations in the United States.* San Francisco, CA: Jossey-Bass.

Agency for Healthcare Research and Quality. 2010. Medical expenditure panel survey. Table 3: Total expenses and percent distribution for selected conditions by type of service: United States 2010. Available at: http://meps.ahrq.gov/data_stats/tables_compendia_hh_interactive.jsp?_SERVICE=MEPSSocket0&_PROGRAM=MEPSPGM.TC.SAS&File=HCFY2010&Table=HCFY2010_CNDXP_C&_Debug=. Accessed January 2014.

American Diabetes Association. 2008. Economic costs of diabetes in the U.S. in 2007. *Diabetes Care* 31, no. 3: 1–20.

Bertakis, K.D., et al. 2000. Gender differences in the utilization of health services. *Journal of Family Practice* 49: 147–152.

Brault, M. 2012. Americans with disabilities: 2010. Household economic studies. *Current Population Reports.* Available at: http://www.census.gov /prod/2012pubs/p70-131.pdf. Accessed September 2013.

Breakey, W.R., et al. (1989). Health and mental health problems of homeless men and women in Baltimore. *Journal of the American Medical Association* 262, no. 10: 1352–1357.

Burks, L.J. 1992. Community health representatives: The vital link in Native American health care. *The IHS Primary Care Provider 16*, no. 12: 186–190.

Centers for Disease Control and Prevention (CDC). 1995. *Facts about women and HIV/AIDS.* Atlanta, GA: CDC.

Centers for Disease Control and Prevention (CDC). 1999a. *CDC fact sheet: Recent HIV/AIDS treatment advances and the implications for prevention.* Available at: http://www.cdc.gov/nchstp/hiv_aids/pubs /facts.htm. Accessed December 2010.

Centers for Disease Control and Prevention (CDC). 1999b. *CDC fact sheet: The deadly intersection between TB and HIV.* Available at: http://www.thebody.com /content/art17109.html. Accessed October 13, 2014.

Centers for Disease Control and Prevention (CDC). 2008. *Cases of HIV infection and AIDS in urban and rural areas of the United States, 2006.* HIV/AIDS surveillance supplemental report: 13(2). Atlanta: US Department of Health and Human Services.

Centers for Disease Control and Prevention (CDC). 2010a. Vital signs: Health insurance coverage and health care utilization, United States, 2006–2009 and January–March 2010. *Morbidity and Mortality Weekly Report* 59: 1–7.

Centers for Disease Control and Prevention (CDC). 2010b. Current depression among adults—United States, 2006 and 2008. Available at: http://www .cdc.gov/mmwr/preview/mmwrhtml/mm5938a2 .htm?s_cid=mm5938a2_e%0d%0a. Accessed September 2013.

Centers for Disease Control and Prevention (CDC). 2010d. Mortality slide series. Available at: http:// www.cdc.gov/hiv/pdf/statistics_surveillance_ HIV_mortality.pdf. Accessed September 2013.

Centers for Disease Control and Prevention (CDC). 2010e. National Center for Injury Prevention and Control (NCIP). Web-based injury statistics query and reporting system (WISQARS). Available at: http://www.cdc.gov/injury/wisqars/index.html. Accessed September 2013.

Centers for Disease Control and Prevention (CDC). 2011a. Health insurance coverage: Early release of estimates from the National Health Interview Survey, January–March 2011. Available at: http://www.cdc.gov/nchs/data/nhis/earlyrelease /insur201109.htm. Accessed September 2013.

Centers for Disease Control and Prevention (CDC). 2011b. *HIV surveillance report: diagnoses of HIV infection and AIDS in the United States and dependent areas, 2011.* Vol. 23. Atlanta, GA: US Department of Health and Human Services.

Centers for Disease Control and Prevention (CDC). 2012a. Deaths: Leading causes for 2009. *National Vital Statistics Reports* 61, no. 7.

Centers for Disease Control and Prevention (CDC). 2012b. Youth Risk Behavior Surveillance—United States, 2011. *Morbidity and Mortality Weekly Report* 61: SS-4.

Centers for Disease Control and Prevention (CDC). 2012c. HIV surveillance by race/ethnicity. Available at: http://www.cdc.gov/hiv/pdf/statistics_ surveillance_raceEthnicity.pdf. Accessed September 2013.

Centers for Disease Control and Prevention (CDC). 2012d. HIV among pregnant women, infants, and children in the United States. Fact Sheet. Available at: http://www.cdc.gov/hiv/pdf/risk_WIC .pdf. Accessed September 2013.

Centers for Disease Control and Prevention (CDC). 2012e. Estimated HIV incidence among adults and adolescents in the United States, 2007–2010. *HIV Surveillance Supplemental Report 2012* 17, no. 4.

Centers for Disease Control and Prevention (CDC). 2013a. *HIV/AIDS surveillance report, 2011.* Vol. 23. Available at: http://www.cdc.gov/hiv/library /reports/surveillance/2011/surveillance_Report_ vol_23.html. Accessed September 2013.

Centers for Disease Control and Prevention (CDC). 2013b. HIV among women. Fact Sheet. Available at: http://www.cdc.gov/hiv/pdf/risk_women.pdf. Accessed September 2013.

Centers for Disease Control and Prevention (CDC). 2013c. HIV infection among heterosexuals at increased risk—United States, 2010. *Morbidity and Mortality Weekly Report* 62, no. 10: 183–188.

Centers for Disease Control and Prevention (CDC). 2013d. Social determinants of health among adults with diagnosed HIV infection in 18 areas, 2005– 2009. *HIV Surveillance Supplemental Report* 18, no. 4.

Congressional Budget Office. 2012. *Updated estimates for the insurance coverage provisions of the Affordable Care Act.* Washington, DC: Government Printing Office.

Cooper, E.R., et al. 2000. Combination antiretroviral strategies for the treatment of pregnant HIV-1-infected women and prevention of perinatal HIV-1 transmission. *Journal of Acquired Immune Deficiency Syndromes* 29, no. 5: 484–494.

Finkelstein, E.A., et al. 2009. Annual medical spending attributable to obesity: Payer-and service-specific estimates. *Health Affairs* 28, no. 5: w822–w831.

General Accounting Office. 2000. Oral health: Dental disease is a chronic problem among low-income populations. Report GAO/HEHS-00-72. Available at: http://www.gao.gov/products/GAO/HEHS-00-72. Accessed January 2014.

Gift, H.C., et al. 1992. The social impact of dental problems and visits. *American Journal of Public Health* 82: 1663–1668.

Greene, J. 1976. The health professions educational assistance act if 1976: a new prescription? *Fordham Urban Law Journal* 5, no. 2: 279–302. Available at: http://ir.lawnet.fordham.edu/cgi/viewcontent.cgi?article=1485&context=ul. Accessed January 2015.

Gross, E.J., and M.H. Larkin. 1996. The child with HIV in day care and school. *Nursing Clinics of North America* 31, no. 1: 231–241.

Guttmacher Institute. 2013. Insurance coverage of contraceptives. Available at: http://www.guttmacher.org/statecenter/spibs/spib_ICC.pdf. Accessed September 2013.

Health Care for the Homeless. 2012. Client demographics. Available at: http://www.hchmd.org/demographics.shtml. Accessed September 2013.

Health Resources and Services Administration (HRSA). 2013a. HIV/AIDS Bureau. FY2010–FY2013 appropriations by program. Available at: http://hab.hrsa.gov/data/reports/funding.html. Accessed September 2013.

Health Resources and Services Administration (HRSA). 2013b. Shortage designation: Health professional shortage areas and medically underserved areas/populations. Available at: http://www.hrsa.gov/shortage/. Accessed September 2013.

Health Resources and Services Administration (HRSA), Bureau of Health Professions. 2013. Mental Health HPSA Designation Criteria. Available at: http://bhpr.hrsa.gov/shortage/hpsas/designationcriteria/mentalhealthhpsacriteria.html. Accessed September 2013.

Health Resources and Services Administration (HRSA), Bureau of Health Professions. 2014. Shortage designation: health professional shortage areas & medically underserved areas/populations. Available at: http://www.hrsa.gov/shortage/. Accessed January 2014.

Health Resources and Services Administration (HRSA), Bureau of Primary Health Care. 2012a. 2011 National Migrant Health Data. Available at: http://bphc.hrsa.gov/uds/view.aspx?fd=mh&year=2011. Accessed September 2013.

Health Resources and Services Administration (HRSA), Bureau of Primary Health Care. 2012b. Special Populations. Available at: http://bphc.hrsa.gov/about/specialpopulations/. Accessed September 2013.

Health Resources and Services Administration (HRSA), Maternal and Child Health Bureau. 2005. *The National Survey of Children's Health 2003.* Rockville, MD: US Department of Health and Human Services.

Health Resources and Services Administration (HRSA), Maternal and Child Health Bureau. 2011. *Women's Health USA 2011.* Rockville, MD: US Department of Health and Human Services.

Health Resources and Services Administration (HRSA), National Health Service Corps. 2013. About the NHSC. Available at: http://nhsc.hrsa.gov/corpsexperience/aboutus/index.html. Accessed September 2013.

Health Resources and Services Administration (HRSA), Office of Rural Health Policy. 2007. The 2007 report to the secretary: Rural health and human services issues: The national advisory committee on rural health and human services. Available at: http://www.hrsa.gov/advisorycommittees/rural/2007secreport.pdf

Herzog, D.B., and P.N. Copeland. 1985. Medical progress: Eating disorders. *New England Journal of Medicine* 313, no. 5: 295–303.

Ikeda, J. 1990. *Food Habits of Farmworker Families. Tulare County. California. 1989.* Visalia: University of California Cooperative Extension Service.

Indian Health Service (IHS). 1999a. *Fact sheet: Comprehensive health care program for American Indians and Alaskan Natives.* Washington, DC: Public Health Service.

Indian Health Service (IHS). 1999b. *A quick look.* Washington, DC: Public Health Service.

Indian Health Service (IHS). 2009. *Trends in Indian health, 2002–2003 edition.* Washington, DC: Government Printing Office.

Indian Health Service (IHS). 2010a. *Indian health disparities*. IHS fact sheet. Washington, DC: Public Health Service.

Indian Health Service (IHS). 2010b. *IHS year 2010 profile*. IHS fact sheet. Washington, DC: Public Health Service.

Indian Health Service (IHS). 2013. Agency Overview. Available at: http://www.ihs.gov/aboutihs /overview/. Accessed September 2013.

Institute for Children, Poverty & Homelessness. 2011. *Profiles of risk: Education*. Research Brief No. 2. Available at: http://www.icphusa.org /PDF/reports/ICPH_FamiliesAtRisk_No.2.pdf. Accessed September 2013.

Jasinski, J.L. 2005. *The experience of violence in the lives of homeless women: A research report*. Available at: https://www.ncjrs.gov/pdffiles1/nij /grants/211976.pdf. Accessed January 2014.

Kaiser Commission on Medicaid and the Uninsured (Kaiser). 2012a. *The uninsured and the difference health insurance makes*. Washington, DC: Kaiser Commission on Medicaid and the Uninsured.

Kaiser Commission on Medicaid and the Uninsured (Kaiser). 2012b. *The uninsured: A primer*. Washington, DC: Kaiser Commission on Medicaid and the Uninsured.

Kaiser Family Foundation. 2013a. *Health reform: Implications for women's access to coverage and care*. Available at: http://kaiserfamilyfoundation.files .wordpress.com/2012/03/7987-03-health-reform -implications-for-women_s-access-to-coverage -and-care.pdf. Accessed September 2013.

Kaiser Family Foundation. 2013b. Medicaid enrollment and spending on HIV/AIDS. Available at: http://kff .org/hivaids/state-indicator/enrollment-spending- on-hiv-fy2009/#notes. Accessed September 2013.

Kaiser Family Foundation. 2013c. Mental health care health profession shortage areas (HPSAs). Available at: http://kff.org/other/state-indicator /mental-health-care-health-professional-shortage- areas-hpsas/. Accessed September 2013.

Kerker, B.D., et al. 2011. A population-based assessment of the health of homeless families in New York City, 2001–2003. *American Journal of Public Health* 101, no. 3: 546–553.

Kessler, R.C., et al. 2005. Prevalence, severity, and comorbidity of twelve-month *DSM-IV* disorders in the National Comorbidity Survey Replication (NCS-R). *Archives of General Psychiatry* 62, no. 6: 617–627.

Kraus, L.E., et al. 1996. *Chartbook on disability in the United States, 1996. An InfoUse Report*. Washington, DC: US National Institute on Disability and Rehabilitation Research.

Kung, H.C., et al. 2008. Deaths: Final data for 2005. *National Vital Statistics Reports*. 56, no. 10.

Lam, N., and K. Liu. 1994. Spread of AIDS in rural America, 1982–1990. *Journal of Acquired Immune Deficiency Syndrome* 7, no. 5: 485–490.

Larson, A., and L. Plascencia. 1993. *Migrant enumeration study*. Washington, DC: Office of Minority Health.

Larson, S. L., and J.A. Fleishman. (2003). Rural-urban differences in usual source of care and ambulatory service use: Analyses of national data using Urban Influence Codes. *Medical care*, III65–III74.

Lloyd-Jones, D., et al. 2009. American Heart Association Statistics Committee and Stroke Statistics Subcommittee. Heart disease and stroke statistics—2009 update: A report from the American Heart Association Statistics Committee and Stroke Statistics Subcommittee. *Circulation* 119: e21–181.

Manderscheid RW, and J.T. Berry, eds. *Mental Health, United States, 2004*. Rockville, MD: US Department of Health and Human Services, Substance Abuse and Mental Health Services Administration, Center for Mental Health Services.

McCurdy, S.A., et al. 1997. Tuberculin reactivity among California Hispanic migrant farm workers. *American Journal of Industrial Medicine* 32, no. 6: 600–505

McGrath, J., et al. 2008. Schizophrenia: A concise overview of incidence, prevalence, and mortality. *Epidemiologic Review*, no. 1: 67–76.

McLean, C.P., et al. 2011. Gender differences in anxiety disorders: Prevalence, course of illness, comorbidity and burden of illness, *Journal of Psychiatric Research* 45, no. 8: 1027–1035.

Merson, M.H. 1996. Returning home: Reflections on the USA's response to the HIV/AIDS epidemic. *Lancet* 347, no. 9016: 1673–1676.

Migrant Health Promotion. 2014. Farmworkers in the United States. Available at: http://mhpsalud.org /who-we-serve/farmworkers-in-the-united-states. Accessed January 2015.

Misra, D., ed. 2001. *Women's health data book: A profile of women's health in the United States*, 3rd ed. Washington, DC: Jacobs Institute of Women's Health and the Henry J. Kaiser Family Foundation.

Nardin, R., et al. 2013. The uninsured after implementation of the Affordable Care Act: A demographic and geographic analysis. Health Affairs Blog. Available at: http://healthaffairs.org/blog/2013/06/06/the-uninsured-after-implementation-of-the-affordable-care-act-a-demographic-and-geographic-analysis/. Accessed September 2013.

National Alliance to End Homelessness. 2012. *The state of homelessness in America 2012. Homelessness Research Institute*. Available at: http://msnbcmedia.msn.com/i/MSNBC/Sections/NEWS/z-pdf-archive/homeless.pdf. Accessed September 2013.

National Association of Rural Health Clinics (NARHC). 2007. About us. Available at: http://narhc.org/?page_id=1410. Accessed January 2014.

National Center for Chronic Disease Prevention and Health Promotion. 2010. *The power of prevention: Chronic disease ... the public health challenge of the 21st century*. Available at: http://www.cdc.gov/chronicdisease/pdf/2009-Power-of-Prevention.pdf. Accessed January 2011.

National Center for Health Statistics (NCHS). 2010. *Health, United States, 2009*. Hyattsville, MD: Department of Health and Human Services.

National Center for Health Statistics (NCHS). 2011. *Health, United States, 2010*. Hyattsville, MD: Department of Health and Human Services.

National Center for Health Statistics (NCHS). 2012. *Health, United States, 2011*. Hyattsville, MD: Department of Health and Human Services.

National Center for Health Statistics (NCHS). 2013. *Health, United States, 2012*. Hyattsville, MD: Department of Health and Human Services.

National Institutes of Health (NIH). 2002. NHLBI stops trial of estrogen plus progestin due to increased breast cancer risk, lack of overall benefit. News release. Available at: http://www.nhlbi.nih.gov/news/press-releases/2002/nhlbi-stops-trial-of-estrogen-plus-progestin-due-to-increased-breast-cancer-risk-lack-of-overall-benefit.html. Accessed December 2006.

National Institutes of Health (NIH). 2012. *Guidelines for the use of antiretroviral agents in HIV-1-infected adults and adolescents*. Department of Health and Human Services. Available at: http://aidsinfo.nih.gov/contentfiles/lvguidelines/AdultandAdolescentGL.pdf. Accessed September 2013.

National Law Center on Homelessness and Poverty. 2004. *Homelessness in the United States and the Human Right to Housing*. Available at: http://www.mplp.org/Resources/mplpresource.2006-06-13.0349156065/file0. Accessed January 2015.

National Women's Law Center. 2011. Closing the wage gap is especially important for women of color in difficult times. Available at: http://www.nwlc.org/resource/closing-wage-gap-especially-important-women-color-difficult-times. Accessed September 2013.

Newcomer, R., T. Kang, M. LaPlante, and S. Kaye. (2005). Living quarters and unmet need for personal care assistance among adults with disabilities. *Journals of Gerontology Series B: Psychological Sciences and Social Sciences* 9, no. 4: S205–S213.

O'Neill, J.E., and D.M. O'Neill. 2009. *Who are the uninsured? An analysis of America's uninsured population, their characteristics and their health*. New York, NY: Employment Policies Institute.

Organista, K.C., and P.B. Organista. 1997. Migrant laborers and AIDS in the United States: A review of the literature. *AIDS Education and Prevention* 9, no.1: 83–93.

Ostir, G.V., et al. 1999. Disability in older adults 1: Prevalence, causes, and consequences. *Behavioral Medicine* 24: 147–154.

Patton, L., and D. Puskin. 1990. *Ensuring access to health care services in rural areas: A half century of federal policy*. Washington, DC: Essential Health Care Services Conference Center at Georgetown University Conference Center.

Regier, D.A., et al. 1988. One month prevalence of mental disorders in the United States: Based on five epidemiologic catchment area sites. *Archives of General Psychiatry* 45, no. 11: 977–986.

Regier, D.A., W.E. Narrow, and D.S. Rae. 1993. The de facto mental and addictive disorders service system. Epidemiologic catchment area prospective 1-year prevalence rates of disorders and services. *Archives of General Psychiatry* 50, no. 2: 85–94.

Rosenbaum, S., and P. Shin. 2005. *Migrant and seasonal farmworkers: Health insurance coverage and access to care*. Kaiser Commission on Medicaid and the Uninsured. Available at: http://kaiserfamilyfoundation.files.wordpress.com/2013/01/migrant-and-seasonal-farmworkers-health-insurance-coverage-and-access-to-care-report.pdf. Accessed September 2013.

Rust, G.S. (1990). Health status of migrant farmworkers: A literature review and commentary. *American Journal of Public Health* 80, no. 10: 1213–1217.

Salganicoff, A., et al. 2005. *Women and health care: A national profile*. Menlo Park, CA: Henry J. Kaiser Family Foundation.

Schackman, B.R., et al. 2006. The lifetime cost of current human immunodeficiency virus care in the United States. *Medical Care* 44, no. 11: 990–997.

Schutt, R.K., and S.M. Goldfinger. 1996. Housing preferences and perceptions of health and functioning among homeless mentally ill persons. *Psychiatric Services* 47, no. 4: 381–386.

Sechzer, J.A., et al. 1996. *Women and mental health.* New York, NY: Academy of Sciences.

Sheller, B., et al. 1997. Diagnosis and treatment of dental caries–related emergencies in a children's hospital. *Pediatric Dentistry* 19: 470–475.

Shi, L., and G. Stevens. 2010. *Vulnerable Populations in the United States.* 2nd ed. San Francisco, CA: Jossey-Bass.

Shortell, S.M., et al. 1996. *Remaking health care in America.* San Francisco, CA: Jossey-Bass.

Solis, J.M., et al. 1990. Acculturation, access to care, and use of preventive services by Hispanics: Findings from HHANES 1982–84. *American Journal of Public Health* 80 (Suppl): 11–19.

Substance Abuse and Mental Health Services Administration (SAMHSA). 2012a. *Mental health, United States, 2010.* HHS Publication No. (SMA) 12-4681. Rockville, MD: Substance Abuse and Mental Health Services Administration.

Substance Abuse and Mental Health Services Administration (SAMHSA). 2012b. *Results from the 2011 National Survey on Drug Use and Health: Mental health findings.* NSDUH Series H-45, HHS Publication No. (SMA) 12-4725. Rockville, MD: Substance Abuse and Mental Health Services Administration.

Summer, L. 1991. *Limited access: Health care for the rural poor.* Washington, DC: Center on Budget and Policy Priorities.

UNAIDS. 2010. *UNAIDS report on the global AIDS epidemic 2010.* Available at: http://www.unaids.org/globalreport/Global_report.htm. Accessed December 2010.

United Nations (UN). 2013. *The state of the world's children 2013.* Available at: http://www.unicef.org/sowc2013/report.html. Accessed September 2013.

United States Conference of Mayors. 2011. *Hunger and homelessness survey.* Available at: http://usmayors.org/pressreleases/uploads/2011-hhreport.pdf. Accessed September 2013.

US Bureau of Labor Statistics (BLS). 2012. *Labor force characteristics by race and ethnicity, 2011.* Washington, DC: Government Printing Office.

US Census Bureau. 2009. *The 2010 census questionnaire: Informational copy.* Available at: https://www.census.gov/2010census/pdf/2010_Questionnaire_Info.pdf. Accessed January 2015.

US Census Bureau. 2010a. *2010 Census. Profile of general population and housing characteristics.* Washington, DC: Government Printing Office.

US Census Bureau. 2010b. *Current population survey, 2010 annual social and economic supplement.* Washington, DC: Government Printing Office.

US Census Bureau. 2010c. *2007–2009 American Community Survey, 3-year estimates.* Washington, DC: Government Printing Office.

US Census Bureau. 2011a. *Overview of race and Hispanic origin: 2010.* Washington, DC: Government Printing Office.

US Census Bureau. 2011b. *The Hispanic population: 2010.* 2010 Census Briefs. Washington, DC: Government Printing Office.

US Census Bureau. 2011c. *Income, poverty, and health insurance coverage in the United States: 2010.* Washington, DC: Government Printing Office.

US Census Bureau. 2011d. *The American Indian and Alaska Native population: 2010.* 2010 Census Briefs. Washington, DC: Government Printing Office.

US Census Bureau. 2011e. *Current population survey annual social and economic supplements.* Washington, DC: Government Printing Office.

US Census Bureau. 2011f. American Community Survey, American FactFinder, Table B18135. Available at: http://factfinder2.census.gov. Accessed September 2013.

US Census Bureau. 2012. *Statistical Abstract of the United States: 2012.* Washington, DC: Government Printing Office.

US Department of Health and Human Services. 2001. *Mental health: Culture, race, and ethnicity—a supplement to mental health: A report of the Surgeon General.* Rockville, MD: US Department of Health and Human Services, Substance Abuse and Mental Health Services Administration, Center for Mental Health Services.

US Department of Housing and Urban Development (HUD). 2012. *The 2011 Annual Homeless Assessment Report to Congress.* Available at: https://www.onecpd.info/resources/documents/2011AHAR_FinalReport.pdf. Accessed September 2013.

US Department of Labor. 2011. *Changing characteristics of US farm workers: 21 years of findings from the National Agricultural Workers Survey*. Available at: http://migrationfiles.ucdavis.edu/uploads/cf /files/2011-may/carroll-changing-characteristics .pdf. Accessed September 2013.

US Department of Veteran Affairs. 2014. *Fact sheet: VA programs for homeless veterans*. Available at: http:// www.va.gov/HOMELESS/for_homeless_veterans .asp. Accessed November 2014.

US Public Health Service. 2000. *Report of the Surgeon General's Conference on Children's Mental Health: A National Action Agenda*. Washington, DC: Department of Health and Human Services.

Villarejo, D., et al. 2000. *Suffering in silence: A report on the health of California's agricultural workers*. Davis: California Institute of Rural Study, California Endowment.

Villarino, M.E., et al. 1994. Purified protein derivative tuberculin and delayed-type hypersensitivity skin testing in migrant farm workers at risk for tuberculosis and HIV coinfection. *AIDS* 8, no. 4: 477–481.

Ward, B.W., and J.S. Schiller. 2013. Prevalence of multiple chronic conditions among US adults: Estimates from the National Health Interview Survey, 2010. Available at: http://www.cdc .gov/pcd/issues/2013/12_0203.htm. Accessed September 2013.

Wenzel, M. 1996. A school-based clinic for elementary school in Phoenix, Arizona. *Journal of School Health* 66, no. 4: 125–127.

Witters, D., and S. Agrawal. 2011. Unhealthy US workers' absenteeism costs $153 billion. Available at: http://www.gallup.com/poll/150026 /unhealthy-workers-absenteeism-costs-153 -billion.aspx. Accessed January 2014.

World Health Organization (WHO). 2004. *Antiretroviral drugs for treating pregnant women and preventing HIV infection in infants. Guidelines on care, treatment and support for women living with HIV/AIDS and their children in resource-constrained settings*. Available at: http://www.who.int/hiv/pub/mtct/en/arvdrugs womenguidelinesfinal.pdf. Accessed September 2013.

World Health Organization (WHO). 2012. Years lived with disability (YLDs) for 1160 sequelae of 289 diseases and injuries 1990–2010: A systematic analysis for the Global Burden of Disease Study 2010. *Lancet* 380: 2163–2196.

Yu, S.M., et al. 2004. Health status and health services utilization among US Chinese, Asian Indian, Filipino, and other Asian/Pacific Islander children. *Pediatrics* 113, no. 1 part 1: 101–107.

CHAPTER 26

Introduction to Ethics

George D. Pozgar

I expect to pass through this world but once. Any good therefore that I can do, or any kindness I can show to any creature, let me do it now. Let me not defer it, for I shall not pass this way again.

—STEPHEN GRELLET

CHAPTER OBJECTIVES

1. Explain what ethics is, its importance, and its application to ethical dilemmas.

2. Describe the concepts of morality, codes of conduct, and moral judgments.

3. Understand relevant ethical theories and principles.

4. Describe virtue ethics and values and how they more clearly describe one's moral character.

5. Understand how religious ethics can affect one's moral character.

6. Explain the concept of situational ethics and how changes in circumstances can alter one's behavior.

7. Understand the importance of reasoning in the decision-making process.

INTRODUCTION

Good can triumph over evil.

—*Author Unknown*

This chapter provides the reader with an overview of ethics, moral principles, virtues, and values. The intent here is not to burden the reader with the philosophical arguments surrounding ethical theories, morals, and principles; however, as with the study of any new subject, "words are the tools of thought." The reader who thoroughly absorbs and applies the content of the theories and principles of ethics discussed herein will have the tools necessary to empathize with and guide patients through the conflicts they will face when making difficult care decisions. Therefore, some new vocabulary is a necessary tool, as a building block for the reader to establish a foundation for applying the abstract theories and principles of ethics in order to make practical use of them.

Theories, principles, virtues, and values are a necessary beginning point for the study of ethics. Words are merely labels for ideas and best used for helping the reader to wire his or her mind to think through difficult dilemmas more easily. The directions on a map are of little value until we make the journey. So it is with ethics; we must begin to make the journey inward with a lot of hard mind work so that we can more easily make the right decisions when faced with ethical dilemmas. The learning process for ethics becomes a more enjoyable and rewarding journey as we grasp the ideas, build upon them, and practice all the good we learn by helping all the people we can as long as we can.

ETHICS

How we perceive right and wrong is influenced by what we feed on.

—*Author Unknown*

Ethics is the branch of philosophy that seeks to understand the nature, purposes, justification, and founding principles of moral rules and the systems they comprise. Ethics and morals are derivatives from the Greek and Latin terms (roots) for custom. The etymology of the words ethics and morality are derived from the roots ethos and mos, which both convey a meaning describing customs or habits. This etymology supports the claims of anthropologist Ruth Benedict that all values are rooted in customs and habits of a culture because the words moral and ethics themselves were essentially created to describe these topics.[1]

Ethics deals with values relating to human conduct. It focuses on the rightness and wrongness of actions, as well as the goodness and badness of motives and ends. Ethics encompasses the decision-making process of determining ultimate actions—what should I do and is it the right thing to do. It involves how individuals decide to live with one another within accepted boundaries and how they live in harmony with the environment as well as one another. Ethics is concerned with human conduct as it ought to be, as opposed to what it actually is.

Microethics involves an individual's view of what is right and wrong based on one's personal life teachings, tradition, and experiences. *Macroethics* involves a more global view of right and wrong. Although no person lives in a vacuum, solving ethical dilemmas involves consideration of ethical issues from both a micro and macro perspective.

Man's duty is to improve himself; to cultivate his mind; and, when he finds himself going astray, to bring the moral law to bear upon himself.

—*Immanuel Kant*

The term *ethics* is used in three distinct but related ways, signifying (1) *philosophical ethics*, which involves inquiry about ways of life and rules of conduct; (2) a *general pattern or way of life*, such as religious ethics (e.g., Judeo-Christian ethics); and (3) a *set of rules* of conduct or "moral code" (e.g., professional codes for ethical behavior).

The scope of health care ethics encompasses numerous issues, including the right to choose or refuse treatment and the right to limit the suffering one will endure. Incredible advances in technology and the resulting capability to extend life beyond what would be considered a reasonable quality of life have complicated the process of health care decision making. The scope of health care ethics is not limited to philosophical issues but embraces economic, medical, political, social, and legal dilemmas.

Bioethics addresses such difficult issues as the nature of life, the nature of death, what sort of life is worth living, what constitutes murder, how we should treat people who are especially vulnerable, and the responsibilities that we have to other human beings. It is about making better decisions when faced with diverse and complex circumstances.

Why Study Ethics?

We study ethics to help us make sound judgments, good decisions, and right choices; if not right choices, then better choices. To those in the health care industry, it is about anticipating and recognizing health care dilemmas and making good judgments and decisions based on universal values that work in unison with the laws of the land and our constitution. Where the law remains silent, we rely on the ability of caregivers to make sound judgments, guided by the Wisdom of Solomon to do good. Doing the right thing by applying the universal morals and values described in this text (e.g., the 10 Commandments) will help shield and protect all from harm.

MORALITY

The three hardest tasks in the world are neither physical feats nor intellectual achievements, but moral acts: to return love for hate, to include the excluded, and to say, "I was wrong."

—*Sydney J. Harris*

The following news clippings portray how a deficiency in the morality of society can lead to a betrayal of humanity. Lawlessness and heartless actions run rampant in a land void of courage and compassion. The reader who thoroughly absorbs, understands, and practices the virtues and values discussed in the pages that follow will spring forth hope in what often seems a desperate and hopeless world.

Trek of tears describes many horrible historic events, from broken treaties with American Indians to an African Journey of horror, where people would flee together as a village to escape the barbaric slaughter of men, women, and children as the remainder of the world stood cowardly by watching the death and starvation of hundreds of thousands of people. Human atrocities committed by humans. Is it not time to stand up and be counted on to do what is right and leave all excuses behind for our complacency toward the genocide that continues throughout the world?

—*GP*

There are those who have been brainwashed into believing, in the name of religion, that if they blow themselves up in public places, killing innocent people, that they will be rewarded in the afterlife. This is not religion and it is not culture; it is evil people brainwashing young minds to do evil things.

—*GP*

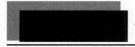

Vietnam—Terror of War

Fire rained down on civilians. Women and children ran screaming. Ut snapped pictures. A little girl ran toward him, arms outstretched, eyes shut in pain, clothes burned off by Napalm. She said, "Too hot, please help me!"

1973 Spot News, Newseum, *Washington, DC*

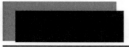

Ethiopian Famine (1985 Feature)

People searched everywhere for food. Some 30,000 tons of it, from the United States, had been held up by an Ethiopian government determined to starve the countryside into submission. And starve the people it did—half a million Ethiopians, many of them children so hungry their bodies actually consumed themselves.

I'll never forget the sounds of kids dying of starvation.

Newseum, *Washington, DC*

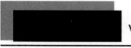

Waiting Game for Sudanese Child ...

Carter's winning photo shows a heartbreaking scene of a starving child collapsed on the ground, struggling to get to a food center during a famine in the Sudan in 1993. In the background, a vulture stalks the emaciated child.

Carter was part of a group of four fearless photojournalists known as the "Bang Bang Club" who traveled throughout South Africa capturing the atrocities committed during apartheid.

Haunted by the horrific images from Sudan, Carter committed suicide in 1994 soon after receiving the award.

A Pulitzer-Winning Photographer's Suicide, National Public Radio (NPR), *March 2, 2006*

Aim above morality. Be not simply good; be good for something.

—Henry David Thoreau

Morality describes a class of rules held by society to govern the conduct of its individual members. It implies the quality of being in accord with standards of right and good conduct. Morality is a code of conduct. It is a guide to behavior that all rational persons should put forward for governing their behavior. Morality requires us to reach a decision as to the rightness or wrongness of an action. *Morals* are ideas about what is right and what is wrong; for example, killing is wrong, whereas helping the poor is right, and causing pain is wrong, whereas easing pain is right. Morals are deeply ingrained in culture and religion and are often part of its identity. Morals should not be confused with religious or cultural habits or customs, such as wearing a religious garment (e.g., veil, turban). That which is considered morally right can vary from nation to nation, culture to culture, and religion to religion. In other words, there is no universal morality that is recognized by all people in all cultures at all times.

Code of Conduct

A *code of conduct* generally prescribes standards of conduct, states principles expressing responsibilities, and defines the rules expressing duties of professionals to whom they apply. Most members of a profession subscribe to certain "values" and moral standards written into a formal document called a code of ethics. Codes of conduct often require interpretation by caregivers as they apply to the specific circumstances surrounding each dilemma.

Michael D. Bayles, a famous author and teacher, describes the differences between standards, principles, and rules:

- *Standards* (e.g., honesty, respect for others, conscientiousness) are used to guide human conduct by stating desirable traits to be exhibited and undesirable ones (dishonesty, deceitfulness, self-interest) to be avoided.
- *Principles* describe responsibilities that do not specify what the required conduct should be. Professionals need to make a judgment about what is desirable in a particular situation based on accepted principles.
- *Rules* specify specific conduct; they do not allow for individual professional judgment.

Moral Judgments

Moral judgments are those judgments concerned with what an individual or group believes to be the right or proper behavior in a given situation. Making a moral judgment is being able to choose an option from among choices. It involves assessing another person's moral character based on how he or she conforms to the moral convictions established by the individual and/or group. A lack of conformity can result in moral disapproval and possibly ridicule of one's character.

Morality Legislated

When it is important that disagreements be settled, morality is often legislated. Law is distinguished from morality by having explicit rules and penalties, as well as officials who interpret the laws and apply penalties when laws are broken. There is often considerable overlap in the conduct governed by morality and that governed by law. Laws are created to set boundaries for societal behavior. They are enforced to ensure that the expected behavior happens.

Moral Dilemmas

Moral dilemmas in the health care setting often arise when values, rights, duties, and loyalties conflict. Caregivers often find that there appears to be no right or wrong answer when faced with the daunting task of deciding which decision path to follow. The best answer when attempting to resolve an ethical dilemma includes the known wishes of the patient and other pertinent information, such as a living will, that might be available when the patient is considered incompetent to make his or her own choices. The right answer is often elusive when the patient is in a coma and there are no known documents as to a patient's wishes and there are no living relatives. However, an understanding of the concepts presented here will help the caregiver in resolving complex ethical dilemmas.

ETHICAL THEORIES

> Ethics, too, are nothing but reverence for life. This is what gives me the fundamental principle of morality, namely, that good consists in maintaining, promoting, and enhancing life, and that destroying, injuring, and limiting life are evil.
>
> —*Albert Schweitzer*

Ethics seeks to understand and to determine how human actions can be judged as right or wrong. Ethical judgments can be made based on our own experiences or based upon the nature of or principles of reason.

Ethical theories and principles introduce order into the way people think about life. They are the foundations of ethical analysis and provide guidance in the decision-making process. Various theories present varying viewpoints that assist caregivers in making difficult decisions when faced with ethical dilemmas that affect the lives of others. The more commonly discussed ethical theories are presented here.

Metaethics is the study of the origin and meaning of ethical concepts. Metaethics seeks to understand ethical terms and theories and their application. "Metaethics explores as well the connection between values, reasons for action, and human motivation, asking how it is that moral standards might provide us with reasons to do or refrain from doing as it demands, and it addresses many of the issues commonly bound up with the nature of freedom and its significance (or not) for moral responsibility."[2]

Normative Ethics

Normative ethics is prescriptive in that it attempts to determine what moral standards should be followed so that human behavior and conduct may be morally right. Normative ethics is primarily concerned with establishing standards or norms for conduct and is commonly associated with investigating how one ought to act. It involves the critical study of major moral precepts, such as what things are right, what things are good, and what things are genuine. One of the central questions of modern normative ethics is whether human actions are to be judged right or wrong solely according to their consequences.

The determination of a universal moral principle for all humanity is a formidable task and most likely not feasible due to the diversity of people and their cultures. However, there is a need to have a commonly held consensus as to right and wrong to avoid chaos. Thus, there are generally accepted moral standards around which laws are drafted.

Normative Ethics and Assisted Suicide

Oregon's Death with Dignity Act of 1997 allows terminally ill state residents to end their lives through the voluntary self-administration of a lethal dose of medications prescribed by a physician.[3] Although this act was voted upon by the Oregon state legislature and agreed upon by referendum, there are those who disagree with the law from a religious or moral standpoint. The Oregon act is controversial at best and has placed morality and the law in conflict. In the middle of the continuing controversy is the terminally ill patient who must make the ultimate decision of life versus death. It could be argued that it is morally wrong to take one's own life regardless of the law or it can be argued that ending one's life is a morally permissible right because the law provides the opportunity for terminally ill patients to make end-of-life decisions that include the right to self-administer a lethal dose of medications.

As there is a diversity of cultures, there is diversity of opinions as to the rightness and wrongness of the Oregon act. From a microethics point of view as it relates to the Oregon law, each individual must decide what is the right thing to do.

Normative ethics prescribes how people should act and descriptive ethics describes how people act. Both theories have application in the Oregon act. The controversial nature of physician-assisted suicide in the various states is but one of many health care dilemmas caregivers will experience during their careers (e.g., abortion, euthanasia).

Descriptive Ethics

Descriptive ethics, also known as comparative ethics, is the study of what people believe to be right and wrong and why they believe it. Descriptive ethics describes how people act, whereas normative ethics prescribes how people ought to act.

Applied Ethics

Applied ethics is "the philosophical search (within western philosophy) for right and wrong within controversial scenarios."[4] *Applied ethics* is the application of normative theories to practical moral problems, such as abortion, euthanasia, and assisted suicide.

Consequential Ethics

> The end excuses any evil.
>
> *–Sophocles, Electra (c. 409 B.C.)*

The *consequential theory* of ethics emphasizes that the morally right action is whatever action leads to the maximum balance of good over evil. From a contemporary standpoint, theories that judge actions by their consequences have been referred to as consequential ethics. Consequential ethical theories revolve around the premise that the rightness or wrongness of an action depends on the consequences or effects of an action. The theory of consequential ethics is based on the view that the value of an action derives solely from the value of its consequences. The consequentialist considers the morally right act or failure to act is one that will produce a good outcome. The goal of a

consequentialist is to achieve the greatest good for the greatest number. It involves asking such questions as:

- What will be the effects of each course of action?
- Who will benefit?
- What action will cause the least harm?
- What action will lead to the greatest good?

These questions should be applied when answering the questions in the following *reality check*.

Reality Check: No Good Deed Goes Unpunished

Matt was assigned to survey "Community Medical Center" (CMC) in Minnesota with a team of three surveyors and one observer. He related to me his experience of surveying the children's dental clinic.

Following his tour of CMC's dental clinic, Matt reviewed with the clinic's staff the dental program, which served the city's underserved children. He also reviewed the care rendered several patients based on common and complex diagnoses, as well as the clinic's performance improvement activities. During the survey Dr. Seiden, the clinic director asked, "Are surveyors trained about the importance of dental care in disease prevention? As you know, dentistry is often a stepchild when it comes to allocation of scarce resources. Departments like surgery and radiology often receive the lion's share of funds." Matt responded by describing a film sponsored by the American Dental Association that was shown when he was in training to become a surveyor. The film presented a man whose dental care had

been sorely neglected throughout his life and not been addressed prior to replacement of a heart valve. The patient developed a systemic infection following surgery, which led to deterioration of the heart valve and the patient's ultimate death. The film described the lessons learned and opportunities for performance improvement that included the need for a dental evaluation by a dentist prior to valve replacement. Dr. Seiden was pleased to learn that the importance of dentistry is included in surveyor training.

Following Matt's survey of the dental clinic, the staff relayed to him their concern that the clinic was going to be closed for lack of funds. Cheryl, the clinic manager, explained, "I sometimes feel the importance of the dental clinic to the underserved population is not well understood." A bit emotional, Cheryl said, "Matt, have you surveyed other dental clinics?" Matt replied, "Yes, several well-funded clinics that come to mind were in Philadelphia and New York." Cheryl then asked, "Matt,

(continues)

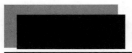

Reality Check: No Good Deed Goes Unpunished (continued)

do you have any ideas as to how we can save our clinic from closing?" Matt replied, "I have some time before lunch and I can share a few ideas with you." Cheryl replied, "The staff will be eager to listen." The staff proceeded to place several chairs in a semicircle and brainstormed with Matt a variety of ideas for saving the clinic. The staff discussed several fund-raising activities including a car wash by children to bring awareness to Any Town's dental clinic. Matt looked at his watch and said, "I need to get back to my survey team, but I want to leave you with one other thought to ponder that could be applicable to any department in the hospital. I was surveying a veteran's hospital physical therapy department and noticed on their bulletin board the staff's dream plan for renovation of their department. I asked the physical therapy staff about the plan. They related how their vision of a new physical therapy department had been sketched out and placed on their bulletin board. Several weeks later, a veteran who had been sitting in the waiting area became curious about their dream. After studying the board during his visits for therapy, he walked to the reception desk on his last visit and asked about their vision for physical therapy. They explained it was a $200,000 dream. Gary looked at the staff at the reception desk and said, "It is no longer a dream. I don't have much, but what I do have is enough to make your dream come true." And, so he did. Matt continued, "You see, if people know your dreams, something as small as a bulletin board can make all the difference." Dr. Seiden smiled and said, "I see where this

is going, community awareness as to the need to fund the clinic. It's really not merely about a car wash, it's about a concept of how the hospital can save not only the dental clinic but other programs earmarked for closing." Matt smiled, as the staff regained hope. Dr. Seiden, seeing that Matt had little time for lunch, stood up, extended his hand and said, "Matt, you gave us hope when we believed there was none. Thank you so much. I will be sure to discuss this with administration."

Matt presented his observations the following morning to the organization's leadership, which included his round table discussion with the staff. He was however cut short in his presentation by the surveyor team leader, Brad, who later reported to Victor, Matt's manager, that Matt should not be discussing how to save a dental clinic by opening a car wash. Matt received a reprimand from Victor and was removed at the end of day 4 of a 5-day survey without explanation.

—*Anonymous*

Discussion

1. Discuss Matt's approach to addressing the staff's concerns for saving the children's dental clinic.

2. If Matt's round table session led to saving the clinic, was Matt's reprimand worth the risk if he could have foreseen the resulting reprimand?

3. The goal of a consequentialist is to achieve the greatest good for the greatest number. Discuss how this applies in this reality check.

Utilitarian Ethics

> Happiness often sneaks in a door you did not think was open.
>
> —*Author Unknown*

The utilitarian theory of ethics involves the concept that the moral worth of an action is determined solely by its contribution to overall usefulness. It describes doing the greatest good for the most people. It is thus a form of consequential ethics, meaning that the moral worth of an action is determined by its outcome, and, thus, the ends justify the means. The utilitarian commonly holds that the proper course of an action is one that maximizes utility, commonly defined as maximizing happiness and reducing suffering, as noted in the following *reality check.*

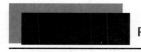

Reality Check: Maximizing Happiness and Reducing Suffering

Daniel was the last of five interviews for the CEO's position at Anytown Medical Center. During the interview, a member of the finance committee asked, "Daniel, how would maximize an allocation of $100,000 to spend as you wished for improving patient care, aside from capital budget and construction projects?" Bishop Paul, the board chairman added, "Daniel, think about the question. I will give you five minutes to form an answer." Daniel responded, "Bishop Paul, I am ready now to answer your question." The trustees looked somewhat surprised, as Bishop Paul with a smile quickly responded, "You may proceed with your answer." Daniel replied, "An old Chinese proverb came to mind as quickly as the question was asked: 'Give a man a fish and you feed him for a day. Teach a man to fish and you feed him for a lifetime.' You are interviewing me as CEO of your hospital. I see my job as assuring you that employees are thoroughly trained to care for the patients the hospital serves. I will maximize the value of each and every dollar by determining the staff skill sets that are lacking and retrain staff in the areas deficiencies are noted." Bishop Paul looked around the long oval table at the trustees, "This has been a long day and a grueling interview process for Daniel. Are there any other questions you would like to ask him." There was silence, as the trustees nodded their heads no. Bishop Paul looked at Daniel and thanked him for his interest in becoming the hospital's next CEO.

As Daniel began to leave the boardroom, Bishop Paul smiled and turned his swivel chair around as Daniel was walking towards the exit and asked, "Daniel, could you not leave the building just yet. If you could, just wait outside the room and have a seat in the doctors' lounge area." After about 20 minutes, a trustee went into the lounge where Daniel was sitting and asked him to return to the boardroom. As he entered the room, Bishop Paul stood up and looked at Daniel straight in his eyes and said, "Daniel, you were the last to be interviewed because you were on the 'short list' of candidates selected to be interviewed. Speaking for the board, your response to the last question was merely icing on the cake confirming our interest in you joining our staff. Both the Board of Trustees and members of the Medical Executive Committee unanimously have recommended you as our CEO, with which I unconditionally concur! Welcome to Anytown hospital." The trustees stood and clapped their hands. The bishop turned to the trustees and said, "Wow, that's a first."

—*Anonymous*

(continues)

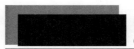

Reality Check: Maximizing Happiness and Reducing Suffering
(continued)

Discussion

1. Discuss how Daniel's response to the trustee's question of how he would spend the $100,000 fits the utilitarian theory of ethics.

2. Did Daniel, metaphorically speaking, succeed in maximizing happiness in the eyes of the board? Discuss your answer.

Deontological Ethics

Act in such a way that you always treat humanity, whether in your own person or in the person of any other, never simply as a means, but always at the same time as an end.

—*Immanuel Kant*

Deontological ethics is commonly attributed to the German philosopher Immanuel Kant (1724–1804). Kant believed that although doing the right thing is good, it might not always lead to or increase the good and right thing sought after. It focuses on one's duties to others and others' rights. It includes telling the truth and keeping your promises. Deontology ethics is often referred to as duty-based ethics. It involves ethical analysis according to a moral code or rules, religious or secular. *Deon* is derived from the Greek word meaning "duty." Kant's theory differs from consequentialism in that consequences are not the determinant of what is right; therefore, doing the right thing may not always lead to an increase in what is good.

Duty-based approaches are heavy on obligation, in the sense that a person who follows this ethical paradigm believes that the highest virtue comes from doing what you are supposed to do—either because you have to, e.g., following the law, or because you agreed to, e.g., following an employer's policies. It matters little whether the act leads to good consequences; what matters is "doing your duty."[5]

The following *reality check* illustrates how duty-based ethics focuses on the act and not the consequences of an act.

Reality Check: Duty Compromises Patient Care

At 33 years of age, I was the youngest administrator in New York State and was about to learn that adhering to company policy sometimes conflicts with the needs of the patient. In this case it was a 38-year-old employee who had been diagnosed with cancer. I remember the day well, even though it was more than 30 years ago. My secretary alerted me that Carol, a practical nurse and employee, had been admitted to the 3-North medical-surgical unit, where she worked. Without delay, I left my office and went to the nursing unit and inquired as to what room Carol was in. Beth, the unit's nurse manager, overheard my question.

She walked up to me and asked, "Daniel, could I please talk to you for a moment before you visit with Carol?" I looked at her and nodded my head yes and without thought we both walked to her office. She closed the door and said, "As you know, we are self-insured and the health insurance program we have does not cover Carol's chemotherapy treatments. She cannot bear the cost. Is there anything you can do to help her?" I replied that I would make an inquiry with our human resources director to see what could be done.

Beth asked, "Would you mind if I went with you to Carol's room for a few minutes." Daniel compassionately replied, "Of course you can."

They walked to Carol's room. Her husband and children had just left. Beth stayed for a few minutes while Daniel remained behind chatting with Carol for a few moments and said he would be back to talk with her more.

Daniel went to speak with Christine, the human resources director for his hospital. There were two other hospitals in the multihospital system. He explained Carol's financial situation and her lack of funds for chemotherapy treatment. Christine replied, "Daniel, this is corporate policy that is applicable to all three hospitals with which we must comply." Following much discussion, Daniel said, "Christine, Carol is an employee and I realize there are conflicting duties here. One is to follow corporate policy or choose to do, as I see it, what is right for Carol. If you prefer, I can request an exception to the rule. To me, right trumps duty." Christine looked at Daniel and said, "Daniel, I will see what I can do. I have a good relationship with the corporate vice president for human resources. If anyone can make an exception, he can make it happen. I know you would do the same for me and any other employee."

—*Anonymous*

Discussion

1. Discuss the potential long-term effect of granting an exception for Carol.

2. Do you believe that duty should be trumped by good? Discuss your answer.

3. Would you describe Daniel as consequentialist because he favors evaluating the outcome of an act rather than the act itself? Discuss your answer.

4. Discuss how deontological ethics in this case is in conflict with consequential thinking.

Nonconsequential Ethics

The *nonconsequential ethical theory* denies that the consequences of an action are the only criteria for determining the morality of an action. In this theory, the rightness or wrongness of an action is based on properties intrinsic to the action, not on its consequences. In other words, the nonconsequentialist believes right or wrong depends on the intention not the outcome.

Ethical Relativism

The theory of *ethical relativism* holds that morality is relative to the norms of the culture in which an individual lives. In other words, right or wrong depends on the moral norms of the society in which it is practiced. A particular action by an individual may be morally right in one society or culture and wrong in another. What is acceptable in one society may not be considered as such in another. Slavery may be considered an acceptable practice in one society and unacceptable and unconscionable in another. The administration of blood may be acceptable as to one's religious beliefs and not acceptable to another within the same society. The legal rights of patients vary from

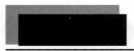

Reality Check: Bad Outcome, Good Intentions

Chelsea was preparing to drape Mr. Smith's leg in OR 6 for surgery, when she was approached by Nicole, the nurse manager, asked, "Chelsea, please come to OR 3. We have an emergency there and urgently need your skills to assist the surgeon." Chelsea turned to Daniel, the surgical technician, and asked him to continue prepping Mr. Smith's leg for surgery. Daniel prepped the leg prior to the surgeon entering the room. The surgeon entered the room a few minutes later and asked, "Where is Chelsea?" Daniel replied, "She was called away for an emergency in OR 3. Karen will be in shortly to assist us."

Following surgery, Mr. Smith was transferred to the recovery room. While he was in the recovery room a nurse was looking at the patient's medical record as to the notes regarding the patient's procedure during surgery. She noticed that surgery was conducted on the wrong leg.

Although there was heated discussion between the surgeon and nursing staff, each member of the staff had good intentions but the outcome was not so good. Nonconsequentialists believe that right or wrong depends on the intention. They generally focus more on deeds and whether those deeds are good or bad. In this case the intentions were good but the outcome was bad. It should be noted that nonconsequentialists do not always ignore the consequences. They accept the fact that sometimes good intentions can lead to bad outcomes. In summary nonconsequentialists focus more on character as to whether someone is a good person or not. Nonconsequentialists believe that right or wrong depends on the intention. Generally, the consequentialist will focus more on outcomes as to whether or not they are good or bad.

Discussion

1. Describe how the nonconsequential theory of ethics applies in this case.
2. What questions might the consequentialist raise after reviewing the facts of this case?

state to state, as is well borne out, for example, by Oregon's Death with Dignity Act. Caregivers must be aware of cultural, religious, and legal issues that can affect the boundaries of what is acceptable and what is unacceptable practice, especially when delivering health care to persons with beliefs different from their own. As the various cultures of the world merge together in communities, the education and training of caregivers become more complex. The caregiver must not only grasp the clinical skills of his or her profession but also have a basic understanding of what is right and what is wrong from both a legal and ethical point of view. Although decision making is not always perfect, the knowledge gained from this text will aid the reader in making better decisions.

PRINCIPLES OF ETHICS

> You cannot by tying an opinion to a man's tongue, make him the representative of that opinion; and at the close of any battle for principles, his name will be found neither among the dead, nor the wounded, but the missing.
>
> —*E.P. Whipple (1819–1886)*

> An army of principles can penetrate where an army of soldiers cannot.
>
> —*Thomas Jefferson*

Ethical principles are universal rules of conduct, derived from ethical theories that provide a practical basis for identifying what kinds of actions, intentions, and motives are valued. Ethical principles assist caregivers in making choices based on moral principles that have been identified as standards considered worthwhile in addressing health care–related ethical dilemmas. As noted by the principles discussed in the following sections, caregivers, in the study of ethics, will find that difficult decisions often involve choices between conflicting ethical principles.

Autonomy

> No right is held more sacred, or is more carefully guarded, by the common law, than the right of every individual to the possession and control of his own person, free from all restraint or interference of others, unless by clear and unquestioned authority of law.
>
> —*Union Pacific Ry. Co. v. Botsford*
> *[141 U.S. 250, 251 (1891)]*

The principle of *autonomy* involves recognizing the right of a person to make one's own decisions. "Auto" comes from a Greek word meaning "self" or the "individual." In this context, it means recognizing an individual's right to make his or her own decisions about what is best for him or herself. Autonomy is not an absolute principle. The autonomous actions of one person must not infringe upon the rights of another. The eminent Justice Benjamin Cardozo, in *Schloendorff v. Society of New York Hospital*, stated:

> Every human being of adult years and sound mind has a right to determine what shall be done with his own body and a surgeon who performs an operation without his patient's consent commits an assault, for which he is liable in damages, except in cases of emergency where the patient is unconscious and where it is necessary to operate before consent can be obtained.[6]

Each person has a right to make his or her own decisions about health care. A patient has the right to refuse to receive health care even if it is beneficial to saving his or her life. Patients can refuse treatment, refuse to take medications, and refuse invasive procedures regardless of the benefits that may be derived from them. They have a right to have their decisions adhered to by family members who may disagree simply because they are unable to let go. Although patients have a right to make their own choices, they also have a concomitant right to know the risks, benefits, and alternatives to recommended procedures.

Autonomous decision making can be affected by one's disabilities, mental status, maturity, or incapacity to make decisions. Although the principle of autonomy may be inapplicable in certain cases, one's autonomous wishes may be carried out through an advance directive and/or an appointed health care agent in the event of one's inability to make decisions.

What happens when the right to autonomy conflicts with other moral principles, such as beneficence and justice? Conflict can arise, for example, when a patient refuses a blood transfusion considered necessary to save his or her life whereas the caregiver's principal obligation is to do no harm. What is the right thing to do when the spouse decides to have the physician withhold from his wife her true diagnosis?

This true life case raises numerous questions, often resulting in conflicts among ethics, the law, patient rights, and family wishes. From a professional ethics point of view, the American Medical Association provides in its *Principles of Medical Ethics* that:

> IV. A physician shall respect the rights of patients, colleagues, and other health professionals, and shall safeguard patient confidences and privacy within the constraints of the law.[7]

Legally, pursuant to the Patient Self-Determination Act of 1990, patients have a right to make their own health care decisions, to accept or refuse medical treatment, and to execute an advance health care directive. Practically speaking, as discussion of this *reality*

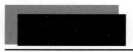

Reality Check: Spouse's Grief Leads to Withholding the Truth

Annie, a 27-year-old woman with one child, began experiencing severe pain in her abdomen while visiting her family in May. After describing the excruciating pain to her husband Daniel, he scheduled Annie for an appointment with Dr. Sokol, a gastroenter-ologist, who ordered a series of tests. While conducting a barium scan, a radiologist at Community Hospital noted a small bowel obstruction. Dr. Sokol recommended surgery to which both Annie and Daniel agreed.

After the surgery, on July 7, Dr. Brown, the operating surgeon, paged Daniel over the hospital intercom as he walked down a corridor on the ground floor. Daniel, hearing the page, picked up a house phone and dialed zero for an operator. The operator inquired, "May I help you?" "Yes," Daniel replied. "I was just paged." The operator replied, "Oh, yes. Dr. Brown would like to talk to you. I will connect you with him. Hang on. Don't hang up." (Daniel's heart began to pound.) Dr. Brown asked, "Is this you, Daniel?" Daniel replied, "Yes, it is." Dr. Brown replied, "Well, surgery is over. Your wife is recovering nicely in the recovery room." Daniel was relieved but for a moment. "That's good." Daniel sensed Dr. Brown had more to say. Dr. Brown continued, "I am sorry to say that she has carci-noma of the colon." Daniel replied, "Did you get it all?" Dr. Brown reluctantly replied, "I am sorry, but the cancer has spread to her lymph nodes and surrounding organs." Daniel, with the tears in his eyes, asked, "Can I see her?" Dr. Brown replied, "She is in the recovery room." Before hanging up, Daniel told Dr. Brown, "Please do not tell Annie that she has cancer. I want her to always have hope." Dr. Brown agreed, "Don't worry, I won't tell her. You can tell her that she had a narrowing of the colon."

Daniel hung up the phone and proceeded to the recovery room. After entering the recovery room, he spotted his wife. His heart sank. Tubes seemed to be running out of every part of her body. He walked to her bedside. His immediate concern was to see her wake up and have the tubes pulled out so that he could take her home.

Later, in a hospital room, Annie asked Daniel, "What did the doctor find?" Daniel replied, "He found a narrowing of the colon." "Am I going to be okay?" "Yes, but it will take a while to recover." "Oh, that's good. I was so worried," said Annie. "You go home and get some rest." Daniel said, "I'll be back later," as Annie fell back to sleep.

Daniel left the hospital and went to see his friends, Jerry and Helen, who had invited him for dinner. As Daniel pulled up to Jerry and Helen's home, he got out of his car and just stood there, looking up a long stairway leading to Jerry and Helen's home. They were standing there looking down at Daniel. It was early evening. The sun was setting. A warm breeze was blowing, and Helen's eyes were watering. Those few moments seemed like a lifetime. Daniel discovered a new emotion, as he stood there speechless. He knew then that he was losing a part of himself. Things would never be the same.

Annie had one more surgery 2 months later in a futile attempt to extend her life. In November 2002, Annie was admitted to the hospital for the last time. Annie was so ill that even during her last moments she was un-aware that she was dying. Dr. Brown entered the room and asked Daniel, "Can I see you for a few moments?" "Yes," Daniel replied. He followed Dr. Brown into the hallway. "Daniel, I can keep Annie alive for a few more days, or we can let her go." Daniel, not responding,

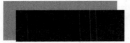

Reality Check: Spouse's Grief Leads to Withholding the Truth
(continued)

went back into the room. He was now alone with Annie. Shortly thereafter, a nurse walked into the room and gave Annie an injection. Daniel asked, "What did you give her?" The nurse replied, "Something to make her more comfortable." Annie had been asleep; she awoke, looked at Daniel, and said, "Could you please cancel my appointment to be sworn in as a citizen? I will have to reschedule. I don't think I will be well enough to go." Daniel replied, "Okay, try to get some rest." Annie closed her eyes, never to open them again.

Discussion

1. Do you agree with Daniel's decision not to tell Annie about the seriousness of her illness? Explain your answer.

2. Should the physician have spoken to Annie as to the seriousness of her illness regardless of Daniel's desire to give Annie hope and not a death sentence? Explain your answer.

3. Describe the ethical dilemmas in this case (e.g., how Annie's rights were violated).

4. Place yourself in Annie's shoes, the physician's shoes, and Daniel's shoes, and then discuss how the lives of each may have been different if the physician had informed Annie as to the seriousness of her illness.

---

check illustrates, one shoe does not fit all. Both legal and ethical edicts have often served to raise an unending stream of questions that involve both the law and ethics. Although discussed later, a case here has been made for the need of a well-balanced ethics committee to help caregivers, patients, and family come to a consensus in the decision-making process.

Life or Death: The Right to Choose

A Jehovah's Witness executed a release requesting that no blood or its derivatives be administered during hospitalization. The Connecticut Superior Court determined that the hospital had no common law right or obligation to thrust unwanted medical care on the patient because she had been sufficiently informed of the consequences of the refusal to accept blood transfusions. She had competently and clearly declined that care. The

hospital's interests were sufficiently protected by her informed choice, and neither it nor the trial court in this case was entitled to override that choice.

Beneficence

Beneficence describes the principle of doing good, demonstrating kindness, showing compassion, and helping others. In the health care setting, caregivers demonstrate beneficence by providing benefits and balancing benefits against risks. Beneficence requires one to do good. Doing good requires knowledge of the beliefs, culture, values, and preferences of the patient—what one person may believe to be good for a patient may in reality be harmful. For example, a caregiver may decide to tell a patient frankly, "There is nothing else that I can do for you." This could be injurious to the patient if the patient really wants encouragement and information about care options from the caregiver. Compassion here requires the caregiver to tell the patient, "I am not aware of new treatments for your illness; however, I have some ideas about how I can help treat your symptoms and make you more comfortable. In addition, I will keep you informed as to any significant research that may be helpful in treating your disease processes."

Paternalism

Paternalism is a form of beneficence. People sometimes believe that they know what is best for another and make decisions that they believe are in that person's best interest. It may involve, for example, withholding information, believing that the person would be better off that way. Paternalism can occur due to one's age, cognitive ability, and level of dependency.

CPR and Paternalism in Nursing Homes

Some nursing homes have implemented facilitywide no CPR policies, as noted in the following Centers for Medicare and Medicaid Services Memorandum Summary. Nursing home patients have a right to make their own care decisions. To eliminate that option in the nursing home setting by having a policy of no resuscitation measures is a paternalistic approach to patient care and is a clear violation of patient rights and autonomous decision making. Such policies are unconditionally morally and legally wrong.

Memorandum Summary

- **Initiation of CPR**—Prior to the arrival of emergency medical services (EMS), nursing homes must provide basic life support, including initiation of CPR, to a resident who experiences cardiac arrest (cessation of respirations and/or pulse) in accordance with that resident's advance directives or in the absence of advance directives or a Do Not Resuscitate (DNR) order. CPR-certified staff must be available at all times.

- **Facility CPR Policy**—Some nursing homes have implemented facilitywide no CPR policies. Facilities must not establish and implement facilitywide no CPR policies.

- **Surveyor Implications**—Surveyors should ascertain that facility policies related to emergency response require staff to initiate CPR as appropriate and that records do not reflect instances where CPR was not initiated by staff even though the resident requested CPR or had not formulated advance directives.[8]

Physicians and Paternalism

Medical paternalism involves making decisions for patients who are capable of making their own choices. Physicians often find themselves in situations where they can influence a patient's health care decision simply by selectively telling the patient what he or she prefers based on personal beliefs. This directly violates patient autonomy. The problem of paternalism involves a conflict between the principles of autonomy and beneficence, each of which may be viewed and weighed differently, for example, by the physician and patient, physician and family member, or even the patient and a family member.

Employment-Related Paternalism

Employment-related paternalism at its best is a shared and cooperative style of management in which the employer recognizes and considers employee rights when making decisions in the workplace. Paternalism at its worst occurs when the employer's style of management becomes more authoritarian, sometimes arbitrary, and unpredictable, as noted in the *reality check* presented next. In this scenario the employer has complete discretion in making workplace decisions and the individual employee's freedom is subordinate to the employer's authority. Here the employer requires strict obedience to follow orders without question. The employer in this case lacks respect and consideration for the employee.

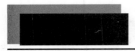

Reality Check: Paternalism and Breach of Confidentiality

Nina traveled with her husband, Dan, to a work assignment in Michigan. While visiting with her brother in Michigan, Nina believed that her potassium was low, which was a frequent occurrence with her for many years. Nina's brother suggested she could have her blood tested at a local blood drawing station. Dan later learned Nina's potassium was low.

Later that morning, while at work, Joan, Dan's colleague, called Bill, Dan's supervisor, to discuss Nina's health. Bill, however, had overslept and had not yet arrived at work. Joan decided to speak to the supervisor on call. After that conversation, Joan, being led by three staff members from the organization, tracked Dan down on several occasions that morning. On the first occasion, at approximately 10:15 A.M., Dan was surveying the organization's family practice center when Joan arrived. She rudely called Dan aside, excusing the organization's staff from the immediate area. Joan said, with surprise, "Dan, you are working?" Dan, even more surprised at the question, "Yes, I have been working." Joan replied, "Well, anyway, the corporate office wants to speak to you." Dan said he would call during lunch hour. Joan, somewhat agitated, walked away.

Joan again tracked Dan down with an entourage of the organization's staff at 11:30 A.M. She located Dan while he was in the organization's transfusion center. Again she rudely entered the conference room where Dan was discussing the care being rendered to a cancer patient. She once again asked in a stern tone of voice, "Could everyone please leave the room. I need to talk to

Dan." The organization's staff left the room and the nurse said, "I finally reached Bill and he wants you to call him." Dan inquired, "Is he pulling me off this assignment?" The nurse replied, "Yes, he is. I spoke to Bill, and he has decided that out of concern for Nina you should be removed from this particular assignment. He wants you to call him." Dan replied, "I don't understand why you did this, calling Bill and continuously interrupting my work and sharing with others confidential information about my wife. I will wrap up with the staff my review of this patient and call Bill." As Joan left the conference room Dan said, "I trusted you and you shared confidential information about my wife?" Joan, realizing that she had no right to share the information, quickly walked away.

Dan called Bill during his lunch break. During that call Bill said, "I am going to remove you from your assignment because I think your wife's health needs should be addressed, and this could be disruptive to the survey." Dan replied, "The only disruption has been the nurse tracking me down with staff from the organization and not conducting her work activities." Bill said, "My decision stands. You can opt to take vacation time for the remainder of the week."

Discussion

1. Discuss what examples of paternalism you have gleaned from this case.

2. Do you think Dan was treated fairly? Discuss your answer.

3. Discuss the issues of trust, confidentiality, and fairness as they relate to this case.

At present, our federal employment discrimination laws fail to provide uniform and consistent legal protection when an employer engages in applicant-specific paternalism—the practice of excluding an applicant merely to protect that person from job-related safety and/or health risks uniquely attributable to his or her federally protected characteristic(s). Under Title VII of the Civil Rights Act of 1964, the courts and the Equal Employment Opportunity Commission (EEOC)

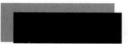

Can a Physician "Change His or Her Mind"?

Walls had a condition that caused his left eye to be out of alignment with his right eye. Walls discussed with Shreck, his physician, the possibility of surgery on his left eye to bring both eyes into alignment. Walls and Shreck agreed that the best approach to treating Walls was to attempt surgery on the left eye. Before surgery, Walls signed an authorization and consent form that included the following language:

- I hereby authorize Dr. Shreck . . . to perform the following procedure and/or alternative procedure necessary to treat my condition . . . of the left eye.

- I understand the reason for the procedure is to straighten my left eye to keep it from going to the left.

- It has been explained to me that conditions may arise during this procedure whereby a different procedure or an additional procedure may need to be performed, and I authorize my physician and his assistants to do what they feel is needed and necessary.

During surgery, Shreck encountered excessive scar tissue on the muscles of Walls's left eye and elected to adjust the muscles of the right eye instead. When Walls awoke from the anesthesia, he expressed anger at the fact that both of his eyes were bandaged. The next day, Walls went to Shreck's office for a follow-up visit and adjustment of his sutures. Walls asked Shreck why he had operated on the right eye, and Shreck responded that "he reserved the right to change his mind" during surgery.

Walls filed a lawsuit. The trial court concluded that Walls had failed to establish that Shreck had violated any standard of care. It sustained Shreck's motion for directed verdict, and Walls appealed. The court stated that the consent form that had been signed indicated that there can be extenuating circumstances when the surgeon exceeds the scope of what was discussed presurgery. Walls claimed that it was his impression that Shreck was talking about surgeries in general.

Roussel, an ophthalmologist, had testified on behalf of Walls. Roussel stated that it was customary to discuss with patients the potential risks of a surgery, benefits, and the alternatives to surgery. Roussel testified that medical ethics requires informed consent.

Shreck claimed that he had obtained the patient's informed consent not from the form but from what he discussed with the patient in his office. The court found that the form itself does not give or deny permission for anything. Rather, it is evidence of the discussions that occurred and during which informed consent was obtained. Shreck therefore asserted that he obtained informed consent to operate on both eyes based on his office discussions with Walls.

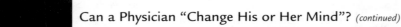

Can a Physician "Change His or Her Mind"? *(continued)*

Ordinarily, in a medical malpractice case, the plaintiff must prove the physician's negligence by expert testimony. One of the exceptions to the requirement of expert testimony is the situation whereby the evidence and the circumstances are such that the recognition of the alleged negligence may be presumed to be within the comprehension of laypersons. This exception is referred to as the "common knowledge exception."

The evidence showed that Shreck did not discuss with Walls that surgery might be required on both eyes during the same operation. There was evidence that Walls specifically told Shreck he did not want surgery performed on the right eye.

Expert testimony was not required to establish that Walls did not give express or implied consent for Shreck to operate on his right eye. Absent an emergency, it is common knowledge that a reasonably prudent health care provider would not operate on part of a patient's body if the patient told the health care provider not to do so.

On appeal, the trial court was found to have erred in directing a verdict in favor of Shreck. The evidence presented established that the standard of care in similar communities requires health care providers to obtain informed consent before performing surgery. In this case, the applicable standard of care required Shreck to obtain Walls's express or implied consent to perform surgery on his right eye.

Walls v. Shreck, 658 N.W.2d 686 (2003)

Ethical and Legal Issues

1. Discuss the conflicting ethical principles in this case.

2. Did the physician's actions in this case involve medical paternalism? Explain your answer.

reject such paternalism, demanding that the applicant alone decide whether to pursue (and accept) a job that poses risks related to his or her sex, race, color, religion, or national origin.[9]

Nonmaleficence

Nonmaleficence is an ethical principle that requires caregivers to avoid causing patients harm. It derives from the ancient maxim *primum non nocere*, translated from the Latin, "first, do no harm." Physicians today still swear by the code of Hippocrates, pledging to do no harm. Medical ethics require health care providers to "first, do no harm." A New Jersey court in *In re Conroy*,[10] found that "the physician's primary obligation is ... First do no harm." Telling the truth, for example, can sometimes cause harm. If there is no cure for a patient's disease, you may have a dilemma. Do I tell the patient and possibly cause serious psychological harm, or do I give the patient what I consider to be false hopes? Is there a middle ground? If so, what is it? To avoid causing harm, alternatives may need to be considered in solving the ethical dilemma.

The caregiver, realizing that he or she cannot help a particular patient, attempts to avoid harming the patient. This is done as a caution against taking a serious risk with the patient or doing something that has no immediate or long-term benefits.

Peninsula Child Psychiatrist William Ayres Sentenced to Eight Years for Molesting Patients

REDWOOD CITY—As one victim after another testified, calling William Ayres a monster and a serial child-abuser who robbed them of their innocence, the once-renowned child psychiatrist sat stoically Monday as a judge sentenced him to eight years in prison for molesting his former patients.

• • •

Ayres used his work with boys having trouble at school, at home or with the law as a setting to abuse them, the victims said. His position of authority allowed him to deflect suspicions about his sexual interest in boys and keep parents from believing their sons' complaints, victims said.

Joshua Melvin, San Jose Mercury News, *August 27, 2013*[11]

Law and Ethics Intersect

The patients described in the news clipping were harmed because the physician who was trained to do good did wrong by taking advantage of the patients' weaknesses. The beneficent person does good and not harm (nonmaleficence). The law in the news clipping is clear. If a person with intent and action causes harm to the patient, that person will be punished.

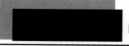

Reality Check: Patient Questions Physical Exam

Dear Sir:

I was a patient on your short-term acute-care psychiatric unit. It was a voluntary admission as is with all patients on that unit. Dr. X was my psychiatrist. Although he was very good as a psychiatrist, I was somewhat disturbed in the way he conducted my physical examination. He had come to my room on the day of my admission and said that he needed to perform a physical exam. He had already conducted a thorough history of my physical ailments and thoroughly reviewed my family history as far back as I could remember.

We were in the room alone when he entered. He had a gown in his hand and asked me to put it on. He then walked out of the room and said he would be back in a few minutes, as soon as I was gowned. When he returned he began his physical examination. Early on in the exam he asked when I had my last breast examination. I told him that I was 28 and never had one. He said, "Well, I better do one." I thought it was a bit odd that he conducted the exam without a female nurse present. I became more concerned when he touched my breasts in what I considered a sensual manner. It was uncanny. It seemed to be a bit more than what I would've expected during a breast examination. He seemed to be caressing my breasts, as opposed to examining them.

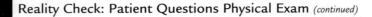

Reality Check: Patient Questions Physical Exam *(continued)*

I don't know if this is a routine procedure, but I was very uncomfortable in the situation. I think it would be better if you considered having a female nurse present when conducting female examinations in a patient room on a psychiatric unit or on any other unit for that matter.

Thanks for listening to my concerns.

Anonymous

Administrator

I called Dr. X into my office and discussed the patient's concerns with him. He said this is what physicians are trained to do. "We are trained to conduct both history and physical examinations." He had brought with him a letter from one of his professional associations that stated psychiatrists are permitted to perform physical examinations on their patients. I asked him why he did not have someone in the room with him when he examined the

patient. He stated, "I generally do but I was extremely busy and the staff was swamped with other patients. It was just a hectic day."

Discussion

1. Discuss how you would respond to the patient.

2. Describe how you would resolve this issue with the physician; assuming this was the first complaint that you had received regarding his care.

3. Explain what policy decisions you would implement.

4. Knowing that the physician is in a position of trust with his patient, discuss what action the physician should take to prevent complaints of this nature from recurring.

One of the many lessons in the preceding *reality check* teaches the reader that one may have good intent but that intent can lead to a perceived wrong and thus be damaging to one's good character and possibly his or her career path.

The intersection of "law" and "ethics" is clear. Deviation from either can lead to unsatisfactory outcomes for both physicians and patients. Although a caregiver may be trained to conduct a physical examination, the question may not be "can I do it" but "should I do it."

Nonmaleficence and Ending Life

The principle of nonmaleficence is defeated when a physician is placed in the position of ending life by removing respirators, giving lethal

injections, or writing prescriptions for lethal doses of medication. Helping patients die violates the physician's duty to save lives. In the final analysis, there needs to be a distinction between killing patients and letting them die. It is clear that killing a patient is never justified.

Justice

Justice is the obligation to be fair in the distribution of benefits and risks. Justice demands that persons in similar circumstances be treated similarly. A person is treated justly when he or she receives what is due, is deserved, or can legitimately be claimed. Justice involves how people are treated when their interests compete with one another.

Distributive justice is a principle requiring that all persons be treated equally and fairly. No one person, for example, should get a disproportional share of society's resources or benefits. There are many ethical issues involved in the rationing of health care. This is often a result of limited or scarce resources, limited access as a result of geographic remoteness, or a patient's inability to pay for services combined with many physicians who are unwilling to accept patients who are perceived as "no-pays" with high risks for legal suits.

Senator Edward M. Kennedy, speaking on health care at the John F. Kennedy Presidential Library in Boston, Massachusetts, on April 28, 2002, stated:

> It will be no surprise to this audience that I believe securing quality, affordable health insurance for every American is a matter of simple justice. Health care is not just another commodity. Good health is not a gift to be rationed based on ability to pay. The time is long overdue for America to join the rest of the industrialized world in recognizing this fundamental need.

Later, speaking at the Democratic National Convention on August 25, 2008, Kennedy said:

> And this is the cause of my life—new hope that we will break the old gridlock and guarantee that every American—North, South, East, West, young, old—will have decent, quality health care as a fundamental right and not a privilege.

Although Kennedy did not live to see the day his dream would come true, President Barack Obama signed into law the final piece of his administration's historic health care bill on March 23, 2010.

The costs of health care have bankrupted many, and research dollars have proven to be inadequate, yet many members of Congress elected to address the needs of the country have elected to continue their bipartisan bickering while they "enjoy" the lowest acceptance ratings in the nation's history. They have, however, ensured that their health care needs are met with the best of care in the best facilities with the best doctors. They have taken care of themselves. Their pensions are intact, whereas many Americans have to face such dilemmas as which medications they will take and which they cannot afford. Many often have to decide between food and medications. Is this justice or theft of the nation's resources by the few incompetents who have been elected to protect the American people? Unfortunately, these problems continue to this day as Congress continues to wrangle over national health insurance.

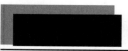 **He Won His Battle With Cancer. Thus, Why Are Millions of Americans Still Losing Theirs?**

For an increasing number of cancer activists, researchers and patients, there is too much death and too much waiting for new drugs and therapies. They want a greater sense of urgency, a new approach that emphasizes translational research over basic research—turning knowledge into therapies and getting them to patients pronto. The problem is, that's not the way our sclerotic research paradigm—principally administered by the National Institutes of Health and the National Cancer Institute (NIH/NIC)—is set up. "The fact that we jump up and down when cancer deaths go from 562,000 to 561,000, that's ridiculous. That's not enough," says Lance Armstrong, the cyclist and cancer survivor turned activist, through his Lance Armstrong Foundation (LAF).

Time, *September 15, 2008*

Justice and Government Spending

Scarce resources are challenging to the principles of justice. Justice involves equality; nevertheless, equal access to health care, for example, across the United States does not exist. How should government allocate a trillion dollars? Consider the following questions:

- Should the money be distributed equally among families?
- Should the money be distributed equally among all citizens?
- Should the money be invested and saved for a rainy day?

- Should the money be used to improve educational programs, build libraries, build state-of-the-art hospitals, or fund after-school programs for disadvantaged youths?
- Should the money include both savings for that rainy day and funding for the programs described previously?
- What would be the greater good for all?
- Should health care be rationed based on one's ability to pay?
- Should those individuals found to be ethically corrupt be condemned to poverty and stand in the same food lines as the poorest of Americans?

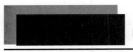

Reality Check: States Have Double Standards

It is no secret that states have had double standards over the years, one for health care organizations and one for physicians and investors, who often duplicated the financially more lucrative hospital services, while referring Medicaid patients and no-pays to hospital programs for care. As administrator of one hospital, allow me to give you a few examples.

1. A radiology group was able to purchase their own Computed Tomography (CT) scanner, while I had to jump through hoops to be able to purchase one.

2. A group of surgeons and private investors established a surgery center in direct competition with my hospital without scrutiny. At the same time, I was required to justify the hospital's proposed surgery center. The hospital was required to complete lengthy questionnaires and gather supporting documentation to justify construction and operation of an outpatient surgery center.

3. The hospital had to justify opening an outpatient rehabilitation program within the hospital in order to provide a continuum of care for patients needing physical therapy services. While I was busy justifying the need for an outpatient rehabilitation program, orthopedic surgeons were busy setting up their own outpatient programs to compete with the hospital.

I remember walking to my car one day after work and one of my orthopedic surgeons caught up to me and said, "You know Dan, I have made enough money in the 3 years that I have been on your staff to buy your hospital."

Discussion

1. Discuss the issues of justice as they apply to this scenario.

2. Discuss the issues of fairness and how physician competition with hospitals can affect the quality of patient care.

Injustice for the Insured

> Even if you're insured, getting ill could bankrupt you. Hospitals are garnishing wages, putting liens on homes and having patients who can't pay arrested. It's enough to make you sick. Think You're Covered? Think Again.
>
> —*Sara Austin, Self, October 2004*

Hospitals are receiving between $4 million and $60 million annually in charity funds in New York City alone, according to Elizabeth Benjamin, director of the health law unit of the Legal Aid Society of New York City; however, even the insured face injustice. In 2003, almost 1 million Americans declared bankruptcy because of medical issues, accounting for nearly half of all of the bankruptcies in the country. When an insured patient gets ill and exhausts his or her insurance benefits, should the hospital be able to:

- Withhold the money from the patient's wages?
- Place a lien on the patient's home?
- Arrest the patient?
- Block the patient from applying for the hundreds of millions of dollars in government funds designated to help pay for care for those who need it?

Age and Justice

- Should an 89-year-old patient get a heart transplant, rather than a 10-year-old girl, just because he or she is higher on the waiting list?
- Should a 39-year-old single patient, rather than a 10-year-old boy, get a heart transplant because he or she is higher on the waiting list?
- Should a 29-year-old mother of three get a heart transplant, rather than a 10-year-old girl, because she is higher on the waiting list?
- Should a 29-year-old pregnant mother with two children, rather than a 10-year-old boy, get a heart transplant because she is higher on the waiting list?

Justice and Emergency Care

When two patients arrive in the emergency department in critical condition, consider who should receive treatment first. Should the caregiver base his or her decision on the:

- First patient who walks through the door?
- Age of the patients?
- Likelihood of survival?
- Ability of the patient to pay for services rendered?
- Condition of the patient?

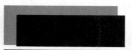

New Kidney Transplant Rules Would Favor Younger Patients

The nation's organ transplant network is considering giving younger, healthier people preference over older, sicker patients for the best kidneys.

Some also complain that the new system would unfairly penalize middle-aged and elderly patients at a time when the overall population is getting older.

If adopted, the approach could have implications for other decisions about how to allocate scarce resources, such as expensive cancer drugs and ventilators during hurricanes and other emergencies.

Rob Stein, The Washington Post, *February 24, 2011*

Patients are to be treated justly, fairly, and equally. What happens, however, when resources are scarce and only one patient can be treated at a time? What happens if caregivers decide that age should be the determining factor as to who is treated first? One patient is saved, and another dies. What happens if the patient saved is terminal and has an advance directive in his wallet requesting no heroic measures to save his life? What are the legal issues intertwined with the ethical issues in this case?

The principle of distributive justice raises numerous issues, including how limited resources should be allocated. For example, when there is a reduction in staff in health care organizations, managers are generally asked to eliminate "nonessential" personnel. In the health care industry, this translates to those individuals not directly involved in patient care (e.g., maintenance and housekeeping employees). Is this fair? Is this just? Is this the right thing to do?

In Search of Economic Justice

Avery Comarow, in his article "Under the Knife in Bangalore" (*U.S. News and World Report*, May 12, 2008), wrote that the high cost of U.S. hospital care is motivating patients to travel to places like India and Thailand for major procedures. There would be no need for uninsured patients to go abroad if the prices they were quoted in the United States were more in line with what insurers and Medicare pay. The uninsured often pay full price for medical procedures in the United States. For example, a self-pay patient will pay between $70,000 and $133,000 for coronary bypass surgery, whereas Medicare will pay between $18,609 and $23,589. Commercial insurance plans often get up to a 60% discount off the list cost of medical procedures. In India, the same surgery will cost the patient $7,000, and in Thailand, it will be $22,000.

To avoid bankruptcy and loss of assets, maybe their homes, Americans risk the unknowns of going abroad for health care.

Reality Check: Boomer Bubble "Bioeconomics"

As baby boomers become Medicare eligible, there is likely to be a huge strain on the federal budget. Is this dramatically increased cost justified, beneficial, and necessary to the country as a whole?

The revenue from working, taxpaying baby boomers over the past 4 decades has fueled unprecedented prosperity. That revenue has made many entitlements possible, but it is going to diminish drastically as boomers retire and become recipients instead of contributors to the revenue base. Advances in medical technology have increased longevity dramatically, and boomers therefore are likely to be on the receiving end of entitlements for a long time. Medical advances, however, also can increase productivity as well as longevity. Boomers with a lifetime of work experience can be a valuable resource if they are kept healthy enough to remain gainfully employed at some level. Maintenance of a skilled American workforce is essential for future prosperity and economic stability. Boomers are a substantial resource of experienced skilled workers. It is a political necessity that they are encouraged to stay productive. The government's

(continues)

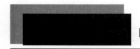

Reality Check: Boomer Bubble "Bioeconomics" *(continued)*

subsidizing health care through Medicare and other programs is therefore an investment that can facilitate this worthwhile goal. Additional incentives may even be appropriate. Even on an ethical basis, boomers that fueled our economy for so long deserve to be taken care of in their later years. Hopefully,

many of them will be healthy enough and willing enough to continue being productive beyond the usual retirement age. Thus, from a political perspective, the healthful, moral, and ethical choice may also turn out to be the profitable choice for our society.

—*Physician*

VIRTUE ETHICS AND VALUES

Virtue ethics focuses on the inherent character of a person rather than on the specific actions he or she performs. A *virtue* is a positive trait of moral excellence. Virtues are those characteristics that differentiate good people from bad people. Virtues such as courage, honesty, and justice are abstract moral principles. A morally virtuous person is one who does the good and right thing by habit, not merely based on a set of rules of conduct. The character of a virtuous person is naturally good,

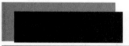

Reality Check: Resilience of the Health Caregiver Spirit

I've been in leadership roles for two sister hospitals in southeast Louisiana, with each experiencing the devastation of hurricane damage twice in the past 3 years. The first experience was temporarily suspending normal operations in New Orleans, and recently, history repeated itself at the sister hospital in Houma, Louisiana.

In both instances, I was stunned at the determination and strength of health care teams to rebuild. Both hospitals needed to resort to MASH-type tent hospitals to allow rebuilding of the hospitals. Health care for the communities was not interrupted. Back-to-basics care ensued, but not without close attention to needed regulatory compliance standards. The regulatory agencies were called and involved from the get-go, and the caregiver teams and support service staff flourished with

enthusiasm to survive and care for the patients in need. Was this because of the nonprofit nature of our state-sponsored hospitals? I don't think so. The human spirit takes over when it comes to patient care, no matter what.

I am happy to say that both New Orleans and Houma are back on track, with care being provided in top-quality hospitals. This is only due to the diligence of all, including facilities management, housekeeping, and multiple direct and indirect caregiver departments. What is the ethical issue here? There is no issue. Support for the art of care-giving will never be disappointed—at least not in southeast Louisiana. I stand in awe of what I have seen and look forward to growing with this team of devoted professionals.

—*Nurse*

as exhibited by his or her unswerving good behavior and actions.

> *Values* are standards of conduct. They are used for judging the goodness or badness of some action. A *moral value* is the relative worth placed on some virtuous behavior.
>
> Values are rooted in customs and habits of a culture because the words moral and ethics themselves were essentially created to describe these topics.[12]

Values are the standards by which we measure the goodness in our lives. *Intrinsic value* is something that has value in and of itself (e.g., happiness). *Instrumental value* is something that helps to give value to something else (e.g., money is valuable for what it can buy).

Values may change as needs change. If one's basic needs for food, water, clothing, and housing have not been met, one's values may change such that a friendship, for example, might be sacrificed if one's basic needs can be better met as a result of the sacrifice. As mom nears the end of her life, a financially well-off family member may want to take more aggressive measures to keep mom alive despite the financial drain on her estate. Another family member, who is struggling financially, may more readily see the futility of expensive medical care and find it easier to let go. Values give purpose to each life. They make up one's moral character.

All people make value judgments and make choices among alternatives. Values are the motivating power of a person's actions and necessary to survival, both psychologically and physically.

The relationship between abstract virtues (principles) and values (practice) is often difficult to grasp. The virtuous person is one who does good, and his or her character is known through the values he or she practices consistently by habit.

We begin our discussion here with an overview of those virtues commonly accepted as having value when addressing difficult health care dilemmas. The reader should not get overly caught up in the philosophical morass of how virtues and values differ but should be aware that virtues and values have been used interchangeably. This text is not about memorizing words; it is about applying what we learn for the good of all whose lives we touch.

Whether we call compassion a virtue or a value or both, the importance for our purposes in this text is to understand what compassion is and how it is applied in the health care setting.

Pillars of Moral Strength

> I am part of all I have met.
>
> —*Alfred Tennyson*

There is a deluge of ethical issues in every aspect of human existence. Although cultural differences, politics, and religion influence who we are, it is all of life experiences that affect who we have become. If we have courage to do right, those who have influenced our lives were most likely courageous. If we are compassionate, it is most likely because we have been influenced by the compassionate.

The *Pillars of Moral Strength* illustrated in **Figure 26-1** describes a virtuous person. What is it that sets each person apart? In the final analysis, it is one's virtues and values that build moral character. Look beyond the words and ask, "Do I know their meanings?" "Do I apply their concepts?" "Do I know their value?" "Are they part of me?"

Courage as a Virtue

> Courage is the greatest of all virtues, because if you haven't courage, you may not have an opportunity to use any of the others.
>
> —*Samuel Johnson*

Courage is the mental or moral strength to persevere and withstand danger. Courage can be characterized as the ladder upon which all the other virtues mount. Courage is the strength of character necessary to continue in the face of fears and the challenges in life. It involves

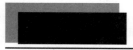 **FIGURE 26-1** Pillars of moral strength.

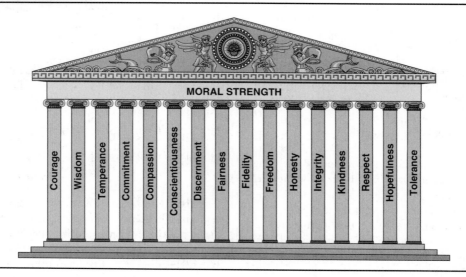

MORAL STRENGTH

Courage · Wisdom · Temperance · Commitment · Compassion · Conscientiousness · Discernment · Fairness · Fidelity · Freedom · Honesty · Integrity · Kindness · Respect · Hopefulness · Tolerance

balancing fear, self-confidence, and values. Without courage, we are unable to take the risks necessary to achieve the things most valued. A courageous person has good judgment and a clear sense of his or her strengths, correctly evaluates danger, and perseveres until a decision is made and the right goal that is being sought has been achieved.

Courage, in differing degrees, helps to define one's character (the essence of one's being) and

Reality Check: My Journey–How Lucky Am I?

No words can be scripted to say what I have been through, so I will just speak from my heart and off the cuff. From the day the Dr. said to me, "Denise, you have a rare cancer and we are sorry there is nothing we can do." I did not waver in my faith in God. He was in me, he was thru me and he was around me. I just asked the Dr., "What do I do?" And yet, although he said a whole bunch of words, I wasn't focused so much on what was being said. It's like a calmness was over me, not much worry, just a feeling of I will never be ALONE on this new journey I'm about to experience. I felt calm. Not until I looked at my loved ones FACES did I realize, oh my, this can be bad. But again, a feeling came over me that I will not face this ALONE. God has plans for me and I will surrender in his grace and as time past [sic], I realized how lucky and blessed I am, for most people who may feel that death may be close by, I didn't feel that way. What I felt was WOW!! Everyone gets to show me their love in the NOW and not in the later when I am no longer HERE. How lucky am I.

—Denise

offers the strength to stand up for what is good and right. It crosses over and unites and affects all other values. Courage must not be exercised to an extreme, causing a person to become so foolish that his or her actions are later regretted.

When the passion to destroy another human being becomes such an obsession that one is willing to sacrifice the lives of others, that person has become a bully and a coward and not a person of courage. History is filled with men and women who have hidden their fears by inciting others to do evil. Such people are not the models of character that we wish to instill thoughts of in the minds of our children.

Wisdom as a Virtue

> True wisdom comes to each of us when we realize how little we understand about life, ourselves, and the world around us.
>
> —*Socrates*

> We can learn from history how past generations thought and acted, how they responded to the demands of their time and how they solved their problems. We can learn by analogy, not by example, for our circumstances will always be different than theirs were. The main thing history can teach us is that human actions have consequences and that certain choices, once made, cannot be undone. They foreclose the possibility of making other choices and thus they determine future events.
>
> —*Gerda Lerner (Pioneer of Women's History)*

Wisdom is the judicious application of knowledge. Wisdom begins first by learning from the failures and successes of those who have preceded us. Marcus Tullius Cicero (106–43 BC), a Roman philosopher and politician, is reported to have said, "The function of wisdom is to discriminate between good and evil." In the health care setting, when the patient's wishes and end-of-life preferences are unknown, wisdom with good judgment without bias or prejudice springs forth more easily.

Temperance as a Virtue

> Being forced to work, and forced to do your best, will breed in you temperance and self-control, diligence and strength of will, cheerfulness and content, and a hundred virtues which the idle will never know.
>
> —*Charles Kingsley*

Temperance involves self-control and restraint. It embraces moderation in thoughts and actions. Temperance is evidenced by orderliness and moderation in everything one says and does. It involves the ability to control one's actions so as not to go to extremes. The question arises, without the ability to control oneself from substance abuse, for example, how can a person possibly live the life of a virtuous person. The old adage, "the proof is in the pudding" lies in one's actions. A virtuous person stands out from the crowd by actions and deeds.

Commitment

> Unless commitment is made; there are only promises and hopes; but no plans.
>
> —*Peter F. Drucker*

> I know the price of success: dedication, hard work, and an unremitting devotion to the things you want to see happen.
>
> —*Frank Lloyd Wright*

Commitment is the act of binding oneself intellectually or emotionally to a course of action (e.g., pursue a career, adhere to a religious belief) or person (e.g., marriage, family, patient care). It is an agreement or pledge to do something. It can be ongoing, such as in a marriage, or a pledge to do something in the future, such as an engagement as a commitment to marry a particular person.

Compassion

> Compassion is the basis of morality.
>
> —*Arthur Schopenhauer*

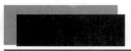

The Fear Factor and Patient Satisfaction

Nurses tend to score highly on measures of empathy, care, and compassion. . . . Here is some specific advice about what hospitals can do to help nurses improve at calming their patients' fears.

Encourage nurses to be sensitive to the level of fear their patients experience when they're admitted to the hospital. Empathy and communication are key. . . .

Set nurses up for success through training and support. In many instances, it is easy to deal with safety concerns by providing detailed protocols, policies, and procedures.

Rick Blizzard, D.B.A., Gallup, *August 6, 2013*[13]

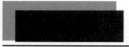

Hospital Video Shows No One Helped Dying Woman

A shocking video shows a woman dying on the floor in the psych ward at Kings County Hospital, while people around her, including a security guard, did nothing to help. After an hour, another mental patient finally got the attention of the indifferent hospital workers, according to the tape obtained by the *New York Daily News*.

Worse still, the surveillance tape suggests hospital staff may have falsified medical charts to cover the utter lack of treatment provided to Esmin Green before she died.

John Marzulli, Daily News, *June 30, 2008*

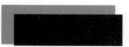

Elderly Patient Hit by Motorcycle Dies in Japan After Being Rejected by 14 Hospitals

After getting struck by a motorcycle, an elderly Japanese man with head injuries waited in an ambulance as paramedics phoned 14 hospitals, each refusing to treat him.

He died 90 minutes later at the facility that finally relented—one of thousands of victims repeatedly turned away in recent years by understaffed and overcrowded hospitals in Japan.

Maria Yamaguchi, Associated Press, *February 5, 2009*

Compassion is the deep awareness of and sympathy for another's suffering. The ability to show compassion is a true mark of moral character. There are those who argue that compassion will blur one's judgment. Caregivers need to show the same compassion for others, as they would expect for themselves or their loved ones.

Compassion is a moral value expected of all caregivers. Those who lack compassion have a weakness in their moral character. In 1996, Dr. Linda Peeno, featured in Michael Moore's 2007 film *Sicko*, testified before Congress (Important issue facing House-Senate conference on health care reform, House of Representatives—March 28, 2000—Page: H1465) to discuss her prior work for Humana, where she worked as a claims reviewer for several health maintenance organizations (HMOs). Dr. Peeno showed compassion as she testified before the Committee on Commerce on May 30, 1996. Here is her story in part:

> I wish to begin by making a public confession. In the spring of 1987, I caused the death of a man. Although this was known to many people, I have not been taken before any court of law or called to account for this in any professional or public forum. In fact, just the opposite occurred. I was rewarded for this. It brought me an improved reputation in my job and contributed to my advancement afterwards. Not only did I demonstrate that I could do what was asked, expected of me, I exemplified the good company employee. I saved a half a million dollars.

> Since that day, I have lived with this act and many others eating into my heart and soul. The primary ethical norm is do no harm. I did worse, I caused death. Instead of using a clumsy bloody weapon, I used the simplest, cleanest of tools: my words. This man died because I denied him a necessary operation to save his heart. I felt little pain or remorse at the time. The man's faceless distance soothed my conscience. Like a skilled soldier, I was trained for the moment. When any moral qualms arose, I was to remember, "I am not denying care; I am only denying payment."

Duty-based ethics required Dr. Peeno to follow the rules of her job. In so doing, a life was lost. Although Dr. Peeno eventually came forward with her story, the irony here lies in the fact that Dr. Peeno lacked the courage, integrity, and compassion to report her story sooner. The lack of compassion for others plagues the health care industry in a variety of settings.

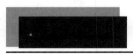

Teaching Doctors to Care

> At Harvard and other medical schools across the country, educators are beginning to realize that empathy is as valuable to a doctor as any clinical skill ... doctors who try to understand their patients may be the best antidote for the widespread dissatisfaction with today's health care system.
>
> *Nathan Thornburgh*, Time, *March 29, 2006*

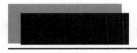

Reality Check: Policy Ruled—Compassion Missing

> Mr. Jones was trying to get home from a long trip to see his ailing wife. Mrs. Jones had been ill for several years, suffering a great deal of pain. His flight was to leave at 7:00 pm. Upon arrival at the airport in New York at 4:30 pm, he inquired at the ticket counter, "Is there an earlier flight that I can take to Washington?" The counter agent responded, "There is plenty

(continues)

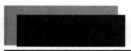

Reality Check: Policy Ruled—Compassion Missing *(continued)*

of room on the 5:00 pm flight, but you will have pay a $200 change fee." The passenger inquired, "Could you please waive the change fee? I need to get home to my ailing wife." The ticket agent responded, "Sorry, your ticket does not allow me to make the change. You can, however, try at the gate."

The passenger made a second attempt at the gate to get on an earlier flight, but the manager at the gate was unwilling to authorize the change, saying, "I don't make the rules."

Mr. Jones decided to give it one more try. He called the airline's customer service center. The customer service agent responded to Mr. Jones's plea: "We cannot overrule the agent at the gate. Sorry, you just got the wrong supervisor. He is going by the book."

—*Anonymous*

Discussion

1. Should rules be broken for a higher good? Discuss your answer.

2. Do the rules seem to be consistently or inconsistently applied in this *reality check*? Discuss your answer.

Detachment

Detachment, or lack of concern for the patient's needs, often translates into mistakes that result in patient injuries. Those who have excessive emotional involvement in a patient's care may be best suited to work in those settings where patients are most likely to recover and have good outcomes (e.g., maternity units). As with all things in life, there needs to be a comfortable balance between compassion and detachment.

> Never apologize for showing feeling. When you do so, you apologize for the truth.
>
> —*Benjamin Disraeli*

Conscientious

> The most infectiously joyous men and women are those who forget themselves in thinking about and serving others.
>
> —*Robert J. McCracken*

A *conscientious* person is one who has moral integrity and a strict regard for doing what is considered the right thing to do. An individual acts conscientiously if he or she is motivated to do what is right, believing it is the right thing to do. Conscience is a form of self-reflection on and judgment about whether one's actions are

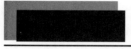

Reality Check: Kill the Messenger

Frank, working as a hospital inspector, found a number of things wrong in his recent building inspection. At first glance the building looked clean and polished—Frank was amazed by how the floors sparkled in the old building. But then, as Frank always does, he asked to look behind a corridor door. Behind the door, Frank found a small storage closet

Reality Check: Kill the Messenger *(continued)*

with medical records strewn on the floor and others stored in cardboard boxes. The records had been soaked by water and floor wax that had seeped under the door when the corridors where cleaned. Entries on the records were blurred, making them difficult to read, and the records appeared to have black mold growing on them.

Behind another door was a medical equipment repair room. Dust balls floated on the floor as the door was opened. There was food on the floor, and a can of soda had been spilled and allowed to dry. Equipment parts were also scattered on the floor.

The staff complained about Frank's findings. Before he left, the staff corrected the issues he had noted and asked, "Frank, could you remove these comments from your report. We cleaned the room and it is spotless. In addition, we stored the records in the medical records department." Frank replied, "I could not in good conscience remove my findings. Yes, the room may be

clean but what about the information that had been recorded on the medical records that is not readable. Further, our process for inspecting your facility is a sampling process. I did not look behind every door and I am not sure what we would find if we did. I would suggest, as we discussed earlier, that a written plan of action be prepared and implemented to address the issues I identified. More important, your action plan should be implemented facilitywide. For example, no boxes should be stored on the floors, including medical supplies, as well as medical records."

—*Anonymous*

Discussion

1. Should Frank have overlooked his findings, as the staff pressed him not to report them? Discuss your answer.

2. Assuming you were Frank, would you have deleted the findings from your report? Explain your answer.

---

right or wrong, good or bad. It is an internal sanction that comes into play through critical reflection. This sanction often appears as a bad conscience in the form of painful feelings of remorse, guilt, shame, disunity, or disharmony as the individual recognizes that his or her acts were wrong.

Discernment

Get to know two things about a man—how he earns his money and how he spends it—and you have the clue to his character, for you have a searchlight that shows up the innermost recesses of his soul. You know all you need

to know about his standards, his motives, his driving desires, and his real religion.

—*Robert J. McCracken*

Discernment is the ability to make a good decision without personal biases, fears, and undue influences from others. A person who has discernment has the wisdom to decide the best course of action when there are many possible actions to choose from.

Fairness

Do all the good you can, By all the means you can, In all the ways you can, In all the places

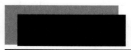

Reality Check: 9/11 Value Judgment

James had been scheduled to fly Monday evening, September 10, 2001, from Ronald Reagan Washington National Airport to New York LaGuardia Airport, and then rent a car and drive to Greenwich, Connecticut, where he was assigned to inspect a hospital. As luck would have it, there was one flight cancellation after another. After the last flight to LaGuardia was canceled, he went to the ticket counter and scheduled the first flight out Tuesday morning, September 11, 2001, at 6:00 AM.

The following morning James flew into LaGuardia, picked up his car, and drove to Connecticut to work with an assigned team led by Dr. Matthews. Not long after he arrived at the hospital, the first plane hit the World Trade Center. Shortly after the second plane crashed into the World Trade Center, the corporate office called and asked if the hospital wanted to reschedule the survey. The hospital opted to continue the survey.

On Thursday, the last day of the survey, a hospital staff member approached Dr. Matthews and asked if he and his survey team would like to attend a short memorial service in the lobby at noon for the victims and workers of 9/11. Without hesitation, Dr. Matthews replied, "No, we really have to finish our reports."

—*Anonymous*

Discussion

1. Did the team leader make an appropriate decision? Discuss your answer.
2. Describe the various virtues and values that come into play in this case.
3. Discuss how you would have addressed the hospital's request to attend the memorial service.
4. Realizing that hindsight is 20/20, could you defend the decision not to attend the ceremony? Explain your answer.

you can, At all the times you can, To all the people you can, As long as you ever can.

—*John Wesley*

In ethics, *fairness* requires each person to be objective, unbiased, dispassionate, impartial, and consistent with the principles of ethics. Fairness is the ability to make judgments free from discrimination, dishonesty, or one's own bias. It is the ability to be objective without prejudice or bias. We often tolerate mediocrity. We sometimes forget to thank those who just do their jobs, and we often praise the extraordinary, sometimes despite questionable faults. To be fair, it is important to see the good in all and to reward that good.

Questions of fairness in the Affordable Care Act have led to lawsuits in a number of the nation's top hospitals including the Mayo Clinic in Minnesota and Cedars-Sinai in Los Angeles because they are cut out of most insurance plans sold on the exchange.

Although care is generally cheaper at community-based hospitals than academic medical centers, the quality of that care often comes into question, as noted in the following *reality check.*

So where are we as it relates to fairness in the delivery of health care? Is it true that people coming out of the ranks of the uninsured don't care about the Mayo Clinic, Cleveland

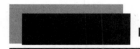

Health Costs Cut by Limiting Choice

"Exchanges exclude, doctors, hospitals; in backlash, some providers file lawsuits"

The result, some argue, is a two-tiered system of health care: Many of the people who buy health plans on the exchanges have fewer hospitals and doctors to choose from than those with coverage through their employers.

• • •

Insurers "looked at the people expected to go on the exchanges and thought: 'these are people coming out of the ranks of the uninsured. They don't care about the Mayo Clinic or the Cleveland Clinic. They will go to community providers,'" explained Robert Laszewski, a consultant to the health-care industry.

Sandhya Somashekhar and Ariana Eunjung Cha, The Washington Post, *August 21, 2013*

Clinic, the Lahey Hospital and Medical Center, or the Massachusetts General Hospital, to name but a few? Or do they care but just don't know the quality differences from one hospital to the next? Or is it a question of accessibility in remote areas of the country? Do we need hospital selection exchanges more then we need insurance exchanges? If one has money or connections is he or she more likely to get a higher quality of medical care than a poorer patient? Who determines what routine care is? Is routine care based on each patient's needs and comorbidities? Should those who have a financial interest in where a patient is treated be excluded from the decision-making process? Cheaper is not always better and providing care very well may not be enough. Although fairness in the delivery of health is a laudable value, it is most likely unachievable. The disparity as to who holds the nation's

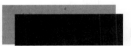

Reality Check: Community Hospital vs. Respected Medical Center

My closest friend Nick was admitted to a small community hospital for what was described as a minor surgical procedure. During surgery, the surgeon unknowingly nicked the large bowel, which went unknown for several days. Nick, as a result, developed a methicillin-resistant *Staphylococcus aureus* (MRSA) infection. Further surgeries were conducted, complicating an already botched surgery. One evening a nurse called his family aside and said, although I am jeopardizing my job, "I would get Nick out of here if I was you." The family decided to move Nick to a major teaching medical center several hours away from his hometown. Following an extended stay at the medical center and discharged home under hospice care, I visited Nick at his home. He looked intensely straight at me with deep sadness and said, "They took my life from me." He told another friend, "My life is over."

—Anonymous

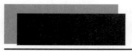

Of the 1%, by the 1%, for the 1%

Americans have been watching protests against oppressive regimes that concentrate massive wealth in the hands of an elite few. Yet in our own democracy, 1 percent of the people take nearly a quarter of the nation's income—an inequality even the wealthy will come to regret.

Joseph E. Stiglitz, Vanity Fair, *May 2011*

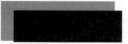

World's Richest 1% Own 40% of All Wealth, UN Report Discovers

The richest 1% of adults in the world own 40% of the planet's wealth, according to the largest study yet of wealth distribution. The report also finds that those in financial services and the internet sectors predominate among the super rich.

Europe, the US and some Asia Pacific nations account for most of the extremely wealthy. More than a third live in the US. Japan accounts for 27% of the total, the UK for 6% and France for 5%.

James Randerson, The Guardian, *December 2006*

wealth continues to widen, as noted in the news clippings here. With so much wealth in the hands of the few, fairness in the delivery of high-quality health care for all is unlikely. However, the human race must continue to strive to meet the needs of all.

Fidelity

Nothing is more noble, nothing more venerable, than fidelity. Faithfulness and truth are the most sacred excellences and endowments of the human mind.

—Cicero

Fidelity is the virtue of faithfulness, being true to our commitments and obligations to others. A component of fidelity, veracity, implies that we will be truthful and honest in all our endeavors. It involves being faithful and loyal to obligations, duties, or observances. The opposite of fidelity is infidelity, meaning unfaithfulness.

Freedom

You can only protect your liberties in this world by protecting the other man's freedom. You can only be free if I am free.

—Dorothy Thompson

Freedom is the quality of being free to make choices for oneself within the boundaries of law. Freedoms enjoyed by citizens of the United States include the freedom of speech, freedom of religion, freedom from want, and freedom from physical aggression (**Figure 26-2**).

Honesty/Trustworthiness/Truth Telling

A lie can travel halfway around the world while the truth is still putting on its shoes.

—Mark Twain (American humorist, writer, and lecturer, 1835–1910)

Honesty and trust involve confidence that a person will act with the right motives. It is

FIGURE 26-2 Freedom speaks.

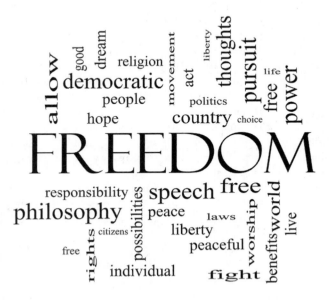

© Keith Bell/Shutterstock, Inc.

the assured reliance on the character, ability, strength, or truth of someone or something. To tell the truth, to have integrity, and to be honest are most honorable virtues. *Veracity* is devotion to and conformity with what is truthful. It involves an obligation to be truthful.

Truth telling involves providing enough information so that a patient can make an informed decision about his or her health care. Intentionally misleading a patient to believe something that the caregiver knows to be untrue may give the patient false hopes. There is always apprehension when one must share bad news; the temptation is to play down the truth for fear of being the bearer of bad news. To lessen the pain and the hurt is only human, but in the end, truth must win over fear.

> Speaking the truth in times of universal deceit is a revolutionary act.
>
> —*George Orwell*

Declining Trust in the Health Care System

The declining trust in the nation's ability to deliver high-quality health care is evidenced by a system caught up in the quagmire of managed care companies, which have in some instances inappropriately devised ways to deny health care benefits to their constituency. In

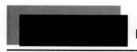

Reality Check: 36,000 Feet over Texas

A few weeks before Frank was to travel to Dodge City, Texas, for a work assignment, he received a call from Dr. Layblame: "Hi Frank. This is Dr. Layblame. Can you be ready for an early afternoon departure from Dodge City on Friday?" Frank replied, "Well you know we have been instructed not to leave early, and the last flight leaves at 4:30 P.M. Anyway, I don't mind flying out Saturday morning." Dr. Layblame replied, "Well, it's only an hour early. If you write most of your report the night before and during lunch on Friday, we should be able to finish up work by 2:30 P.M. The airport is small and close to the hospital. Besides, my team has to drive to Louisiana and we would like to get there so we can go out to dinner and enjoy evening. I am the tour leader, so it should not be a problem." Frank said OK and scheduled a 4:30 P.M. return flight.

While Frank was in a flight to Washington, DC, following his work assignment, Ronald, Frank's supervisor was dictating a voicemail message to him. When Frank returned home at about 10:30 that evening, he retrieved his voice-mail messages. Ronald had left Frank a message at 4:30 P.M. earlier that day asking Frank, "Call me as soon as you get this message. I will be in my office until about 5:30 P.M. If you miss me, you can reach me over the weekend. My cell phone number is xxx/xxx-xxxx."

Frank called Ronald that evening and the next morning; however, Ronald never answered, nor did he return his call. Frank called Ronald Monday morning. As luck would have it, Ronald was out of the office for the day. Frank called Ronald again on Tuesday morning and Ronald answered. Frank asked, "Ronald, you called?" He replied, "Yes, I did. How were you able to get to the airport on Friday and catch a 4:30 P.M. flight without leaving

your job early? I had your flight schedule and you left the survey early. You could not possibly have traveled to the airport in time to catch your flight without leaving early."

Frank replied, "I did not schedule the exit time from the survey. The physician team leader determined the time of the exit. He said that he was conducting a system tour and would like to get the exit briefing started as soon as possible. He asked for everybody to be ready to exit by having draft reports ready the night before." Ronald replied, "Dr. Layblame told me the team had to exit early because you scheduled an early flight."

Frank asked, "Just one question, Ronald. Why would you leave a message for me at 4:30 P.M. to call you by 5:30 P.M. when you knew I was 36,000 feet high in the sky? And why didn't you call the team leader at the beginning of the assignment and not after it was completed? Since you know flight schedules, why would you wait until the assignment was completed to raise this issue? Sounds a bit peculiar, don't you think? Sort of like observing a protocol not being followed in the OR and then chastising the OR team after the surgery is completed for not following protocol. This is a serious business we are in. You need to ask yourself why you would allow an event to occur if you believed it to be wrong."

Discussion

1. Discuss the ethical issues involved in this case.

2. Discuss what you would do if you found yourself in Frank's situation.

3. What should Frank have said if his manager said, "You should have reported Dr. Layblame"?

4. How would you describe Ronald's management style?

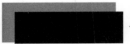

Cancer Doctor Allegedly Prescribed $35 Million Worth of Totally Unnecessary Chemotherapy

A Michigan oncologist has been charged with giving $35 million in needless chemotherapy to patients—some of whom didn't even have cancer, The Today Show reported.

Popular physician Farid Fata, who had more than 1,000 patients, allegedly misdiagnosed people with cancer just so he could bill Medicare.

He's also accused of giving chemo to "end-of-life" patients who wouldn't benefit and had to endure the treatment's nasty side effects during their final days.

Christina Sterbenz, Business Insider, *August 15, 2013*

addition, the continuing reporting of numerous medical errors serves only to escalate distrust in the nation's political leadership and the providers of health care.

Physicians find themselves vulnerable to lawsuits, often because of misdiagnosis. As a result, patients are passed from specialist to specialist in an effort to leave no stone unturned. Fearful to step outside the boundaries of their own specialties, physicians escalate the problem by ineffectively communicating with the primary care physician responsible for managing the patient's overall health care needs. This can also be problematic if no one physician has taken overall responsibility to coordinate and manage a patient's care.

Politics and Distrust

Lies or the appearance of lies are not what the writers of our Constitution intended for our country—it's not the America we salute every Fourth of July, it's not the America we learned about in school, and it is not the America represented in the flag that rises above our land.

—Anonymous

Truthfulness is just one measure of one's moral character. Unfortunately, politicians do not always set good examples for the people they serve. The following news clipping is an

example of how political decisions can lead to distrust in government.

Integrity

Nearly all men can stand adversity, but if you want to test a man's character, give him power.

—Abraham Lincoln

Integrity involves a steadfast adherence to a strict moral or ethical code and a commitment not to compromise this code. A person with integrity has a staunch belief in and faithfulness to, for example, his or her religious beliefs. Patients and professionals alike often make health care decisions based on their integrity and their strict moral beliefs. For example, Jehovah's Witnesses generally refuse blood transfusions because it is contrary to their religious beliefs, even if such refusal may result in death. A provider of health care may refuse to participate in an abortion because it is against the provider's moral beliefs. A person without personal integrity lacks sincerity and moral conviction and may fail to act on professed moral beliefs.

Medical Integrity and Patient Autonomy

The integrity of the medical profession is not threatened by allowing competent patients to decide for themselves whether a

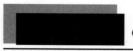

Cheney's Staff Cut Testimony on Warming

In a letter to Sen. Barbara Boxer (D-Calif.), former EPA deputy associate administrator Jason K. Burnett said an official from Cheney's office ordered last October that six pages be edited out of the testimony of Julie L. Gerberding, director of the Centers for Disease Control and Prevention. Gerberding had planned to say that the "CDC considers climate change a serious public health concern."

Juliet Eilperin, The Washington Post, *July 9, 2008*

Discussion

1. Discuss how headlines such as this affect your opinion of politicians.
2. Assuming a cover-up, discuss how the principles of beneficence and nonmaleficence apply.
3. At the end of our days, the most basic principles of life—trust and survival—are on trial. What is your verdict, if indeed there was a cover-up?

particular medical treatment is in their best interests. Patient autonomy sets the foundation of one's right to bodily integrity, including the right to accept or refuse treatment. Those rights are superior to the institutional considerations of hospitals and their medical staffs. A state's interest in maintaining the ethical integrity of a profession does not outweigh, for example, a patient's right to refuse blood transfusions.

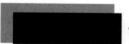

Wrong-Operation Doctor

Hospitals find it hard to protect patients from wrong-site surgery

Last year a jury returned a $20 million negligence verdict against Arkansas Children's Hospital for surgery on the wrong side of the brain of a 15-year-old boy who was left psychotic and severely brain damaged. Testimony showed that the error was not disclosed to his parents for more than a year. The hospital issued a statement saying it deeply regretted the error and had "redoubled our efforts to prevent" a recurrence.

"Healthcare has far too little accountability for results. . . . All the pressures are on the side of production; that's how you get paid," said Peter Pronovost, a prominent safety expert and medical director of the Johns Hopkins Center for Innovation in Quality Patient Care, who added that increased pressure to turn over operating rooms quickly has trumped patient safety, increasing the chance of error.

Sandra G. Boodman, Kaiser Health News, The Washington Post, *June 20, 2011*

Discussion

1. Discuss the issues of integrity in this case.
2. Should criminal charges be a consideration in this case, if accurately reported? Discuss your answer.

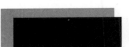

Reality Check: Behind the Smiles

Jeff well remembers what happened after Bill left the hospital boardroom. He, however, remembers more clearly how Bill, a consultant, was treated while he was in the room after presenting his organizational improvement report to the hospital's leadership. Bill was treated with kindness and assurances as to how well he took an educational approach to his audit findings with the staff and how employees appreciated his suggestions for improvement.

Prior to exiting the conference room, Bill asked whether there were any questions about his report. No questions, just smiles, accolades, and goodbyes. Jeff thought to himself, wow, it is good to see good people take suggestions and be so willing to make the changes that Bill suggested.

Oops, hold on, it turns out Bill wasn't as wonderful as the leadership described. The organization's leadership was now disgruntled about Bill's report. Bill was gone and now vilified. Jeff, a consultant not scheduled to finish his assignment for another 2 weeks, asked, "Why didn't you ask questions while Bill was here?" Carol, the finance director replied, "I spent 2 weeks with Bill. He just made up his mind. There was just no changing his mind."

Jim said, "Are you saying that you disagree with Bill's report?" Carol, replied, "Yes, I do disagree with it." Jeff continued, "But you did not state that while he was here. You told him you liked his suggestions and that you were already in the process of implementing them." Carol replied, "That's true, but since we made the suggested changes while he was here, he did not have to include them in his written report." Bill replied, "It speaks well of leadership that you have done so; however, it is the hospital board that asked for the audit. We must report what we found." Carol, disgruntled, remained silent. Jim thought to himself, integrity includes being honest and truthful and surely not criticizing a person after leaving the conference room.

—*Anonymous*

Discussion

1. Should Bill have left his findings off the report? Explain your answer.
2. Discuss why Bill's integrity in reporting the deficiencies he found and reported were important to both ABC consulting and the hospital board, which had contracted with ABC to conduct the audit.

Reality Check: Employee Satisfaction Survey

The human resources department manager was reporting on an employee satisfaction survey at a leadership roundtable session with the organization's employees. To maintain employee confidentiality, a third-party consulting firm had conducted the survey. Approximately 49% of employees had responded to the survey, compared with 47% 3 years earlier. The HR manager commented that it is was the first satisfaction survey conducted

(continues)

Reality Check: Employee Satisfaction Survey *(continued)*

in 3 years and that the results were excellent, with a 4.2% rise in overall employee satisfaction. Management was all smiles as they sat listening to the report. The HR manager had actually briefed the organization's leadership prior to the roundtable session. Following the report, she asked if there were any questions. The silence was deadly—no one responded. Finally, one employee, Richard, placed his hands on the table to stand up, but he felt a nudge on his right shoulder from Phil, a physician friend. Phil whispered, "Richard, are you sure you want to ask any questions? There is nothing to gain here." Richard, looking down with a smile, said, "I agree, but I can't help myself." Richard then stood up and asked he HR manager, "Do you know what the employee turnover rate has been during the past 3 years?" She responded,

"Well, ugh, yes, it was about 30%." Richard replied, "So, then, does this report reflect that we have had a 30% turnover?" The manager replied, "Good point, I will have to get back to you on that." When he returned to his seat, Phil said, "Do you really think you will ever hear back an answer to your question?" Richard smiled and replied, "Not really." Richard was right; she never did get back to him.

Discussion

1. Discuss why employees are often reluctant to ask questions when their questions are solicited by leadership.

2. Knowing that the HR manager never followed up with Richard, should he have followed up with the manager as to the validity of the survey data? Explain your answer.

Kindness

> When you carry out acts of kindness, you get a wonderful feeling inside. It is as though something inside your body responds and says, yes, this is how I ought to feel.
>
> —*Harold Kushner*

Kindness involves the quality of being considerate and sympathetic to another's needs. Some people are takers, and others are givers. If you go through life giving without the anticipation of receiving, you will be a kinder and happier person.

Respect

> Respect for ourselves guides our morals; respect for others guides our manners.
>
> —*Laurence Sterne*

Respect is an attitude of admiration or esteem. Kant was the first major Western philosopher to put respect for persons, including oneself as a person, at the center of moral theory. He believed that persons are ends in themselves with an absolute dignity, which must always be respected. In contemporary thinking, respect has become a core ideal extending moral respect to things other than persons, including all things in nature.

Caregivers who demonstrate respect for one another and their patients will be more effective in helping them cope with the anxiety of their illness. Respect helps to develop trust between the patient and caregiver and improve healing processes. If caregivers respect the family of a patient, cooperation and understanding will be the positive

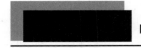

Reality Check: Kindness Is Not Always Returned

The widely known saying "actions speak louder than words" is well demonstrated in this *reality check*. Joe was a health care consultant. He had collected thousands of documents of helpful information to share with health care organizations with which he had worked. His thinking was this: Why should hospitals have to reinvent the wheel? If organizations are willing to share with others, why not disseminate such information for the benefit of other hospitals? His hopes were that larger trade organizations would eventually collect the information and freely share with their constituents. After all, the goal was better care for all wherever they lived. Joe would provide copies of his CD to fellow consultants and encourage them to share the information with others. One day upon arriving at work he noticed that one of the consultants to whom he had given a copy of the CD had four or five newspaper clippings about hospitals spread out on a conference room table. Joe thought they looked interesting and asked, "Could I have a copy of your clippings?" The consultant said, "No, these are proprietary information."

On another occasion, after sharing his CD with an organization, he asked, "Would you be willing to share your '12 Step Addiction Program' with other health care organizations?" A representative from the organization said, "We will share it with you but not others." Joe kindly said, "That's okay. I can accept only what you are willing to share with others."

—*Anonymous*

Discussion

1. Should Joe have asked for his CD back from the consultant and organization? Discuss your answer.

2. Discuss why an organization might not be willing to share program information.

result, encouraging a team effort to improve patient care.

Hopefulness

> Hope is the last thing that dies in man; and though it be exceedingly deceitful, yet it is of this good use to us, that while we are traveling through life, it conducts us in an easier and more pleasant way to our journey's end.
>
> —*Francois de la Rochefoucauld*

Hopefulness in the patient care setting involves looking forward to something with the confidence of success. Caregivers have a responsibility to balance truthfulness while promoting hope. The caregiver must be sensitive to each patient's needs and provide hope. As noted by Brooke's father, we can pass on hope and love to others.

Tolerance

> There is a criterion by which you can judge whether the thoughts you are thinking and the things you are doing are right for you. The criterion is: Have they brought you inner peace? If they have not, there is something wrong with them—so keep seeking! If what you do has brought you inner peace, stay with what you believe is right.
>
> —*Peace Pilgrim*

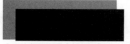 Brooke Greenberg: 20-Year-Old "Toddler's" Legacy of Hope and Love

The baffling case of Brooke Greenberg, a 20-year-old who never developed beyond the toddler stage, may provide clues to help scientists unlock the secrets of longevity and fight age-related disorders, such as Alzheimer's, Parkinson's, and heart disease. Brooke, who passed away last Thursday, had the body and cognitive function of a 1-year-old. She didn't grow after the age of 5—and basically, she stopped aging entirely.

Brooke may have been the only person in the world suffering from a mysterious genetic disease that her doctors called Syndrome X. "Finding out that her DNA makeup is completely different than anyone else brought to our attention that we could help," her father, Howard Greenberg, told Yahoo Shine in a previous interview. "So eventually, at the end of the rainbow, there will be something that comes out of all this. I believe everyone is here for a reason."

Sarah B. Weir, Healthy Living, *October 29, 2013*[14]

Tolerance can be viewed in two ways, positive or negative. *Positive tolerance* implies that a person accepts differences in others and that one does not expect others to believe, think, speak, or act as he or she does. Tolerant people are generally free of prejudice and discrimination. Recognizing this fact, Thomas Jefferson incorporated theories of tolerance into the U.S. Constitution. *Negative tolerance* implies that one will reluctantly put up with another's beliefs. In other words, he or she merely tolerates the views of others.

Although tolerance can be viewed as a virtue, however, not all tolerance is virtuous nor is all intolerance necessarily wrong. An exaggerated tolerance may amount to a vice, whereas intolerance may sometimes be a virtue. For example, tolerating everything regardless of its repugnance (e.g., persecution for religious beliefs) is no virtue, and having intolerance for that which should not be tolerated and is evil is no vice (e.g., mass executions).

Cooperation and Teamwork

If we do not hang together, we will all hang separately.

—*Benjamin Franklin (1706–1790)*

Cooperation is the process of working with others. In the health care setting, caregivers must work together to improve patient outcomes. The health care worker today works in an environment where change is the norm. Those unwilling to accept change and work in unity will eventually be working alone. Change is the only constant in today's workplace and society in general. Technological change is occurring at a pace faster than the human mind can absorb, thus requiring teamwork between individuals with a wide variety of skills sets. Congress, as noted in the following news clipping, is an example of how little can be accomplished when its members are dysfunctional and unwilling to cooperate and work together towards common goals.

Failure to cooperate has a rippling effect in any setting. The failure of Congress to cooperate and resolve funding issues for the Federal Aviation Administration (FAA) before taking its summer recess in 2011 left 74,000 people out of work, costing the nation nearly a billion dollars for the month of August. Failure of the few to cooperate and act responsibly not only affected employees placed on a leave of absence but also placed a financial hardship on their families, not to mention the effect it

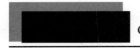

Congress Gets Stuck Again—Over FAA

Parties Blame Each Other in Funding Dispute and Partial Shutdown

A dispute over funding for the Federal Aviation Administration has left an estimated 74,000 people out of work for a dozen days and tossed Congress into the throes of yet another interparty battle.

Now, with lawmakers leaving town or already on recess, there seems to be little hope of a resolution on the horizon.

Ashley Halsey III, The Washington Post, *August 4, 2011*

---

has had on the communities where they live. In addition, passenger safety on airline flights was placed in jeopardy. If hospitals operated in this manner, there would be even more recorded bad outcomes. Teamwork is effective only as long as each member of the team cooperates and fulfills the duties assigned. High-quality patient care is more likely to be better in those organizations where respect and cooperation abounds.

Tying together the Patient Protection and Portable Care Act, commonly referred to as Obamacare, as a prerequisite to approving the national budget has merely resulted in name-calling by government officials, which has stirred bitterness between citizens of varying beliefs. Pundits and politicians alike fill the airways with contemptuous remarks that stoke the flames of division. The need to win one's point of view has selfishly become the norm and more important than the nation itself. Pride and self-appointed power brokers are the hallmarks of those responsible for crisis after crisis. Change comes when the players learn to cooperate for the common good.

Forgiveness

Forgiveness is a virtue of the brave.

—*Indira Gandhi*

Forbearing one another, and forgiving one another, if any man have a quarrel against any: even as Christ forgave you, so also do ye.

—*Colossians 3:13 KJV*

Forgiveness is a virtue and a value. It is the willingness to pardon someone who has wronged you in some way. It is also a form of mercy. Forgiveness is to forgive and let lose the bonds of blame. It is a form of cleansing souls of both those who forgive and those who accept the forgiveness offered.

The following *reality check* is an excerpt of a Facebook discussion between two friends involving courage and forgiveness by two very special people.

RELIGIOUS ETHICS

The Great Physician: Dear Lord, You are the great physician. I turn to you in my sickness, asking you for help. I place myself under Your loving care, praying that I may know Your healing grace and wholeness. Help me to find love in this strange world and to feel your presence by my bed both day and night. Give my doctors and nurses wisdom, that they may understand my illness. Steady and guide them with your strong hand. Reach out Your hand to me and touch my life with Your peace. Amen.

—*University of Pennsylvania Health System*

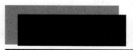

Reality Check: Courage and Forgiveness

7:38 am

    Scotty: Did you see this link http://www
.josieking.org/page.cfm?pageID=10 on the
Internet?

7:38 am

    Diane: Reading it now

    Josie was 18 months old.... In January
of 2001 Josie was admitted ... after suffering
first and second degree burns from climbing
into a hot bath. She healed well and within
weeks was scheduled for release. Two days
before she was to return home she died of
severe dehydration and misused narcotics ...

    Josie spent 10 days in the PICU. I [Josie's
mother] was by her side every day and night.
I paid attention to every minute detail of the
doctors' and nurses' care, and I was quick to
ask questions. I bonded with them and was in
constant awe of the medical attention she received.... She was sent down to the intermediate care floor with expectations of being sent
home in a few days. Her three older siblings
prepared for her welcome home celebration ...

    The following week her central line had
been taken out. I began noticing that every
time she saw a drink she would scream for it,
and I thought this was strange. I was told not
to let her drink. While a nurse and I gave her a
bath, she sucked furiously on a washcloth. As
I put her to bed, I noticed that her eyes were
rolling back in her head. Although I asked the
nurse to call the doctor, she reassured me that
oftentimes children did this and her vitals were
fine. I told her Josie had never done this and
perhaps another nurse could look at her. After
yet another reassurance from another nurse
that everything was fine, I was told that it was
okay for me to sleep at home. I called to check
in two times during the night and returned to

the hospital at 5:30 am. I took one look at
Josie and demanded that a doctor come at
once. She was not fine. Josie's medical team
arrived and administered two shots of Narcan.
I asked if she could have something to drink.
The request was approved, and Josie gulped
down nearly a liter of juice. Verbal orders were
issued for there to be no narcotics given. As
I sat with Josie, I noticed that the nurse on
morning duty was acting very strangely. She
seemed nervous, overly demonstrative and in a
hurry. Uneasy, I asked the other nurses about
her and they said she had been a nurse for a
long time. Still worried, I expressed my concern
to one of the doctors, and he agreed that she
was acting a bit odd. Meanwhile, Josie started
perking up. She was more alert and had kept
all liquids down. I was still scared and asked
her doctors to please stay close by. At 1:00 the
nurse walked over with a syringe of metha-
done. Alarmed, I told her that there had been
an order for no narcotics. She said the orders
had been changed and administered the drug.

    Josie's heart stopped as I was rubbing her
feet. Her eyes were fixed, and I screamed for
help. I stood helpless as a crowd of doctors
and nurses came running into her room. I was
ushered into a small room with a chaplain.

    The next time I saw Josie she had been
moved back up to the PICU. Doctors and
nurses were standing around her bed. No
one seemed to want to look at me. She was
hooked up to many machines, and her leg was
black and blue. I looked into their faces, and
said to them, "You did this to her now YOU
must fix her." I was told to pray. Two days
later Jack, Relly, and Eva were brought to the
hospital to kiss their beloved Josie goodbye.
Josie was taken off of life support. She died in

Reality Check: Courage and Forgiveness *(continued)*

our arms on a snowy night in what's considered to be one of the best hospitals in the world. Our lives were shattered and changed forever.

　　Josie died from severe dehydration and misused narcotics. Careless human errors. On top of our overwhelming sorrow and intense grief we were consumed by anger. They say anger can do one of two things to you. It can cause you to rot away or it can propel you forward. There were days when all I wanted was to destroy the hospital and then put an end to my own pain. My three remaining children were my only reason for getting out of bed and functioning. One day I will tell them how they saved my life. My husband Tony and I decided that we had to let the anger move us forward. We would do something good that would help prevent this from ever happening to a child again.

7:43 am

Diane: I've experience first hand human error in the hospital. I was told by my Dr. it could have been critical and I would have died.

7:45 am

Diane: The nurses don't like him and he told me to write a letter to file a complaint, but the thing is, the nursing staff was so good to me before and after that incident. Evidently when it was happening he yelled at the staff without me knowing. I had no clue what had happened till days later the nurse involved apologized to me profusely.

7:46 am

Diane: But I was so ill I didn't give it much

thought you ever heard of tpn? Its a sugar mixture via iv cuz i couldn't eat. Supposedly it was supposed to be infused in me I think over a 12 hr period?

7:47 am

Diane: But the nurse put it for 4 hrs. I could have gone into diabetic shock. I do remember trying to wake up but I couldn't open my eyes and I heard a lot of movement in my room with the nurses. I yelled out. I can't open my eyes and I'm dretched in sweat. I had no idea wat was happening. I was then put on insulin.

7:50 am

Scotty: I must say you are an amazing young lady.

—Anonymous Patient

Discussion

1. This young lady forgave the nurse and suggested that when the nurse was setting the timing for the TPN, she may have distracted the nurse, and she blamed herself for the wrong setting. Discuss how courage and forgiveness were displayed in this case.

2. Discuss the similarities in values that Josie's mother and the young lady on the Internet have in common.

3. Discuss your thoughts as to how human errors can be prevented, including what roles patients, families, caregivers, hospitals, and regulatory agencies should play in preventing similar errors.

Religious ethics serve a moral purpose by providing codes of conduct for appropriate behavior through revelations from a divine source. These codes of conduct are enforced through fear of pain and suffering in the next life and/or reward in the next life for adhering to religious codes and beliefs. The prospect of divine justice helps us to tolerate the injustices in this life, where goodness is no guarantee of peace, happiness, wellness, or prosperity.

FIGURE 26-3　Religious influence on ethics.

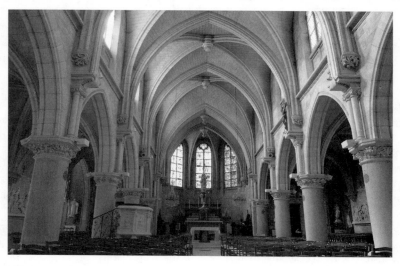

© Pack-Shot/Shutterstock, Inc.

Religion should be a component of the education, policy development, and consultative functions of ethics committees. There is a need to know, for example, how to respond to Jehovah's Witnesses who refuse blood transfusions. Some hospitals provide staff with materials that describe various religious beliefs and how those beliefs might affect the patient's course of care while in the hospital.

Religion is often used as a reason to justify what otherwise could be considered unjustifiable behavior. Political leaders often use religion to legitimize and consolidate their power. Leaders in democratic societies speak of the necessity to respect the right to "freedom of religion."

Political leaders often use religion to further their political aspirations. They have often used religion to justify their actions. Religious persecution has plagued humanity from the beginning of time.

The world today, with the aid of the news media, is able to see firsthand the results of what can happen to innocent people in the name of religion. The atrocities of evil people strapping bombs to the mentally deficient with the purpose of blowing themselves up in public places, killing and maiming men, women, and children, are but a few of the numerous atrocities of what has occurred throughout the ages.

Spirituality implies that there is purpose and meaning to life; spirituality generally refers to faith in a higher being. For a patient, injury and sickness are frightening experiences. This fear is often heightened when the patient is admitted to a hospital or nursing facility. Health care organizations can help reduce patient fears by making available to them appropriate emotional and spiritual support and coping resources. It is a well-proven fact that patients who are able to draw on their spirituality and religious beliefs tend to have a more

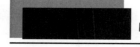

Many Think God's Intervention Can Revive the Dying

When it comes to saving lives, God trumps doctors for many Americans. An eye-opening survey reveals widespread belief that divine intervention can revive dying patients. And, researchers said, doctors "need to be prepared to deal with families who are waiting for a miracle."

Lindsey Tanner, USA Today, *August 18, 2008*

comfortable and often improved healing experience. To assist both patients and caregivers in addressing spiritual needs, patients should be provided with information as to how their spiritual needs can be addressed.

Difficult questions regarding a patient's spiritual needs and how to meet those needs are best addressed on admission by first collecting information about the patient's religious or spiritual preferences. Caregivers often find it difficult to discuss spiritual issues for fear of offending a patient who may have beliefs different from their own. If caregivers know from admission records a patient's religious beliefs, the caregiver can share with the patient those religious and spiritual resources available in the hospital and community.

A variety of religions are described next for the purpose of understanding some of the basic tenets of these religions. They are presented here to note the importance of better understanding why patients differ in decision-making processes and how religion affects their beliefs and to encourage further study of how each religion affects the decision-making process. Hospitals should maintain a directory of the various religions that includes contacts for referral and consultation purposes.

Judaism

Jewish Law refers to the unchangeable 613 mitzvot (commandments) that God gave to the Jews. Halakhah (Jewish Law) comes from three sources: (1) the Torah (the first five books of the Bible); (2) laws instituted by the rabbis; and (3) longstanding customs. The Jewish People is another name for the Children of Israel, referring to the Jews as a nation in the classical sense, meaning a group of people with a shared history and a sense of a group identity rather than a specific place or political persuasion.[15]

Judaism is a monotheistic religion based on principles and ethics embodied in the Hebrew Bible (Old Testament). The notion of right and

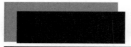

Syrian Rebels Combat al-Qaeda Force

The ISIS extremists "have not the support of the people because they treated them badly. They were cutting off people's heads all of the time to scare them in the name of religion," said Col. Qassim Saadeddine, spokesman for the Revolutionary Front.

Liz Sly, The Washington Post, *January 6, 2013*

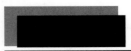

Surgeon Uses Ministry in Medical Practice

DALLAS—At 83, Carl Smith found himself facing quadruple bypass surgery and the real possibility that he might not survive.

Within hours on this spring morning, Dr. Daniel Pool would temporarily bring Smith's heart to a stop in an attempt to circumvent its blocked passages.

And to help his patient confront the uncertainty, Pool did something unusual in his profession: He prayed with him.

The power of healing: Medicine and religion have had their day, and they haven't always been able to coexist. But as today's medical treatment becomes more holistic, doctors are increasingly taking spirituality into account.

Marc Ramirez, Altoona Mirror, *August 9, 2013*

Discussion

1. Discuss the pressure, if any, placed on the patient in responding to the suggestion of prayer prior to surgery.

2. Describe how you, as the surgeon, would address a patient's religious or spiritual needs if the risks of a complex surgical procedure appear to be threatening.

wrong is not so much an object of philosophical inquiry as an acceptance of divine revelation. Moses, for example, received a list of 10 laws directly from God. These laws were known as the 10 Commandments. Some of the 10 Commandments are related to the basic principles of justice that have been adhered to by society since they were first proclaimed and published. For some societies, the 10 Commandments were a turning point, where essential commands such as "thou shalt not kill" or "thou shalt not commit adultery" were accepted as law. The 10 Commandments (King James Version of the Bible) are as follows:

1. Thou shalt have no other gods before me.
2. Thou shalt not make unto thee any graven image, or any likeness of anything that is in heaven above, or that is in the earth beneath, or that is in the water under the earth. Thou shalt not bow down thyself to them, nor serve them.
3. Thou shalt not take the name of the Lord thy God in vain.
4. Remember the Sabbath day, to keep it holy.
5. Honor thy father and thy mother: that thy days may be long upon the land which the Lord thy God giveth thee.
6. Thou shalt not kill.
7. Thou shalt not commit adultery.
8. Thou shalt not steal.
9. Thou shalt not bear false witness against thy neighbor.
10. Thou shalt not covet thy neighbor's house, thou shalt not covet thy neighbor's wife, nor his manservant, nor his maidservant, nor his ox, nor his ass, nor anything that is thy neighbor's.

When caring for the dying, family members will normally want to be present and prayers will be spoken. If a rabbi is requested, the patient's own rabbi should be contacted first.

Hinduism

Hinduism is a polytheistic religion with many gods and goddesses. Hindus believe that God is everything and is infinite. The earliest known Hindu Scriptures were recorded around 1200 BC. Hindus believe in reincarnation and that one's present condition is a reflection of one's virtuous behavior or lack thereof in a previous lifetime.

When caring for the dying, relatives may wish to perform rituals at this time. In death, jewelry, sacred threads, or other religious objects should not be removed from the body. Washing the body is part of the funeral rites and should be carried out by the relatives.[16]

Buddhism

Buddhism is a religion and philosophy encompassing a variety of traditions, beliefs, and practices, based largely on teachings attributed to Prince Siddhartha Gautama (563–483 BC), son of King Suddhodana and Queen Mayadevi, who lived in the present-day border area between India and Nepal. He had gone on a spiritual quest and eventually became enlightened at the age of 35, and from then on, he took the name Buddha. Simply defined, Buddhism is a religion to some and a philosophy to others that encourages one "to do good, avoid evil, and purify the mind."

When caring for the dying, Buddhists like to be informed about their health status in order to prepare themselves spiritually. A side room with privacy is preferred.[17]

Falun Gong

Falun Gong, also referred to as *Falun Dafa*, is a traditional Chinese spiritual discipline belonging to the Buddhist school of thought. It consists of moral teachings, a meditation, and four exercises that resemble tai chi and are known in Chinese culture as *qigong*. Falun Gong does not involve physical places of worship, formal hierarchies, rituals, or membership and is taught without charge. The three principles practiced by the followers are truthfulness, compassion, and forbearance/tolerance toward others. The followers of Falun Gong claim a following in 100 countries.

Zen

Zen evolved from Buddhism in Tibet. It emphasizes dharma practice (from the master to the disciple) and experiential wisdom based on learning through the reflection on doing, going beyond scriptural readings. In Zen, Buddhism learning comes through a form of seated meditation known as *zazen*, where practitioners perform meditation to calm the body and the mind and experience insight into the nature of existence and thereby gain enlightenment.

Taoism

Taoists believe that ultimate reality is unknowable and unperceivable. The founder of Taoism is believed to be Lao Tzu (6 BC). Taoist doctrine includes the belief that the proper way of living involves being in tune with nature. Everything is ultimately interblended and interacts.

Christianity

Christianity is based on the Bible's New Testament teachings. Christians accept both the Old and New Testament as being the word of God. The New Testament describes Jesus as being God, taking the form of man. He was born of the Virgin Mary, sacrificed his life by suffering crucifixion, and after being raised from the dead on the third day, he ascended into Heaven from which he will return to raise the dead, at which time the spiritual body will be united with the physical body. His death, burial, and resurrection provide a way of salvation through belief in Him for the forgiveness of sin. God is believed to be manifest in three persons: the Father, Son, and Holy Spirit.

The primary and final authority for Christian ethics is found in the life, teachings, ministry, death, and resurrection of Jesus Christ. He clarified the ethical demands of a God-centered life by applying the obedient love that was required of Peter. The 10 Commandments are accepted and practiced by both Christians and Jews.

Christians, when determining what is the right thing to do, often refer to the Golden

Rule, which teaches us to "do unto others as you would have them do unto you," a common principle in many moral codes and religions.

There have been and continue to be numerous interpretations of the meaning of the scriptures and their different passages by Christians over the centuries. This has resulted in a plethora of churches with varying beliefs. As noted later, such beliefs can affect a patient's wishes for health care. However, the heart of Christian beliefs is found in the book of John:

> For God so loved the world, that he gave his only begotten Son, that whoever believeth in him should not perish, but have everlasting life.
>
> — *King James Version, John 3:16*

The Apostle Paul proclaimed that salvation cannot be gained through good works but through faith in Jesus Christ as savior. He recognized the importance of faith in Christ over good works in the pursuit of salvation.

> That if thou shalt confess with thy mouth the Lord Jesus, and shalt believe in thine heart that God hath raised him from the dead, thou shalt be saved.
>
> — *King James Version, Romans 10:9*

The Apostle Paul, however, did not dismiss the importance of good works. Works are the fruit of one's faith. In other words, good works follows faith.

Anointing of the Sick

When caring for the dying, services of the in-house chaplain and/or one's religious minister should be offered the patient. A Catholic priest should be offered when last rites need to be administered to those of the Catholic faith.

Islam

The Islamic religion believes there is one God: Allah. Muhammad (570–632 AD) is considered to be a prophet/messenger of God. He is believed to have received revelations from God.

These revelations were recorded in the Qur'an, the Muslim Holy Book. Muslims accept Moses and Jesus as prophets of God. The Qur'an is believed to supersede that of the Torah and the Bible. Muslims believe that there is no need for God's grace and that their own actions can merit God's mercy and goodness. Humans are believed to have a moral responsibility to submit to God's will and to follow Islam as demonstrated in the Qur'an. The five pillars of the practice of Islam are believing the creed, performing five prayers daily, giving alms, fasting during Ramadan, and making a pilgrimage to Mecca at least once in a lifetime.

When caring for the dying, patients may want to die facing Mecca (toward the southeast) and be with relatives. In death, many Muslims follow strict rules in respect of the body after death.

Religious Beliefs and Duty Conflict

Religious beliefs and codes of conduct sometimes conflict with the ethical duty of caregivers to save lives. For example, Jehovah's Witnesses, believe that it is a sin to accept a blood transfusion because the Bible states that we must "abstain from blood" (Acts 15:29). Current Jehovah's Witness doctrine, in part, states that blood must not be transfused. In order to respect this belief, bloodless surgery is available in a number of hospitals to patients who find it against their religious beliefs to receive a blood transfusion.

Every attempt should be made to resolve blood transfusion issues prior to any elective surgery. The transfusion of blood to an emergent unconscious patient may be necessary to save the patient's life. Because some Jehovah's Witnesses would accept blood in such situations, most courts would most likely find such a transfusion acceptable. When transfusion of a minor becomes necessary and parental consent is refused, it may be necessary to seek a court order to allow for such transfusions. Because time is of the essence in many cases, it is important for hospitals to work out such issues in advance with legislative bodies and the judicial

Code of Hammurabi

5

If a judge try a case, reach a decision, and present his judgment in writing; if later error shall appear in his decision, and it be through his own fault, then he shall pay twelve times the fine set by him in the case, and he shall be publicly removed from the judge's bench, and never again shall he sit there to render judgment.

194

If a man give his child to a nurse and the child die in her hands, but the nurse unbeknown to the father and mother nurse another child, then they shall convict her of having nursed another child without the knowledge of the father and mother and her breasts shall be cut off.

215

If a physician make a large incision with an operating knife and cure it, or if he open a tumor (over the eye) with an operating knife, and saves the eye, he shall

receive ten shekels in money.

217

If he be the slave of some one, his owner shall give the physician two shekels.

218

If a physician make a large incision with the operating knife, and kill him, or open a tumor with the operating knife, and cut out the eye, his hands shall be cut off.

219

If a physician make a large incision in the slave of a freed man, and kill him, he shall replace the slave with another slave.

221

If a physician heal the broken bone or diseased soft part of a man, the patient shall pay the physician five shekels in money.

system in order to provide legal protection for caregivers who find it necessary to transfuse blood in order to save a life. In those instances in which the patient has a right to refuse a blood transfusion, the hospital should seek a formal signed release from the patient.

SECULAR ETHICS

Unlike religious ethics, *secular ethics* is based on codes developed by societies that have relied on customs to formulate their codes. The Code of Hammurabi, for example, carved on a black Babylonian column 8 feet high, now located in the Louvre in Paris, depicts a mythical sun god presenting a code of laws to Hammurabi, a great military leader and ruler of Babylon (1795–1750 BC). Hammurabi's code of laws is an early example of a ruler proclaiming to his people an entire body of laws. The preceding excerpts are from the Code of Hammurabi.

ATHEISM

Atheism is the rejection of belief in any god, generally because atheists believe there is no scientific evidence that can prove God exists. They argue that there is no objective moral standard for right and wrong and that ethics and morality are the products of culture and politics, subject to individual convictions.

Those of various religious faiths, however, believe there is overwhelming evidence that there is reason to believe that God does exist and that the evidence through historical documents, archeological finds, and the vastness of space and time clearly supports and confirms the existence of God. Christians often refer to the Old Testament and cite the book of Isaiah:

It is He that sitteth upon the circle of the earth . . .

—Isaiah 40:22 (King James Version)

Christians argue when citing this verse that Isaiah could not possibly know that the earth is the shape of a circle. He presents no magical formula or scientific argument in his writings as to why the earth is round. Furthermore, Isaiah does not belabor the fact that the earth is round. The argument continues in the book of Job:

> He stretcheth out the north over the empty place, and hangeth the earth upon nothing.
>
> —*Job 26:7 (King James Version)*

The obvious question then arises, how did Job know, 3,000 years before it became a scientific, verifiable fact, the earth hangs upon nothing?

SITUATIONAL ETHICS

> Be careful how you judge others… . As Scottish author J.M. Barrie said, "Never ascribe to an opponent motives meaner than your own." We tend to judge others based on their behavior, and ours based on our intent. In almost all situations, we would do well to recognize the possibility—even probability—of good intent in others … sometimes despite their observable behavior.
>
> —*Stephen M. R. Covey, The Speed of Trust* (*Free Press*)

Situational ethics is concerned with the outcome or consequences of an action in which the ends can justify the means. It refers to those times when a person's beliefs and values can change as circumstances change. Why do good people behave differently in similar situations? Why do good people sometimes do bad things? The answer is fairly simple: One's moral character can sometimes change as circumstances change; thus the term *situational ethics*. A person, therefore, may contradict what he believes is the right thing to do and do what he morally considers wrong. For example, a decision not to use extraordinary means to sustain the life of an unknown 84-year-old may result in a different decision if the 84-year-old is one's mother.

The news clipping that follows illustrates how far society can regress when there are no common rules, values, or boundaries to guide us.

Have we lost our way? Have we lost our sense as to what is right and what is wrong? We say we have become a melting pot with some common themes but uncommon beliefs. In religion, there are those who sometimes seek a place of worship not always because one seeks what is right but because unconsciously it supports an individual's beliefs of what is right and wrong. Sometimes one's ever-changing choice of lifestyle contradicts earlier beliefs and can often result in a change in place of worship.

The values held ever so strongly in one situation may conflict with the same values given a different fact pattern. To better understand the concept of situational ethics, consider the desire to live and the extreme measures one will take in order to do so, remembering that ethical decision making is the process of determining the right thing to do when faced with moral dilemmas.

Consider the account of the plane crash on October 13, 1972, high in the Andes Mountains. The survivors of the crash, until the day they were rescued, were faced with difficult decisions in order to survive. Of the original 40 passengers and 5 crewmembers, 16 emerged alive 72 days later to tell the story of the difficult ethical dilemmas and survival decisions they had to make.

Those who wished to survive had to eat the flesh of those who did not survive. They realized that to survive, they would have to deviate from their beliefs that teach it is morally wrong to eat the flesh of another human being. Given a different fact pattern, where there would have been an abundance of food at the site of the plane crash, the survivors would have found it reprehensible to eat human flesh. This is a gruesome story indeed, but it illustrates how there are no effective hard and fast rules or guidelines to govern ethical behavior when faced with-life-or death decisions. The reader here should consider here how one's beliefs, decisions, and/or

Viet Cong Execution

"And out of nowhere came this guy who we didn't know." Gen. Nguyen Ngoc Loan, chief of South Viet Nam's national police, walked up and shot the prisoner in the head. His reason: The prisoner, a Viet Cong lieutenant, had just murdered a South Vietnamese colonel, his wife, and their six children.

The peace movement adopted the photo as a symbol of the war's brutality. But

Adams, who stayed in touch with Loan, said the photo wrongly stereotyped the man. "If you're this general and you caught this guy after he killed some of your people ... how do you know you wouldn't have pulled that trigger yourself? You have to put yourself in that situation.... It's a war."

1969 Spot News, Newseum, *Washington, DC*

---

actions can change as circumstances change. Such is the case in the patient care setting where individual differences emerge based on needs, beliefs, and values.

ABSENCE OF A MORAL COMPASS

> The world is a dangerous place. Not because of the people who are evil; but because of the people who don't do anything about it.
>
> —*Albert Einstein*

The nation's health care system is off course as noted by the absence of a moral compass. Trust in the health care system continues to decline when those who are entrusted with providing health care prescribe unnecessary procedures (e.g., cardiac catheterizations, hysterectomies, tonsillectomies), molest our children, secretly record photographic pictures of patients while they are receiving physical examinations, commit numerous fraudulent billing scams costing the nation billions of dollars annually, tamper with chemotherapy agents by diluting them (unbeknown by patients who trust they are being treated by caregivers with integrity), allow unwarranted delays in high-risk life-saving treatment for our veterans and falsification of records, and the list of unethical behavior

continues to grow, seemingly unabated. The failure of government and those in leadership roles have failed to reset the nation's moral compass. The present path to better health care for all continues on an unacceptable course of corruption and is increasingly becoming a disturbing public concern.

Political corruption, antisocial behavior, declining civility, and rampant unethical conduct have heightened discussions over the nation's moral decline and decaying value systems in the delivery of health care. The numerous instances of questionable political decisions and numbers-cooking executives with exorbitant salaries, including health care executives working for both profit and nonprofit organizations, have all contributed to the nation's moral decline.

The continuing trend of consumer awareness of declining value systems mandates that the readers of this text understand ethics and the law and how they intertwine. Applying the generally accepted ethical principles (e.g., do good and not harm) and the moral values (e.g., respect, trust, integrity, compassion) described in this chapter will help sit a better course for those who are guided by a moral compass. It is the responsibility of every person to participate

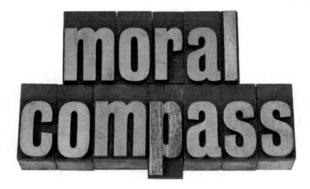

© marekuliasz/Shutterstock

in resetting the moral compass, in our nation and in the world at large.

SUMMARY THOUGHTS

Be careful of your thoughts, for your thoughts inspire your words. Be careful of your words, for your words precede your actions. Be careful of your actions, for your actions become your habits. Be careful of your habits, for your habits build your character. Be careful of your character, for your character decides your destiny.

—Chinese Proverb

Although you cannot control the amount of time you have in this lifetime, you can control your behavior by adopting the virtues and values that will define who you are and what you will become and how you will be remembered or forgotten.

Become who you want to be and behave how you want to be remembered. The formula is easy and well described previously in what has been claimed to be a Chinese proverb. Read it. Reread it. Write it. Memorize it. Display it in your home, at work, and in your car, and most of all, practice it, always remembering that it all begins with thoughts.

Control your thoughts, and do not let them control you. As to words, they are the tools of thought. They can be sharper than any double-edged sword and hurt, or they can do good and heal.

It is never too late to change your thoughts, as long as you have air to breathe. Your legacy may be short, but it can be powerful. Remember the Gettysburg address. In the final analysis:

People are often unreasonable, illogical and self-centered; forgive them anyway. If you are kind, people may accuse you of selfish, ulterior motives; be kind anyway. If you are successful, you will win some false friends and some true enemies; succeed anyway. What you spend years building, someone may destroy overnight; build anyway. The good you do today, people will often forget tomorrow; do good anyway. Give the world the best you have, and it may never be enough; give the world the best you have anyway. You see, in the final analysis, it is between you and God; It was never between you and them anyway.

—Author Unknown

CHAPTER REVIEW

1. *Ethics* is the branch of philosophy that seeks to understand the nature, purposes,

justification, and founding principles of moral rules and the systems they compose.

   a. *Microethics* involves an individual's view of what is right and wrong based on his or her life experiences.
   b. *Macroethics* involves a more generalized view of right and wrong.

2. *Bioethics* addresses such difficult issues as the nature of life, the nature of death, what sort of life is worth living, what constitutes murder, how we should treat people who are especially vulnerable, and the responsibilities we have to other human beings.

3. We study ethics to aid us in making sound judgments, good decisions, and right choices.

4. Ethics signifies a general pattern or way of life, such as religious ethics; a set of rules of conduct or "moral code," which involves professional ethics; or philosophical ethics, which involves inquiry about ways of life and rules of conduct.

5. *Morality* is a code of conduct. It is a guide to behavior that all rational persons would put forward for governing the behavior of all moral agents.

6. There is no "universal morality." Whatever guide to behavior that an individual regards as overriding and wants to be universally adopted is considered that individual's morality.

7. *Moral judgments* are those judgments concerned with what an individual or group believes to be the right or proper behavior in a given situation.

8. Morality is often legislated when differences cannot be resolved because of conflicting moral codes with varying opinions as to what is right and what is wrong (e.g., abortion). Laws are created to set boundaries for societal behavior, and they are enforced to ensure that the expected behavior is followed.

9. *Ethical theories* and principles introduce order into the way people think about life. *Metaethics* seeks to understand ethical terms and theories and their application. The following are ethical theories:

   a. *Normative ethics* is the attempt to determine what moral standards should be followed so that human behavior and conduct may be morally right.
   b. *Descriptive ethics*, also known as comparative ethics, deals with what people believe to be right and wrong.
   c. *Applied ethics* is the application of normative theories to practical moral problems. It is the attempt to explain and justify specific moral problems such as abortion, euthanasia, and assisted suicide.
   d. The *consequential theory* emphasizes that the morally right action is whatever action leads to the maximum balance of good over evil. The consequential theory is based on the view that the value of an action derives solely from the value of its consequences.
   e. *Utilitarian ethics* involves the concept that the moral worth of an action is determined solely by its contribution to overall utility, that is, its contribution to happiness or pleasure as summed among all persons.
   f. *Deontological ethics* focuses on one's duties to others. It includes telling the truth and keeping your promises. Deontology is an ethical analysis according to a moral code or rules.
   g. The *nonconsequential ethical theory* denies that the consequences of an action or rule are the only criteria for determining the morality of an action or rule.
   h. *Ethical relativism* is the theory that holds that morality is relative to the norms of one's culture.

10. Common principles of ethics include:

    a. *Autonomy* involves recognizing the right of a person to make his or her own decisions.

    b. *Beneficence* describes the principle of doing good, demonstrating kindness, showing compassion, and helping others.

        i. *Paternalism* is a form of beneficence. It may involve withholding information from a person because of the belief that doing so is in the best interest of that person.

        ii. *Medical paternalism* involves making choices for (or forcing choices on) patients who are capable of choosing for themselves. It directly violates patient autonomy.

    c. *Nonmaleficence* is an ethical principle that requires caregivers to avoid causing harm to patients.

    d. *Justice* is the obligation to be fair in the distribution of benefits and risks.

        i. *Distributive justice* is a principle that requires treatment of all persons equally and fairly.

11. *Virtue ethics and values*

    a. *Virtue* is normally defined as some sort of moral excellence or beneficial quality. In traditional ethics, virtues are characteristics that differentiate good people from bad people.

    b. *Virtue ethics* focuses on the inherent character of a person rather than on the specific actions he or she performs.

    c. *Value* is something that has worth. Values are used for judging the goodness or badness of some action.

        i. *Ethical values* imply standards of worth.

        ii. *Intrinsic value* is something that has value in and of itself.

        iii. *Instrumental value* is something that helps to give value to something else (e.g., money is valuable for what it can buy).

        iv. Values may change as needs change.

12. *Religious ethics* serves a moral purpose by providing codes of conduct for appropriate behavior through revelations from a divine source.

13. *Secular ethics* is based on codes developed by societies that have relied on customs to formulate their codes.

14. *Situational ethics* describes how a particular situation may influence how one's reaction and values may change in order to cope with changing circumstances.

15. The acceptance, understanding, and application of the ethical and moral concepts learned in this chapter will provide a *moral compass* to guide the reader through life's journey.

DISCUSSION QUESTIONS ⎯⎯⎯⎯⎯

1. What is ethics?

2. Why should one study ethics?

3. What is morality?

4. Describe the ethical theories presented in this chapter.

5. What is ethical relativism? What is the relevance of this concept to individuals of various cultures living in the same society?

6. Describe the various ethical principles reviewed and how they might be helpful in resolving health care ethical dilemmas.

7. Describe virtue ethics and values. How do virtues and values differ?

8. Discuss why courage could be considered as the greatest of all virtues.

9. Discuss how religion can affect one's character.

10. Describe the principle of justice and how it can affect the decision-making process.

11. Explain how you would allocate scarce resources in the provision of health care?

12. What is situational ethics? Why do people behave differently in different situations?

NOTES _____

1. http://www.bukisa.com/articles/15091_the -root-of-ethics-and-morality.

2. Ayer, A. J., 1946. "A Critique of Ethics," in *Language, Truth and Logic*, London: Gollanz, pp. 102–114.

3. http://public.health.oregon.gov/ProviderPartner Resources/EvaluationResearch/Deathwith DignityAct/Pages/index.aspx.

4. http://www.ethicsmorals.com/ethicsapplied. html.

5. http://smallbusiness.chron.com/workplace -example-duty-based-ethics-11972.html

6. 105 N.E. 92, 93 (N.Y. 1914).

7. http://www.ama-assn.org/ama/pub/physician -resources/medical-ethics/code-medical-ethics /principles-medical-ethics.page

8. http://www.healthlawyers.org/Members /PracticeGroups/PALS/emailalerts/Documents /131111_SurveyandCertLetter.pdf.

9. Craig Robert Senn, Fixing Inconsistent Paternalism Under Federal Employment Discrimination Law 58 UCLA L. Rev. 947. http://uclalawreview .org/?p=1679.

10. 464 A.2d 303, 314 (N.J. Super. Ct. App. Div. 1983).

11. http://www.mercurynews.com/san-mateo-county -times/ci_23948856/peninsula-child-psychiatrist -william-ayres-sentenced-eight-years?source =rss&cid=dlvr.it.

12. http://www.bukisa.com/articles/15091_the-root -of-ethics-and-morality.

13. http://www.gallup.com/poll/7288/Fear-Factor -Patient-Satisfaction.aspx.

14. http://shine.yahoo.com/healthy-living/brooke -greenberg-20-old-8220-toddler-8217-8221 -185100345.html.

15. Tracey R. Rich, "Halakhah: Jewish Law," http: //www.jewfaq.org/halakhah.htm (accessed October 13, 2010).

16. *Id.*

17. *Id.*

Advanced Practice Nursing: The Nurse–Patient Relationship and General Ethical Concerns

Pamela J. Grace

© A-R-T/Shutterstock

> Our privileges can be no greater than our obligations. The protection of our rights can endure no longer than the performance of our responsibilities.
>
> —John F. Kennedy, "The Educated Citizen," Vanderbilt University 90th Convocation Address, May 18, 1963

CHAPTER OBJECTIVES

1. Identify which individual and environmental factors interfere with ethical nursing actions.

2. Describe ethical issues that can occur when obtaining one of the three types of informed consent.

3. Discuss proxy decision making and advance directives.

4. Understand the role of social media as it pertains to privacy and confidentiality in healthcare settings.

INTRODUCTION

An estimated 24 countries have nurses practicing in advanced roles (Nieminen, Mannevaara, & Fagerström, 2011). Where possible, the expertise of colleagues from countries outside the United States has been solicited to help understand and account both for similarities and differences in ethical issues faced by persons who are in a variety of roles and designations.

For North America, the acronym APN stands for advanced practice nurses to avoid confusion because the acronym for advanced nursing practice (ANP)—the term used by the International Council of Nurses (ICN)—denotes specialty certification as an adult nurse practitioner in the United States, which is just one of many possible advanced practice designations globally.

Here it is important to consider the essence of the advanced practice role. Are there commonalities across countries and settings? Contemporarily, there is wide interest in describing the scope and boundaries of such roles, and deriving a coherent internationally acceptable definition is seen as a necessary step in professional development to meet the needs of diverse patients and communities across country boundaries. Hanson and Hamric (2003) have synthesized a definition of advanced practice nursing from several important resource documents and their own experiences of the development of advanced practice: "Advanced nursing practice is the application of an expanded range of practical, theoretical, and research-based therapeutics to phenomena experienced by patients within a specialized clinical area of the larger discipline of nursing" (p. 205). The ICN's publication on advanced practice nursing (Schober & Affara, 2006) cites the 2002 ICN definition of the advanced practice nurse as:

> a registered nurse who has acquired the expert knowledge base, complex decision-making skills and clinical competencies for expanded practice, the characteristics of which are shaped by the context and/or country in which s/he is credentialed to practice. [Further the ICN recommends] a masters degree… for entry level (practice). (Schober & Affara, 2006, p. 210)

Advanced nursing roles have existed for several decades in many countries, for example, midwifery and health visitors in the United Kingdom and other countries and nurse anesthetists in the United States. However, the first officially designated advanced practice role in the United States was that of nurse practitioner (NP) in the mid-1960s (Schober & Affara, 2006). Ketefian, Redman, Hanucharurnkul, Masterson, and Neves (2001) identified several critical factors that have been conducive to the development of these roles internationally. These are "environment; the health needs of society; the health workforce supply and demand; governmental policy and support; intra- and interprofessional collaboration; the development of nursing education; and documentation of effectiveness of the advanced role" (p. 152).

The APN role is nevertheless a nursing role that is distinguishable from other nursing roles only by the breadth and depth of responsibility to patients implied by the term *advanced practice*. This means, for example, that APNs often oversee a patient's total care in a given practice setting (e.g., primary care, anesthesia, midwifery, gerontology), and in alternate settings they also have expanded responsibilities. For example, in acute care they may be responsible for handling emergencies and ordering and carrying out invasive interventions. For this reason and in this sense, their moral responsibilities can sometimes seem more complex and onerous "than those of nurses who share [patient] oversight with other health-care professionals" (Grace, 2004b, pp. 321–322). Effective exploration of ethical issues faced in advanced practice, then, should reflect the implications of these broad role obligations. That is, although the ethical substance of situations may not differ from that faced by nurses in nonexpanded roles, advanced practice nursing ethics account for the more extensive duties incurred in these roles.

The following inquiry focuses on a variety of ethical problems and concerns that are common across many advanced practice settings. Such concerns are also discussed in general nursing ethics textbooks and will not be unfamiliar to the seasoned clinician. Here, however, the implications of these issues are discussed specifically in terms of the APN's augmented responsibilities. Illustrative examples are drawn from a variety of advanced practice sources and from my experiences as an APN, as well as from cases shared by nurses in the master's level ethics course I teach. Because it is not feasible to cover all issues that an APN is likely to encounter, it is suggested that any troubling issues that the student or graduated APN faces that are not directly addressed in this text be brought up for in-class exploration with faculty and peers or explored with colleagues using the insights and strategies provided here or in other resources. Other helpful resources include clinical ethicists, philosophers who have ethics expertise, ethics websites, and networking groups.

An appropriate start to the next section is a comprehensive discussion of the demands of the nurse–patient relationship. Characteristics discovered to be essential for consistently good patient care and decision making are explored, with suggestions for the development of these. These qualities are sometimes called virtues and include the use of both intellect (thinking) and affect (emotions and motivation) in decision making and ensuing action. Certain philosophers, such as Aristotle and more contemporarily Alasdair MacIntyre (2007), have argued that virtues can be developed through habitual practice. A person who develops a virtuous personality through habitual practice is predisposed to consistently engage in "good" actions. It is debatable whether all persons can become virtuous in this way or even that people who might be considered "good" persons always act in "good" ways. It is useful to focus on developing existing qualities that facilitate professional–patient relationships and equally useful to be mindful that circumstances can sometimes get in the way of this focus. Examples of important qualities are discussed in more depth later in the chapter; they include such characteristics as empathy, veracity, transparency of purpose, cultural sensitivity, motivation to act, courage to act, and perseverance in carrying an act through.

A further important issue for all clinical and research settings is that of adequately informing patients (or their surrogate decision makers) about their options for care, treatments, and procedures. Thus, the parameters and demands of informed consent are explicated in this chapter with the exception of informed consent in human subjects' protection. Problems associated with the adequacy of informed consent to the provision of care and therapeutics include the issue of patients who lack decision-making capacity for a variety of reasons, persons who are difficult to engage with, and people who are making decisions that seem to be at odds with their own values. A further topic investigated is that of privacy and confidentiality related to patients' health information. In this highly technological age, it is becoming increasingly difficult to adequately protect patient information from entities that do not necessarily have a patient's best interests in mind when seeking it. Additionally, inadvertent breaches of confidentiality can occur via the use of social media. Unethical use of social media can also lead to loss of trust in the involved profession (an example of this is provided later). The protection of information is multifaceted. One important aspect is transparency. The person at risk should be told for what purposes the data are required and to what uses they will be put, and insofar as these are known, the risks and benefits of sharing the data. This is in addition to being careful about who can have access to a person's data.

Additionally, APNs often have concerns about how to maintain their personal integrity. Sometimes this is related to patient or peer requests to engage in something that is at odds with a nurse's values, or it may be related to conflicts within the healthcare system, such as managed care or institutional pressures to limit care. Some of the sources of these concerns, along with strategies to address them, are presented. Finally, because some practice problems end up as complex and extremely difficult to sort out, the issue of preventive ethics is woven throughout this section. Many so-called dilemmas actually can be prevented or diffused by good communication or an early understanding of the likelihood that unaddressed problems might cause critical difficulties for the patient in question and/or the patient's significant others.

VIRTUE ETHICS: THE CHARACTERISTICS OF GOOD APNs

Many people are attracted to the nursing profession because they see it as a practice that contributes to individuals, as well as the greater societal good. This is true not just at the undergraduate level but also for those who choose nursing as a second career and take an accelerated route to ANP. Thus, the personal values of nurses are often congruent with the values of the nursing profession—for example, nascent nurses are drawn to the idea of contributing to the well-being of others. The desire to contribute to the welfare of others is often considered a virtue (as opposed to the desire to hurt someone, which would be considered a vice). As Feldman (1978) writes, in acknowledging that something is good, we are noting its qualities "relative to some class of comparison… some feature of that thing in virtue of which [we] hold it to be good. This feature is its virtue, or good-making characteristic" (p. 234). This section explores the issue of virtue ethics as it relates to good APNs, where *good* is taken to be synonymous with ethical. Virtue ethics in healthcare practice is essentially the idea that a person can cultivate certain characteristics (virtues) that will predispose him or her to good actions related to the profession's predetermined goals.

Contemporary proponents of virtue ethics almost all trace their influences back to Aristotle, although ideas about virtue can also be discovered in ancient texts on Eastern philosophy. Aristotle's idea is that a good or virtuous person is someone who possesses practical wisdom or prudence. The Greek term for this is *phronesis*. Practical wisdom permits a man (in ancient times women were considered subordinate to men) to understand both what is a good way to live and that living a good life necessarily means developing mutually beneficial relationships with others. To act well, a man must learn to habitually moderate emotional impulses by using reasoning. This is what is required to achieve the desired purpose of living a good life. Eventually, a person will habituate himself to always engaging in good action—he will become a good or virtuous person. The desirable or virtuous purpose of all human beings, according to Aristotle, is to live in accordance with their human nature. The essential characteristic of human nature—that which distinguishes human nature from the nature of all other beings—is rationality. The ability of human beings to use logical reasoning gives human beings purpose, and that purpose is the pursuit of a satisfying life. The Greek term for this is *eudaimonia*, often also referred to as happiness, although it loses something in the translation and does not mean happiness in any superficial sense of the term (Hutchinson, 1995).

Practical reason acts as a constraint on emotional and instinctual drives that can result in harmful actions on the one hand and on the other hand in a lack of needed action or in inadequate action. Reason mediates a balance between extremes of action. For example, according to Aristotle, courage is a virtue. Unrestrained courage can cause unnecessarily risky behavior, which is therefore irrational. Alternatively, timidity in the face of doing something important is problematic and also requires reason to moderate action. Practicing the development of virtue eventually leads to the formation of a virtuous character. Additionally, a satisfying life is necessarily lived within society and in relationships with others and facilitates harmony in these relationships. It is noteworthy that for Aristotle being virtuous has a self-focus, but nonetheless a harmonious society is also requisite for a satisfying life. Thus, the actions of a virtuous man have the serendipitous result of contributing to the good of others.

How does this explanation of virtue pertain to the current project of understanding what characteristics are necessary for good practice? The answer is that contemporary moral philosophers, such as Elizabeth Anscombe (1958/1981), Bernard Williams (1985), and Alasdair MacIntyre (2007), have been interested in resurrecting the idea of virtue as a way to understand peoples' relationships to each other and to inform provider–patient relationships. This move represents, in part at least, a way around the problem that deontological and consequentialist ethical theories do not account for the contextual and relationship-dependent nature of human life in situations where moral decision making is needed. Neither do these theories always capture contingencies of healthcare providers' multifaceted and relationally oriented roles.

MacIntyre's work, although not resulting in a theory that can be applied directly to action, does provide some unifying ideas about virtues (Sellman, 2000, p. 27). The constituents of virtue, or those characteristics that make a person virtuous in MacIntyre's view, are context dependent. Thus, virtues may be "seen as supporting and maintaining particular ends" (Sellman, 2000, p. 27). Because virtues are seen as those characteristics necessary to support a particular end, goal, or practice, some common objections to the idea that a virtue ethic is helpful in healthcare practice are overcome (Armstrong, 2006; Begley, 2005; Sellman, 2000). Criticisms of virtue ethics include the observation that what is virtuous in one situation or in a given culture may not be considered virtuous in another. Therefore, there is no stable footing for the idea of a virtuous person, and neither is there a list of virtues a person must possess to be virtuous.

An additional and potentially serious criticism is that there is no external criterion (within virtue theory) for judging whether the actions of a virtuous person are actually good. There is no "gold standard" for good actions. Additionally, the actions of someone who is thought to be virtuous will not necessarily always be good; that is, they may not meet a predetermined goal. Many factors can interfere with a good person's ability to do good actions, as listed in **Table 27-1**.

However, if certain virtues are viewed as pertaining to a particular professional practice and necessary for meeting the goals of that practice, then it is possible to evaluate a given action based on how well it addresses those goals. Because nursing is a practice profession with relatively well articulated goals, it is possible to agree that persons who possess certain characteristics are more likely than those who do not to routinely engage in good practice to be willing to address practice structures that interfere with good actions. A further consequence is that, as a profession, nursing must continue to investigate what the characteristics of a good nurse are and then nurture these traits in the education and mentoring of nurses. A big question for the profession itself is whether all prospective nurses are capable of developing the characteristics of good nurses. If not, what is the profession's responsibility (assumed by its educators) to "weed out" those who are incapable of being good nurses?

Virtues of Nursing

Nursing practice and the fulfillment of nursing goals, then, can be understood as requiring the development of certain facilitative characteristics. Indeed, by exploring what is needed to provide good nursing care to patients—as outlined in the literature and in codes of ethics—relatively quickly, it becomes possible to compose a list of virtues that it would be good for nurses to cultivate. Additionally, nursing curricula should nurture these characteristics (Haggerty & Grace, 2008). Begley (2005) has composed such a list; it includes compassion, integrity,

TABLE 27-1	Factors That Interfere with Ethical Nursing Action

Locus	Factors
Agent related	Level of moral development
	Capacity to recognize ethical content. Chambliss (1996) discusses the phenomenon "routinization of disaster."
	Openness to reflection
	Personal or emotional issues
	Energy levels
	Creativity
	Locus of control (powerfulness/powerlessness)
	Unable to connect with patient
	Fear of disapproval (peer or other)
	Disapproval of patient's choice
	Time of day—complexity of preceding workload or decisions
	Level of knowledge related to the issue
	Subconscious cognitive processes—effects of unexamined "universal" cognitive biases—overreliance on intuitions (Doris & the Moral Psychology Research Group, 2010; Kahnemann, 2011)
Environmental	Pressures from peers—supervisors
	Competing demands (peers/patients/relatives/institution)
	Social sanction
	Economic and institutional conditions
	Time or resource constraints
	Conflicts of interest
	Job insecurity
	Catastrophic conditions

honesty, patience, tolerance, courage, imagination, perception, perseverance, self-reflection, and many more. For her dissertation, *Optimizing Stewardship: A Grounded Theory of Nurses as Moral Leader in the Intensive Care Unit*, Breakey (2006) studied characteristics of nurses who reportedly engaged successfully in end-of-life (EOL) decisions. Salient characteristics for this important nursing role included understanding the professional obligations of the role, the ability to empathize with others, and willingness to understand an issue in detail and to support others in their decision making using expertise and knowledge. The possession and exercise of any virtue within a nursing care setting will also rely on other interrelated virtues, the clinician's knowledge, and skills pertinent to the practice domain. Compassion for a cancer patient's suffering, for instance, without knowledge of how to mitigate it or the motivation to alleviate it is an empty virtue. However, theoretical knowledge of pain management without experience in patient assessment, planning, delivery, and evaluation or without understanding the meaning that suffering holds for the patient is also problematic.

Two studies of my own (currently in the publication stages), focused on understanding nurses' views of the characteristics of a "good" nurse, support these ideas. One study analyzed essays ($N = 42$) from a graduate nursing ethics class, and the other interviewed nurses from a variety of settings who had been identified by others as "good nurses" ($N = 11$). The major characteristics of "good" nurses are dependent on having a certain level of knowledge and expertise relevant to the setting. Roughly, they include perceptiveness, engagement, understanding of the nursing role as having obligations, good communication, the ability to collaborate, the ability to support others, and moral courage (the courage to act for the patient and/or family in the face of obstacles). Additionally, beginning data analyses from our CERN (Clinical Ethics Residency for Nurses) project, along with course discussions, support the assumption that being a "good" nurse requires nurses to understand and act on their obligations to patients, patients' families, and those the nurses supervise. These studies are examples of descriptive ethics. *Descriptive ethics* portrays what people think are good actions and good characteristics. It is differentiated from *normative ethics*, which mandates certain types of behaviors. Where a code of ethics provides the normative aspects—that is, what nurses should do and how they should do it—descriptive ethics paints a picture of what is actually happening in practice or what nurses perceive as their obligation and appropriate action and what sorts of things get in the way of providing, or ensuring the provision of, "good" patient care. The two types of ethics taken together provide a bigger picture of what changes in education, environment, or policy may be necessary for good patient care.

For APNs, who are often required to supervise, mentor, or collaborate with others, virtues such as leadership, cooperation, and discernment of the different needs of those with whom they interact are important to cultivate in order to meet professional duties. The next section examines the idea that certain virtues are needed for interacting with patients who are faced with making decisions about their care. Patients give their consent to care, implicitly, verbally, or in written form, depending on the invasiveness or risk of the proposed action. APNs are in the privileged position of assisting or empowering the patient to make healthcare decisions that by their nature have some sort of effect on that patient's life. With this privilege comes added responsibility.

INFORMED CONSENT

The principle of autonomy underlies the idea of informed consent. Because human beings have the capacity to reason, decide, and act and because they might be presumed to know better than anyone else what their interests are, all things being equal, they have the right to make decisions concerning their health care. They should (barring any incapacitating factors) be free from the interference of others, at least as far as personal decision making is concerned. This translates into the right of patients to accept or refuse healthcare treatments, regardless of risk, given the possession of decision-making capacity and an adequate understanding of the risks of refusal and the potential benefits of treatment. This right was legislated in the United States under the Patient Self-Determination Act (PSDA), ratified in 1991 (as part of the Omnibus Budget Reconciliation Act [OBRA], 1990), which is discussed in more detail shortly. In the United Kingdom, the right to make autonomous care decisions is protected by the Mental Capacity Act (2005), and in several other countries the right is also legally protected. Regardless of whether there are legal protections for the healthcare professional in helping patients understand their human rights related to health care, understanding the generally accepted and fundamental right of persons to make their own decisions provides a strong foundation for advocating that patients' real needs are evaluated and met, including the need for information tailored to their level of understanding and preferences.

Types of Consent

People give three types of consent in permitting healthcare professionals to evaluate and act on their health needs. The first is implicit consent, the second is verbal consent, and the third is written consent. When a patient is unable to consent, as discussed later, then an informed proxy makes a decision on the patient's behalf and with the patient's best interests (where this is knowable) in mind. Informed consent, then, is the process of interaction between a healthcare provider and person in which necessary information is exchanged and an appropriate level of understanding is gained to enable that person to make a decision about acceptable care, treatment, interventions, or courses of action in light of his or her preexisting values, beliefs, and lifestyle. One critical message implicit in this idea is that consent is not a static concept. Evaluation of current circumstances, patient understanding, and continued willingness to participate or proceed requires that consent be, for the most part, an ongoing process.

Implicit Consent

In presenting to a healthcare delivery setting in search of assistance for health needs, a person is implicitly consenting, at minimum, to be evaluated for those needs. If the setting is an inpatient or institutional setting such as a hospital, the person might sign a form giving consent for certain routine evaluations. However, this form is general and does not detail all aspects of the

evaluation, which may include tests and manual assessments such as a physical examination. Moreover, typically the admitting personnel charged with obtaining signatures have no or little medical or nursing knowledge. Thus, implicit consent is not usually very informed, and patients may well not understand what rights they have.

In primary care sites, those who present for care do not necessarily understand the customary routines of the practice site—nor are they required to accept them, although frequently both ancillary staff and clinic nurses do not act as if they understand this. For these reasons, nurses need to be ready to ascertain what the patient has understood and what it would be helpful for him or her to know. If a patient objects to some aspects of routine care, nurses are responsible for discovering what underlies the objection, how important it is to gather the data in question, and whether acceptable alternatives may be offered. For example, a faculty colleague who is also a women's health NP reported that she was doing a breast exam on a patient as part of the patient's yearly checkup. She asked the woman if she did monthly breast exams on herself. The woman replied, "No, I don't like to touch my breasts, and for that matter I don't like anyone else to touch them either—not even my husband." At that point, my colleague realized both that she had not asked permission and had not sought to understand what, if any, meaning this particular act of assessment held for the woman. She apologized and the patient said she understood that it was part of the exam and had to be done. But my colleague wished she had thought to ask permission. She felt that this might have allowed the patient to discuss the issue with her, but the opportunity was lost. Touching someone without that person's permission is also a legal consideration and may subject a nurse to legal charges such as battery or assault.

The preceding scenario, which happened early in my colleague's professional life, made her more sensitive to the idea that patients can have good reasons for refusing even routine care and that they have a right to refuse it. However, nurses also have a responsibility to ensure that patients understand the implications of refusing evaluations, tests, or treatments and try to lessen any risks from this refusal by reformulating an acceptable plan of care. To illustrate this point, I give an example from my practice experience. A slightly overweight woman in her early twenties came to my primary care setting for treatment of a sore throat. It was her first visit. The office assistant, a nurse's aide, told her she had to be weighed as part of the "new patient" routine. The young woman refused. The aide tried to persuade her but to no avail.

I heard arguing in the hall, went to investigate, and saw a very upset young woman. I brought her right away into an empty room, acknowledged how upset she was, and asked her what happened. She said, "I really hate being weighed—I don't see why it is necessary—they used to do that at the other clinic." I explained that measuring a person's weight is in many cases a very useful assessment and had become a routine, but I realized from her reaction that we might need to rethink this policy. In the course of our interaction, and because she could see that I took her concern seriously, she confided that she used to be weighed weekly by her mother when she was a teenager and was physically punished for gaining weight. This opened an opportunity to help her further, and she eventually got counseling for unresolved issues with her mother.

After this, we changed our office policy and educated the medical assistants and aides about a patient's right to accept or refuse some of the routines that were not important for the given patient's care. If the routine was important, for example, weighing a patient with chronic heart failure, then rationale should be given. Alternatives, such as self-weighing and reporting significant changes, can be negotiated. Also, there are, of course, some cases when weighing a patient becomes crucial. For example, some drug dosages are calculated based on weight. In surgical operating areas, intensive care units, and pediatric settings, accurate weights may be crucial to avoid the harms (nonmaleficence) of over- or underdosing patients with essential therapeutics. In such cases nurses remain responsible for anticipating and minimizing any possible harms, including psychological distress.

Verbal Consent

Although for many patients a host of routines covered by implicit consent neither cause distress nor affect their care in any perceptible way, in the cases described earlier, informed consent to care was important both for the patients' immediate well-being and for determining whether follow-up care was necessary or desired. Gaining informed verbal consent permitted the nurse to understand what else might be required to provide good care. Sound clinical judgment facilitates identification of the patient's particular needs, which in both cases proved to be more extensive than initially understood. Obtaining verbal consent to care—including evaluation, tests, therapeutics, and decisions about the best ways of managing chronic conditions—is synonymous with good APN practice in direct patient care and is dependent on establishing a nurse–patient relationship that is concerned with understanding the patient's vulnerability and needs and then addressing these.

Written Consent

The third type of informed consent is a written consent. Written consent "is intended to protect patients from… ethical or legal breaches and make formal their right to all relevant information, tailored specially to them" (Grace & McLaughlin, 2005, p. 79). Experienced nurses practicing in institutional settings are mostly familiar with *informed consent* as it relates to invasive medical procedures and perhaps to patients who are participating in research studies. In their definition of the term, Beauchamp and Childress (2009) acknowledge that "informed consent occurs if and only if a person or subject, with substantial understanding and in the absence of substantial control by others, intentionally authorizes a professional to do something" (p. 78). Although Beauchamp and Childress are explicitly discussing the necessary criteria for written and verbal informed consent rather than implicit consent, these criteria are also relevant for implicit consent.

In the case of proposed invasive procedures or surgery, the person responsible for carrying out or supervising the intervention is the one responsible for obtaining written consent. This is usually a physician, although increasingly it may be an APN. APNs who are qualified to carry out procedures or perform anesthesia are responsible for obtaining written consent. Staff nurses have responsibilities for ensuring that their patients are in a position to adequately understand what they are agreeing to. This has implications for the clinical nurse specialist (CNS) or nurse manager who serves as a floor resource, mentor, and educator and who sets the tone for the staff nurses on his or her unit.

INFORMED CONSENT: ETHICAL PROBLEMS

Informed consent, however, is a complex and tricky concept. For each person, the information needed for the person's consent to be *substantially informed* is different. For procedures or interventions that involve more than minimal risk (risk that is encountered in daily life), informing the patient should be viewed as a process because, for the most part, those faced with invasive procedures are already upset and anxious. Information processing under conditions of anxiety and stress is difficult, and studies have shown that patients do not retain information well under such conditions (Broadstock & Michie, 2000; Charles, Gafni, & Whelan, 1999; Kegley, 2002). The informing process involves understanding certain things

about the patient. Nurses need to understand the patient's beliefs, including culturally based beliefs, values, and goals; the patient's ability to process information; and psychological, physiological, or environmental factors that might interfere with or facilitate processing of information.

Kegley (2002) notes that the "subjective substantial disclosure rule" (p. 461) is a standard that is starting to be used to understand what information is needed related to genetic testing and other complex decision-making scenarios. It "requires a substantial degree of knowledge about the patient, her context, and what is important to her" (p. 461). This represents a change from previous tests used in law to evaluate the adequacy of information given to a patient. The standards used in legal systems as a measure of adequacy either compared the knowledge possessed by the person in question against that of a knowledgeable group of physicians or against conceptions of what a reasonable person should know. Neither standard took into account the particular needs of a patient within the context of his or her life.

Patient-related psychological factors that can interfere with information processing are such things as psychological denial of a physical illness or diagnosis, loss of hope, unreasonable expectations of an intervention, a desire to please a provider or significant others, lack of energy to think through possible options and how they relate to goals, and cognitive problems. Physical factors include pain, sedation, fever, and poor cerebral perfusion, among others. Provider-related problems include inadequate knowledge about a procedure and its potential side effects (for example, a lack of understanding of the full range of implications related to genetic testing); an inability to connect with a particular person, which can interfere with the project of tailoring information to that person's specific needs and abilities; lack of understanding of the origins or meaning of any cultural factors; lack of knowledge about existing options or objections to providing the full range of options (for example, provider beliefs about the moral status of emergency contraception); and self-knowledge related to prejudice or bias. Additionally, certain situations are fraught with communication difficulties. Examples of such situations include language barriers, hearing impairments, and patients who are perceived as "difficult."

This discussion focuses on three important complicating factors related to appropriately informing patients: (1) the provider's appeal to conscience in not providing patients with the full range of options legally available, (2) cultural considerations in informing patients, and (3) the issue of difficult patients. Early identification of potential communication problems and attempts to anticipate and address these problems has been termed *preventive ethics*. One important professional problem is that of withholding information or not offering the available range of options for a patient's situation because it is against the provider's conscience. The next section addresses this issue.

Conscience and Personal Integrity

The issue of healthcare professionals' refusal to provide patients with certain information or services has recently received publicity in the popular press in the United States. There are reports also from Europe of movements to protect healthcare providers who refuse care or limit information to patients based on conscience (Catholics for Choice, 2012). In 2010, the Parliamentary Assembly of the Council of Europe (PACE) debated the issue of the right of healthcare providers to conscientious objection (resolution #1763), urging states to provide patients timely access to legally permissible options (PACE, 2010). In opposition, the Swedish parliament has urged that their delegates work to change this resolution, reportedly because they overwhelmingly find it problematic that providers can withhold legally available options (Protection of Conscience

Project, 2012). The ethical implications of refusing to disclose legally available options or to offer a full range of services have elicited renewed scrutiny on the part of moral philosophers, ethicists, and scholars in the various healthcare professions (Wicclair, 2011). Appeals to conscientious refusal to provide certain options are usually based on one of the following arguments: (1) although legally available, the healthcare provider finds the option morally objectionable based on religious grounds or on the basis of other personal beliefs; (2) the provider believes certain options to be congruent with his or her beliefs, and others are not, and there is no obligation to reveal this bias to the patient; or (3) the provider believes some available options are inferior or have too many side effects, and thus the provider is saving the patient from confusion.

As an example of the first argument, Jacobson (2005) highlights the case of registered nurse Andrea Nead, who did not want to "administer emergency contraception" (p. 27) as part of her role responsibilities. She claimed that she did not get a position she sought in a university health clinic because of her religious beliefs. Other examples (of the second and third arguments) from advanced practice settings include a colleague who referred patients in need of mental health services only to a Christian mental health facility, and another colleague who neglected to offer a variety of therapeutic options available for labor pains by encouraging patients to "have an epidural—it is a woman's best friend." In palliative care settings, refusal to provide adequate pain relief may result from providers' beliefs that they are contributing to a person's death.

The preservation of personal integrity is very important. It enables nurses to provide for a patient's good, sometimes against sturdy barriers and sometimes against the "generally accepted view" of what is permissible. Integrity means maintaining a sense of self as a whole. It is tied into ideas of personal identity (Benjamin,

1990). Loss of a sense of self and personal integrity has been associated with the experience of moral uncertainty and moral distress, especially when a nurse is unable to ensure that a patient receives the care that clinical judgment reveals is needed. These experiences can lessen an APN's confidence and resolve related to decision making. Provision 5 of the American Nurses Association's (ANA, 2001) *Code of Ethics for Nurses with Interpretive Statements* upholds nurses' needs to care for the self, asserting, "The nurse owes the same duties to self as to others, including the responsibility to preserve integrity and safety, to maintain competence, and to continue personal and professional growth." Additionally, many U.S. state laws (45 states) have conscience clauses that allow providers to refuse treatment or recuse themselves from participating in care based on philosophical or religious objection.

Charo (2005) notes that conscience clauses in U.S. state law result from "the abortion wars" in the United States (p. 2471). That is, conscience clauses are "laws that balance a physician's conscientious objection to perform an abortion with the profession's obligation to afford all patients non-discriminatory access to services" (Charo, 2005, p. 2471). These laws are often broad enough to protect other professionals from the legal consequences of conscientious objection to certain procedures or treatments.

However, legal protection is not a good reason for a person to impose his or her beliefs and values on someone else. In fact, refusing to provide care because of personal beliefs requires that the nurse carefully consider the situation and understand the implications of this refusal. This is especially important when the nurse is in a strong (powerful) position relative to the person who is seeking legally available information or treatment. A nurse's ethical responsibilities for good care may often include following the considered wishes of patients for something with which the nurse does not agree because it is not what the nurse herself would want, because

the nurse does not think it is in the patient's best interests, or because the nurse thinks it is misguided. However, it is important to keep in mind that a healthcare decision should not be based on a provider's preferences; ideally, decisions should be based on the lifestyle, culture, beliefs, and values of the person that they will most affect. Thus, nurses must understand whether they have the facts straight, to what extent they are likely to be affected by going against what they believe, and how enduring the insult to their sense of identity is likely to be.

Moral distress is the feeling of disequilibrium experienced by nurses when they either cannot give the care needed or are asked to participate in care that they feel is wrong or harmful. The experience of moral distress and its residue (Webster & Baylis, 2000) can have long-lasting effects on nurses' practice. Some nurses leave the profession, whereas others may end up distancing themselves from certain patients because of repeated or serious experiences of emotional or ethical conflict. The question, then, is, "How do nurses preserve integrity while fulfilling their professional duties related to informed consent?" First, it is crucial to remember the almost inevitable inequality of any provider–patient relationship. Patients are vulnerable because of a lack of knowledge, skills, resources, or capacities in regard to meeting their health needs. They present to a provider trusting that their concerns will be taken seriously, the healthcare provider will be honest and transparent, and the healthcare provider will not either deliberately or unthinkingly hide available options or potential resources. In a sense, healthcare providers can be said to "hold the keys" to a wide variety of not easily available pieces of knowledge and to have the necessary skills of interpretation for making distinctions clear. Such privileges should not be abused. The ANA (2006) position statement *Risk and Responsibility in Providing Nursing Care* provides important guidance. "The nurse who decides not to take part on the grounds of conscientious objection must communicate

BOX 27-1	Criteria for the Acceptance of Conscientious Objection

When the following criteria are met, conscientious objection ought to be accepted:

1. Providing health care would seriously damage the health professional's moral integrity by
   a. Constituting a serious violation...
   b. ... of a deeply held conviction.
2. The objection has a plausible moral or religious rationale.
3. The treatment is not considered an essential part of the health professional's work.
4. The burdens to the patient are acceptable and small:
   a. The patient's condition is not life-threatening.
   b. Refusal does not lead to the patient not getting the treatment or to unacceptable delay or expenses.
   c. Measures have been taken to reduce the burdens to the patient.
5. The burdens to colleagues and healthcare institutions are acceptable and small.

In addition, the claim to conscientious objection is strengthened if:

6. The objection is founded in medicine's own values.
7. The medical procedure is new or of uncertain moral status.

Source: Courtesy of Magelssen, M. (2012). When should conscientious objection be accepted? *Journal of Medical Ethics, 38,*18–21.

this decision in appropriate ways. Whenever possible, such refusal should be made known in advance and in time for alternate arrangements to be made for patient care." This position statement includes criteria for determining what level of personal risk is acceptable and what further responsibilities fall to the nurse involved. Magelssen (2012) has also provided a set of criteria for conscientious objection (see **Box 27-1**).

Several integrity-preserving options are open to APNs in difficult situations. First, self-reflection should reveal the source and strength of the objection and whether the APN has a thorough grasp of the state of the science involved. For example, many objections to emergency contraception are based on inaccurate information related to how it works. The APN's objection may stand even after researching the facts involved; nevertheless, fact gathering is a professional responsibility.

Second, the APN should answer the following questions: "If I needed information about a healthcare issue with which I was unfamiliar, what would I want from the specialist? How would I feel if I discovered the provider had selectively withheld options or information from me?" If the APN on answering these questions remains strongly opposed to participation in a legally available procedure or to providing certain types of information, the reason for not discussing options or not providing the requested care must be communicated to the patient. The patient should be enlightened about the fact that resources are available and/or should be referred to another provider who is willing to discuss the range of options or undertake the procedure. APNs should clearly communicate that there are other options but that the APN's own beliefs do not permit him or her to discuss them.

Further, if the APN personally does not object to providing certain types of information or interventions but is restrained by the institution or practice (e.g., in a setting that is managed by a religiously based organization) from discussion of options or undertaking the procedure, this should be acknowledged and appropriate resources provided.

Culturally Based Communication Issues

Other issues that serve as obstacles to obtaining substantially informed consent are related to culture differences and lack of fluency in the patient's language or the patient's lack of fluency in the language of the context. Although in Western cultures the idea of autonomy is valued, in many other cultures decision-making responsibility belongs to the head of the household or is a family affair. Trying to understand the beliefs and values of someone from another culture can be a perplexing and frustrating task. It can be difficult to separate issues of coercion and undue influence from the cultural norm. Additionally, the cultural norm in some cultures can be oppressive for one group such as women or, less commonly, may be age related.

What are the APN's responsibilities in such circumstances? There are no ready answers to such questions. It is an obligation of practice to learn more about a culture if members of that culture are seen frequently in the APN's practice environment. In some cultures where there is evidence to show that certain practices are harmful, for example, female circumcision, the nurse can join with concerned others to understand more about the practice, the underlying assumptions of the practice, and what others have done to either change it or provide appropriate care for its subjects. Most important, maintaining a nonjudgmental but interested affect is probably the most helpful both in ascertaining a person's needs and providing assistance.

For language difficulties, certain considerations are important. Does the APN have a good interpreter? Are there ways to validate understanding and ensure that the interpreter has translated the intent of the APN's evaluation or information sharing? The following are some helpful hints synthesized from a variety of sources, including my own professional experiences.

In line with viewing informed consent as a process, time and patience are needed. More than one appointment or session may be required. It is helpful to speak in short units and have all parties take turns speaking—the nurse, the interpreter, and the patient. For exchanges involving complex information, the nurse should request the interpreter to report what the patient understood the information to mean for himself or herself in addition to conveying the patient's responses. This permits identification of areas of concern and facilitates patient understanding.

The nurse should look at the patient while speaking and be aware of the patient's body language and appearances of confusion or discomfort. The nurse must also validate with the patient if the nurse's perception is accurate and respond accordingly. Speaking directly to the patient is important, as in, "This will mean that you…" The interpreter will interpret everything, so the nurse should be careful not to say to the interpreter something that he or she does not want shared with the patient. Explanations should be supplemented with visual materials when possible. Practices may want to invest in video presentations in the patient's language as an adjunct, but this does not substitute for a fuller process of information gathering and giving. The focus should be on meeting the patient's needs, and not on any inconvenience or discomfort that the nurse feels.

It is best not to use family members for interpretation service (except for mundane matters such as what kind of food they like), especially not children. It can be a temptation to rely on a person's children because they may be more fluent in English (or the language of the provider) than their elders are, but interpreting is a heavy responsibility to place on them and inappropriately shifts family roles. A case study outlined in the *Hastings Center Report* (2004) describes the case of a 15-year-old daughter of a Chinese male immigrant. Her father was admitted with a cardiac problem. Circumstances were such that a Cantonese translator could not be found easily. The physician wondered if he should allow the daughter to translate for her father, among other things, the seriousness of his condition. This sketch is included at the end of the chapter, along with questions for discussion.

Difficult Patients

All nurses have encountered patients whom they perceive as difficult in some way. Wolf and Robinson-Smith (2007) define difficult patients "as those whom nurses perceive consume greater periods of time than their condition suggests; they impede the work of the nursing staff with demands, complaints, and lack of co-operation" (p. 74). Sometimes it is not the patient so much as the patient's family that is perceived as difficult. Patients may seem or be difficult for a variety of reasons. Nurses may experience a dislike for them for unknown reasons. Perhaps the patient reminds the nurse of someone of his or her acquaintance with whom the nurse argues, or the patient questions the nurse's knowledge or expertise. Perhaps the patient is violent, abusive, or argumentative. Patients may be difficult because of the complexity of their issues or the perceived hopelessness of their situations. Additionally, certain patients may be stigmatized by their lifestyle, obesity, or disease.

Whatever the reason, APNs are still responsible for trying to meet these patients' needs. Wolf and Robinson-Smith's (2007) study investigates strategies that are used by CNSs in "difficult clinician–patient situations" (p. 74). Two frequently used strategies were demonstrating "respect for the patient" and "focusing on the issue at hand" (pp. 79–80). This includes avoiding labeling the patient and CNSs setting an example to others. Both of these strategies avoid bias and are aimed at trying to understand who the patient is and what underlies the patient's actions and affect in order to meet the patient's needs. In addition to the preceding problems related to assessing the patient's particular needs, the provider may also be subtly influenced to emphasize some aspects of information over others, as discussed next.

OTHER INFLUENCES ON THE INFORMING PROCESS

Conflicts of Interest

Ensuring that patients' decision making is adequately informed for their needs also requires nurses to reflect on which other factors may be subtly influential, such that they are not readily recognized. The ethos of the practice environment, economic or time constraints, the influence of drug company practices, and pressures from colleagues all have the potential to cause a subtle skewing of the information given to patients. Conflicts of interest (COIs) are pervasive in healthcare practice, regardless of profession. A COI exists any time there is pressure or temptation to act in a way that a given patient's interests are not held as primary. COIs in professional nursing practice can be of several types: economic, for example, the financial pressures on a clinic or healthcare institution can shift the primary focus off patient "good"; interpersonal, for example, a battle between providers for control of a situation can cause loss of focus on mutual goals; environmental, for example, others not noticing that there is a problem and putting pressure on nurses to go along with the status quo; appropriate resources/referring physicians are not available; in psychiatric and counseling practices, sexual or boundary-related issues can arise. Studies show, for example, that drug companies have been quite successful in influencing prescribing practices in the United States (Angell, 2004; Kassirer, 2005; Steinman, Harper, Chren, Landefeld, &

Bero, 2007). An example from my experience is that of the drug company representative who provides dinner for the local APN association. He brings his samples to the office and urges us to try them with patients (Kassirer, 2005). Several studies have confirmed the suspicion that drug company gifts influence prescribing patterns (Coyle, 2002; Steinman et al., 2007; Wazana, 2000). Kassirer's book urges physicians to divorce themselves altogether from accepting drug company gifts. NP prescribing practices are perhaps not as amenable to study as physicians' are but probably would mirror those of physicians.

As discussed earlier, ensuring that patients are well informed is a difficult task that must not be taken for granted. Ongoing self-reflection and reflection on nursing practice are crucial, as is remaining aware that conflicts of interest are ever present and may result in subconscious biases that do not serve the patient well. Understanding the important elements of the process, as well as likely problem areas, necessitates vigilance. The other side of the problem has to do with the obstacles that exist for patients in apprehending and processing the information they need for decision making. The next section explores a concern related to informed consent, that of determining decision-making capacity. APNs in different roles and across specialties may be faced with the responsibility of determining whether a patient is reasonably capable of making an informed decision.

DECISION-MAKING CAPACITY

How does an APN know when a patient is not able to make an informed decision? In some cases, the answer to the question is relatively easy. It is obvious, for example, that a comatose patient, a neonate, or a patient with an advanced dementing illness cannot process information or communicate his or her wishes directly to a provider. For such patients, an alternate decision maker is necessary. This person acts as a proxy either to convey what the person's wishes

would probably have been, given knowledge of the person's beliefs, values, and life goals, or to ensure the patient's probable best interests where no knowledge is possible (neonates) or available. The issue of decision-making capacity is especially pervasive in mental health settings.

In other cases, determinations of decision-making capacity may be more difficult. Buchanan and Brock (1989) note that decision making in healthcare settings is almost always for the purposes of accomplishing a task and occurs along a continuum. In the United States, the issue of decision-making capacity was explored in-depth by the President's Commission for the Study of Ethical Problems in Medicine and Biomedical and Behavioral Research, a group assembled by President Carter in 1978. This commission was formed in response to the increasing complexity of problems caused by biological and technological advances. Examples of such problems include how and when to determine death when it is possible to indefinitely prolong life artificially. What is the range of possible effects caused by the application of genetic innovations in health care? What can APNs do about health disparities? And, important for the purposes of this discussion, how do nurses ensure that patients are capable of making their own medical decisions and are not subject to undue interference by interested others who may or may not hold a person's best interests as primary? The commission's report (President's Commission for the Study of Ethical Behavior in Medicine and Biomedical and Behavioral Research, 1982) concluded that minimal capacities for decision making are "1. Possession of a set of values and goals, 2. the ability to communicate and to understand information, and 3. the ability to reason and deliberate about one's choices" (p. 57).

These criteria are made more stringent when the risks are high and the patient seems to be making a choice that is not in concert with his or her own values and goals. Beauchamp and Childress (2009) note that in cases where

Jenny is a 33-year-old woman brought into the emergency room from a homeless shelter by shelter staff. She is evaluated by Pauline Hill, an emergency department NP, who, after evaluating Jenny, determines that Jenny's provisional diagnosis is pneumonia accompanied by dehydration. Jenny is also confused and keeps saying, "How did I get here?" The shelter staff person tells Pauline that Jenny completed detoxification for alcohol and unspecified drug abuse just 2 weeks ago, was staying sober, and had just gotten a job. Currently, she is febrile with a temperature of 103.5°F and RR 36. Pauline determines that intravenous fluids and antibiotics are necessary because Jenny is in danger of sepsis. Jenny refuses treatment; she says, "I am trying to stay clean. I want to get my kids back." Pauline talks to Jenny about her worries, tells her of the proposed plan, and reassures her that she is not receiving anything that will set her rehabilitation back. At first Jenny seems to understand and acquiesces, but when it is time to insert the cannula, Jenny starts crying and yelling, "No, I don't want it! I can't have it!" When questioned further, it becomes obvious that Jenny has not retained the information that Pauline discussed with her, nor does she see the connection between treatment and achieving her goals. Pauline realizes that Jenny is not capable of making this decision because she keeps misunderstanding what is proposed.

the risk of action or inaction is relatively high (the possibility of serious harm exists), it is also important to assess for the voluntariness of the decision. That is, nurses should evaluate whether some internal or external influence is pressuring the person to make a particular decision (see the section "Informed Consent: Ethical Problems" earlier in this chapter). The Case Study is provided as an example of considerations related to decision-making capacity.

There is a lot more that could be said about this case, including responsibilities to try to improve Jenny's ability to process information (oxygen, or a respiratory treatment) or to consider alternative courses of action that might achieve the purpose of resolving Jenny's immediate physical needs without further distressing her. However, the purpose of Jenny's case is to illustrate a problem with decision-making capacity for the task at hand. The risks of not treating are high and do not serve Jenny's goals of becoming physically capable of having her children returned to her and being able to care for them. Therefore, the nurse does need to treat the pneumonia and dehydration because not to do so could result in Jenny's harm, perhaps even her death. Thus, the point is that, paradoxically, in treating her against her will, which could be seen as not honoring her autonomy, the nurse is actually facilitating autonomous future decision making. A person cannot exercise autonomy when she is not alive to do so.

Proxy Decision Making

Proxy decision making is the act of deciding what healthcare actions are permissible for someone who temporarily or permanently has lost decision-making capacity, never had decision-making capacity (profound cognitive deficits), or is not yet considered to have sufficient maturity to make health-care decisions (children). When children are involved, the proxy decision maker is usually a parent or guardian who makes decisions on the child's behalf. If developmentally appropriate, children may assent or dissent to a course of treatment. However, a child's dissent may be overruled by a parent or guardian when the risk of not treating is high.

Types of Proxy Decision Making

In clinical ethics literature and practice, a hierarchy of three levels of proxy decision making is used to determine appropriate treatment for those who are or have become incapacitated. The first level is based on the principle of autonomy and aims to reproduce as nearly as possible what an incapacitated person's wishes would have been. The person may have previously formulated a written directive (also known as a living will or advance directive [AD]) or may have appointed a person who could accurately represent those wishes. When these formal arrangements do not exist, the healthcare team may be able to discern what a patient's wishes would likely be by gathering information about the patient from family members and friends. The second level is often called the best interests standard. Beauchamp and Childress (2009) note that sometimes "the patient's relevant preferences cannot be known" (p. 138). In such cases a surrogate decision is made based on quality of life (QOL). Thus actions are favored if they are likely to provide the highest net benefits in terms of QOL. The best interest standard may permit overriding a surrogate decision maker's directions for treatment when the proposed treatment does not seem capable of benefiting the patient or may cause more harm than benefit. The third level is that of the reasonable person standard. It is used when neither level one nor two is applicable. For example, it is not possible to discern from neonates or profoundly cognitively disabled persons what they would want for themselves. In such cases a decision is made

based upon what a "reasonable" person would want. This third level is problematic because it is hard to determine who is "reasonable" when there are a host of contextual factors involved in any decision-making process (Beauchamp & Childress, 2009; Grace, 2004b).

Legal Aspects

In the United States, what is accepted as legal surrogate decision making differs from state to state. This necessitates that APNs familiarize themselves with the laws of the state (or country) in which they practice. This section outlines some general issues associated with APNs' role in assisting their patients to be prepared for a variety of possibilities related to decision making.

Proxy decision making in health care may be needed for everyday healthcare decisions, for decisions related to an acute illness, and for end-of-life (EOL) issues. Although many APNs do not work in a hospital setting, understanding a little about legislation related to EOL decision making, such as the PSDA (OBRA, 1990) in the United States, provides clarity about the reasons for such legislation and likely related issues. The PSDA applies to institutions that receive federal funding (almost all U.S. hospitals and long-term care facilities) and was meant to improve patient decision making especially around (although not limited to) EOL decisions. It was meant to improve providers' as well as patients' knowledge about patients' rights to accept or refuse therapeutics and interventions and providers' obligations to provide appropriate information. It was also hoped that providers would assist patients to think about what they would want in the event that they lost decision-making capacity.

Advance Directives

It is, of course, generally better for patients to have considered in advance what sort of care they would like and who might best serve as a good proxy decision maker on their behalf. Although such decisions may be made when patients are already critically ill, this is not optimal (Hiltunen, Medich, Chase, Peterson, & Forrow, 1999; Marshall, 1995; Wolf et al., 2001). Time, a low-pressure environment, and the assistance of a trusted health provider are probably the best conditions under which to process information. Thus, good APN practice means taking the opportunity to raise questions and provide necessary information related to the idea of proxy decision making if a patient appears receptive. Additionally, recent research (Parks et al., 2011) questioning prospective proxies and those for whom they were to make decisions found that "spousal proxies were more accurate in their substituted judgment than adult children, and proxies who perceive higher degree of family conflict [within their family] tended to be less accurate than those with lower family conflict" (p. 179). From my experiences in both critical care and primary care settings and from the research cited, it is very difficult to discuss such issues when a person is gravely ill, already receiving highly technical care, and in a noisy and hectic environment. Proxy decision making can be an arduous task at the best of times but is made even more difficult with the potential loss of a loved one looming and when the decision maker may already be overwhelmed with circumstances and lack of needed clinical knowledge. Preventive ethics strategies include providers making routine a practice of discussing patient preferences at primary care or regular provider visits; helping patients to select an appropriate surrogate—one who can separate personal desires and wishes from the preferences of the person in question; and encouraging patients to provide written instructions for their proxy. A reminder is needed that a proxy only makes healthcare decisions for another person in the event of that person's loss of decision-making capacity. When a proxy is obviously not making decisions that are in the patient's best interests, the proxy can legally be relieved of proxy duties.

Discussion about ADs need not be limited to the older population. McAliley, Hudson-Barr, Gunning, and Rowbottom (2000) studied adolescent attitudes toward living wills or, as they are alternatively known, ADs. Of the 107 participants in the study, the majority felt that it was "somewhat important" or "very important" for someone of their age to have a living will (p. 471). A study of young adults living with chronic illness also supported the idea that conversations about advanced care planning (ACP) are desirable (Wiener et al., 2008). The advent of ADs or living wills is relatively new. According to Clarke (1998), the term *living will* was invented in 1967 by Louis Kutner, a human rights lawyer and cofounder of Amnesty International, "in a law journal proposal" (p. 92). Kutner, having gone through a disturbing EOL scenario with a close friend, wanted to ensure the right of patients to determine how their last days should unfold in the event of a catastrophe.

THE PATIENT SELF-DETERMINATION ACT: INTERNATIONAL IMPLICATIONS

The PSDA in the United States (OBRA, 1990) was conceptualized as a result of several landmark right-to-die cases. It relies on state laws related to EOL care and "was designed to encourage communication about end-of-life issues" (Grace, 2004b, p. 310). It requires institutions that receive Medicare and Medicaid funds (U.S. government funds), which includes essentially all healthcare institutions in the United States, to inform patients in writing of their rights to accept or refuse care. It was meant to increase healthcare provider knowledge and thus affect current EOL problems arising in tertiary care institutions.

The PSDA has not been as effective as hoped, and there are many documented reasons for this. A large study undertaken to understand prognoses and preferences for outcomes and risks of treatment conducted over several years and initially involving observation but later adding interventions aimed at improving the communication of patients' wishes failed to show that patients' preferences were respected. Marshall (1995) and others have argued that this is because institutional hierarchies and power structures had not significantly changed as a result of the PSDA.

Others have noted a variety of concerns about ADs that might make some people reluctant to draft them and some healthcare providers reluctant to comply with them. The concerns include the idea that people do not like to imagine themselves experiencing serious illness or death. Accurately predicting what might be needed given a wide array of possibilities is difficult. Patients are afraid they might change their minds, but not in time to change their AD, or that not accepting certain interventions might lead to their abandonment by caregivers (Teno, Gruneir, Schwartz, Nanda, & Wetle, 2007; Wolf et al., 2001). Additionally, there are cultural and minority fears about the untrustworthiness of predominantly white middle-class healthcare professionals (Baker, 2002); see the next section for further discussion.

Regulations related to the use of ADs, whether in the written form or in the form of an appointed proxy, vary from country to country. Regardless of the existence of regulations enforcing or supporting patients' previously articulated wishes, it is a healthcare professional's responsibility to help patients and those close to them to think through what care and interventions they might wish for in the event of a loss of decision-making capacity. This permits advocacy and honors autonomy. Durbin, Fish, Backman, and Smith (2010) reviewed available research on the influence of educational interventions in improving AD completion. They found (perhaps not unsurprisingly) that a two-pronged approach—providing written and oral information—had the best effects on completion, but the results were not strongly compelling. More interventional research is needed.

Despite concerns about ADs, many professionals and ethicists who are involved in EOL

care think that with time and custom more people will become involved in the process of advance planning for the event of lost decision making. The most effective plan is probably a two-part initiative: the appointment of a trustworthy representative who may or may not be a relative, and written instructions to assist the proxy. Understanding both the benefits and criticisms of formal ADs enables APNs to assist patients in thinking about their specific advance planning wishes. In advanced practice, nurses are key to interpreting a variety of EOL scenarios in terms that are tailored to a particular patient's needs and level of understanding.

ADVANCED CARE PLANNING: MINORITY AND CULTURAL ISSUES

Although ACP is generally thought to be a good thing, facilitative of an individual's choices, there are historical and cultural reasons for certain groups to view ACP with uncertainty and fear. Indeed, such fears coupled with the ones noted earlier may be in part responsible for the slow progress made in preparing and educating the public about the potential benefits of ACP. Johnstone and Kanitsaki (2009) draw attention to the problem in the United States and Australia in particular; it is likely that in other multicultural societies certain groups feel disenfranchised by society as well. "Emerging international research suggests that in multicultural countries, such as Australia and the United States, there are significant disparities in end-of-life care planning and decision making by people of minority ethnic backgrounds compared with members of mainstream English-speaking background populations" (p. 405).

Moreover, public policies in these countries are not always sensitive to this problem. Johnstone and Kanitsaki (2009) note that the few studies that have looked at differences between cultural majority and cultural or linguistic minority groups within a society related to ACP reveal several tendencies on the part of minority cultures: a smaller number complete ADs, family involvement in discussions about decision making is preferred, ADs are viewed as an intrusive and legalistic mechanism that has no place in health care, and aggressive treatment is preferred, especially when patients have experienced prior mistreatment or bias (Bito et al., 2007, p. 260). In ethical terms, these patients' prior experiences, distrust of the system, and fears about undertreatment can paradoxically lead to greater harms (a nonmaleficence problem) from overtreatment or treatment that is futile for the intended purpose and that causes unnecessary suffering. Strategies for APNs include engaging patients in dialogue about their cultural values, their prior experiences, and their fears. Planning for the future includes understanding what patients' goals are given a variety of scenarios and helping them to envision desirable courses of action.

VERACITY AND TRANSPARENCY

Veracity is an ethical principle underlying the idea of trust and fiduciary relationships. "Veracity or truthfulness in giving patients information about their health-care needs facilitates autonomous choice and enhances patient decision making" (Grace, 2004b, p. 315). However, veracity is a more difficult concept to apply than it appears on the surface. It is fair to say that in ordinary life people are rarely completely truthful with friends, family, and strangers. People hold information back, either because they feel it could come back to haunt them or because to be completely truthful may well hurt another person. Yet "truthfulness has long been regarded as fundamental to the existence of trust" (Fry & Grace, 2007, p. 287), and as noted earlier, trust is fundamental to the nurse–patient relationship. Patients are vulnerable because of their healthcare needs and must rely on nurses to help them. If APNs are not able to gain a certain level of trust with patients, then their data-gathering activities are likely to be frustrated. This, in turn, lessens the likelihood that nurses will be able to give holistic care, which in turn means that nursing goals are not met.

However, being too honest or giving patients more information than necessary for their decision-making purposes can also frustrate the project of attending to their needs. Clinical judgment is required to make determinations about acceptable levels of information for a given patient; that is, what will permit the patient's participation in decision making. For example, to the family nurse practitioner (FNP) caring for Ms. Jones, a 60-year-old in a rural family practice clinic, it has become obvious that her patient needs to add an antihypertensive drug to her care plan. Although for several years Ms. Jones has, with the FNP's help, managed to control her blood pressure by increasing her exercise regimen, reducing stress, and being careful with her diet, her blood pressure is starting to show a pattern of persistent elevation above recommended levels. Ms. Jones does not want to start taking blood pressure pills, but the FNP has done a good job of educating her about long-term effects of poorly controlled hypertension, so she is willing to start taking them. What drug the FNP tries initially and how much information she gives Ms. Jones depends on what the FNP knows about Ms. Jones. Discussion of the side effects Ms. Jones is most likely to experience and how these match her lifestyle and preferences will facilitate a first choice. Explanation of likely side effects will also be tailored to her needs. However, transparency about the extensiveness of what is known related to the drug and the amount of information the FNP gives are also important. These are all clinical judgments based on knowledge of the patient and, like many clinical judgments, they have some element of uncertainty. With Ms. Jones, it might be beneficial to discuss major side effects, whether these effects are acceptable to her, and what she should report to the FNP. Additionally, the FNP should acknowledge that there are possible side effects that Ms. Jones may not experience and that the best way to deal with this is to remain accessible for questions Ms. Jones may have if she experiences unexpected changes.

In palliative care or EOL care settings, problems of veracity can occur when relatives pressure nurses and others to withhold the truth about a condition from patients. Veracity has some implications in the care of patients from cultures where the patient is traditionally protected from knowledge of the criticality of the condition. "Decision making about whether to honor [the demands] of veracity in such cases must take into consideration what is known about the culture, the particular patient, the strength of his or her personal and cultural beliefs, and whether there is evidence about what sort of things the patient would like to know" (Grace, 2004b, p. 316). If a patient is asking questions about his or her condition, then nurses need to respond accordingly. Nurses need to draw on what is known or has been discovered (evidence) related to a person's needs to come to terms with his or her condition and nearness to death. But nurses also may need to assist the family with their needs to fulfill cultural responsibilities. Resources may be found within the cultural community.

In pediatric settings, the issue of veracity is also complicated. Questions arise about how to communicate information in age- or developmentally appropriate ways. How do APNs interact with parents or guardians who seem overly protective or are working in ways that seem at odds with what is known about the child?

PRIVACY AND CONFIDENTIALITY

The healthcare principles of privacy and confidentiality are also derivations of the ethical principle of autonomy. The terms *privacy* and *confidentiality* are often lumped together as if they mean the same thing. Privacy, however, is "the broader concept and includes the right to be free from the interference of others" (Grace, 2004a, p. 33) and freedom to grant or

withhold access to information about oneself. Justification for the right to privacy, as noted by Beauchamp and Childress (2009), "flow[s] from fundamental rights to life, liberty, and property" (p. 295). Confidentiality is related more specifically to the protection of a person's information, particularly the person's healthcare information. Beauchamp and Childress (2009) note that in healthcare settings, the right to privacy is most often a control right of sorts: it is the right to control both access to and distribution of information.

For Beauchamp and Childress (2009), a helpful distinction can be made between privacy and confidentiality in terms of the status of violations of these. Confidentiality is violated when one person discloses information about another person, whereas when privacy is violated, one person gains access to another person's personal data. Rights to privacy and confidentiality in healthcare settings are contemporary recognitions. The reason for recognition of these rights is that a person's healthcare information can be used in negative ways that cause harm. In nonhealthcare situations, the status of confidentiality is considered so important that it is protected by privilege and is "shielded from exposure by the legal system" (Grace, 2005, p. 114). For example, the clergy-supplicant privilege prevents courts from forcing clergy to reveal confidential information entrusted to them by congregants.

Limitations on the Right to Privacy

For healthcare providers, honoring privacy, which includes the maintenance of patient confidentiality, is important but does not supersede all other considerations. There may be occasions when an APN should break confidentiality to prevent serious harm to another person. The difficulty, however, lies in making the assessment of dangerousness—how imminent it is and how severe the likely consequences are.

The well-known *Tarasoff* case set a precedent in the United States related to limitations in provider–patient privilege. In October 1969, Prosenjit Poddar killed Tatiana Tarasoff. Poddar had been seeing a psychiatrist and told the therapist he was going to kill a woman, who was easily identifiable as Tatiana. At the time of Poddar's statement to his therapist, Tatiana was out of the country in Brazil. The therapist sought to have Poddar committed but was unsuccessful because Poddar appeared rational. No one warned Tatiana or her family of the threat, and on her return Poddar killed her. The courts, in this case, aligning against the idea that psychiatrist–patient privilege is absolute, concluded that "once a therapist does in fact determine, or under applicable professional standards reasonably should have determined, that a person poses a serious danger of violence to others, he bears a duty to exercise reasonable care to protect the foreseeable victim of that danger" (*Tarasoff v. Regents of University of California*, 1976).

Beauchamp and Childress (2009) note three main areas where limits on privacy might require a "balancing of privacy interests against other interests" (p. 297). These areas are "(1) screening and testing for HIV infection, (2) ensuring effective treatments for patients with active tuberculosis (TB), and (3) human genetics" (p. 297). Contemporary issues of dangerousness to others include the deliberate dissemination to, or careless exposure of, others by someone with a transmissible disease, such as HIV or TB. For example, recently there was a highly publicized case of a patient with extensively drug-resistant TB who traveled across the continent on public airliners.

The Meaning of Privacy in Health Care

The concept of privacy is important to the preceding discussion of informed consent, although this was not explicitly stated. Essentially, the privacy principle means two things: (1) patients should have a say in who is allowed access to their bodies or, for the purposes of evaluation and treatment, other information; and (2) unless the patient gives explicit permission, there is a proscription against healthcare personnel sharing information gained, except for the purposes of helping that patient. In contemporary society, privacy and confidentiality concerns are exacerbated by the pervasive nature of electronic media, as discussed in more detail shortly. The ease with which information, including photographs, can be transmitted via cell phones and other devices, and the ubiquitous use of social media such as Facebook, Twitter, and so on, can lead to the careless exposure of patient information. For example, a mother in the neonatal infant care unit takes a photo of her baby and posts it on Facebook; inadvertently she has included the baby in the next incubator and the visiting parents.

The protection of a patient's privacy has a variety of implications, both in institutional settings and in primary care. It requires nurses to think carefully about their actions related to patients, including what they tell referral sources, how they transfer information, and what the implications of testing are related to privacy and protection. It is a reminder not to take privileged access to sensitive patient information for granted. Respecting a patient's right to privacy means that when a student APN interacts with a patient as part of gaining clinical expertise, the student status should be revealed. In patient rounds, persons in the rounding group should be clearly identified. Patients can waive this right but should be made aware of it.

The principle of privacy has other numerous implications; for the most part, concern for the delivery of good patient care will ensure that a patient's privacy is respected. For example, the privacy principle means that providers protect those who are not capable of protecting themselves from the intrusion of others, perhaps because they are not aware of the possibility that sharing personal information can affect such opportunities as job prospects and the ability to have health insurance. Providers in the United States should be aware of the so-called Privacy Rule and its impact on their practice. This rule is explored in more detail in the following section. It is impossible in this text to discuss the regulations surrounding privacy concerns in all countries that have such regulations; however, the implications of the privacy rule and ethical considerations concerning privacy and confidentiality are pertinent regardless of country of practice.

HIPAA and the Privacy Rule in the United States: History

According to Beauchamp and Childress (2009), "Privacy received little attention in the law or legal theory until the late 19th century" (p. 294), and then it was concerned with protecting family life, child-rearing practices, and other areas of personal choice. Confidentiality as a subcategory of privacy refers to patient rights to have their healthcare information safeguarded. The irony of confidentiality is that in order to receive care, highly personal information has to be revealed to those who will be providing that care. Those providing direct care may sometimes need to share patient information with others whose expertise is important in meeting patient needs. Thus, illness itself makes a person vulnerable, and in trying to address illness a person also becomes vulnerable, to those who have access to that personal information.

Prior to 1996, rights to privacy and confidentiality were protected by state or country laws, professional ethical codes, and ethical deliberation. The advent of large electronic databases for storing medical records, however, jeopardized providers' ability to protect their patients' records. Most who have been involved in health care in the United States, whether patients or providers, have become familiar with the Health Insurance Portability and Accountability Act (HIPAA); however, much confusion about this act remains (Anderson, 2007). HIPAA was enacted in 1996. Before HIPAA,

if a person lost his or her job, they often also lost health insurance coverage, because health insurance in the United States for the most part is attached to a particular place of employment. HIPAA ensured that a person could continue coverage until regaining employment, at which point new coverage would begin with the work-associated health insurance company. HIPAA was also supposed to expand coverage. Another section of HIPAA, the "Privacy Rule," was meant to standardize the use of health information across the country while providing privacy protection. Suggestions had been made for the development of a megadatabase that could track almost everyone's health care in the United States from birth to death. Thus, HIPAA was supposed to accomplish two somewhat contradictory tasks: (1) allow for the flow of information that would enable research and access to patient care records for the purposes of improving care and public health, and (2) act as a brake on covered entities' free use of medical information enabled by such a database. A *covered entity* is a person, practice, clinic, pharmacy, or institution covered by HIPAA. Essentially, a covered entity is anyone providing patient care services or undertaking research on human subjects.

Subsequently, a privacy rule was attached to HIPAA (U.S. Department of Health and Human Services, Office for Civil Rights, 2003). The Privacy Rule specifically covers all individually identifiable information, including written, oral, and computerized. This went into effect in 2003. An important point to note is that if state rules about privacy are more stringent than HIPAA, then the more stringent standard applies. That is, state regulations trump HIPAA if they are more rigorous than HIPAA standards.

The problem with the Privacy Rule, as noted earlier, and the problem with maintaining privacy and confidentiality based purely on ethical considerations (i.e., without such a rule) is that it is impossible to delineate all imaginable scenarios related to privacy infringements, so clinical judgment, including ethical reflection, is still needed for its interpretation in specific situations. "A rule of thumb for health care professionals related to sharing information with others is to disclose only as much information as is necessary to permit optimal care and only information that is pertinent to the situation" (Grace, 2005, p. 115). Additionally, prudence and mindfulness are required when other people's healthcare records are in the APN's hands.

Anderson (2007) provides tips for ensuring that patient information is not overheard or overseen. Importantly, care must be taken not to leave information lying around and not to discuss patients in public places, and the nurse must consider whether an outsider could identify the person being discussed if he or she overheard the conversation. In rural settings, maintaining confidentiality can be especially difficult. Providers are often members of the small communities in which they practice. It is not unusual for an APN to be asked about the status of a family member or friend's health in a grocery store or other local gathering place. Additionally, in rural settings office staff may have access to the records of family members or friends. Part of the APN's responsibilities in such settings is educating the staff about the implications of accessing information to which they neither have a need nor a right to access.

In a recent *American Journal of Nursing* article offered for continuing education credit, Anderson (2007), the privacy officer for her institution, provided and answered some questions that may be helpful in understanding the intent of the Privacy Rule; some of these suggestions also have utility outside of the Privacy Rule. Anderson posed some common questions to highlight confusions and to illustrate common-sense answers.

- Is it permissible to call or write to a community provider when referring a patient? Yes, if the disclosure is for treatment purposes.

- Am I allowed to e-mail a diagnostic report to another provider for treatment or consultation purposes? Yes, but encryption is strongly encouraged.

- May I videotape or photograph patients for teaching purposes? Yes, but consent should be obtained or patients should be "de-identified." (Anderson, 2007, p. 67)

Additional insights into experiences of APNs related to privacy and confidentiality are provided by Deshefy-Longhi, Dixon, Olsen, and Grey (2004). They conducted a series of studies aimed at describing the views of APNs and their patients related to the protection of healthcare data. Of nine issues identified in focus group explorations, six were identified by both patients and nurses. One of these mutual concerns was the issue of "breaches in privacy occurring through carelessness" (p. 387). Examples given included phone conversations that could be overheard, conversations about patient information that took place in public spaces, and patient information lying around or viewable on computer screens. Additionally, both groups worried that excessive regulation prevented needed information from being communicated to appropriate resources. Even the need to leave a telephone message for a patient at home posed concerns. Nurses wondered how much, if any, information to leave. Additional concerns of the APN group were abuses of privacy related to the use of computers and problems attending to the privacy concerns of adolescents.

Hidden Privacy and Confidentiality Hazards of Electronic and Social Media

A very contemporary threat to privacy and confidentiality is the widespread use of social media. A stable definition of social media is difficult because of the continual metamorphosis of the forms available. Boyd and Ellison (2007), information specialists, propose a tentative definition for a social networking site: "web-based services that allow individuals to (1) construct a public or semi-public profile within a bounded system, (2) articulate a list of other users with whom they share a connection, and (3) view and traverse their list of connections and those made by others within the system" (para. 4). Such sites facilitate information sharing that would otherwise be difficult or nonexistent.

Social media is very promising for healthcare professionals as a way of reaching more people with health information, assisting self-help health promotion groups, permitting patient access to results and records, enrolling research subjects, carrying out surveys, and so on. Additionally healthcare professionals use social media for personal reasons. The danger, as noted earlier, is that in the course of a healthcare professional's private discussions patient information might be revealed. Furthermore, unprofessional behavior that is publicly accessible can undermine public trust in an institution or in the profession. For example, a nursing student was conversing on Facebook with a medical student. They had both spent a couple of days in the same clinic as part of their unrelated clinical practices. They were making fun of a patient they had seen. What if the patient had been identified? Perhaps even more seriously, such behavior can undermine public trust in the professions.

The ANA (2011) has provided tips for engaging with social media and for avoiding problems. They include guarding confidentiality, maintaining professional boundaries, remembering that postings are widely viewable, and reporting unethical behavior of others or calling it to the attention of the writer. Nurses can avoid problems by thinking through the possible ramifications of actions. Nurses can also help patients and visitors think about their actions before posting pictures or videos—Is anyone else inadvertently shown in the picture? Is any confidential material being exposed? Questions to ask include, "Would I be okay if what I am posting appeared on the front page of the local newspaper? Could what I am saying be misconstrued as disrespectful or dehumanizing? Could what I am saying as a private citizen reflect on my professional standing? Should I be engaging with a patient this way? Does this cross professional boundaries?"

SUMMARY

This chapter discusses characteristics that are important for good nursing care and good decision making in APN settings. It presents an argument for the APN to engage in ongoing professional and personal development in the interests of good patient care. The possession of certain nursing virtues is necessary both for facilitating patient decision making and protecting patient information. These virtues are not all or nothing—there are barriers to practicing well. Mindfulness allows the APN to maintain focus.

The discussion in this chapter reinforced the idea that professional nursing practice at the advanced level is still good nursing practice. All healthcare practice that involves individual human beings is ethical in nature because of professional goals. The broad importance of honoring the ethical principle of autonomy was the underlying assumption for the topics of this chapter. Patients have the right to make personal decisions both about what care will or will not be accepted and who may have access to personal information and for what purposes. The APN has responsibilities to help patients safeguard these rights.

Unfortunately, as hard as APNs work to secure information, insurance companies that are privy to the private information of their subscribers are not always so scrupulous.

DISCUSSION QUESTIONS _____

1. A case study outlined in the *Hastings Center Report* (2004) describes the case of a 15-year-old daughter of a Chinese immigrant man

who was admitted with a cardiac problem. Circumstances were such that the physician could not get a Cantonese translator in the middle of the night, and he wanted the daughter to translate for her father, among other things, the seriousness of the man's condition.

a. What are the implications of asking an adolescent to interpret for a family member?

b. What information would an APN need to decide appropriateness?

c. What risks are involved?

d. How would you resolve this issue for this current situation? In the future?

2. Have you cared for a patient who you would describe as difficult? Explore the situation you encountered with classmates or colleagues. Identify assumptions that you made about the patient. What is the basis for these assumptions? Did you think the patient was responsible for the characteristic that made him or her difficult? In what ways was he or she responsible? How would you have liked the person to have acted? Have you ever been considered difficult or felt that you were misunderstood?

3. Joe, a 17-year-old patient, is scheduled for a sports physical at your clinic. After examining him, you decide to draw a complete blood count because he complains of feeling a bit "more than usually tired" after 30 minutes of shooting hoops. Joe asks you to tell his dad what you are doing because "he gets antsy when he has to wait." You bring Joe's dad into your office to talk to him, and he asks you to draw extra blood for drug testing and not to tell Joe what you are doing. He says, "I just know he is taking something."

a. What is the main issue in this case?

b. What are the APN's responsibilities?

c. What are the implications of the Privacy Rule?

d. Discuss with classmates or peers how this situation should be addressed.

4. What is the relevance of discussing ADs with your population of patients? (Neonatal intensive care unit nurses may have to imagine caring for another population.)

a. Do you have an AD? Why or why not?

b. What innovative approaches to educating patients about ADs might be used?

c. What obstacles would you anticipate (e.g., personal, environmental, time constraints, cultural)?

5. Have you seen unethical conversations about patients or practices on a social media site? As an APN and leader, how would you address such issues in your setting?

REFERENCES

American Nurses Association. (2001). *Code of ethics for nurses with interpretive statements*. Washington, DC: Author.

American Nurses Association. (2006). *Risk and responsibility in providing nursing care*. Retrieved from http://www.nursingworld.org/MainMenuCategories/Policy-Advocacy/Positions-and-Resolutions/ANAPositionStatements/Position-Statements-Alphabetically/RiskandResponsibility.pdf

American Nurses Association. (2011). *Principles for social networking and the nurse*. Silver Spring, MD: Nurse Books.

Anderson, F. (2007). Finding HIPAA in your soup: Decoding the Privacy Rule. *American Journal of Nursing, 107*(2), 66–71.

Angell, M. (2004). *The truth about drug companies: How they deceive us and what to do about it*. New York, NY: Random House.

Anscombe, G. E. M. (1958/1981). Modern moral philosophy. In *Ethics religion and politics: Collected Papers, Vol. 3* (pp. 1–19). Minneapolis: University of Minnesota Press. Reprinted from *Philosophy, 33*(124), 1958.

Armstrong, A. E. (2006). Towards a strong virtue ethics for nursing practice. *Nursing Philosophy, 7*, 101–124.

Baker, M. (2002). Economic, political and ethnic influences on end-of-life decision-making: A decade in review. *Journal of Health and Social Policy, 14*(3), 27–39.

Beauchamp, T. L., & Childress, J. F. (2009). *Principles of biomedical ethics* (6th ed.). New York, NY: Oxford University Press.

Begley, A. M. (2005). Practising virtue: A challenge to the view that a virtue centered approach to ethics lacks practical content. *Nursing Ethics, 12*(6), 622–637.

Benjamin, M. (1990). *Splitting the difference.* Lawrence, KS: Lawrence University Press.

Bito, S., Matsumura, S., Singer, M. K., Meredith, L. S., Fukuhara, S., & Wenger, N. S. (2007). Acculturation and end-of-life decision making: Comparison of Japanese and Japanese American focus groups. *Bioethics, 21,* 251–262.

Boyd, D. M., & Ellison, N. B. (2007). Social network sites: Definition, history, and scholarship. *Journal of Computer-Mediated Communication, 13*(1), 210–230. Retrieved from http://onlinelibrary.wiley.com/doi/10.1111/j.1083-6101.2007.00393.x/abstract

Breakey, S. (2006). Optimizing stewardship: A grounded theory of nurses as moral leaders in the ICU. Unpublished dissertation. Boston College, William F. Connell School of Nursing. ProQuest document 3221256. Retrieved from http://search.proquest.com.proxy.bc.edu/docview/304913628/13D564FA2C2BC814F8/1?accountid=9673

Broadstock, M., & Michie, S. (2000). Processes of patient decision making: Theoretical and methodological issues. *Psychology and Health, 15,* 191–204.

Buchanan, A. E., & Brock, D. W. (1989). *Deciding for others: The ethics of surrogate decision making.* New York, NY: Cambridge University Press.

Catholics for Choice. (2012). In good conscience. Retrieved from http://www.catholicsforchoice.org/documents/InGoodConscience–Europe.pdf

Chambliss, D. F. (1996). *Beyond caring: Hospitals, nurses, and the social organization of ethics.* Chicago, IL: University of Chicago Press.

Charles, C., Gafni, A., & Whelan, T. (1999). Shared decision-making in the medical encounter: What does it mean? (or it takes at least two to tango). *Social Science and Medicine, 44,* 681–692.

Charo, R. A. (2005). The celestial fire of conscience—refusing to deliver medical care. *New England Journal of Medicine, 352*(24), 2471–2473.

Clarke, D. B. (1998). The Patient Self-Determination Act. In J. F. Monagle & D. C. Thomasma (Eds.), *Health care ethics for the 21st century* (pp. 92–116). Gaithersburg, MD: Aspen.

Coyle, S. L. (2002). Physician–industry relations. Part I: Individual physicians. *Annals of Internal Medicine, 136*(5), 396–402.

Deshefy-Longhi, T., Dixon, J. K., Olsen, D., & Grey, M. (2004). Privacy and confidentiality issues in primary care: Views of advanced practice nurses and their patients. *Nursing Ethics, 11*(4), 378–393.

Doris, J. M., & the Moral Psychology Research Group. (2010). *The moral psychology handbook.* New York, NY: Oxford University Press.

Durbin, C. R., Fish, A. F., Backman, J. A., & Smith, K. V. (2010). Systematic review of educational interventions for improving advance directive completion. *Journal of Nursing Scholarship, 14*(2), 234–241.

Feldman, F. (1978). *Introductory ethics.* Englewood Cliffs, NJ: Prentice Hall.

Fry, S. T., & Grace, P. J. (2007). Ethical dimensions of nursing and healthcare. In J. L. Creasia & B. J. Parker (Eds.), *Conceptual foundations: The bridge to professional practice* (4th ed., pp. 273–299). St. Louis, MO: Mosby Elsevier.

Grace, P. J. (2004a). Ethical issues: Patient safety and the limits of confidentiality. *American Journal of Nursing, 104*(11), 33–37.

Grace, P. J. (2004b). Ethics in the clinical encounter. In S. K. Chase (Ed.), *Clinical judgment and communication in nurse practitioner practice* (pp. 295–332). Philadelphia, PA: F. A. Davis.

Grace, P. J. (2005). Ethical issues relevant to health promotion. In C. Edelman & C. L. Mandle (Eds.), *Health promotion throughout the lifespan* (6th ed., pp. 100–125) St. Louis, MO: Elsevier/Mosby.

Grace, P. J., & McLaughlin, M. (2005). When consent isn't informed enough: What's the nurse's role when a patient has given consent but doesn't fully understand the risks? *American Journal of Nursing, 105*(4), 79–84.

Haggerty, L. A., & Grace, P. J. (2008). Clinical wisdom: Approximating the ends of individual and societal health. *Journal of Professional Nursing, 24*(4), 235–240.

Hanson, C. M., & Hamric, A. B. (2003). Reflections on the continuing evolution of advanced practice nursing. *Nursing Outlook, 51*(5), 203–211.

Hastings Center Report. (2004). A fifteen-year-old translator. *Hastings Center Report, 34*(3), 10–13.

Hiltunen, E. F., Medich, C., Chase, C., Peterson, L., & Forrow, L. (1999). Family decision making for end-of life-treatment: The SUPPORT nurse narratives. *Journal of Clinical Ethics, 10*(2), 126–134.

Hutchinson, D. S. (1995). Ethics. In J. Barnes (Ed.), *The Cambridge companion to Aristotle* (pp. 195–232). New York, NY: Cambridge University Press.

Jacobson, J. (2005). When providing care is a moral issue. *American Journal of Nursing, 105*(10), 27–28.

Johnstone, M. J., & Kanitsaki, O. (2009). Ethics and advance care planning in a culturally diverse society. *Journal of Transcultural Nursing, 20*(4), 405–416.

Kahnemann, D. (2011). *Thinking, fast and slow*. New York, NY: Farrar, Strauss and Giroux.

Kassirer, J. P. (2005). *On the take: How medicine's complicity with big business can endanger your health.* New York, NY: Oxford University Press.

Kegley, K. A. (2002). Genetics decision-making: A template for problems with informed consent. *Medicine and Law, 21,* 459–471.

Ketefian, S., Redman, R. W., Hanucharurnkul, S., Masterson, A., & Neves, E. P. (2001). The development of advanced practice roles: Implications in the international nursing community. *International Nursing Review, 48*(3), 152–163.

MacIntyre, A. (2007). *After virtue* (3rd ed.). Notre Dame, IN: Notre Dame University Press.

Magelssen, M. (2012). When should conscientious objection be accepted? *Journal of Medical Ethics, 38,* 18–21.

Marshall, P. A. (1995). The SUPPORT study: Who's talking? *Hastings Center Report, 25*(6), S9–S11.

McAliley, L. G., Hudson-Barr, D. C., Gunning, R. S., & Rowbottom, L. A. (2000). The use of advance directives with adolescents. *Pediatric Nursing, 26*(5), 471–482.

Mental Capacity Act of 2005. Retrieved from http://www.legislation.gov.uk/ukpga/2005/9/contents

Nieminen, A. L., Mannevaara, B., & Fagerström, L. (2011). Advanced practice nurses' scope of practice: A qualitative study of advanced clinical competencies. *Scandinavian Journal of Caring Sciences, 25*(4), 661–670.

Omnibus Budget Reconciliation Act. (1990). PL 100-508, 42 U.S.C. § 4206.

Parks, S. M., Winter, L., Santana, A. J., Parker, B., Diamond, J. J., Rose, M., & Myers, R. E. (2011). Family factors in end-of-life decision-making: Family conflict and proxy relationship. *Journal of Palliative Medicine, 14*(2), 179–184.

Parliamentary Assembly of the Council of Europe. (2010). *Women's access to lawful medical care: The problem of unregulated use of conscientious objection.* Doc. 123. Rapporteur Ms. Christine McCafferty. Retrieved from http://eclj.org/pdf/EDOC 12347doc20juillet.pdf

President's Commission for the Study of Ethical Behavior in Medicine and Biomedical and Behavioral Research. (1982). *Making health care decisions.* PB 83236703. Washington, DC: U.S. Government Printing Office.

Protection of Conscience Project. (2012). Homepage. Retrieved from http://www.consciencelaws.org/

Schober, M., & Affara, F. (2006). *International Council of Nurses: Advanced nursing practice.* Malden, MA: Blackwell.

Sellman, D. (2000). Alasdair MacIntyre and the professional practice of nursing. *Nursing Philosophy, 1*(1), 26–33.

Steinman, M. A., Harper, G. M., Chren, M. M., Landefeld, C. S., & Bero, L. A. (2007). Characteristics and impact of drug detailing for Gabapentin. *PLOS Medicine, 4*(5), e134. Retrieved from http://www.plosmedicine.org/article/info%3Adoi%2F10.1371%2Fjournal.pmed.0040134

Tarasoff v. Regents of University of California. (1976, July 1). California Supreme Court 131. *California Reporter, 14.*

Teno, J. M., Gruneir, A., Schwartz, Z., Nanda, A., & Wetle, T. (2007). Association between advance directives and quality of end-of-life care: A national study. *Journal of the American Geriatrics Society, 55*(2), 189–194.

U.S. Department of Health and Human Services, Office for Civil Rights. (2003). *Summary of the HIPAA Privacy Rule.* Retrieved from http://www.hhs.gov/ocr/privacy/hipaa/understanding/summary/privacysummary.pdf

Wazana, A. (2000). Physicians and the pharmaceutical industry: Is a gift ever just a gift? *Journal of the American Medical Association, 283,* 373–380.

Webster, G. C., & Baylis, F. (2000). Moral residue. In S. B. Rubin & L. Zoloth (Eds.), *Margin of error: The ethics of mistakes in the practice of medicine* (p. 208). Hagerstown, MD: University Publishing Group.

Wicclair, M. (2011). *Conscientious objection in healthcare: An ethical analysis.* New York, NY: Cambridge.

Wiener, L., Ballard, E., Brennan, T., Battles, H., Martinez, P., & Pao, M. (2008). How I wish to be remembered: The use of an advance care planning document in adolescent and young adult populations. *Journal of Palliative Medicine, 11*(10), 1309–1313.

Williams, B. (1985). *Ethics and the limits of philosophy.* London, England: Fontana.

Wolf, S. M., Boyle, P., Callahan, D., Fins, J., Jennings, B., Lindemann Nelson, J.,... Emanual, L. (2001). Sources of concern about the Patient Self-Determination Act. In W. Teays & L. Purdy (Eds.), *Bioethics, justice and health care* (pp. 411–419). Belmont, CA: Wadsworth Thompson Learning. Reprinted from *New England Journal of Medicine, 325*(23), 1666–1671.

Wolf, Z. R., & Robinson-Smith, G. (2007). Strategies used by clinical nurse specialists in "difficult" clinician–patient situations. *Clinical Nurse Specialist, 21*(2), 74–84.

PART 6

Leadership and Role Transition for the Advanced Practice Nurse

The last three chapters of this book take a different perspective on the role of the advanced practice nurse, looking at personal development of the reader for assuming a new role and leadership in the profession.

In Chapter 28, Barker identifies the importance of having a mentor and suggests how to select a mentor and how the relationship may develop over time. The checklist for selecting a mentor presented in this chapter is a helpful tool for the reader,

Conventional wisdom for all leaders states that to be successful, the individual needs to lead a balanced life. To achieve this goal, both time and stress management are central. However, the author suggests that a slightly different perspective be considered: energy management with time and stress management being strategies. Chapter 29 suggests relevant strategies related to these aspects of self-care and offers tools to assist readers in assessing their own skills and developing strategies to capitalize on their strengths and note opportunities for improvement.

In Chapter 30, Beauvais discusses role transitions for advanced practice registered nurses. She outlines the pathway from novice to expert and reviews important strategies for career development, including interviewing skills, portfolio and curriculum vitae development, and involvement in professional organizations. The author's expertise in executive administration lends itself well to her discussion of organizational fit, continued professional development, and credentialing and obtaining hospital privileges.

CHAPTER 28

Developing Leadership Skills for the Advance Practice Nurse Through Mentorship

Anne M. Barker

CHAPTER OBJECTIVES

1. Discuss the benefits of having a mentor to transition to and grow in the role of an advanced practice nurse.

2. Assess issues to consider when selecting and working with a mentor.

3. List the stages of the mentor–mentee relationship.

4. Distinguish between mentoring, precepting, networking, and coaching,

5. Recognize one's responsibilities to mentor less experienced nurse colleagues.

INTRODUCTION

A mentor is an experienced, influential person who guides and nurtures a less experienced person (the mentee). The mentor is someone who inspires, instructs, nurtures, and encourages the mentee to reach professional and personal goals. Further, the mentor has a respected reputation in the organization and profession and can access the resources and connections to help advance the career of the mentee.

Research regarding mentorship shows that individuals who have a mentor, as compared to those not having a mentor, have

- Increased job satisfaction
- Higher salaries
- Enhanced self-esteem and confidence
- Greater opportunities for promotion and advancement
- Enhanced role socialization
- A definitive career plan (Grindell, 2003)

MENTORSHIP: THE BARKER–SULLIVAN MODEL

Figure 28-1 illustrates the Barker–Sullivan model of mentorship (Barker, Sullivan, & Emery, 2006), which was devised through a review of the literature and through personal experiences of having a mentor and being a mentor. The relationship between the mentor and mentee can best be described as a partnership. In this partnership there is a congruency between the expertise and organizational connections of the mentor and the learning needs of the mentee. As a result of the relationship and interactions between the two, the mentee is energized for self-reflection, learning, and action, leading to professional role development and growth.

At the heart of this relationship there is mutual trust, respect, and open communications (Klein, 2002). Since the mentee will likely be disclosing sensitive information, exposing weaknesses, and discussing development of skills and competence in job-related areas, the mentee needs to be open and honest and, in return, can expect confidential, nonjudgmental, and sensitive feedback from the mentor.

STAGES OF THE MENTOR–MENTEE RELATIONSHIP

Because mentorship is a relationship that exists over a long period of time, the relationship goes through several stages (Anderson et al., 2002; Grossman, 2013).

Stage 1: Initiation: Selecting a Mentor and Determining Expectations

At the heart of the mentor–mentee relationship is an attraction of both people whose personality and values fit. Mentor–mentee relationships happen because both the mentor and the mentee wish to work together and they share mutual respect and admiration. (Mentorship and preceptor relations are compared and contrasted later in this chapter.)

There are several guidelines to assist the advanced practice nurse to identify an appropriate individual to serve as a mentor. First, one may find that there are several people to consider as mentors. Each of these individuals might bring something different to one's professional growth and development; therefore, one should not rule out having more than one mentor. However, more than likely, most people have only one mentor at any one point in time.

| FIGURE 28-1 | Barker-Sullivan Model of Mentor Partnerships |

Open, Honest, Discreet Communications

Mutual Attraction

Based on similarity of values characterized by trust and respect

Mentor
- Expertise in role competencies
- Transformational leader
- Skills as a mentor

Mentee
- Learning needs for developing role competencies and leadership skills

Energized

- Self-reflection
- Learning
- Action

Second, the mentor should not be a direct supervisor or a potential supervisor. There are several reasons for this. Most importantly, since the supervisor serves as an evaluator, the mentee may be reluctant to share weaknesses for fear that these will be included in an official evaluation or in decisions regarding advancement. This means that an honest conversation about developmental needs will not happen. On the other hand, to be an effective advanced practice nurse, the nurse does need to establish an effective and appropriate relationship with one's supervisor.

A third consideration is whether to ask someone within or outside the organization to serve as a mentor. The pros of having an internal mentor are that the person knows the organization, can help make connections, can observe behaviors and outcomes, and may get feedback about the mentee's performance from others. A mentor external to an organization, however, can offer new insights and different ways of doing things and can help make connections outside the organization.

A final consideration is whether to use a peer mentor or someone in an advanced position other than the supervisor position. The advantages of having a mentor from among peers are that the person is experiencing the issues and needs of the role in a similar way. That person's network of connections may be more appropriate. A mentor at a higher level in the organization, however, can provide a broader view of the organization and a different level of connections with others.

Table 28-1 is a checklist for nurses to use in selecting a mentor. The first six questions focus on the person's skills and role expertise. If the answer to any of these questions is "no," then the advanced practice nurse might want to consider whether this person would be the best mentor. However, that person might have several important skills the mentee wishes to learn, and the assessment might make clear what the potential mentor can and cannot offer. The last

five questions relate to the person's ability to be an effective mentor. A negative response suggests the need to clarify expectations in the relationship or to seek someone else to be a mentor.

After using the checklist to select a mentor, the next step is to establish ground rules. Borges and Smith (2004) provide a set of strategies to set up expectations for the relationship in the very early stage. First, they suggest setting up the details of when, where, and how long meetings will take place and which other forms of communication, such as email, should be used. Second, the mentee should write down long-term career goals and visions and use this information as a starting point for discussion and planning. The last strategy is to develop specific professional learning goals and personal goals. In this process the mentee should also consider life goals such as salary, health, family, spiritual needs, and so forth. Advanced practice nurses must lead balanced and happy lives to be effective. A mentor can help the advanced practice nurse pay attention to personal goals while at the same time balancing them with professional goals.

Stage 2: Cultivation Stage

In stage 2, the mentee works on goals by engaging in specific learning activities to develop competencies as an advanced practice nurse with the guidance and support of the mentor. The mentor serves as teacher, advisor, facilitator, coach, and sounding board (Anderson et al., 2002). During this time the mentor connects the mentee to appropriate people both inside and outside the organization and helps the mentee develop the skills, knowledge, and attitudes to be effective.

Stage 3: Growing Independence

As time progresses, the mentee grows in confidence, gains the necessary knowledge and skills to be an effective advanced practice nurse, and demonstrates the attainment of the role competencies. At this point the mentee begins to seek

TABLE 28-1   Mentor Selection Checklist

	Yes	No	Don't Know
1. Does the person have the expert knowledge and skills in the competencies that you need to develop?	☐	☐	☐
2. Is the person a leader by action and by example?	☐	☐	☐
3. Does this person have the ability to guide, coach, and teach you?	☐	☐	☐
4. Is the person respected in the organization?	☐	☐	☐
5. Does the person have access to important organizational information and can he or she help you to direct attention on important issues?	☐	☐	☐
6. Does the person have a network of influential people and is he or she willing to assist you to be visible, credible, and accepted by others in the organization?	☐	☐	☐
7. Is the person willing to work collaboratively with you?	☐	☐	☐
8. Is the person willing to spend the time and energy required for the development of this relationship?	☐	☐	☐
9. Are you comfortable with this person and do you trust this person to hold confidentiality?	☐	☐	☐
10. Is the person able to provide you with negative as well as positive feedback?	☐	☐	☐
11. Can the person help you identify what you need to learn and provide the structure for learning activities?	☐	☐	☐

independence, and the mentor role changes to consultant, giving advice only when asked (Anderson et al., 2002).

Stage 4: The Redefinition of the Relationship

In the last stage, the mentee is ready to move on from the relationship and no longer needs the mentor's advice and support. However, often an enduring friendship and colleagueship evolve and are maintained over the course of many years (Anderson et al., 2002).

OTHER SUPPORT SYSTEMS

Mentorship is a support system that requires much time and commitment from one person for another person's professional growth. Often people commit to being a mentor because someone had been a meaningful mentor for them and they are "paying it forward." Others commit to being a mentor because of their commitment to the profession. However, other professional relationships exist that provide an adjunct, not a replacement, to having a mentor.

Preceptorship

Some organizations have formal, structured programs, which may mistakenly be called mentorship programs, whose purpose is to assist employees, primarily new hires, in developing into a new role. These programs are better called preceptorship. A preceptor is assigned by the organization, and the relationship lasts a defined period of time, usually a shorter time than a mentorship. The purpose is to meet established objectives for knowledge and skill acquisition and socialization. The benefits of formal preceptorship programs is that they provide structured and well-defined expectations for both parties, as well as deploy organizational resources, particularly time, for the ongoing development of the relationship (Anderson et al., 2002). If the organization offers such a program, the advanced nurse practitioner should take full advantage of this resource, but this does not preclude having a mentor as well.

Networking

Networking is connecting with many influential individuals within and outside the organization to share ideas, to keep current, and to give and get advice. Networking is mutually beneficial to both parties. In contrast to mentoring and precepting, networking is less sustained and less structured and there are fewer interactions with others. Having a network of people is as important for professional success as it is to have a mentor.

For internal networking to be effective, advanced practice nurses must reflect on networking needs and set up processes to ensure that they interact with people who can contribute to their professional growth and development. First of all, one should think about people in the organization who can provide good insights about the organization, whose personality and values are similar to one's own, whose communication style is compatible, and who might be willing to share. In turn, the advanced practice nurse should think about people in the organization with whom to share experiences and ideas. One can think about this broadly and include other disciplines and peers. Next, the advanced practice nurse needs to make contact with these people by asking them to have coffee or lunch or to stay after a meeting for a few minutes just to talk or to give advice about a specific issue. As nurses establish a relationship with others, phone calls and email can assist them in maintaining contact even when busy. The key here is to be attentive about developing and sustaining networks rather than just letting relationships emerge.

Besides having a network within the organization, a network of contacts external to the organization is important for professional growth. Most often this occurs through professional organizations and meetings. The same thought process for establishing an internal network can be used for establishing a network of people outside the organization. Contact with others can be made and can be easily maintained over time using the current technology available.

Coaching

In the past few years, coaching has become another popular approach to assist one's professional development. This is a paid relationship between a person needing a sounding board and advice from a person with organizational expertise. Since coaches do not have direct observation of one's performance their advice is limited to what they are told by their client versus what they directly observe. A good coach has insight and knowledge that transcends any one organization or individual; rather, the coach understands organizational behavior. The relationship, similar to mentoring, is based on trust and confidentiality.

PAYING IT FORWARD

A core value of the nursing profession is to help others to develop for the good of patients, communities, and society. The previous sections of this chapter discuss a variety of connections with others to assist the advanced practice nurse to grow professionally. At times the focus of making such connections may seem self-serving. However, on the other side of the coin, it is equally important for the advanced practice nurse to be a mentor, preceptor, and networker to help novice advanced practice nurses.

DISCUSSION QUESTIONS

1. Identify several individuals you know who may be a good mentor for you. Use Table 28-1 to assess these individuals. Which one would you choose as a mentor and why?

2. Discuss your experiences of being a mentor and/or mentee. What were the advantages of the relationship for you?

REFERENCES

Anderson, M., Kroll, B., Luoma, J., Nelson, J., Sheman, K., & Surdo, J. (2002). Mentoring relationships. *Minnesota Nursing Accent, 74*(4).

Barker, A., Sullivan, D. T., & Emery, M. (2006). *Leadership competencies for clinical managers: The renaissance of transformational leadership.* Sudbury, MA: Jones and Bartlett.

Borges, J. R., & Smith, B. C. (2004, June). Strategies for mentoring a diverse nursing workforce. *Nurse Leader*, 45–48.

Grindell, C. G. (2003). Mentor managers. *Nephrology Nursing Journal, 30*(5), 517–522.

Grossman S. (2013). *Mentoring in nursing: A dynamic and collaborative process* (2nd ed.). New York, NY: Springer.

Klein, E. (2002). Missing something in your career? *Reflections on Nursing Leadership, 30*(1), 41–42.

CHAPTER 29

Managing Personal Resources: Time and Stress Management

Anne M. Barker

CHAPTER OBJECTIVES

1. Consider how to manage personal resources by managing energy.
2. Appreciate the need to balance efficiency and effectiveness.
3. Assess and reflect on time and stress management strategies to be a successful advanced practice nurse.

INTRODUCTION

Schippers and Hogenes (2011) propose a contemporary view of managing personal resources as energy management with time and stress management being strategies. For the purpose of this chapter, energy is defined as one's capacity for sustained activity, be it mental or physical, characterized by enthusiasm and focused effort. This chapter presents several tools to assess and reflect on time and stress management. By completing the self-assessment activities in this chapter, reflecting on the findings using the self-reflection model, and adopting new ways to manage time and stress, the reader can be more productive, have more energy, prevent burnout, and be more satisfied.

TIME MANAGEMENT

Covey (1989) suggests in his classic, best-selling book that one of the seven habits of effective people is to "put first things first." He further proposes that the current understanding about time management as it has evolved over the past decades is now focused on managing oneself versus managing time.

Managing time in today's health care organizations is more difficult than it was a decade ago because of the complexity of the industry and the need to respond to the external environment to decrease costs while at the same time providing quality care. Balancing efficiency and effectiveness is perhaps the biggest challenge in managing time. Being efficient means completing tasks on time and with a quality output. Being effective means working with others to sustain the goals of the organization. Since this involves building trust, developing high-performance teams, and making changes that will last, being effective while at the same time being efficient is a challenge. Certainly there is no one solution to this challenge, but by being reflective and self-aware, understanding the conflict, and applying some of the strategies discussed here, the goal to balance efficiency and effectiveness can be achieved.

Compounding the issue may be that time management is not the organization's priority (Schippers & Hogenes, 2011). In today's technological environment there is frequently an organizational value that people are immediately available through email, text, and social media, leading to distractions and interruptions that are the major causes of wasting time. As the advanced practice nurse develops increased expertise and assumes more responsibilities in the health care organization, it becomes increasingly more difficult to balance work life and personal life. Although it is difficult, it is essential for health, personal, and professional satisfaction and a sense of well-being to achieve this balance. The good news is that people can find additional time to be both more effective and efficient in their lives by assessing how they manage time and by adopting specific strategies to capture wasted time. The newfound time can then be deployed to work on strategic initiatives to meet personal and organizational goals. Research supports that long-term success is determined by the amount of time an individual spends on the most important goals on a weekly basis (Schippers & Hogenes, 2011).

Benefits of Managing Time

Managing one's time has many benefits (Barker, 2013):

- *Conserving personal energy.* By assessing personal energy levels while keeping a time log, one can learn to expend energy when it is most effective.

- *Having clarity of mind.* Managing time well leads to having a clear, calm mind when confronted with multiple demands. In the confusion and disorder of daily activities and crises, the advanced practice nurse still must pay attention to long-term strategic goals for both oneself and the organization. If one is struggling to accomplish daily tasks and to keep on top of work demands, one will not have the peace of mind to reflect, engage with others, and act proactively.

- *Nonverbal messaging about significance.* How a person spends time sends a message to others about what is important and what is not important. It is in essence "walking the talk" by spending time on important, strategic activities.

- *Contributing to feelings of well-being and happiness.* When individuals effectively manage time, they feel more in control of life, less stressed, and less likely to experience burnout. In fact, personal success can be measured by how a person spends time on activities that bring meaning, satisfaction, and joy to life.

Consequences of Poor Time Management

The consequences of not managing time well include the following (Barker, 2013):

- *Reflecting poorly on one's performance.* Missed deadlines and poor quality work do not reflect a nurse's best work, thus possibly leading to being overlooked for advancement and receiving poor performance evaluations.

- *Negatively affecting others.* Others in the workplace can be negatively affected if someone does not complete work and projects on time. People often rely on others' input and work to complete their work. It is simply unfair to others not to be timely in submission of one's own work.

■ *Burnout.* People who are burned out are emotionally and often physically exhausted. Burnout can occur when one feels overwhelmed by demands and a constant pressure of not completing work on time or completing it poorly. Burnout is an extreme form of stress leading to lack of motivation, low personal satisfaction, and adoption of bad habits.

Time Management: Self-Assessment

This section presents two approaches for assessing time management skills. The first is a self-assessment survey of best practices in time management. Many of these practices are further explained later in this chapter. The second assessment, and the most effective, is to keep a time log. The author suggests completing the survey and log prior to reading the rest of this chapter; but before you analyze the log, read the rest of the chapter to help with a meaningful self-assessment.

The following conditions are symptoms of poor self-management and should alert the reader to complete the two self-assessments and reflect on behaviors.

■ Regularly exceeding the number of required hours spent on the job

■ Regularly taking work home and working in the evenings and on weekends

■ Feeling resentful about the amount of time that one must devote to the job

■ Having no clarity of mind and an inability to focus

■ Constantly feeling rushed and out of control

■ Not having time for personal reflection and growth

■ Not achieving long-term personal and professional goals

The good news is that people can gain control over their time. When individuals assess how time is spent and adopt the suggested techniques, they should be able to capture wasted time for more meaningful, strategic, and important activities.

The first self-assessment activity is to complete a brief self-report survey. (See **Table 29-1**.) These practices are described in more detail later, and the results of the survey can guide where readers can pay particular attention.

The second self-assessment is to keep a time log for at least 1 week. This should be done for a "routine" week. This is a more detailed and time-consuming assessment but is well worth the effort. It is best to keep a time management log for both organizational time and personal time, since the goal is to have a balance between both aspects of life.

Table 29-2 is a time log format that can be used for completing this activity. Column 1 identifies the beginning and ending times for an activity. There should be an entry for every activity switch. In column 2, the individual completing the log states what the activity is and who else is involved in this activity. In column 3, the purpose of the activity is recorded. Next, one's energy level is noted in column 4 using the following scheme: L for low, M for medium, and H for high. In column 5, the individual notes interruptions while completing the activity. Indicate who interrupted, the time the interruption took, and whether the interruption was important or urgent.

The last column is to be used to analyze the log. This can be done at the end of each day. First look at each column and ask the following:

Column 1: Time

■ Did I spend too much or not enough time on the activity? Was I able to complete the task?

Column 2: Activity/People

■ Was this activity directly related to my role in the organization and/or to ensuring positive patient outcomes?

■ Could the task have been done in a better way or delegated?

TABLE 29-1 Assessment Tool for Time Management

Use the following scoring system for each answer below.

1 = Never

2 = Rarely

3 = Occasionally

4 = Usually

5 = Always

Place an X in the appropriate column.

	1	2	3	4	5
1. I feel calm and in control of my time.	☐	☐	☐	☐	☐
2. I am aware of fluctuations in my energy level and perform my most challenging tasks when my energy level is at its highest.	☐	☐	☐	☐	☐
3. I spend the majority of my time in meaningful work that contributes to positive work in the workplace.	☐	☐	☐	☐	☐
4. I spend the majority of my time in activities that I find satisfying.	☐	☐	☐	☐	☐
5. I complete my paperwork and projects on time.	☐	☐	☐	☐	☐
6. I follow through on promises I make to colleagues.	☐	☐	☐	☐	☐
7. I have written daily goals.	☐	☐	☐	☐	☐
8. I delegate tasks to others in my clinical unit.	☐	☐	☐	☐	☐
9. I assess tasks for their importance and their urgency.	☐	☐	☐	☐	☐
10. I keep a to-do list and schedule time to complete the tasks on the list.	☐	☐	☐	☐	☐
11. I set aside time each week to complete paperwork and other tasks.	☐	☐	☐	☐	☐
12. I am able to control interruptions.	☐	☐	☐	☐	☐
13. I embrace the philosophy "do today instead of putting off until tomorrow."	☐	☐	☐	☐	☐
14. I set aside time each day for planning.	☐	☐	☐	☐	☐
15. I have written long-term goals.	☐	☐	☐	☐	☐

TABLE 29-2   Time Management Log

Times	Activity/ People	Purpose	Energy Level	Interruptions	Effectiveness of the Time Spent

Column 3: Purpose

- Was the activity a mundane task or not meaningful?
- Was the activity related to long-term or short-term goals?

Column 4: Energy Level

- Was the task performed at the right time in relation to my energy level?

Column 5: Interruptions

- How many times were you interrupted during the day?
- By whom?
- For how long?

Column 6: Effectiveness of the Time Spent

- Overall how effective and efficient was the activity

At the end of the week, the advanced nurse practitioner performs an analysis of the entire week looking for themes and areas of improvement where less time could be wasted, activities could be more effective and efficient, and items could be delegated to others. In addition to the preceding questions, the advanced practice nurse can ask these questions:

- What percentage of time is spent in work, family and home, social, spiritual, and physical activities? Is there a balance?

- What percentage of time is spent in activities that are important or urgent?
- Are the people interacting on a daily basis appropriate to reaching individual and organizational goals?
- What are the main interruptions? Assess the percentage of time interruptions fall into each of the categories: very important, important, not important. Can the number of interruptions be reduced? How? (Note: This analysis may have the biggest impact on better use of time.)
- What are the biggest time wasters?
- Are there any activities that can be reduced or eliminated?
- What can be delegated to others?
- Were there any tasks that had been put off and then became urgent/a crisis to complete?

Strategies for Managing Time

Time management is not easy, and everyone will experience setbacks and days when they will not feel they have managed their time well. Keeping a time log can be completed annually or more often if a time management tune-up is needed. It will help identify areas of improvement and suggest what else can be done in the future. It takes constant care and attention to be a good manager of time. But there are strategies that can be adopted and when practiced regularly can improve one's time management skills. Based on the self-assessment survey and the findings from the time management log, the reader should focus on the strategies discussed in this section that are most applicable to provide leverage in managing time.

Goal Setting and Planning

Most time management experts agree that goal setting and planning are the premier time management strategies. In this section, ways to plan for goal achievement are suggested.

First, individuals should write down short-term and long-term goals. The goals should be readily available electronically on the device most often carried by the advanced nurse practitioner or in a written format on a calendar or planner. Practitioners should do two complementary things with these documented goals. First, they should look at the goals daily to keep them fresh. By doing so, practitioners will be more sensitive to opportunities that will help them reach their goals. Second, at the beginning of each day, individuals should have a list of activities to accomplish that day to move toward their written goals. It is not easy to set realistic daily goals; at first it is common to plan more than one can accomplish, but as time progresses most people get better at this task. Most important, people should not get frustrated if they do not accomplish every task every day. In fact, one time management principle suggests that a task will consume the time that has been allotted for it. Therefore, planning an aggressive schedule is a good strategy as long as the person does not get frustrated about not accomplishing everything he or she set out to do.

Barker (2013) suggests a number of guidelines to follow when setting goals:

- Goals should include all aspects of life, including work, family, social, financial, spiritual, physical, and psychological areas.
- Goals should be measurable and achievable, yet challenging.

- In determining realistic goals, organizational constraints, resources, and personal strengths and skills should be considered.
- Time frames for goal completion should be realistic but should not allow for procrastination.
- Time lines can be reassessed, new deadlines set, old goals dropped when they are no longer appropriate, and new goals added as needed.
- Individuals should reward themselves upon completion of goals.
- People should pursue goals with enthusiasm, even when they are not feeling enthusiastic.

Strategy: Scheduling Time to Achieve Goals Today most individuals use a smart phone and or an e-calendar to schedule meetings. These devices can also be used to block out time to accomplish tasks, keep written goals, and have an ongoing "to do" list. Blocking out time to complete both short- and long-term work on important activities is one of the top time management strategies and leads to peace of mind. When one knows that there is time set aside to complete the activity, one can decrease worrying about the activity until the scheduled time. Blocking out time also provides a picture of what is needed when and supports "saying no" when a time is set aside for a certain activity and someone wants to intrude on this time.

Prioritizing Tasks: Urgent Versus Important

A useful way of prioritizing daily, weekly, and monthly goals and tasks is to consider whether activities are important or not important and whether they are urgent or not urgent. This schema can also be used for assessing interruptions in the time management log. Urgency has to do with an immediate need to take some action. On the other hand, important activities are generally those that contribute to short- and long-term goal attainment.

FIGURE 29-1 Assessing Tasks for Importance and Urgency

URGENCY		
High ↑	Quadrant III Low Importance High Urgency	Quadrant I High Importance High Urgency
Low ↓	Quadrant IV Low Importance Low Urgency	Quadrant II High Importance Low Urgency
	Low ← Importance	→ High

Figure 29-1 provides a template to assess the importance and urgency of tasks. On the vertical axis is a rating of urgency from low to high; on the horizontal axis is a rating of importance from low to high. The grid can be used in two ways: in the short term to make a decision about how to use one's time, and for the long term to view how much time one is spending in each quadrant. For the short term, a task can assessed to determine its urgency and importance and to decide whether to engage in the activity. In the longer term the advanced practice nurse can use the grid to reflect on how much time is spent in each quadrant.

Covey (1989) suggests that highly effective people who are able to self-manage spend most of their time in Quadrant II paying attention to developing, implementing, and evaluating strategic plans, vision, and values. Since these matters are often important (the most important work of the organization), but not urgent, there may be a tendency to procrastinate and spend time and energy on the urgent. A cautionary note is that spending too much time in Quadrant I, high urgency and high importance, is crisis management mode and may be a symptom that Quadrant II work was "put off" with important, nonurgent work suddenly becoming urgent. This can lead to increased stress and burnout.

Controlling Interruptions

Controlling interruptions is not only one of the most lucrative ways to gain time but it is also one of the hardest. Sykes (2011) reports that an average of 2 hours per day is spent addressing unplanned tasks, which results in an employee's inability to focus and taking more time to complete tasks and making more errors than employees who are not distracted. Therefore, controlling interruptions has great potential for capturing time to work on important activities. The advanced practice nurse should go back over the time log and identify patterns in the interruptions, the time spent dealing with them, and whether there are people who interrupt more than others do. After this analysis, the nurse can then implement strategies to decrease interruptions. For example, if one person interrupts more than others, it might be necessary to routinely schedule time with this person and ask that individual to have a list of items to discuss rather than ask for time "on the fly."

Allowing Oneself Private Time

An oft-spoken value for which people take great pride is having an open-door policy. However, there is a difference between having an open-door policy (meaning being accessible and listening) and having the door open all the time. In order to control interruptions one can schedule and set aside time every week to literally "close the door" and to work on the important activities. Two ways to accomplish this are to have a regularly scheduled time to close the door and request no interruptions and to review one's calendar at the beginning of each week and find 2 to 4 hours within the week to block off time for quiet time and individual work.

Avoid Multitasking

The term *multitasking* is derived from the ability of computers to process more than one task at a time and in parallel. It is now used to describe the human activity of doing two or more things simultaneously, moving back and forth from one task to another or moving quickly from task to task. For instance, a person can read and write emails while attending a meeting, take a phone call while at composing a written document, and so forth. Multitasking is a form of interruption that can be managed to find more time.

The American Psychological Association (2006), after considering research about multitasking, stated that "multitasking may seem efficient on the surface but may actually take more time in the end and involve more error. . . . Even brief mental blocks created by shifting between tasks can cost as much as 40 percent of someone's productive time." Further, multitasking in the presence of others sends a message that one is not mentally or emotionally present with those with whom one is face to face and is not fully listening to or engaged with them.

Delegation

Delegation is an important skill that enables one to accomplish one's work and goals. As readers will appreciate in this section, delegation is a fine art with many things to consider and approaches to take. Depending on the role and reporting structure in the organization, some advanced practice nurses may not have others to whom they can formally delegate. However, there may be others in the organization who do not have a formal reporting structure but who can assist nonetheless, such as graduate teaching assistants, program assistants/secretaries, and patient care technicians.

Before a person can successfully delegate to others, however, that person needs to reflect on his or her attitude and values about delegating. Too often one hears "I'd rather do it myself" or "It is faster to do it myself than to tell someone else how to do it." These statements imply that there are others in the organization to whom one can delegate, yet those individuals are not ready or able to give up control. And, indeed, it might in the short term be faster to complete a task alone, but, in the long term, once someone has successfully accomplished a delegated task it becomes easier and easier for the delegator and the delegatee.

Delegation has many advantages:

- Delegation is a trust-building activity.
- Delegation builds the confidence and self-esteem of others.
- Delegation unburdens one from routine, mundane tasks to provide the time for important activities and relationship building.
- Delegation helps others to grow, learn, and become leaders as they see more of the big picture.
- Delegation is an important tool in succession planning.
- Delegation can match the right person with the right expertise to the right job.

The process of delegation involves looking at the task(s) the advanced practice nurse plans to delegate and the skills of the delegatee. Some tasks should not be delegated. This includes important organizational functions and meetings where one's presence is needed and noted. Human resources matters such as rewarding people, disciplining people, and managing conflict also cannot be delegated. Eliminating these tasks from the delegation possibilities leaves the nurse with a substantial number of routine tasks that can be delegated.

The next step is to consider the individuals to whom one might delegate. The advanced practice nurse should judge the expertise, strengths and weaknesses, knowledge, interests, skills, and attitudes of the potential delegatee. These should match the job to be done.

When delegating, one also needs to be sensitive to the workload of the person to whom one is delegating. Giving the person the ability to negotiate what the scope of the task will be and when it will be done is essential for success. There is a fine line between individuals' perception that they are being trusted to complete an important task and the perception they are being "dumped on." To accentuate the positive and minimize the negative, involvement of the person who is being asked to do the task, open communication, negotiation, and lots of praise are required.

Further, the process used to delegate is important. First, the person who is being assigned a task needs to understand its importance and urgency, why it is being delegated, and what the requirements and guidelines are. The delegatee needs appropriate information and resources such as time, space, and money to complete the task. The person should be aware of dates for task completion and periodic evaluation if the task extends over a long time period. As difficult as this may be to accept, the results of the assignment are more important than the means by which the person completes it, as long as he or she completes the task consistent with organizational policies and works with others in a positive manner.

Throughout the process of task completion, the person who assigned the task must be available to give advice, support, and guidance. Once the task is completed the delegatee should be provided feedback and recognition and an appropriate reward.

Procrastination and Perfectionism

Procrastination—delaying what needs to be done until the last minute—is often referred to as "putting off until tomorrow what I should have done today." Procrastination can take several forms, including knowingly doing something other than what needs to be done; starting to work on a project, but then stopping work on it, only to have to complete it at the last minute; or doing less difficult tasks rather than the required one (Seaward, 2004). Being aware of a tendency toward procrastination is important in understanding time management skills and strategies. Scheduling, maintaining to-do lists, and adhering to the list can help break this habit.

A different but parallel problem is being a perfectionist. Perfectionists generally get caught up in the details and never see the whole picture; thus they waste time (Seaward, 2004). Further, believing that one can be perfect is detrimental to one's self-esteem. No one is or can be perfect. To moderate this is to consider "what is good enough?" while at the same time holding high standards and expectations of oneself and others.

Managing Communications

Email   The problem with emails is that they convert issues that are not important or urgent to having an aura of being urgent and important. Many people in organizations are connected to their email full time. For example, someone may send an email noting he or she will be late for a meeting that is starting in a half hour and expect it to be read.

Reading and responding to email can consume a large portion of time. Here are several hints for making the task more meaningful and less time consuming:

- Read emails one to two times per day, depending on one's schedule and the volume received. Prescheduling time for this rather than trying to fit the emails in between other tasks means one can focus better.
- Turn off email when doing other tasks on the computer to avoid constant interruptions.
- Keep the inbox uncluttered by reading and responding to messages and then moving those emails to an appropriate folder if they need to kept. Otherwise, immediately delete emails that do not need to be saved.

- For emails that need a short response, respond and delete. This is an example of an old time adage, "handle each piece of paper once."

- Read emails that are marked as urgent first. However, what the sender thinks is urgent is not necessarily what is truly urgent, and the urgent/important grid can be used to assess the response.

- Use the From button at the top of the Inbox to sort email by sender versus by date. This then lumps all emails in one chain of correspondence and makes the communication easier to follow. Further, for emails from senders that do not require reading, you can delete all the messages at once.

- If one cannot respond to an email quickly and one does not have time to answer it, schedule time for composing a response later.

Phone Calls   Managing phone calls is another important time management technique. Phone conversations can be much more pertinent and personal than emails. However, common advice is to keep phone conversations to less than 5 minutes. One of the downsides of phone calls is that of playing "phone tag," which can be a time waster. When leaving a voice mail, specify a good time for the person to reach you, which can increase the possibility being available when the person returns the call.

If the advanced practice nurse has a support person who answers the phone, instructions for how to handle phone calls are needed. Whoever is taking calls should be able to screen calls and refer the caller to the appropriate person. The support person can find out when a convenient time is to return the call or can schedule a phone appointment. The advanced practice nurse can also instruct the support person on how to communicate availability. For example, saying "she is not on the unit" is a different message from saying "she is at *x* meeting, and I expect her back in an hour."

STRESS MANAGEMENT

Advanced practice nurses are already familiar with the physiology of stress and stress-related diseases. The focus of this section in on the causes of occupational stress. The premise of the discussion is that stress cannot be avoided or eliminated, but how one reacts to stressors can be altered.

No doubt most advanced practice nurses already use many different techniques to reduce their own stress. In the section, the author reviews some well-known, conventional techniques. These techniques will discuss both cognitive and biochemical strategies to manage stress.

Occupational Stress

The National Safety Council (Seaward, 1994) lists many causes of job stress. How someone experiences and reacts to these stressors varies from person to person. **Table 29-3** can be used to assess job-related stress based on the reasons identified by the National Safety Council. After completing the assessment, the advanced practice nurse can look at each item rated at 3 or more to reflect on their occupational stress.

STRESS MANAGEMENT TECHNIQUES

This section provides a review of techniques to manage stress both cognitively and biochemically. The cognitive approach to self-management of stress has been the primary focus over the past several decades, but there is new evidence of the effectiveness of techniques to change biochemistry. The goal is to manage one's energy through self-assessment and self-reflection.

Cognitive Approach

The cognitive stress management techniques fall into four categories: (1) altering one's thinking, (2) avoiding stress, (3) adapting to the stress, and (4) accepting stress (Miller, 2013).

TABLE 29-3	Assessment Tool for Occupational Stress

Use the following scoring system for each answer below.

1 = Never

2 = Rarely

3 = Occasionally

4 = Usually

5 = Always

Place an X in the appropriate column.

	1	2	3	4	5
1. I have too much responsibility with little or no authority.	☐	☐	☐	☐	☐
2. The organization sets unrealistic expectations and deadlines that I am unable to meet.	☐	☐	☐	☐	☐
3. I do not feel adequately trained for my position.	☐	☐	☐	☐	☐
4. I do not feel appreciated.	☐	☐	☐	☐	☐
5. I am not able to voice concerns.	☐	☐	☐	☐	☐
6. I have too much to do with too few resources.	☐	☐	☐	☐	☐
7. I lack a clear understanding of what is expected of me.	☐	☐	☐	☐	☐
8. I have a difficult time keeping pace with technology.	☐	☐	☐	☐	☐
9. The physical environment in which I work has poor lighting, a lot of noise, and poor ventilation.	☐	☐	☐	☐	☐
10. There is the possibility of workplace violence.	☐	☐	☐	☐	☐
11. People in the organization have experienced sexual harassment and racial discrimination.	☐	☐	☐	☐	☐
12. The organization has recently downsized or restructured.	☐	☐	☐	☐	☐
13. Creativity and autonomy are not valued.	☐	☐	☐	☐	☐

Altering Techniques

Many stressors cannot be eliminated, but techniques can be used to alter how one deals with stress more effectively:

- *Problem solving:* This allows a better understanding of the stressor and thinking about it differently. By doing this, one may be able to better accept what one cannot control and "let it go."

- *Communication:* The purpose is to make sure that people know in a respectful way how one is feeling about a situation. This prevents building up resentment and feeling one's voice has not been heard.

- *Having the right information:* Given how information sometimes get distorted in an organization, having the right information may elucidate the issue and decrease stress.
- *Time management, priority setting, and planning:* These activities provide clarity of mind.

Avoidance Techniques

A second set of strategies to deal with stress suggests ways to avoid stress rather than altering one's reactions to it:

- *Use an assertive communication style.* Respectfully state one's point of view and stand up for what one believes in. After this is done, one should once more "let go," content in the realization that one's opinion had been expressed.
- *Say "no" and walk away.* This is very difficult to do. The most direct way is to simply say "no" to a request. However, other approaches may be to (1) reflect on other priorities currently needing time, (2) suggest someone else who might be more appropriate for the task, and (3) delay the request for a better time, particularly if this activity is important and exciting for you.
- *Avoid people, situations, and hot-button topics that increase stress.*

Adapting Techniques

Adapting techniques call for the person to adapt to the change:

- *Reframe the picture.* Look at the issue from another's point of view, try to gain a better understanding, and look at the positive aspects.
- *Consider how important the issue is in the long run.* Will it really matter in a month from now? Think back on similar stressors and recognize how much meaning they had in the long term.
- *Adjust expectations.* Similar to a negative impact on one's time management, perfectionism can be a cause of stress. Adjust expectations without compromising values and visions and accept "good enough."

Acceptance Techniques

Acceptance techniques enable one to recognize there are many stressors outside one's control and that one must accept this and change how one reacts to the stress.

- Let go and recognize what one cannot control.
- Look for how the issue is helping you to grow, develop, and perhaps gain new competencies.
- Share your feeling with others who are neutral and objective.
- Write down one's viewpoint and concerns as means for venting.

Stress Management Techniques to Adjust Biochemical Response to Stress

Although it is beyond the purpose of this text to summarize the pathophysiology of stress, neuroendocrine hormones play a crucial role in the human response to stress and in its management. In a review of the evidence to reduce stress and promote health, Varvogli and Darviri (2011) suggest the following techniques for managing stress. A person can learn these techniques by working with trainers, through additional reading including Web resources, from audiotapes, and on one's own:

- Progressive muscle relaxation is the alternate tensing and relaxing of major muscle groups.
- Autogenic training is a self-relaxation technique.
- Relaxation response uses the repetition of a word and concentration.
- Biofeedback monitors reactions using instrumentation.
- Guided imagery uses a person's images to reduce stress and improve health.
- Diaphragmatic breathing is deep breathing characterized by expansion of the abdomen rather than the chest.
- Transcendental meditation is a meditation technique in which a person repeats a mantra.

DISCUSSION QUESTIONS _____

1. Based on the assessments in this chapter, what time and stress management strategies were you already using? How effective have they been? What new ones will you adopt and why? Do you have other techniques you use that have been useful for you?

2. If you completed a time management log, what were your findings and what strategies will you adopt to improve your time management skills?

3. Review the information regarding stress management. Realistically, how much stress are you experiencing? Which strategies will you try to help you cope with stress?

REFERENCES _____

American Psychological Association. (2006, March 20). Multitasking: Switching costs. Retrieved from https://www.apa.org/research/action/multitask.aspx

Barker, A. M. (2013). Managing personal resources: Time and stress management. In S. M. DeNisco & A. M. Barker (Eds.), *Advanced practice nursing: Evolving roles for the transformation of the practice* (2nd ed., pp. 595–606). Burlington, MA: Jones & Bartlett.

Covey, S. R. (1989). *The 7 habits of highly effective people: Powerful lessons in personal change.* New York, NY: Simon and Schuster.

Miller, H. S. (2013). Stress management for you. Retrieved from http://www.millergroup.com/wp-content/uploads/2013/12/Stress-Management-for-You-V1.0-12.03.13-FINAL.pdf

Schippers, M. C., & Hogenes, R. (2011, May 3). Energy management of people in organizations: A review and research agenda. *Journal of Business Psychology, 26,* 193–203.

Seaward, B. L. (1994). *National Safety Council's stress management.* Sudbury, MA: Jones and Bartlett.

Seaward, B. L. (2004). *Managing stress: Principles and strategies for health and well-being* (4th ed.). Sudbury, MA: Jones and Bartlett.

Sykes, E. R. (2011). Interruptions in the workplace: A case study to reduce their effects. *International Journal of Information Management, 31,* 385–394.

Varvogli, L., & Darviri, C. (2011). Stress management techniques: Evidence-based procedures that reduce stress and promote health. *Health Sciences Journal, 5*(2), 74–89.

CHAPTER 30

Role Transition: Strategies for Success in the Marketplace

Audrey Beauvais

CHAPTER OBJECTIVES

1. Discuss strategies to facilitate role transition for advanced practice nurses.

2. Conduct a personal, marketplace, and organizational analysis when transitioning to the job market.

3. Identify components of a professional portfolio.

4. Develop a curriculum vitae.

5. Review interviewing skills and techniques.

6. Recognize opportunities to foster professional development and life-long learning.

INTRODUCTION

The Institute of Medicine (2010) has made recommendations about the role of nursing for the future. Several of these recommendations apply to this chapter and the role transition for advanced practice nurses. These include

- Allow advanced practice registered nurses to practice to the full extent of their education and training.

- Expand opportunities for nurses to lead and diffuse collaborative improvement efforts.

- Ensure that nurses engage in lifelong learning.

- Prepare and enable nurses to lead change to advance health.

If advanced practice nurses are to meet the recommendations set forth by the IOM, they will need to secure a work setting that enables them to work to the full extent of their education and to collaborate with the other disciplines, that encourages life-long learning, and that supports the role of the nurse to lead and influence change. This chapter is intended to help advanced practice nurses who are entering the job market by addressing how to find employment opportunities, how to complete several different assessments to prepare them for the job market, how to develop a professional portfolio, and how to apply for a job.

Once they are employed, it is essential that advanced practice nurses put structures and strategies in place to promote their growth and development. To this end, the chapter identifies ways to foster professional development.

TRANSITIONING ROLES

The role transition from registered nurse to advanced practice can be a challenging journey (Cleary, Matheson, & Happell, 2009; Spoelstra & Robbins, 2010). Having realistic expectations about new roles and responsibilities can help alleviate the angst associated with this evolution. Experiencing a positive transition between roles will help facilitate the advanced practice nurse's ability to achieve independence, self-sufficiency, and influence over his or her professional practice In addition, it will help foster a sense of worth and identity within the profession of nursing (Cleary et al., 2009).

The role transition from registered nurse to advanced practice nurse begins during educational preparation and goes right through the first few years of practice. Some scholars have proposed that this transition happens in a three-phase composite model of social, cultural, and professional components that involves identity loss, transitional role evolution, and incorporation into clinical practice (Barton, 2007). The following subsections briefly describe the three phases.

Identity Loss Phase

Identity loss happens early in the educational program (Barton, 2007). Students become cognizant that they are both novice advanced practice nurses and experienced, practicing, professional nurses (Barton, 2007; Spoelstra & Robbins, 2010). For students to progress in their transition, it is necessary for them to reexamine and separate from their prior career status. However, advanced practice nursing students often attend school part-time. Hence, it is difficult for them to completely disengage from their previous professional role because they are functioning in that role as part of their ongoing nursing employment. This duality can enhance the feeling of identity loss. The perception of identity loss is advanced through these learning transitions, which enable the students to acquire new knowledge and skills that affect their clinical practice within their current nursing role (Barton, 2007; Lindblad, Hallman, Gillsjo, Lindblad, & Foerstrom, 2010; Spoelstra & Robbins, 2010). Interestingly, during this phase students tend to have intensified consciousness of the anxieties among their colleagues, which can help foster cohesion and a unique group identity (Barton, 2007).

Transitional Role Evolution Phase

The uncertainty of professional identity can grow as students cope with the increasing duality of roles. During the transitional role evolution phase, students experience a sense of role limbo and at times feel invisible and /or inept. Fortunately, during this stage, graduate students have developed a strong sense of community and group identity. This mutual support is critical, as they often experience opposition and aggression from professionals in the healthcare field. The camaraderie and support from fellow peers allows them to become competent in their new skill sets. The transition phase and sense of community often emerge at the midpoint of the academic preparation. After this time, the sense of unity gradually decreases as the students anticipate graduation from the program. This trend helps foster resocialization into the new professional role as students grow individually and develop their new identities. The end of the transition phase is denoted by the students' independence and self-reliance as well as decreased group cohesion (Barton, 2007).

Incorporation Phase

During the incorporation phase, which begins during the latter part of the educational program, students begin to resolve their issues regarding their new role in their practice (Barton, 2007). By the time their studies are completed, advance practice nurses have increased confidence and security in their new role (Lindblad et al., 2010). Throughout this phase, students start to look at practical problems and begin to select role models.

Specifically for nurse practitioners, these role models may be from both the medicine and nursing disciplines, allowing students to take various traits and develop them into the new role construct. During this stage, their relationships with their medical peers change (Barton, 2007). For example, nurse practitioners may begin to describe a reciprocal trust and confidence between themselves and the general medical practitioners who serve as their role models and supervisors. The medical staff become aware of the skills the nurse practitioner has acquired and note those areas in which the individual requires additional guidance (Lindblad et al., 2010). This changing clinical relationship tends to support mutual admiration and increasing collegiality. Students' licensure exam is perceived as the final initiation and source of legitimacy of their new clinical role (Barton, 2007). Although they are still novices who are developing their professional identity in clinical practice, after passing their licensing examination they are qualified nurse practitioners.

STRATEGIES FOR A SUCCESSFUL TRANSITION

A successful transition begins with competent, knowledgeable advanced practice nurses who demonstrate critical thinking, self-awareness, and effective interpersonal and leadership skills. To promote successful role transition, advanced practice nurses should utilize a framework that emphasizes evidence-based practice, research, collaboration, and consultation as a way to inform nursing practice. Additionally, those in advanced nurse practice roles who provide direct care (e.g., nurse practitioners, clinical nurse leaders, midwives, clinical nurse specialists, and nurse anesthetists) must provide patient care that is grounded in evidence and theory while viewing the patient holistically and as deserving of comprehensive treatment. Finally, they need to demonstrate comprehension and exemplification of professional responsibilities. To be successful, advanced practice nurses will need to demonstrate leadership skills grounded in ethical values. Not only will they need to be knowledgeable in their area of clinical practice but also they will have to communicate effectively with others, identify goals, determine effective strategies to accomplish those goals, role-model professional behavior, and collaborate with others to improve patient and financial outcomes (Spoelstra & Robbins, 2010).

Ideally, students' academic programs will implement strategies to help foster the development of the previously mentioned characteristics. However, once students have graduated, it is essential for advanced practice nurses to function within a supportive learning milieu that continues to encourage the synthesis of knowledge and critical thinking (Forbes, While, Mathes, & Griffiths, 2006; Heitz, Steiner, & Burman, 2004).

Advanced practice nurses in direct care roles have a unique set of issues for their transition because of their interaction with physicians and families. They may need to overcome some barriers—such as a lack of knowledge about advanced practice nurses' scope of practice, lack of knowledge about advanced practice nurses' role, negative physician attitudes, lack of respect, poor communication, and patient and family reluctance to accept advanced practice nurse care—if they want to facilitate a positive transition. Fortunately, several useful strategies to overcome these barriers are easily implemented. For example, advanced practice nurses can provide formal and informal education and orientation to physicians and medical students on their scope of practice and roles. In addition, they can develop and utilize integrated collaboration models when establishing a new advanced practice nurse's position within a particular organization or practice. Furthermore, advanced practice nurses can attend interdisciplinary rounds to visibly show the patients and families their involvement with the medical management of care. Moreover, they can advocate for medical students to be exposed to graduate nursing students early in their education as well as advocate for uniformity in advanced practice nurse education and certification. An essential part of overcoming these barriers and, therefore, of ensuring a successful transition is to demonstrate and showcase the positive outcomes that advanced practice nurses can foster, such as decreased length of hospital stay, improved medical management resulting in decreased numbers of unnecessary office visits, more comprehensive patient education, improved health maintenance, and greater patient satisfaction (Clarin, 2007).

A smooth transition can also be fostered by selecting preceptors and mentors who can help ensure sufficient socialization and encourage feelings of self-worth. Mentors can certainly provide additional teaching of skills needed for the job, if needed. Moreover, they can help expose advanced practice nurses to additional aspects of their role and boost their confidence in their capability to assume the role. Novice advanced practice

nurses are more apt to assimilate other facets of their role when they observe their preceptors in action (Hayes, 1998).

Finally, reflective journaling can be used as a strategy for promoting a successful transition. Reflective journaling can help novices transition successfully into an expert role by keeping a written record in which they contemplate their professional experiences and learn from the process (Hamric & Taylor, 1989; Latham & Fahey, 2006). The method used can be as simple as daily written reflections on the following four questions:

1. What happened today?
2. What did I think about that?
3. How do I feel about it?
4. What did I learn?

The act of analyzing thoughts, ideas, and feelings helps to develop metacognitive skills by assisting nurses to self-evaluate and discern what they know versus what they have yet to learn. Such reflection, which addresses their cognitive, psychomotor, and emotional growth, will help identify potential educational strategies to help them advance their professional development. The practice of analyzing one's thoughts and feelings is especially useful for learning how to handle complicated situations that exceed a straightforward right or wrong response. A reflective journal can assist advanced practice nurses in recognizing their capabilities, professional worth, and future educational needs critical to the development of their new role. Reflective journals can also be a positive way to map one's growth and development (Latham & Fahey, 2006).

ENTERING THE JOB MARKET

To complete the transition from students to experts working in the healthcare field, graduating advanced practice nursing students will need to secure their first position. This section discusses some practical aspects to entering the job market, such as how to find open positions. In addition, it reviews the personal, marketplace, organization, and organization fit assessments that can be used to prepare for the job market. Furthermore, it presents practical ideas for developing a portfolio that can be shared with potential employers to highlight one's knowledge and skills. Specifics about applying for a job such as applications and interviews are reviewed.

The Job Market

The statistics for employment of nurses and advanced practice nurses for the next decade are dramatic. In general, the Bureau of Labor Statistics (U.S. Department of Labor, Bureau of Labor Statistics, 2014a) reports that there will be a 19% growth in the demand for registered nurses from 2012 to 2022. Even more astounding is that the employment of nurse anesthetists, nurse midwives, and nurse practitioners is expected to grow 31% from 2012 to 2022 (U.S. Department of Labor, Bureau of Labor Statistics, 2014b). Similarly, the demand for nursing faculty will continue to grow to prepare these nurses for practice and to meet the market demand. According to a report by the American Association of Colleges of Nursing (AACN) in October 2013, there was a national nurse faculty vacancy rate of 8.3% with a total of 1,358 faculty vacancies in higher educational settings. However, most of these vacancies require a doctorate. These statistics bode well for students pursuing education in all of the advanced practice roles in nursing. Additionally, the IOM report previously discussed further suggests that there are many driving forces that will increase the need for advanced educated nurses.

FINDING EMPLOYMENT OPPORTUNITIES

A first step with regard to entering the job market is to locate job openings. There are several sources to find openings via print and online resources, professional memberships, and networking. These strategies are discussed next.

Print and Online Resources

Job openings can be found via multiple media. The traditional way to find jobs has been through printed classified advertisements. Today, however, few practices or organizations post job openings only in printed advertisements, if they publish them in printed form at all. Instead, most job postings appear on the Internet. There are job boards, such as advancedpracticejobs.com, nursepractitionerjobs.com, higheredjobs.com, to name a few, that may be of use. However, nurses must bear in mind that national job boards attract large numbers of job seekers. As a result, the national job boards may not produce the results that one would like. Experts warn that it is difficult for individuals to differentiate themselves online; as such, it is more useful to follow leads through contacts and thorough research (Vilorio, 2011). Many organizations post job openings on their own websites; searching individual websites can be a cumbersome approach but worth the effort if one is familiar with the local market.

Professional Memberships

An initial step in a job search should be to get involved in the appropriate professional organizations at the local, state, and national levels. Actively participating on committees within professional organizations helps job seekers to be visible and known to people who might be making selection decisions.

Networking

Referrals are one of the key ways of finding employment opportunities, even for positions that are not being publicized (Hosking, 2010). In fact, research results indicate that approximately 70% of job postings are never advertised publicly (Owens & Young, 2008). In addition, referrals help raise advanced practice nurses' chances of having their curriculum vitae placed directly in front of employers who are hiring (Hosking, 2010). Practices and organizations are apt to hire individuals with whom they are familiar and who are recommended by someone they trust (Vilorio, 2011). For this reason, it is suggested that advanced practice nurses develop a network of professionals in the healthcare field (Hosking, 2010; Vilorio, 2011). A network involves cultivating relationships that are mutually beneficial. Remember—it is not about who the advanced practice nurse knows but who knows the advanced practice nurse that will make a difference (Owens & Young, 2008).

When meeting individuals, it is imperative that the advanced practice nurse elicit feelings of liking, trust, and knowing to establish a good rapport and relationship. When advanced practice nurses initially interact with individuals, they should ask these persons about themselves and their careers rather than immediately inquiring how they can get a job (Owens & Young, 2008). In addition to the professional healthcare network, advanced practice nurses can utilize other contacts such as professors, alumni networks, former classmates, colleagues, family, friends, and employers both past and present (Mize, 2011a; Vilorio, 2011). Advanced practice nurses should start developing their professional network while they are students. This can be done by becoming active in professional organizations, participating in professional conferences, attending continuing education programs, and partaking in volunteer work (Vilorio, 2011).

One of the benefits of networking is that it allows the chance to create contacts with potential employers as well as to determine the work environment and employee morale in that organization or practice (Critchley, 2003; Vilorio, 2011). One word of caution is in order, however: Professional contacts will become leery if advanced practice nurses talk about specific job opportunities before they have established a good rapport and trusted relationship. This kind of relationship can take some time to

develop and foster. It is important to show genuine interest in each contact and learn about the individual and his or her job. For example, it is appropriate to ask what contacts' responsibilities are, what the most rewarding and challenging aspects of the role are, and what the work environment is like (Vilorio, 2011).

Advanced practice nurses should take care to organize their networks. One suggestion is to keep a file that lists all the contacts and identifies a little something of note about each person. Then, when nurses review an article of interest or need a contact in a certain specialty, the network is at their fingertips. If the network list is short, then a simple tickler file based on a notebook, note cards, or business cards may be helpful (Owens & Young, 2008).

Advanced practice nurses should make a conscious effort to stay in contact with the people in their network. Although underutilized, thank you notes can help set individuals apart. Techniques such as sending a note with a clipping from the paper or a journal relating to the individual's area of interest and sending a link to an appropriate website are strategies to stay in contact (Owens & Young, 2008). Other strategies, such as arranging follow-up meetings over coffee, can also be helpful when trying to establish a mutually beneficial relationship.

ASSESSMENTS TO PREPARE FOR THE JOB MARKET

For advanced practice nurses to promote their success in today's competitive job markets, they need to be prepared (Selph, 1998). Part of that preparation should involve in-depth personal, marketplace, organizational, and organizational fit analyses.

Personal Assessment

Prior to engaging in pursuit of work, advanced practice nurses should complete a comprehensive, honest, affirmative personal assessment (Shapiro & Rosenberg, 2002). This assessment should identify their strengths and weaknesses as well as their goals and objectives (Hosking, 2010; Shapiro & Rosenberg, 2002; Vilorio, 2011). Organizations and practices are seeking the most qualified advanced practice nurses to fill their open positions (Mize, 2011a). If advanced practice nurses want to stand out as the most qualified candidates to potential employers, then they will need to begin with an objective and constructive assessment of their strengths and weaknesses (Selph, 1998). Nurses should highlight the unique qualities that they offer and indicate how they complement the position for which they are applying (Mize, 2011a; Shapiro & Rosenberg, 2002). For example, advanced practice nurses with the ability to speak more than one language may be an asset to the organization or practice (Shapiro & Rosenberg, 2002). As another example, advance practice nurses who do not require a license to practice may want to seek certification in their field to enhance their qualifications before beginning their job search.

Likewise, deficiencies should be noted to provide a realistic description of the individual's performance (Shapiro & Rosenberg, 2002). If job applicants do not have the expertise that will help them stand apart, then they need to consider ways to make improvements to enhance their marketability (Hosking, 2010). In addition advanced practice nurses need to give some thought to their short- and long-term goals (Selph, 1998). Determining these goals will assist in making appropriate decisions about their future employment (Mize, 2011a) and may help to make a decision if more than one job offer is made.

In addition to determining strengths, weaknesses, and goals, the applicant should give thought to personal financial and benefit needs (Selph, 1998). Assessing salary and benefit requirements helps to determine what the bottom line will be in negotiations. Setting acceptable salary ranges prior to negotiations can help advanced practice nurses balance or adjust certain elements to design the best possible benefits package. There are many factors to consider.

Does the organization/practice include malpractice insurance in the benefits package? If this is not the case, advanced practice nurses may wish to negotiate for an increased salary to cover this expense. Sometimes there are other benefits besides salary to consider, such as work hours (on-call, off shifts, required weekends), flexible scheduling, potential for growth, and vacation time (Selph, 1998).

Last, the personal assessment should include an evaluation of the work location and setting as well as the professional environment requirements. Advanced practice nurses need to consider constraints regarding the location. Are they willing to relocate? Do they want to stay in the same location? If they want to stay locally, then do they have limits on the distance they are willing to commute? In addition, in which specialty and setting do they wish to work? With which populations are they qualified to work and enjoy working? Once the location and setting have been determined, job seekers need to assess the time commitments required by the position, the professional development requirements, and the anticipated work environment. Advanced practice nurses must decide how many hours are needed for the role and identify any personal constraints such as the necessity to leave the site at a particular time.

The professional development assessment includes an evaluation of the needs for mentoring and orientation, the amount of autonomy preferred, and continuing education required to maintain licensure, certification, and credentialing. Continuing education time and expenses as well as costs of journals, professional organization membership fees, and licensure and certification should all be assessed. Having this knowledge may assist advanced practice nurses when it comes time to negotiate the benefits package for the position. With regard to the work environment, advanced practice nurses need to assess the specific environment such as office space, support staff, pagers, cell phones, and computer (Selph, 1998).

Once advanced practice nurses have completed the personal assessment, they need to prioritize these elements to determine which are absolutely essential versus which are more flexible. Oftentimes, advanced practice nurses may need to make adjustments based on information obtained from the current marketplace and organizational assessments (Selph, 1998).

Marketplace Assessment

After completing the personal assessment, it is time to begin a marketplace assessment. This assessment comprises an evaluation of the regional and national marketplace and political atmosphere. When evaluating the regional and national marketplace, advanced practice nurses need to take into account the state rules and regulations that guide advanced practice, the need for the roles, the number of qualified nurses, typical financial packages/salary, scope of practice, and chief surrounding competitors (Hupcey, 1993; Selph, 1998).

Organizational Assessment

Once the preceding information is obtained, advanced practice nurses need to assess potential employers to determine specific healthcare organizations they would like to consider. It is important for nurses to find a practice or an organization that they admire and wish to work for. Advanced practice nurses should pursue organizations and practices, not job openings (Vilorio, 2011).

Assessing the qualities of a particular practice or organization requires advanced practice nurses to complete additional research. Some experts maintain that it is inexcusable for applicants not to know the fundamentals of an organization. Thus advanced practice nurses need to know which services their potential employer provides and how the organization compares to its competitors. This information can be found through advanced practice nurses' network contacts if possible; otherwise, nurses can seek it out through newspaper articles, healthcare publications, employer websites, employee blogs, and online discussions (Vilorio, 2011). If possible, advanced practice nurses will want to find out as many details as possible by looking for answers to the following questions (Brox, 2010; Selph, 1998; Shapiro & Rosenberg, 2002; Vilorio, 2011):

- Which population does the organization service?
- What are common diagnoses?
- What are the strengths and weaknesses of the organization/practice?
- What is the average daily census? What is the number of patient visits per day?
- How many outpatient and inpatient facilities does the organization have? Where are they located?
- Is the organization a teaching institution with medical teaching staff? What is the relationship between advanced practice nurses and the medical teaching staff—that is, how is the work shared? Is there clear role delineation?
- What are the reporting mechanisms? Do advanced practice nurses report to the nursing department? If so, are they expected to fulfill other obligations such as participating in annual educational in-service programs?
- Who will be completing the performance evaluation?
- How many advanced practice nurses work in the institution/practice?
- How have they structured their practices and services? Are there specialty practices? Is the practice based primarily on consultation? Are there primary care providers?
- What is the reimbursement scheme and payer mix? Can revenue be generated from the services that the advanced practice nurses can offer?
- What is the organizational structure?
- What is the organizational culture? Is the organization accepting of advanced practice nurses? Are nurses empowered in the organization?

- What is the reputation of the organization in the community and among other professionals?

The preceding information helps advanced practice nurses evaluate specific organizations' and practices' characteristics. This information, paired with the results of the personal assessment, helps advanced practice nurses determine their fit with an organization (Selph, 1998).

Advanced practice nurses who provide direct care should also gather data about the organization's privileging and scope of practice policies, recent political concerns, and the exposure the healthcare team has had to advanced practice roles (Selph, 1998). In addition, they should assess whether there are any competitors for the position or role they are seeking to fill. If they face competition, advanced practice nurses need to develop a strategy to advocate for their specific skills, expertise, and contributions (Selph, 1998).

Advanced Practice Nurse–Organizational Fit Assessment

At this point, it is time to see whether the personal assessment fits with the organizational assessment. This initial evaluation is intended to decide whether a good relationship between the advanced practice nurse and the particular organization is viable. However, advanced practice nurses cannot fully complete the fit assessment until they have had a chance to interview for the position and interact with the particular healthcare environment. In fact, advanced practice nurses will not know for sure whether the fit is a good one until they are employed for some period of time. Organizational fit is essential for a good long-term relationship, as research studies have linked congruence between individual and organizational values (fit) with positive affect (Chatman, 1989; Mount & Muchinsky, 1978; Spokane, 1985) and a greater likelihood of staying with the organization, commitment, satisfaction, and performance (Chatman, 1989; Meir & Hasson, 1982),

Causal mapping and storytelling are two strategies that, when combined, may be helpful in determining advanced practice nurses' organizational fit. Causal mapping in this context entails reflecting on factors that have an effect on advanced practice nurses' fit in an organization. Advanced practice nurses should contemplate which factors determine their fit in an organization. Given that they begin this evaluation before they are actually working at the institution, nurses will want to draw upon their past experiences and determine which factors were most important to them. Through the reflections, advanced practice nurses can begin to learn the particular individual factors that influence their sense of fit in an organization (Billsberry, Ambrosini, Moss-Jones, & March, 2005).

Causal mapping involves creating a graphic depiction of what affects the sense of fit. Advanced practice nurses add to the picture by reflecting on what influences their sense of fit and then what happens to cause that effect. They continue to develop this map by reflecting on additional questions that help them get more specific about what causes the feelings. Advanced practice nurses should continue to reflect until they are unable to come up with additional information. At that point, they should try to recall an individual work experience that influenced fit and tell a story about it.

Some advanced practice nurses may have difficulty determining what has influenced their fit in an organization and, therefore, will have trouble creating a map. In such instances, it is useful to utilize the storytelling technique in which advanced practice nurses recount stories from their work that illustrate how they felt about their employer. These two techniques help advanced practice nurses to reflect on the underlying factors and provide an initial exploration of the sense of fit.

PORTFOLIO DEVELOPMENT

Advanced practice nurses entering the job market need to be able to promote their positive personal and professional qualities to potential employers. Some organizations may not be familiar with the scope of practice and competencies of advanced practice nurses. As a consequence, advanced practice nurses will need to educate prospective employers as they concurrently negotiate for a position (Selph, 1998). For instance the hiring manager for a clinical nurse leader, a relatively new role in nursing and not yet employed in many settings, will need an understanding of the role and evidence of its potential impact on patient outcomes and cost savings.

One strategy advanced practice nurses can utilize to educate key individuals in an organization as well as to develop a strong base for negotiation is a well-prepared career portfolio. A good portfolio must be paired with an attitude of confidence and competence to ensure success. Advanced practice nurses will want all observers to see their positive attitude, which arises from their education, clinical knowledge and skills, adaptability, effective communication skills, and strong conviction in the capability of the advanced practice nurse to contribute to positive patient and financial outcomes. Successful negotiations begin with advanced practice nurses' passionate belief in the worth and benefits of this advanced nursing practice role. If they lack the conviction that advanced practice nurses offer a valuable service, candidates will run the risk of making compromises that undermine their professional and personal goals. It is helpful to have data to support the notion that advanced practice nurses can have a positive impact on practice (Selph, 1998). Such data can be found in the literature, proving evidence is an important strategy in today's healthcare environment.

Professional portfolios can serve two purposes. First, they display evidence of the individual's professional knowledge, skills, expertise, work experiences, clinical experience, professional accomplishments, and scholarly work as well as highlight the contributions the individual can make to the organization. Second, they can be effective means for conveying the significant worth of advanced practice nursing by educating potential employers who are unacquainted with the role and scope of practice (Selph, 1998). In the following discussion, the suggestions for the content of some sections of the portfolio assume that the potential employer is unfamiliar with the role. This obviously needs to be modified depending on the organization and the advanced practice role.

The portfolio may contain the following components: curriculum vitae, professional development and continuing education activities, references, clinical experiences, legal regulations, standards and scope of practice, collaborative practice agreements, reimbursement guidelines, procedures, hospital privileging, job descriptions, scholarly work, advanced practice documentation, and professional expenses (Shapiro & Rosenberg, 2002). The most positive impact occurs when advanced practice nurses present and organize this information in a professional manner while maintaining attention to detail to ensure a polished project.

Curricula Vitae

Some experts recommend that advanced practice nurses include a curriculum vitae as opposed to a résumé. Although the two documents are similar, there are some significant differences. A résumé is typically a one- or two-page document that gives an overview of education, employment history, and achievements (Hinck, 1997). The curriculum vitae, by comparison, is typically longer and more detailed. Such profiles are typically used in academia, although medical and nursing professionals often use them as well.

The curriculum vitae is a practical tool that can highlight advanced practice nurses' abilities, skills, and accomplishments and promote their careers (Hinck, 1997). It is a wonderful opportunity for advanced practice nurses to make a positive impression. Of course, this document can quickly make a negative impression if it is poorly constructed or contains errors. Advanced practice nurses should carefully proofread the curriculum vitae, as misspellings, typographical errors, and grammatical errors will likely give the impression that nurses lack attention to detail and professionalism. In one study, more than 75% of organization leaders interviewed indicated that only one or two typographical errors in the curriculum vitae would eliminate the candidate from consideration for a position (Hosking, 2010).

The curriculum vitae should be printed on high-quality paper, on only one side. Some experts suggest using 10- to 14-point Times New Roman font as it is easy to read. All information in the curriculum vitae must be honest and accurate. Providing false information or embellishing one's accomplishments is not just unethical but also can cause advanced practice nurses great trouble when the information is verified (Hinck, 1997). Advanced practice nurses should modify their curriculum vitae at frequent intervals to ensure inclusion of all accomplishments (Hinck, 1997; Hosking, 2010; Selph, 1998).

When applying for a job, advanced practice nurses should include a cover letter explaining how they could benefit the employer. In addition, the content of the cover letter should express that they are familiar with the organization and explain how they can make an immediate contribution to its success (Hinck, 1997; Hosking, 2010). Cover letters are vitally important as they make the first impression and can offer insight into one's uniqueness and passion that is not conveyed in a curriculum vitae.

The curriculum vitae can be organized in different ways depending on preferences. There are no strict rules that have to be applied (Hinck, 1997). Typically, this document contains the general categories shown in **Figure 30-1** (Critchley, 2003; Hinck, 1997; Selph, 1998).

FIGURE 30-1 Curriculum Vitae Template.

Name, credentials
Home Address:
Work Address: (if desired)
Phone:
Email Address:
Education: (list highest degree first)
Degree
Graduation date
University
University's address
Professional Employment: (list most recent nursing position first)
Dates of employment
Employer
Position title: brief description of responsibilities and achievements

Licensure and Certifications:
List licenses
License number
State(s) where qualified to practice
List certifications
Certification number
Credentialing body
Dates certification is valid
Professional Honors and Recognition: (list most recent first)
Professional and community awards, scholarships, honorary degrees, fellowships, and/or prizes
Name of the award
Presenting organization
Date

(continues)

FIGURE 30-1   Curriculum Vitae Template. *(continued)*

Reason for the award
Research/Grant History:
Research fellowships
Master's theses
Doctoral dissertations
Grants (do not list a project if funding was denied)
Lectures, Courses, and Presentations: (may include presentations given to colleagues, healthcare professionals, or the community)
List of names of course/lecture/presentations
Dates given
Professional Service:
Peer review groups/grant study sections
Journal service: (served as a reviewer for a journal)
 Dates of service
 Journal name
Professional organizations:
 Names of organizations in which current membership is held
 Dates of membership
 Offices held
 Committees served in each organization
Consultative service:
 Names of organizations where salaried consulting work was provided
 Address of the organization
 Type of consulting work
 Dates

Organizational service:
 Dates
 Committees and task forces
 Role on the committee (i.e., member or chairperson)
 If appropriate, note any major accomplishment of the committee
Hospital boards and committees
Public/Community Service:
Community agency where volunteer work was completed
Type of service (e.g., parish nursing, fundraising, educational sessions to nonnursing groups)
Population served
Date
Bibliography: (Use the American Psychological Association format for listing publications; list the publications in chronological order by year. Group types of publications separately, such as by the following groupings.)
Peer-reviewed manuscripts
Case reports, technical notes, letters
Reviews, chapters, books
Papers in press
Peer reviews of presentations
(Note in the footer the date on which the curriculum vitae was last revised.)

Professional Development and Continuing Education Activities

Advanced practice nurses may wish to include information in the portfolio about their professional development or continuing education activities. Doing so highlights their dedication to lifelong learning. In this section, advanced practice nurses should outline any ongoing specialty training that was received (Hinck, 1997). The information can be displayed in a simple table that notes the date and title of the program as well as the organization that provided the education.

References

If advanced practice nurses have letters of support or recommendation available, these can be included in this section of the portfolio. If such letters are not available, advanced practice nurses can either note that references will be available upon request or list people who are willing to serve as references (Hinck, 1997). Advanced practice nurses can ask current or former managers and colleagues if they would be willing to serve as references for them as they enter the job market in the new role of an advanced practice nurse (Hosking, 2010). Nurses should not list people as references before obtaining their permission to do so, as that can increase the risk of the reference not being prepared for the call or giving a negative response to the caller (Hinck, 1997; Hosking, 2010). When listing references, advanced practice nurses should include each reference's name, title, work address, and telephone number (Hinck, 1997).

Experience

Advanced practice nurses in direct care roles should include a section in the career portfolio that underscores their experience. To demonstrate their proficiency, a summary of the types of patients managed, age ranges, diagnoses, procedures performed, preceptorships, and practice settings and locations should be provided (Burgess & Misener, 1997; Selph, 1998). When possible, advanced practice nurses should try to obtain letters of reference to strengthen this section (Selph, 1998). For those in indirect care roles, a discussion of their experiences and accomplishments are included here. Written well, this is an opportunity for the potential employer to learn more about applicants' uniqueness.

Legal Regulations

If the organization has little or no experience with the advanced practice nurse's role in direct care, then nurses will want to be sure to include a section on legal regulations in the portfolio. Advanced practice nurses should begin by including a copy of the state's nurse practice act as well as regulations regarding advanced practice nursing. In addition, documentation should be provided that verifies advanced practice nurses' prescriptive authority if appropriate. If the advanced practice nurse does not yet have prescriptive authority, then the nurse can describe the process of how it is obtained (Selph, 1998). This information indicates that advanced practice nurses are concerned with the legal aspects of their clinical practice while simultaneously educating the employer (Burgess & Misener, 1997; Hravnak & Magdic, 1997; Selph, 1998).

Standards and Scopes of Practice

The portfolio ought to include any professional standards on the scope of practice for the role. (Selph, 1998). In addition, this document serves as the basis for performance evaluation and a quality review program (Burgess & Misener, 1997; Selph, 1998).

Collaborative Practice Agreements

For direct care providers, sample collaborative practice agreements included in the portfolio can be useful for potential employers who are not familiar with this information and would like to review a copy. Collaborative practice agreements are printed contracts among physicians and advanced practice nurses that outline the scope of the collaborative practice. The agreement should note how the two healthcare professional groups will organize and manage care and the breadth or constraints of the APN practice (Shapiro & Rosenberg, 2002).

Reimbursement Guidelines

As appropriate, including reimbursement guidelines in the portfolio helps educate employers regarding the types of payments that are available for nurses in advanced practice roles (Burgess & Misener, 1997; Selph, 1998);

nurses can include current information regarding the guidelines or statutes on reimbursement, as these criteria change frequently. To do so, advanced practice nurses should ascertain the practice payer mix and directly communicate with the payers to determine which APN services they reimburse for. Advanced practice nurses can utilize the resources that are available such as the billing department or practice manager to help determine what is typically billed and how often (what percentage) it uses each provider (Selph, 1998).

Scope of Practice: Procedures

For those in direct care practices, a list of procedures typically performed by advanced practice nurses in that state should be provided in the portfolio. The procedures that advanced practice nurses can perform within their scope of practice are typically noted in the state's nurse practice act. In this section of the portfolio, advanced practice nurses should list which procedures they have performed with supervision and which procedures they are prepared to learn. Advanced practice nurses should highlight any special training received, the number of completed procedures, and outcomes. When possible, they should provide information regarding reimbursement for the procedure, which will help in the negotiation process (Selph, 1998).

Hospital Privileging

If advanced practice nurses are hoping to gain employment in a hospital, they need to be privileged based on the medical staff bylaws and policies for advanced practice nurses. Specific procedures must be followed and documentation must be submitted, which a committee will review and use as the basis for making a recommendation. If the institution has not utilized advanced practice nurses in the past, procedures may not have been established to allow privileging of advanced practice nurses. In this case, advanced practice nurses will want to research best practices for privileging and provide this information in the portfolio. This effort helps prepare advanced practice nurses to assist in developing a plan to implement a procedure (Selph, 1998).

Job Description

Depending on the individual advanced practice nurse's situation, a job description may or may not be included in the portfolio. If advanced practice nurses are well established in the potential employer's institution, then providing job descriptions may not be necessary. However, a sample job description can be a good tool for delineating particular instances in which advanced practice nurses can use knowledge and skills to influence patient care. As such, advanced practice nurses may wish to provide a sample job description that highlights how their skills can positively influence the healthcare environment. The job description should be individualized for the setting in which the advanced practice nurse will be working and include specific roles and responsibilities (Selph, 1998).

Scholarly Work

In this part of the portfolio, advanced practice nurses can demonstrate their writing skills and showcase professional expertise by supplying copies of publications, papers, or abstracts they have written that are germane to the practice setting. These examples illustrate their capability for additional scholarly activities and lay the groundwork for negotiating time for such work and attendance at professional meetings (Selph, 1998).

Protocols

In many states, advanced practice nurses utilize protocols and guidelines to inform their practice. In turn, they may wish to provide in their portfolio a sample protocol for the management of a clinical situation particular to the specialty of interest. Such protocols and guidelines are useful tools to demonstrate the responsibilities advanced practice nurses have in regard to diagnostic reasoning, treatments, and outcomes (Selph, 1998).

Advanced Practice Documentation

In this section of the portfolio, advanced practice nurses can provide affirmation of advanced practice documentation ability by presenting examples of admission notes, history and physicals, orders, progress notes, and discharge summaries. They should remember to remove all identifying patient information from these samples. If possible, the documents should be related to the population with whom the advanced practice nurse intends to work. These examples can serve as powerful testaments of the advanced practice nurses' clinical expertise and can show the distinct abilities that advanced practice nurses can provide within the practice, particularly in healthcare settings where the advanced practice nurse is a new role (Selph, 1998).

Similarly, advanced practice nurses in indirect care roles can present syllabi, performance evaluations from their supervisors, student evaluations, and so forth.

Professional Expenses

This section of the portfolio includes a detailed inventory of advanced practice nurses' expected professional expenses. Advanced practice nurses may choose to hold this information aside until it is time for negotiating a benefits package; nevertheless, it is important to be cognizant of the professional costs. When developing the record of expenses, advanced practice nurses should think about all of their expenses, including one-time costs such as the initial application for a certification or for prescriptive authority, as well as annual costs such as malpractice insurance and fees for license renewal. Other expenses that can be included are the cost of continuing specialty certifications, continuing education expenses,

professional organization memberships, journals, and books. The more detailed the list, the more prepared the advanced practice nurse is to articulate his or her needs and expectations (Selph, 1998).

APPLYING FOR THE JOB

Once advanced practice nurses have completed their personal, marketplace, organizational, and advanced practice nurse–organizational fit assessments, they can present themselves to the employer, feeling empowered with the information provided in the career portfolio (Shapiro & Rosenberg, 2002). The next step in entering the job market is to place an application; this step is followed by the job interview.

Applications

An increasing number of employers are moving to an online application process. Of course, although an online process might be used, there is still a human being at the receiving end who does the hiring. Advanced practice nurses can increase their chances of being hired if they contact the hiring individual instead of relying solely on computer contact. Online processes have increased the number of applications organizations receive. As a result, many organizations utilize software that can somewhat automate the selection process by rejecting candidates based on minimum qualifications or keywords. For this reasons, advanced practice nurses are advised to customize the cover letter, curriculum vitae, and application for each position that they apply to. To avoid being removed by the automatic culling software, they should be sure to include the words in the job posting and to emphasize the connection between their education and skills and the duties necessary for the desired position (Vilorio, 2011).

Experts recommend that advanced practice nurses use extreme caution when posting identifying personal data online, particularly on social media websites such as LinkedIn and Facebook. Many organizations conduct online information checks to evaluate potential hires. Many social media programs have loose privacy settings, which make it easy for members of the public to access users' personal information. One way to manage this access is to search one's own name online to see what information is available to the general public as well as to adjust privacy settings to protect personal information and photos, control what others share about the user, and reduce information that can compromise being hired. All personal data should be kept private; however, advanced practice nurses can certainly share professional accomplishments such as publications or awards or other information that presents a professional image (Hosking, 2010; Vilorio, 2011).

When possible, it is helpful for advanced practice nurses to talk with the hiring manager, as this individual is responsible for choosing candidates and has a vested interest in finding a qualified candidate who can meet the job responsibilities and fulfill the mission of the organization. If advanced practice nurses have existing contacts within the organization, perhaps those individuals might be able to arrange an informational meeting with the hiring manager. Such a meeting can help candidates learn more about the job responsibilities and the institution while also giving them a chance to impress the individual responsible for hiring. During this meeting, advanced practice nurses should be sure to demonstrate initiative while remaining polite and being mindful of the hiring channels (Vilorio, 2011).

After submitting an application and curriculum vitae, advanced practice nurses should follow up with the hiring manager within 2 weeks of sending the application. Experts recommend sending a brief email or calling the organization or practice after submitting the information to confirm one's interest in the post and to offer to respond to any questions the employer might have about the application. This sort of professional attention to detail can set advanced practice nurses apart in this process (Hosking, 2010).

Once advanced practice nurses have submitted an application, they should be prepared to respond when the organization calls. The first impression begins with that call. Sometimes organizations use this initial phone conversation as a screening tool. As a result, advanced practice nurses may wish to let the call go to voicemail so that they have time to adequately prepare and make a polished first impression (Brox, 2010).

Interviewing

Being brought in for an interview indicates that an organization is interested in the applicant's background (Brox, 2010). The interview is a critical time when advanced practice nurses have the opportunity to dazzle the employer and secure a position (Vilorio, 2011). According to experts, the main reason why people are not successful in interviews is a lack of preparation. Role-playing mock interviews with an individual who is knowledgeable about the process can help advanced practice nurses develop and hone their interviewing skills. It may also help advanced practice nurses to correct some potentially damaging behaviors. For example, many people are unaware that they use words and phrases such as "you know," "like," and "um" while speaking. Eliminating this habit can help advanced practice nurses obtain a job. During the interview, advanced practice nurses will want to attempt to work into the conversation all of their career highlights. They should practice both delivering this information in a charming and natural fashion and telling engaging stories that help make what is listed on their curriculum vitae memorable (Brox, 2010).

It might sound simple, but first impressions really do make a difference. The hiring individual wants to know that the candidate will be a good representative on behalf of the organization or practice (Mize, 2011b). As such, advanced practice nurses should show common sense and professionalism in all dealings with the possible new employer (Vilorio, 2011). At the very least, they should be on time, professionally dressed, and polite to all staff regardless of their position (Mize, 2011b; Vilorio, 2011). With any job, advanced practice nurses need to bring a positive "can do and will do" attitude. In particular, they should be prepared to respond to questions that require them to give examples of previous problem-solving and time-management scenarios (Mize, 2011b). Advanced practice nurses should prepare for the interview by developing answers to questions that the employer might potentially ask (Brox, 2010). The employer will certainly ask questions to determine the applicant's knowledge, skills, and interests (Vilorio, 2011). Advanced practice nurses should not be vague when responding to questions but rather should provide the employer with specific details of how they solved problems and brought situations to a positive resolution.

Behavioral interviews are currently in vogue in many larger organizations. In these interviews, applicants are asked about how they behaved previously in given situations. For instance, the hiring manager may ask: "Tell me about a time when you worked effectively with a team to implement a practice change?" (as opposed to questions such as, Are you a good team player?).

The Internet is the best source for sample interview questions and there is information on how to pose behavioral interview questions and how to answer them. Once again, the job posting can provide some hints on what might be asked in the interview. Having one or two stories prepared—just in case—about successes and issues in dealing with patients, team members, bosses, and so forth is helpful.

In other situations or in addition to behavioral questions, interviewers may ask generic questions such as the following (Brox, 2010; Vilorio, 2011):

- What do you see yourself doing in 5 years?
- What are your strengths and weaknesses?
- Why would you like to be employed here?
- How do you handle conflict with peers?

- What do you consider to be your greatest accomplishment?
- What can you tell me about your reasons for leaving your last job?
- What was the most challenging issue you have encountered and how did you deal with it?

In addition, advanced practice nurses should have a list of questions to ask the hiring manager (Vilorio, 2011). If they have not obtained details about the position and its associated responsibilities, then the interview is the time to ascertain this information. Advanced practice nurses should find out details about specific responsibilities. These details will differ based on the role.

The main purpose of the interview is to help the advanced practice nurse and the employer determine whether the candidate is a good fit for the organization (Vilorio, 2011). Advanced practice nurses should be positive and truthful about everything they say, but especially when discussing previous managers and colleagues (Brox, 2010; Vilorio). Advanced practice nurses' interactions should be assertive and courteous while avoiding presumptions and aggression. For example, if advanced practice nurses' have information in their employment history that potentially might be perceived as negative, such as gaps in employment or frequent job changes, then they should succinctly acknowledge the situation and then redirect the discussion toward something positive, such as what has been learned from the experience and constructive actions that have been taken to prepare for the new position (Vilorio, 2011). Advanced practice nurses' need to sell themselves and be clear about what they can bring to the organization (Mize, 2011b).

Finding the right fit is a two-way venture. If the advanced practice nurse is not excited about the organization, foresees issues that might cause problems that are not resolvable, and did not "click" with the manager and the team, then the advanced practice nurse should continue the search for the right employment opportunity. It is better to delay employment than to accept a job in which one is unhappy and leaves after a short period of time.

At the conclusion of the interview the nurse can ask what the next step or steps are and how long the decision-making process may take. Advanced practice nurses should thank the interviewer in person as well as in writing with a thank-you letter. According to experts, it is most effective to hand-write the note, but an email thank-you letter is also considered acceptable. The thank-you note gives advanced practice nurses one more opportunity to emphasize their positive qualifications and skills as well as confirm their interest in the position.

The length of the hiring process can vary greatly between organizations. As such, advanced practice nurses may wish to follow up with a phone call or email to reassert their interest in the position (Vilorio, 2011).

Salary Negotiation

Many organizations' human resources departments have guidelines and structures in place to help determine what the starting pay level will be. As a result, negotiations may not yield the results nurses wish for (Mize, 2011b). However, there is generally a salary range for a particular position, and some managers may start nearer the bottom of the range, leaving room to negotiate. Beginning salary dictates the salary for the rest of the time the nurse is employed—except if he or she is promoted. When assessing compensation, however, advanced practice nurses need to consider the entire benefits package, which includes such items as life insurance, health insurance, dental and vision care, vacation, and retirement/pension plans. In addition, advanced practice nurses should consider whether the organization will provide compensation for professional memberships, continuing education opportunities, and travel expenses. It is important to consider these factors in conjunction with the salary (Mize, 2011b).

FOSTERING DEVELOPMENT

Once advanced practice nurses are in their new roles, they need to continue their education and foster their growth and development. Advanced practice nurses begin their first advanced practice positions as novices and need to put structures and strategies in place to support their growth and development so that they can become experts (Ackerman, Norsen, Martin, Wiedrich, & Kitzman, 1996; Doerksen, 2010). Continuing education and ongoing training are obvious ways to promote development. A few additional strategies are discussed in this section as well.

Formal and Informal Mentorship

Formal and informal mentorship has been noted in the literature as a method to address the professional development needs of advanced practice nurses. Formal mentorship (also referred to a preceptorship) is often offered by an institution/practice with some prescribed components. Each organization goes about the process differently. Ideally, a needs assessment is completed to develop an individualized program that meets the specific needs of new advanced practice nurses. In addition, novice advanced practice nurses may be paired with ones who have agreed to serve in the mentor role. Once an agreement has been reached between the two parties, they can discuss the process to be used as well as goals and expectations. Ground rules and a contract should be established to facilitate a positive experience (see Chapter 28).

Some organizations provide a welcoming package including a directory of potential mentors, which lists the areas of interest and strengths of the individuals (Doerksen, 2010). This tool can be very useful for beginning advanced practice nurses who would like to identify a colleague who can help them develop their professional interests.

Informal mentoring, a mentorship that emerges from an attraction of two people versus assignment of a formal mentor, can also be a useful tool for fostering the development of novice advanced practice nurses (see Chapter 28). Informal mentoring in this context refers to an ongoing relationship with another professional who can offer assistance, provide encouragement, and stimulate growth. Being open and willing to learn and grow is the first step in developing informal mentoring relationships. Informal mentoring is less structured, with advanced practice nurses scheduling their own time with the mentor, perhaps meeting in the office or casually over coffee (Doerksen, 2010).

The ongoing professional development needs of advanced practice nurses will most likely be met through multiple mentors, and these needs will likely change over time. Initially, advanced practice nurses need to learn about the daily ins and outs of their role. New advanced practice nurses may need assistance with specific activities as well as policies and procedure. With time, they will become more comfortable and confident with the daily functions, with their attention for mentoring focusing on additional growth in the role. The need for mentoring regarding research has been identified as a need that will increase for advanced practice nurses over time. On-site mentors for research can be a useful way to meet that need if the facility is lacking in such expertise. Visiting advanced practice nurses from other institutions and practices can help both with conducting research and determining how this role can be implemented in a variety of ways (Doerksen, 2010). Physicians may be able to help nurse practitioners identify gaps in clinical knowledge and help by serving as mentors for research. However, advanced practice nurses need to be cognizant of the professional obligation to further not just medical and healthcare research but nursing research as well.

Experiential Learning and Reflective Narratives

Advanced practice nurses can foster their growth and development via experiential learning embedded in narratives. In this context, experiential learning involves advanced practice nurses actively reflecting on their work experiences with the assistance of written journal entries. Advanced practice nurses' work environments can provide opportunities to acquire new skills and develop new knowledge if they are open to these events, have self-initiative, and are willing to self-evaluate. Making meaning from work experiences requires attention to pertinent occurrences, active reflection on the situation by using analytical skills, consideration of alternative ways to handle the encounter, and development of new ideas from the experience (Cathcart, Greenspan, & Quin, 2010).

Written reflections can help advanced practice nurses recognize the skilled knowledge and accomplishments they have achieved (Cathcart et al., 2010). Without contemplation, advanced practice nurses' achievements or difficulties may be seen as merely isolated occurrences, possibly not remembered until the next time a similar event happens (Benner, 1984; Benner, Sutphen, Leonard, & Day, 2010; Benner, Tanner, & Chesla, 2009; Cathcart et al., 2010). Writing about experiences at work gives advanced practice nurses an opportunity to remember the event and start to understand the importance and implication of the incidents. It also helps them appreciate why the specific incident was important and how their judgment and actions influenced the situation. Written narratives reinforce the notion that advanced practice nurses' professional development is a lifelong process based on constant exposure to a variety of experiences (Cathcart et al., 2010).

Online Listservs

Online listservs are another practical strategy for fostering professional growth and development; they provide advanced practice nurses with a network of support and informal knowledge sharing. In this context, listservs comprise an electronic mailing list management system that lets advanced practice nurses subscribe to a mailing list of other advanced practice nurses or healthcare professionals. Listservs can help advanced practice nurses stay current with the latest changes in their area of expertise, which in turn may assist them in making informed decisions about clinical practice. Listservs provide advanced practice nurses with a professional network to which they can pose questions or ideas regarding their practice, no matter what their role. Advanced practice nurses often gladly share their knowledge, as they feel a sense of obligation if they have been given assistance previously from others or if they hope to receive help in the future. Advanced practice nurses tend to provide information to the listserv because they want to improve patient outcomes and assist their peers by imparting the needed information (Hew & Hara, 2008).

There are some downsides to listservs, however. Notably, advanced practice nurses should be certain to verify the information obtained via a listserv prior to using it in practice. In addition, although listservs can provide some pearls of wisdom, often advanced practice nurses receive redundant messages that can overload their email inboxes.

Grand Rounds

Grand rounds are a useful venue to promote and demonstrate nursing practice as well as foster growth and development. If grand rounds are not available in the institution in which the advanced practice nurse is practicing, then Benner's theoretical framework of skill acquisition can guide this process. Grand rounds are often held quarterly and are expected to connect evidence-based practice literature to practice. In this learning activity, healthcare professionals who provide direct care gather to hear about a clinical issue or particular patient case. For advanced practice nurses, grand rounds serve as a means to improve nursing care by focusing on the educational needs of their clinical practice. In addition, they offer a way to be recognized for clinical knowledge and skills,

foster networking among advanced practice nurses and other healthcare professionals, and provide recognition of the value of nursing's contribution to practice (Furlong et al., 2007). Traditionally, grand rounds have been limited to hospitals, notably academic medical centers. However, the concept of interprofessionals gathering to learn together can happen in any setting, including universities.

Recognition Programs

Recognition programs have been noted in the literature as a way to foster advanced practice nurses' growth and development, as well as that of other members of the interprofessional team. Organizations develop and implement recognition programs as a way to publicly acknowledge contributions to meeting the goals and objectives of the institution. Typically, the goals and objectives in health care involve obtaining positive patient, staff, institutional, and community outcomes. If the advanced practice nurse's institution has not developed a recognition program, he or she might propose developing one to recognize the numerous contributions of the healthcare professionals in that institution, including advanced practice nurses. Such a program can be utilized to acknowledge advanced practice nurses' competency in the role, achievement of goals above and beyond their job expectations, and promotion of nursing practice (Sullivan, Arlington, Madsen, & Guidry, 2006).

SUMMARY

Advanced practice nurses' educational programs are limited in their ability to fully assist students with the transformation that is necessary as they move from pupil, to novice, and eventually to expert. This transition has been described in the recent literature as a process that involves three stages: identity loss, transitional role, and incorporation. Advanced practice nurses' educational programs attempt to facilitate this transition by providing students with a framework that emphasizes evidence-based practice, research, collaboration, and consultation as a way to inform nursing practice (Spoelstra & Robbins, 2010). Although these educational programs may assist students with this process, other strategies to facilitate a positive transition can be implemented as well.

The transition from student to expert cannot be fully achieved until graduating students have secured their first position. As graduating students prepare for the job marketplace, they need to locate job openings and conduct the following assessments: personal, marketplace, organization, and advanced practice nurse–organization fit. In addition, a professional portfolio is helpful to demonstrate the benefits that advanced practice nurses can offer to an employer. Finally, advanced practice nurses need to present themselves favorably in the application and interview processes.

Once advanced practice nurses have begun a new position, it is essential that they develop a lifelong learning plan that includes measures to foster their growth and development. Some suggested methods to promote development are formal and informal mentorships, experiential learning and reflective narratives, online listservs, grand rounds, and recognition programs.

DISCUSSION QUESTIONS

1. As you lay the foundation for professional advanced nursing practice, conduct a personal analysis. What are your strengths and your needs for further development?

2. Which strategies can the novice advanced practice nurse employ to have a successful transition to the professional role?

3. Following a self, marketplace, and organizational assessment, which factors are most important for you to consider when selecting an advanced practice position?

REFERENCES

Ackerman, M. H., Norsen, L., Martin, B., Wiedrich, J., & Kitzman, H. (1996). Development of a model of advanced practice. *American Journal of Critical Care, 5*, 68–73.

American Association of Colleges of Nursing. (2013). Nursing faculty shortage fact sheet. Retrieved from http://www.aacn.nche.edu/media-relations/FacultyShortageFS.pdf

Barton, T. D. (2007). Student nurse practitioners—a rite of passage? The universality of Van Gennep's model of social transition. *Nurse Education in Practice, 7*, 338–347.

Benner, P. (1984). *From novice to expert: Excellence and power in clinical nursing practice.* Menlo Park, CA: Addison-Wesley.

Benner, P., Sutphen, M., Leonard, V., & Day, L. (2010). *Educating nurses: A call for radical transformation.* San Francisco, CA: Jossey-Bass.

Benner, P., Tanner, C., & Chesla, C. (2009). *Expertise in nursing practice* (2nd ed.). New York, NY: Springer.

Billsberry, J., Ambrosini, V., Moss-Jones, J., & March, P. (2005). Some suggestions for mapping organizational members' sense of fit. *Journal of Business and Psychology, 19*(4), 555–570.

Brox, D. (2010). Mastering the interview. *PM Network,* 51–53.

Burgess, S. E., & Misener, T. R. (1997). The professional portfolio: An advanced practice nurses job search marketing tool. *Clinical Excellence for Advanced Practice Nurses, 1*(7), 468–471.

Cathcart, E. B., Greenspan, M., & Quin, M. (2010). The making of a nurse manager: The role of experiential learning in leadership development. *Journal of Nursing Management, 18*, 440–447.

Chatman, J. A. (1989). Improving interactional organizational research: A model of person-organization fit. *Academy of Management Review, 14*(3), 333–349.

Clarin, O. A. (2007). Strategies to overcome barriers to effective nurse practitioner and physician collaboration. *Journal for Advanced Practice Nurses, 3*(8), 538–548.

Cleary, M., Matheson, S., & Happell, B. (2009). Evaluation of a transition to practice programme for mental health nursing. *Journal of Advanced Nursing, 65*(4), 844–850.

Critchley, D. (2003). Moving house or moving jobs: What's the difference? *Nursing Management, 10*(2), 12–14.

Doerksen, K. (2010). What are the professional development and mentorship needs of advanced practice nurses? *Journal of Professional Nursing, 26*(3), 141–151.

Forbes, A., While, A., Mathes, L., & Griffiths, P. (2006). Evaluating MS specialist nurse program. *International Journal of Nursing Studies, 43*, 985–1000.

Furlong, K. M., D'Luna-O'Grady, L., Macari-Hinson, M., O'Connel, K. B., & Pierson, G. S. (2007). Implementing nursing grand rounds in a community hospital. *Clinical Nurse Specialist, 21*(6), 287–291.

Hamric, A. B., & Taylor, J. W. (1989). Role development of CNS. In A. B. Hamric & J. Spross (Eds.), *The clinical nurse specialist in theory and practice* (2nd ed., pp. 41–82). Philadelphia, PA: W. B. Saunders.

Hayes, E. (1998). Mentoring and nurse practitioner student self-efficacy. *Western Journal of Nursing Research, 20*, 521–525.

Heitz, L. J., Steiner, S. H., & Burman, M. E. (2004). RN to nurse practitioner: A qualitative study of role transition. *Journal of Nursing Education, 43*, 416–420.

Hew, K. H., & Hara, N. (2008). An online listserv for nurse practitioner: A viable venue for continuous nursing professional development? *Nurse Education Today, 28*, 450–457.

Hinck, S. (1997). A curriculum vitae that gives you a competitive edge. *Clinical Nurse Specialist, 11*(4), 174–177.

Hosking, R. (2010). Top 10 tips for job seekers. *OfficePro, 70*(2), 5.

Hravnak, M., & Magdic, K. (1997). Marketing the acute care nurse practitioner. *Clinical Excellence Nursing Practice, 1*, 9–13.

Hupcey, J. E. (1993). Factors and work settings that may influence nurse practitioner practice. *Nursing Outlook, 41*, 181–185.

Institute of Medicine. (2010). *The future of nursing: Leading change, advancing health: Report recommendations.* Retrieved from http://www.iom.edu/~/media/Files/Report%20Files/2010/The-Future-of-Nursing/Future%20of%20Nursing%202010%20Recommendations.pdf

Latham, C. L., & Fahey, L. J. (2006). Novice to expert advanced practice nurses role transition: Guided student self-reflection. *Journal of Nursing Education, 45*(1), 46–48.

Lindblad, E., Hallman, E. B., Gillsjo, C., Lindblad, U., & Foerstrom, L. (2010). Experiences of the new role of advanced practice nurses in Swedish primary health care: A qualitative study. *International Journal of Nursing Practice, 16*, 69–74.

Meir, E., & Hasson, R. (1982). Congruence between personality type and environment type as a predictor of stay in an environment. *Journal of Vocational Behavior, 21*, 309–317.

Mize, S. (2011a, March). Future leaders: Finding a job in a tight market. *Parks & Recreation*, 39–40.

Mize, S. (2011b, April). Future leaders: Your first job. *Parks & Recreation*, 41–41.

Mount, M., & Muchinksy, P. (1978). Person-environment congruence and employee job satisfaction: A test of Holland's theory. *Journal of Vocational Behavior, 13*, 84–100.

Owens, L. A., & Young, P. (2008). You're hired! The power of networking. *Journal of Vocational Rehabilitation, 29*(1), 23–28.

Pye, S. (2011). Professional development for an advance practice nursing team. *Journal of Continuing Education in Nursing, 40*(5), 217–222.

Selph, A. M. (1998). Negotiating an acute care nurse practitioner position. *AACN Clinical Issues, 9*(2), 269–276.

Shapiro, D., & Rosenberg, N. (2002). Acute care nurse practitioner collaborative practice negotiations. *AACN Clinical Issues, 12*(3), 470–478.

Spoelstra, S. L., & Robbins, L. B. (2010). A qualitative study of role transition from RN to APN. *International Journal of Nursing Education Scholarship, 7*(1), 1–14.

Spokane, A. (1985). A review of research on person-environment congruence in Holland's theory of career. *Journal of Vocational Behavior, 26*, 306–343.

Sullivan, T., Arlington, R., Madsen, V., & Guidry, V. (2006). Development and implementation of a recognition and development model for advanced practice nurses: An opportunity for professional growth. *Oncology Nursing Forum, 33*(2), 420.

U.S. Department of Labor, Bureau of Labor Statistics. (2014a). *Occupational outlook handbook, 2014-15 edition, nurse anesthetists, nurse midwives, and nurse practitioners.* Retrieved from http://www.bls.gov/ooh/healthcare/nurse-anesthetists-nurse-midwives-and-nurse-practitioners.htm

U.S. Department of Labor, Bureau of Labor Statistics. (2014b). *Occupational outlook handbook, 2014–15 edition, registered nurses.* Retrieved from http://www.bls.gov/ooh/healthcare/registered-nurses.htm

Vilorio, D. (2011). Focused job seeking: A measure approach to looking for work. *Occupational Health Quarterly*, 2–11.

Index

Exhibits, figures, and tables are indicated by exh, f, and t following the page number